Principles and Practice of Obstetric Anaesthesia and Analgesia

ANITA HOLDCROFT
MD, FRCA
Reader in Anaesthesia
Department of Anaesthetics
Royal Postgraduate Medical School
Hammersmith Hospital
London

AND

TREVOR A. THOMAS
MB, ChB, FRCA
Consultant Anaesthetist
Sir Humphry Davy Department of Anaesthesia
Bristol Royal Infirmary and St Michaels Hospital
Bristol

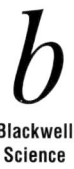
Blackwell
Science

© 2000 by
Blackwell Science Ltd
Editorial Offices:
Osney Mead, Oxford OX2 0EL
25 John Street, London WC1N 2BL
23 Ainslie Place, Edinburgh EH3 6AJ
350 Main Street, Malden
 MA 02148-5018, USA
54 University Street, Carlton
 Victoria 3053, Australia
10, rue Casimir Delavigne
 75006 Paris, France

Other Editorial Offices:
Blackwell Wissenschafts-Verlag GmbH
Kurfürstendamm 57
10707 Berlin, Germany

Blackwell Science KK
MG Kodenmacho Building
7–10 Kodenmacho Nihombashi
Chuo-ku, Tokyo 104, Japan

First published 2000

Set by Graphicraft Ltd,
Hong Kong
Printed and bound in Great Britain
by MPG Books Ltd, Bodmin,
Cornwall

The Blackwell Science logo is a
trade mark of Blackwell Science Ltd,
registered at the United Kingdom
Trade Marks Registry

The right of the Authors to be
identified as the Authors of this
Work has been asserted in
accordance with the Copyright,
Designs and Patents Act 1988.

All rights reserved. No part of
this publication may be reproduced,
stored in a retrieval system, or
transmitted, in any form or by any
means, electronic, mechanical,
photocopying, recording or otherwise,
except as permitted by the UK
Copyright, Designs and Patents Act
1988, without the prior permission
of the copyright owner.

A catalogue record for this title is
available from the British Library

ISBN 0–86542–828–X

Library of Congress
Cataloging-in-publication Data

Holdcroft, Anita.
 Principles and practice of
 obstetric anaesthesia and
 analgesia / Anita Holdcroft,
 Trevor A. Thomas.
   p.   cm.
 Includes bibliographical
 references and index.
 ISBN 0–86542–828–X
 1. Anesthesia in obstetrics.
 I. Thomas, Trevor A.
 II. Title.
 [DNLM: 1. Anesthesia,
Obstetrical.
 2. Analgesia, Obstetrical.
WO 450 H726p   1999]
RG732.H64   1999
617.9′682—dc21
DNLM/DLC
for Library of Congress   99–21230
                            CIP

DISTRIBUTORS

Marston Book Services Ltd
PO Box 269
Abingdon, Oxon OX14 4YN
(*Orders*: Tel: 01235 465500
          Fax: 01235 465555)

USA
Blackwell Science, Inc.
Commerce Place
350 Main Street
Malden, MA 02148-5018
(*Orders*: Tel: 800 759 6102
              781 388 8250
       Fax: 781 388 8255)

Canada
Login Brothers Book Company
324 Saulteaux Crescent
Winnipeg, Manitoba R3J 3T2
(*Orders*: Tel: 204 837 2987)

Australia
Blackwell Science Pty Ltd
54 University Street
Carlton, Victoria 3053
(*Orders*: Tel: 3 9347 0300
         Fax: 3 9347 5001)

For further information on
Blackwell Science, visit our website:
www.blackwell-science.com

Contents

Preface, v

Section 1: Obstetric Anaesthetic Services: Organization and Outcome

1 Maternity Services, 3

2 Maternal and Perinatal Mortality, 20

Section 2: Systematic Physiology and Pathology

3 Cardiovascular System, 31

4 Respiratory System, 57

5 Gastrointestinal System, 86

6 Renal System, 100

7 Hepatobiliary System, 109

8 Nervous System, 116

9 Metabolism and its Disorders in Pregnancy, 137

10 Immunity and Infection, 165

11 Uterine and Placental Function, 188

12 Puerperium, 193

13 Drug Abuse, 198

Section 3: Regional Anaesthesia

14 Anatomy, 213

15 Regional Anaesthetic Techniques, 227

Section 4: General Anaesthesia

16 Anaesthesia for Caesarean Section, 285

17 Anaesthesia for Antepartum and Postpartum Surgery, 326

Section 5: Labour

18 Labour, 335

19 Complications in Labour, 359

Section 6: The Fetus and Neonate

20 Fetal Medicine, 371

21 The High-Risk Fetus: Labour and Delivery, 386

Section 7: Obstetric Complications

22 Hypertensive Disorders in Pregnancy, 403

23 Haemorrhage, Thromboembolism and Amniotic Fluid Embolism, 419

24 Other Complications, 430

Section 8: Appendices

Appendix 1: Reference values, 441

Appendix 2: Pharmacology, 443

Index, 450

Preface

It was an outstanding tribute to the original author of this title, the late Dr Jeffrey Selwyn Crawford, that the publishers were confident to produce a book with a traditional individual textual style rather than a multi-author edited tome. 'Jeff' was an anaesthetist who 'fathered' the subspecialty of obstetric anaesthesia. He will be particularly remembered for his rigorous debating style based on sound scientific principles; for example, his firmly held views on aspects of anaesthetic practice were constantly reconsidered in the light of fresh evidence and new information. His enormous enthusiasm made him a delightful teacher and colleague. This rational approach led him to the informed view that regional techniques for pain relief in labour and anaesthesia for Caesarean section would be of great benefit and safety for mothers.

He championed the cause of obstetric anaesthesia on the political as well as the medical stage. In particular, together with Bruce Scott, he brought to the government's notice the high risks of obstetric anaesthesia revealed in the world's longest running audit project (as it was then) on the triennial series of reports on Confidential Enquiries into Maternal Deaths in England and Wales. This evidence gave our specialty the greatest conceivable encouragement. The identification of the importance of the control of pH of gastric contents and the necessity for a lateral tilt during labour and delivery by Jeffrey Selwyn Crawford created an awareness of these profound risk factors and also the opportunity to improve the safety of obstetric anaesthesia and analgesia through manipulation of physiological mechanisms. The physiological changes of pregnancy make a parturient unique. These physiological alterations are often further modified by pathological processes so that the anaesthetist today not only has to have technical expertise but also an understanding of physiological functions in 'normal' pregnancy plus any additional medical or obstetric complications. These basic scientific principles have provided the foundation for this book. Thus, the text should meet the requirements of those taking professional examinations as well as those with a more profound interest in obstetric anaesthesia.

In compiling this book we have been interrupted by professional duties which, at times, have led to significant chapter developments motivated by specific patient care or trainee interactions. In style, brevity and expansiveness have been in conflict but the final result is considered by us to be a worthwhile compromise which only readers can judge. We wish to thank our publishers for their patience and perseverance with our process of production. It has left those who battled with their word processors short of breath—as does labour.

It has been painful at times too, but cohesion has been maintained by many supporters.

We would wish particularly to thank our spouses for their long suffering tolerance, Ruth Oji for her invaluable contributions to our hard copy and also Stuart Taylor and Audrey Cadogan at Blackwell Science.

Anita Holdcroft
Trevor A. Thomas

Section 1
Obstetric Anaesthetic Services: Organization and Outcome

1: Maternity Services

1.1 International issues

1.1.1 Maternal health

Maternal health and obstetric care are the two factors that contribute to maternal deaths. Maternal health suffers because of a lack of education and poverty. The commonest causes of maternal mortality are the same throughout the developing world: abortion, haemorrhage, mechanical difficulties (obstructed labour), infection and hypertension [1,2]. It is apparent from data in countries with a low mortality that solutions to these problems of maternal health and obstetric care are available. They require the investment of substantial resources in maternity services. This is a luxury denied to most of the developing world, where insufficient money, materials and trained staff limit what can be achieved. Deaths from haemorrhage could be substantially reduced by improving the nutritional status of women. Provision of basic obstetric services or techniques such as antenatal care, instrumental delivery, Caesarean section, manual removal of the placenta, administration of an anaesthetic and blood transfusion are essential. However, in some developing countries, where sepsis and abortion account for more than a third of fatalities, maternal deaths could decline markedly with adequate provision for contraception. Tragically, contributions to international family planning have been severely reduced [3].

It is recognized that not only do medical facilities have to change, but also cultural, social and religious attitudes to women and their role in society [4]. Where there is a lack of access to family planning with barrier contraceptives, the prevalence of sexually transmitted disease is high, and maternal mortality is increasing from acquired immune deficiency disease [5]. A number of these disadvantaged women are delivering in Britain, and they will require a full anaesthetic assessment.

1.1.2 Obstetric interventions

Postal surveys from 1984 and 1989 in England and Wales of interventions during childbirth indicate changes in obstetric practice for which accurate collection of data is required [6]. For instance the percentage of women with episiotomies decreased, whereas the Caesarean section rate increased (Table 1.1).

Caesarean section is an instrumental delivery which overcomes problems related to vaginal delivery. These range from life-threatening obstructed

	1984	1989
Caesarean section	10 (1473)	13 (1491)†
Induction of labour by drugs	26 (1411)	26 (1386)
Artificial rupture of membranes		
Before onset of labour	17 (1419)	11 (1399)‡
After onset of labour	47 (1419)	46 (1399)
Epidural analgesia	22 (1416)	20 (1388)
Episiotomy	43 (1399)	36 (1375)‡
Stitches	74 (1418)	70 (1391)*
Shave	45 (1421)	8 (1386)‡

Table 1.1 Percentage of women receiving interventions during childbirth, based on a postal survey [6]. Figures in parentheses are the total number of women who completed the survey.

* $P < 0.05$; † $P < 0.01$; ‡ $P < 0.001$.

labour or placenta praevia to a social demand to avoid the stress and pain of labour or long-term labour-related perineal problems, such as stress incontinence. Caesarean section rates change with geography, fashion and the population studied. In the United States, the rates for Caesarean section have increased from one in 20 births to one in four in the past 20 years [7]. One of the factors in this increase is the fear of litigation, especially related to the threshold at which a decision is made to diagnose fetal distress or failure to progress. As a consequence, medical defence premiums have become so high that doctors cannot afford to practise low-cost obstetrics. Maternity care for the poor is therefore at risk. However, in Canada, where litigation is not so widespread as in the United States, the Caesarean section rate is as high, and may reflect a doctor-led rather than midwife-led service. The rates have increased for multiple births, breech presentation and low birth weight [8].

Rates for Caesarean section in Europe are more varied. They range from 6–7% in the Netherlands, where there is support for midwifery care in low-risk deliveries, to 10–15% in Norway and Sweden [9]. The Caesarean section rate in Scotland was 14–15% for 1989–91. Rates within the North-West Thames region varied from 9% to 24%, depending on case mix [10]. The outcome results from these variable rates show a clear advantage for very low birth weight infants being delivered by Caesarean section in centres where there was a high birth rate of low-weight infants. For the mother, the higher rates were associated with an increased risk of blood transfusion. A Caesarean section rate of 9% has been proposed as the most reasonable [11], but the circumstances surrounding Caesarean section rates in the United Kingdom are becoming more complex. The report on *Changing Childbirth* [12] and choices introduced by the Patient Charter are producing demands for elective Caesarean delivery as a patient choice, even though no medical indications exist.

Maternal choice may be having an effect on Caesarean section rates elsewhere. Brazil has the highest rate in the world: 38% in public clinics and 75% in private ones [13]. Women have been persuaded that it stops the pain of labour, avoids potential damage to the perineum and allows tubal ligation. It is unfortunate that accurate data are no longer available on the number of Caesarean sections in the United Kingdom. When data were available, emergency but not elective Caesarean section was associated with a significantly increased risk of death compared with that of vaginal delivery [14]. The risk of death is considered to be two to four times greater than that with a vaginal delivery, and patients cannot be legally required to accept a risk to health in order to benefit another [15]. The increased risk of mortality has been professionally accepted both in the United Kingdom and in the United States, where the professional obstetric bodies oppose forced emergency Caesarean sections.

1.2 United Kingdom policies

1.2.1 Anaesthetic service organization

The limited anaesthetic services provided by many small obstetric units with an annual delivery rate of less than 500 mothers prompted the Association of Anaesthetists of Great Britain and Ireland and the Obstetric Anaesthetists' Association to make recommendations for anaesthetic obstetric care [16]. In particular, it was agreed that the response time of an anaesthetist to an obstetric call must be immediate, because any delay may endanger both the mother and baby. Physical distance from an obstetric unit does not allow this ease of access, especially for senior help. Fetal distress requiring anaesthesia for operative delivery requires the start of operative delivery to be within 30 minutes of the call to the anaesthetist [17]. Request for 'on-demand' regional analgesia in labour should be satisfied within 60 minutes, except in exceptional circumstances.

In many centres, the obstetric anaesthetist is involved in the care of more than half the women presenting to our obstetric colleagues. The presence of a trained obstetric anaesthetist contributes to obstetric team care as follows.

Antenatal
- Education. Antenatal classes to discuss methods of pain relief, e.g. transcutaneous electrical nerve stimulation (TENS), opioids, local anaesthetics, regional nerve blocks.
- Consultation. Antenatal clinic or ward to identify and manage pre-existing or pregnancy-related disorders that may complicate anaesthesia.
- Preoperative. Assessment and preparation.

Intrapartum/postpartum
- Pain relief during labour and after delivery.
- Anaesthesia and analgesia for elective/emergency operative interventions.
- Cardiovascular and fluid balance (assessment, management and monitoring).

At all times
- Resuscitation of the:
  Mother (haemorrhage, cardiac arrest).
  Fetus (*in utero*).
  Neonate (if the paediatrician is absent or is in difficulty).

- High-dependency care.
- Intensive care.

Staffing

All consultant units should have a designated consultant anaesthetist to organize the obstetric anaesthesia service. This includes teaching, training, maintaining standards of practice and 24-hour consultant cover. Guidelines on the delivery to consultant ratio have been published [16] and accepted by various professional bodies. Attempts are currently being made to relate consultant sessional allocation more closely to workload, because of the expanding role of the obstetric anaesthetist. Skilled assistance from an adequately trained assistant must be available at all times for anaesthetic procedures.

Close supervision is required for all anaesthetists who have had less than a year of general training. The supervision should be provided in the delivery suite as well as the operating rooms. Procedures such as general anaesthesia in obstetrics are a rarity for many trainees, partly because of the increasing use of regional analgesia but also because of a reduction in trainees' hours of work. Extension of supervision into the second year of training for general anaesthesia in obstetrics may become necessary.

Regional analgesia service

An obstetric unit that offers an 'on-demand' regional analgesia service—for example, epidural or combined spinal and epidural analgesia, e.g. 'mobile epidural'—must also provide a duty anaesthetist to be in the hospital with obstetric consultant anaesthetist supervision, continuous care from a trained midwife and a trained obstetric team.

Guidelines

Guidelines for management are given in the following sections.
- Failed intubation (see Chapter 16, p. 313).
- Haemorrhage (see Chapter 23, p. 420).
- Cardiac arrest (see Chapter 24, p. 431).
- Malignant hyperthermia (see Chapter 9, p. 155).
- Regional analgesia (see Chapter 15, pp. 275–8) and its complications; e.g. epidural blood patch, total spinal block must be available.

Facilities

Labour ward. The labour ward should have at least one fully equipped, dedicated operating theatre, a recovery area and a high-dependency area [17,18]. An emergency electrical supply is essential. Ideally, an obstetric unit should be part of, or close enough to, the main hospital to have easy access to the main theatres, intensive care unit, neonatal unit and other support services.

A comprehensive range of anaesthetic drugs must be available for immediate access. These should include anaesthetic agents and resuscitation drugs, but not opioids. In the operating theatre, the following equipment and monitoring facilities are required:

Equipment
- anaesthetic machine;
- difficult intubation kit;
- defibrillator;
- anaesthetic gas scavenging;
- automatic pulmonary ventilator;
- drug storage with refrigerator;
- blood storage refrigerator.
- resuscitation:
  adult;
  neonatal (with temperature measurement and equipment for maintaining the temperature of the neonate).

Monitoring
- For all anaesthetic procedures:
  electrocardiogram;
  pulse oximeter;
  inspired oxygen concentration (on the fresh gas supply);
  automatic blood pressure (non-invasive) with 1-minute cycles.
- For general anaesthesia:
  end-tidal carbon dioxide measurement;
  peripheral nerve stimulator;
  intravascular central venous and arterial pressure;
  fetal heart rate;
  disconnect alarm.

Department. The department of anaesthesia should be sited beside or close to the labour ward and operating theatre. It should provide secretarial support for administrative, audit, teaching and clinic/consultation bookings. The department should also have appropriate books, journals and computer facilities. Resident staff require quiet, clean areas to rest and sleep, along with catering facilities.

Support services. The support services for obstetric anaesthesia include blood transfusion, radiology, pharmacy, pathology and trained staff to maintain essential clinical physiological monitoring equipment.

For blood transfusion, the equipment on the labour ward should include:
- blood storage refrigerator (with two units of O negative blood);
- pressure infusion bags;
- blood warming device.

In preparation for obstetric haemorrhage, which complicates 6–8% of deliveries, adequate amounts of plasma expanders must be available, and a quantity of group O Rh-ve blood should be held. Rapid infusion of blood requires pressure infusors and blood warming facilities. Supplies of blood must be available on site. The protocol for the management of severe haemorrhage should be readily available on the unit and agreed with all concerned (see p. 420). Laboratory facilities are required that provide biochemical, haematological and coagulation investigations. A haematological opinion with 24-hour cover is essential for adequate management of obstetric haemorrhage.

Transfer. Facilities and support equipment for transfer of the mother or neonate must be available, together with appropriately trained medical and paramedical personnel.

1.2.2 Information

Consent

To meet certain legal standards, patients should be informed whenever possible about any intended procedure, including its nature and purpose. Failure to inform and obtain consent for treatment whenever possible can expose a medical practitioner to a criminal charge of battery. Guidance on patient consent has been produced by the Association of Anaesthetists of Great Britain and Ireland [19], the General Medical Council [20] and the Department of Health [21]. The latter contains the recommended format for consent forms. The latter is worthless unless the proposed treatment and its alternatives have been explained in ways that the patient can understand. A patient has a fundamental right to grant or withhold consent. During labour, it is often difficult to comprehend information, and a woman may also be under the influence of drugs with sedative side effects, such as pethidine. Postoperative recall of information is poor [22], and after epidural insertion in labour more than a quarter of women could not recall any risk information being given [23]. It is therefore recommended that details of the risks explained should be recorded in the patient's notes. Information about the advantages, disadvantages and risks of all forms of pain relief and anaesthesia is best given during antenatal classes (Table 1.2). It can be in the form of written information, videos and interactive computer programs.

Antenatal assessment

Consultant obstetric anaesthetists are involved in the antenatal assessment of patients. Outpatient consultations can be formally arranged with a separate clinic, or on an *ad hoc* basis. In-patient ward rounds provide important obstetric

Table 1.2 Review of information for informed consent.

---

1 Adequate information can be provided to a mother as a result of the anaesthetist answering the following questions:
   Has the purpose of the proposed intervention been explained?
   What are the hoped-for benefits?
   Has the timing been described?
   Has the equipment to be used been explained?
   How serious are the risks?
   What is the inevitable distress or inconvenience?
   What are the alternatives?

2 The choice of methods and aids are listed below:

Methods used in providing information:	*Additional help:*
Check understanding	E.g. question information received, ask for summary from woman
Use diagrams, examples	Use books, posters
Use correct language	Seek interpreter
Allow time, discussion	Address relatives
Elicit fears	Measure VAS* for fear
Formulate preferences	Write a list

---

* VAS, visual analogue scale.

anaesthetic care. The types of patient who require anaesthetic assessment are summarized in Table 1.3. Obstetricians and midwives should be aware of the need for anaesthetic assessment in such cases, so that appropriate referral is not delayed.

At the antenatal assessment, a detailed history and physical examination are obtained, and risk factors should be identified. Options for management and relevant risks can then be discussed with both the patient (and partner) and the obstetrician. If necessary, further investigations and opinions can be sought within an appropriate time period. The details of the assessment and treatment plans should be recorded both in the patient's notes and also on the labour ward, together with the proposed date of delivery. Anaesthesia or analgesia can then be planned to meet the individual patient's needs.

A study from an outpatient obstetric anaesthetic clinic in Ottawa showed that the main reason for antenatal referral was musculoskeletal disorders, in 62% of women [24]. The outcome of epidural analgesia was studied in women who had prior low back pain, spina bifida, or posterior spinal instrumentation. It was found that pain relief was often inadequate in patients who had a history of spinal fixation with rods. Other clinic referrals were for neurological and cardiac disorders, adverse drug reactions and previous difficulties with anaesthesia. After the anaesthetic consultation, the referring obstetrician was advised on anticipated difficulties with either local or general anaesthesia that might affect obstetric decisions.

Table 1.3 Disorders that should be reported antenatally to an anaesthetist.

Disorder	Recognition	Anticipated problems
Anatomical		
Airway	Small mandible Unable to see uvula when looking in mouth	Difficult intubation
Spine	Laminectomy Scoliosis Other spinal injuries	Failed epidural/dural tap
Gross obesity	> 120 kg (?)	Difficult airway Poor respiratory reserve Failure of nerve block
Cardiovascular		
Valvular	History, heart sounds	Hypotension and death
Cardiomyopathy	Short of breath, echocardiogram, ECG	
Ischaemia	Elderly, diabetic	Myocardial infarction
Respiratory		
Severe asthma	Wheezing	Hypoxia
Infection	Cough	
Neurological		
Vascular abnormality	Headache, SAH	Increased intracranial pressure, stroke
Deficits	History	Paralysis
Haematological		
Sickle-cell disease	Routine screen	Sickling crisis
Bleeding diathesis, von Willebrand's Factor	History, clotting	Bleeding-airway -epidural haematoma
Inherited		
Enzyme defects	Family history	
Pseudocholinesterase deficiency		Suxamethonium apnoea
Porphyria	History	Avoid barbiturates
Malignant hyperpyrexia	Pyrexia, increased carbon dioxide	Avoid triggers
Drugs		
Allergies	History	Anaphylaxis
Vomiting	History postoperatively	Aspiration, discomfort, electrolyte imbalance
Placenta praevia		
Severe	Ultrasound	Bleeding
Neonate		
Surgery	Ultrasound	Paediatric anaesthetist

Clinical audit

Audit is required to identify deficiencies in services and correct them whenever possible, so that continuing improvements are made. Five areas can be audited in obstetric anaesthetics [25].

- Workload.
- Clinical practice data.
- Complications.
- Patient satisfaction.
- Research questions.

A minimum data set (Table 1.4) has been accepted by the Obstetric Anaesthetists' Association and requires regular updating. However, the data required to audit all five areas are not included—for example, information on patient satisfaction is lacking. This is an aspect of patient care that is of most interest to purchasers.

Clinical audit should not only record clinical activities and outcomes, but also assist in setting standards against which activities and outcome can be compared. Such standards have to be defined nationally and be evidence-based. Departmental and interdepartmental meetings focus on identified problems. The data needed to analyse particular questions are often not collected routinely [26], and the computerized systems designed for data analysis require finance both for equipment and personnel. They also have to be updated periodically.

Audit is only as accurate as the records kept. A case note audit of missing antenatal records identified 6.4% of notes missing, but these contained the notes for women who had significantly worse delivery outcomes, with a higher incidence of perinatal deaths, preterm labour and low Apgar score babies [27]. Notes may be misplaced, and after emergency admission with obstetric complications the patient may have been transferred with inadequate documentation.

Maternal choices

Standards of care, formulated by a maternity group for the Department of Health, have been proposed for women in a major reorganization of the maternity services in Britain. They allow women to have the choice to give birth at home or in hospital and to have a named midwife responsible for their care. Unfortunately, there was no formal representation from obstetricians or anaesthetists during the preparation of these proposals [12,28]. It is recommended that maternity care should be community-based and that women should have continuity of care; that midwives should more often be the sole provider of maternity care; and that women should have more choice with regard to where and how they deliver their babies. The Cumberledge report, as it is known after the name of its chairwoman, states that the mother 'needs to be fully informed about the options for care available, so that she can with confidence decide what best suits her, including the amount and type of interventions proposed'. Women should be informed at booking of the services, including analgesia, what they can expect during labour and delivery. However, although home birth may be an acceptable option, the appropriate information on which a mother can base her choice is not available [29].

The emergency services mentioned in the report were clearly perceived by mothers not to be so readily at hand in rural areas, yet there were occasions in hospital when an inexperienced obstetric senior house officer responded to calls for emergency help. It was therefore considered that emergency services should be improved both within and outside the hospital by identifying lines of communication, such as to the obstetric consultant, and improving training in neonatal resuscitation.

A joint report resulting from consultations between obstetricians, midwives and general practitioners followed, and examined the future of maternity services [30]. This made specific and general recommendations, based on an

Table 1.4 Obstetric Anaesthetists' Association Minimum Data Set.

A All patients	B Regional analgesia	C General anaesthesia (GA)
General	*Maternal*	*Procedure*
Date of procedure	Previous epidural?	EUA
Hospital number	Indication	*Elective Caesarean section
Grade of anaesthetist(s)	Breech	*Emergency Caesarean section
Type of anaesthetic:	Eclampsia	Forceps
Epidural	Elective Caesarean section	Postpartum
Spinal	Elective instrument delivery	Other
General	Hypertension of pregnancy	
Combined epidural and spinal	Intrauterine death	*Indication*
Other	Maternal request	Antepartum haemorrhage
Elective/emergency*	Multiple pregnancy	Breech
	Premature labour	Cephalopelvic disproportion
Maternal	Postpartum	Diabetes
Age	Trial of labour/scar	Eclampsia
Weight	Other	Fetal distress
Parity	Timing of procedure	Hypertension of pregnancy
ASA physical status	Before ARM	Intrauterine death
	First stage	Previous Caesarean
Neonatal	Second stage	Other
Gestational age	Third stage	
Time of delivery	Length of labour before procedure	*Induction and laryngoscopy*
Apgar at 1 and 5 minutes	< 2 h	Time
Was paediatrician present?	2–8 h	Drug and dose
	> 8 h	Difficulty or ease of intubation
	Site of epidural/spinal	(grades 1–4)
	Depth of epidural space	ETT size
	Total duration of epidural (h)	Failed intubation

(Cont'd)

Table 1.4 (*Cont'd*)

	B Regional analgesia	C General anaesthesia
	Analgesia prior to epidural	*Before delivery*
	Nil	Volatile and concentration
	Inhalational	Opiate drug and dose
	Intramuscular	F_{IO_2}
	Intravenous	Time of uterine incision
	Drug(s), dose and over how long	
		After delivery
	Drugs and mode of administration	Volatile and concentration
	Drug names	Opiate drug and dose
	Concentration and volume (total)	F_{IO_2}
	Total dose given	
	Over how long	*Relaxants/reversal*
	Intermittent or infusion	Drug(s) and dose
	Patient control or not	Time of reversal
	Delivery	*Personnel*
	Mode of delivery	Grade of surgeon(s)
	Spontaneous	Assistant present
	Breech	*Follow-up*
	Caesarean epidural	Was there any dreaming?
	Caesarean spinal	Was the patient 'aware'? If yes,
	Caesarean GA	assess:
	Rotational forceps	Partial recall
	Other instrumentation	Total recall
	Reason for forceps/instrumentation	Aware but no pain
	Fetal distress	Aware and some pain
	Long 1st or 2nd stage	Aware and severe pain
	Elective	
	Antepartum haemorrhage	
	Complications	
	Was epidural resited?	
	Dural tap	
	Headache	
	Backache	
	Neurological problems	
	Urological problems	
	Shivering	
	Follow-up	
	Satisfactory 1st stage	
	Satisfactory 2nd stage	
	For regional Caesarean section:	
	Was it comfortable?	

* These timing classifications are more appropriately 'elective' or 'scheduled', i.e. convenient to all staff; 'urgent', i.e. necessary because of maternal or fetal compromise but not immediately life-threatening; and 'emergency', i.e. life-threatening to the mother or fetus.
ARM, artificial rupture of membranes; ASA, American Society of Anesthesiologists; ETT, endotracheal tube; EUA, examination under anaesthesia.

acceptance of pregnancy and labour as natural phenomena. Shared care with midwives was an important theme. Of interest to anaesthetists is the support given to the policy of letting a woman carry her own notes. If this could be done in all types of anaesthetics, we might be able to identify anaesthetic problems more easily. However, confidential information would not be included in the record. Delivery outside a high-technology setting is attractive to one in eight women at some time prior to labour. As less than one in 100 achieve this, something must happen along the way to dissuade them [31].

The implementation of midwifery-led care is taking many forms, and requires evaluation. Midwives have always delivered the majority of babies in the United Kingdom, but when the dominant place of birth changed from the community to the hospital earlier this century, the role of the independent practitioner midwife declined. The proposed changes seek to reverse this trend. The debate about obstetric safety and choice has not been left to mothers and professionals. A House of Commons select committee recently raised questions about the safety of general-practitioner maternity units [32], and the Social Services Committee raised questions about all small obstetric units in its report of 1978–79 [33]. Access to specialist advice, adequate training and selection of patients have been recognized as important elements of a safe service by most authorities.

1.2.3 Domiciliary obstetrics

Rural and urban practice

Midwives and general practitioners are caring for more women in the community, and this process has been accelerated by the Cumberledge report. Many women positively wish to avoid the high-technology atmosphere of a hospital [34]. In Britain each day, more than 20 women deliver a baby at home, and in about half of these cases, the home birth is unintentional [35]. An inner London domiciliary practice with interested general practitioners and midwives delivered 79% of women booked for home births [36]. Nulliparous women were significantly more likely to require transfer. Emergency transfer was required in 2% of cases for postpartum haemorrhage, retained placenta and large tear. A previous study [37] expected a low-risk group of women scheduled for home birth to need emergency care in 12% of cases. In a rural maternity unit, unplanned transfer to a consultant unit occurred in 12.8% of 530 women, but in all, one-third of women at 'low risk' for complications of delivery required medical support due to delivery or postpartum complications [38]. If this rate can be minimized by providing ready access to a consultant-based service, as occurred in the study, a better outcome for the mother and baby can be expected. Rapid discharge from hospital and transfer back into the care of the general practitioner or midwife are now being practised.

Midwifery skills

The problem of developing and maintaining skills for midwives has been addressed by allowing them to work both within the community and also in hospital, so that a midwife or her professional partner are available for one mother throughout her labour, wherever it is, and postnatally for 28 days [39].

The activities of a midwife [40] include:
- monitoring normal pregnancies;
- diagnosing pregnancies at risk;
- parenthood preparation;
- caring for a mother in labour and appropriately monitoring the fetus;
- conducting spontaneous delivery with episiotomy if necessary, and in urgent cases breech delivery;
- recognizing abnormality and referring and assisting a doctor;
- examining and if necessary resuscitating a newborn baby;
- postnatal care;
- maintaining records.

General practitioner liaison

In domiciliary practice, general practitioners can add two important areas of maternity care that are appreciated by mothers. These are general medical care for the woman and continuity of care and support for the woman and her family. These aspects should be remembered by anaesthetists in their management of obstetric problems, so that the family doctor is aware of any anaesthetic difficulties the patient has experienced and any follow-up that may be appropriate in the community.

Peripartum transfer

Transfer may be required from a patient's home to hospital, or between hospitals—usually from a non-specialist hospital to a more specialist obstetric unit. The main indication for interhospital transfer is premature labour. The factors to be considered in transferring a patient are listed in Table 1.5. A woman who has had a haemorrhage should have a large-bore intravenous cannula with a fluid infusion of crystalloid or colloid set up prior to transfer, oxygen therapy, and be accompanied by a suitably trained medical practitioner. Communication with the receiving hospital should allow the patient's blood group to be known prior to transfer, so that adequate blood is available on arrival. Cardiovascular measurements of pulse and blood pressure and the respiratory rate should be continued throughout the journey.

Transfer of a diabetic mother may require a constant infusion of insulin to be maintained, with monitoring of the conscious state.

Table 1.5 Factors to be considered in parturient transfers.

Transport
Type, e.g. ambulance, helicopter
Duration of journey
Equipment available, e.g. oxygen, monitors, ventilator
Access to patient during transport to allow intubation, delivery etc.

Staff to accompany patient
Medical (consider specialist skills)
Paramedical
Midwife

Monitoring
Mother, especially cardiorespiratory observations
Fetus *in utero*

Medical condition of the patient
Assessment
Treatment

Cardiorespiratory stability and possible interventions
Infusions
Intubation
Ventilation of the lungs

Communication before and during transfer
Advice prior to transfer
Preparation for care on arrival
Ability to relay messages of deterioration in the clinical state of the patient during transfer

Care during labour
Fetal monitoring
Pain relief

A woman with severe pre-eclampsia or eclampsia on transfer may be receiving maintenance doses of antihypertensive and anticonvulsant drugs after the initiation of therapy prior to transfer. The accompanying staff should be familiar with the use of these, and should be able to monitor their effects on the mother. *In utero* transfer is hazardous [41] and is associated with maternal morbidity, especially in women with worsening pre-eclampsia or antepartum haemorrhage. Caesarean section is usually required soon after admission to the specialist hospital, and so the obstetric anaesthetist needs to be involved early in the patient's management.

1.3 Adolescent pregnancy

High rates of poor outcome in pregnancy have been reported in the USA in adolescents [42]—specifically, the number of premature infants and babies with low birth weight and those small for gestational age. Even in the lowest risk group, who were married and had been educated appropriately for their age and attended antenatal clinics, there was a higher risk of poor fetal outcome in adolescents than in similar mothers above 20 years of age. Socioeconomic factors such as low income, insufficient education and lack of antenatal care increase these risks. The risk that a second child will also be premature or of low birth weight is also higher [43], and this finding had an association with a low pre-pregnancy weight in the mother.

1.4 The elderly parturient

The phrase 'elderly primigravida' was formerly used to describe a woman of 35 years or older who became pregnant for the first time. It included women who had delayed childbearing and conceived naturally, and also women who had received fertility treatment to aid conception. A general trend towards later maternity has developed in women who wish to pursue a career or to start a family with a new partner, and it is now no longer unusual for older women to be pregnant.

The effects of ageing on reproductive functions occur earlier than in other systems and affect both the mother and the fetus. Age-related maternal antepartum complications, such as hypertension and carbohydrate intolerance, are more frequent [44]—for example, the presence of chronic hypertension doubles the incidence of hypertension in pregnancy [45]. Serious bleeding complications, such as placenta praevia and abruptio placentae, are more frequent in older women. Premature separation of the placenta is apparently related to the ageing of uterine vessels and to chronic hypertensive disorders. Maternal mortality from haemorrhage increases with age, being four times higher among women of 35–39 years of age than among women of 20–24 years. The increase in antepartum complications is probably responsible for a doubling in the Caesarean section rate.

There has been a substantial reduction in fetal mortality in older women compared with that of women in all age groups, but the rate of stillbirth remains higher than in younger women. The rate is six per 1000 deliveries, and it is probably increased by multiple gestations (e.g. with assisted reproduction techniques, which have a higher fetal rate). Six per 1000 is a lower rate than might be expected if fetal screening in early pregnancy for abnormalities was not highly developed. The incidence of Down syndrome increases by up to 10-fold with advancing maternal age from 35 to 45 years; at age 45, the incidence is one in 32 [46].

Genetic diagnosis and counselling should be available to this group of women, together with appropriate antenatal care in order to ensure a satisfactory maternal and fetal outcome. The contribution of the obstetric anaesthetist to the older parturient begins at the pre-anaesthetic visit—which may often involve in-depth discussion, because of high patient expectations—and continues throughout labour and delivery, with heightened anticipation of obstetric complications developing.

References

1. Papiernik E. Safe motherhood. *Lancet* 1989; **i**: 321.
2. Tonks A. Pregnancy's toll in the developing world: developing countries need integrated programmes devoted to women's reproductive health. *Br Med J* 1994; **308**: 353–4.
3. Potts M. USA aborts international family planning. *Lancet* 1996; **347**: 556.
4. Verkuyl DAA. Two world religions and family planning. *Lancet* 1993; **342**: 473–5.
5. Logie AW, Logie DE. Women's health in Africa. *Lancet* 1994; **343**: 170.
6. Fleissig A. Prevalence of procedures in childbirth. *Br Med J* 1993; **306**: 494–5.
7. Localio AR, Lawthers AG, Bengtson JM *et al*. Relationship between malpractice claims and Cesarean delivery. *JAMA* 1993; **269**: 366–73.
8. Macfarlane A, Chamberlain G. What is happening to Caesarean section rates? *Lancet* 1993; **342**: 1005–6.
9. Notzon FC. International differences in the use of obstetric interventions. *JAMA* 1990; **236**: 3286–91.
10. Joffe M, Chapple J, Paterson C, Beard RW. What is the optimal Caesarean section rate? An outcome-based study of existing variation. *J Epidemiol Community Health* 1994; **48**: 406–11.
11. Savage W, Francome C. British Caesarean section rates: have we reached a plateau? *Br J Obstet Gynaecol* 1993; **100**: 493–6.
12. Expert Maternity Group. *Changing Childbirth*. London: HMSO, 1992.
13. Souza C de M. C-Sections as ideal births: the cultural constructions of beneficence and patient's rights in Brazil. *Cambridge Q Healthcare Ethics* 1994; **3**: 358–66.
14. Department of Health. *Report on Confidential Enquiries into Maternal Deaths in England and Wales, 1982–1984*. London: HMSO, 1989.
15. Dyer C. Colleges say no to forced Caesarean sections. *Br Med J* 1994; **308**: 224.
16. Association of Anaesthetists of Great Britain and Ireland and Obstetric Anaesthetists' Association. *Anaesthetic Services for Obstetrics: a Plan for the Future with Special Reference to the Smaller Obstetric Unit*. London, 1987.
17. Obstetric Anaesthetists' Association. Recommended minimum standards for obstetric anaesthetic services (Obstetric Anaesthetists' Association guidelines). *Int J Obstet Anaesth* 1995; **4**: 125–8.
18. Department of Health. *Report on Confidential Enquiries into Maternal Deaths in the United Kingdom, 1988–1990*. London: HMSO, 1994.
19. *Information and Consent for Anaesthesia*. Association of Anaesthetists of Great Britain and Ireland. London, 1999.
20. *Seeking Patients' Consent: The ethical considerations*. London: General Medical Council, 1999.
21. Department of Health, NHS Management Executive. *Patient Consent to Examination or Treatment*. London: HMSO, 1990. HC(90)22.
22. Robinson G, Merav A. Informed consent: recall by patient tested postoperatively. *Ann Thoracic Surg* 1976; **22**: 209–12.
23. Swan HD, Borshoff DC. Informed consent: recall of risk information following epidural analgesia in labour. *Anaesth Intensive Care* 1994; **22**: 139–41.
24. Roseag OP, Yarnell RW. The obstetrical anaesthesia assessment clinic: a review of six years' experience. *Can J Anaesthesia* 1993; **40**: 346–56.
25. Royal College of Anaesthetists. *Guidance for Purchasers*. London, 1994.

26 Yudkin PL, Redman CWG. Obstetric audit using routinely collected computerised data. *Br Med J* 1990; **301**: 1371–3.
27 Yoong A, Hudson C, Chard T. Medical audit: the problem of missing case notes. *Health Trends* 1993; **25**: 114–16.
28 Walker P. Should obstetricians see women with normal pregnancies? Obstetricians should be included in integrated team care. *Br Med J* 1995; **310**: 36–8.
29 Young G. Uncertainty is likely to persist, but some knowledge would be better than none. In: 'Should there be a trial of home versus hospital delivery in the United Kingdom?' *Br Med J* 1996; **312**: 753–7.
30 *The Future of Maternity Services*. Royal College of Obstetricians and Gynaecologists. London/RCOG Press, 1994.
31 Court C. Britain's maternity services come under the microscope. *Br Med J* 1994; **309**: 1106.
32 Brahams DGP. Maternity units. *Lancet* 1992; **339**: 1407.
33 *Second Report from the Social Services Committee, Session 1979–80, Perinatal and Neonatal Mortality Vol. 1*. London: HMSO, 1980.
34 Taylor A. Maternity services: the consumer's view. *J R Coll Gen Pract* 1986; **36**: 157–60.
35 Chamberlain G. The place of birth: striking a balance. *Practitioner* 1988; **232**: 771–4.
36 Ford C, Iliffe S, Franklin O. Outcome of planned home births in an inner city practice. *Br Med J* 1991; **303**: 1517–19.
37 Dixon EA. Review of maternity patients suitable for home delivery. *Br Med J* 1982; **284**: 1753–5.
38 Baird AG, Jewell D, Walker JJ. Management of labour in an isolated rural maternity hospital. *Br Med J* 1996; **312**: 223–6.
39 Page L, Cooke P. Moving forward on the Cumberledge report: changing childbirth. *J R Soc Med* 1995; **88**: 115P–116P.
40 United Kingdom Central Council for Nursing, Midwifery and Health Visiting. *A Midwife's Code of Practice: for Midwives Practising in the United Kingdom*. London, 1989.
41 Ryan TDR, Kidd GM. Maternal morbidity associated with intrauterine transfer. *Br Med J* 1989; **299**: 1383–5.
42 Fraser AM, Brockert JE, Ward RH. Association of young maternal age with adverse reproductive outcomes. *N Engl J Med* 1995; **332**: 1113–17.
43 Blankson ML, Cliver SP, Goldenberg RL, *et al*. Health behavior and outcomes in sequential pregnancies of black and white adolescents. *JAMA* 1993; **269**: 1401–3.
44 Berkowitz GS, Skovron ML, Lapinski RH, Berkowitz RL. Delayed childbearing and the outcome of pregnancy. *N Engl J Med* 1995; **332**: 659–64.
45 Cunningham FG, Leveno KJ. Childbearing among older women: the message is cautiously optimistic. *N Engl J Med* 1995; **333**: 1002–3.
46 Hook EB. Rates of chromosomal abnormalities at different maternal ages. *Obstet Gynecol* 1981; **58**: 282–5.

2: Maternal and Perinatal Mortality

2.1 Maternal mortality

The magnitude of global maternal mortality cannot be assessed on the basis of maternal mortality in developed countries such as Britain, where it is approximately one in 10 000 maternities. Ninety-nine per cent of the world's maternal deaths are in the developing countries, at a rate of half a million women a year. There is also a difference in infant mortality, such that an infant is 10 times more likely to die in a developing country, while a mother is more than 100 times more likely to die. In Africa, the rate is one in 14 [1], equivalent to one maternal death every minute. It has been calculated that family planning could reduce this figure by 60%. The World Health Organization has convened a Safe Motherhood Initiative to develop strategies to combat high maternal mortality, but it is taking a long time for maternal death to be recognized as a serious health problem [2]. The survival of a mother will, of course, benefit her family. However, women also suffer the long-term effects of obstructed labour and abortion.

Maternal death is one end of the spectrum of a natural process, that of delivering a baby. It is an end point that is easy to define, unlike morbidity, so it has been used to analyse the multiple causes contributing to an adverse outcome of pregnancy. Mortalities from anaesthesia have similar causes from country to country within the developed world. Most of the deaths relate to complications of general anaesthesia, as discussed later in the chapter on general anaesthesia (p. 285). A broader analysis of maternal mortality is presented here, because with the expertise of the obstetric anaesthetist expanding to include the care of the critically ill mother, anaesthesia is increasingly being identified as a factor contributing to maternal deaths due, for example, to hypertension or haemorrhage. Unfortunately, deaths are still being reported that are wholly caused by anaesthesia.

Reports on *Confidential Enquiries into Maternal Deaths* have been produced for three-yearly periods since 1952 in England and Wales (since 1956 Northern Ireland and 1965 in Scotland). A single triennial report has covered the United Kingdom since 1985, because of declining numbers of maternal deaths. It is the best audit of maternal deaths in a clearly defined population, and sets an international standard. The confidentiality of the reports' contents has made possible the inclusion of critical assessment of the quality of care in individual cases. Substandard care related to service provision, staffing and clinical standards can be and are identified. Details of each case are collected from general practitioners, midwives, health visitors, consultant obstetricians

Table 2.1 A definition of terms relating to maternal mortality, with numerical examples [4,5].

Maternal death	Death of a woman while pregnant or within 42 days of termination of pregnancy from any cause related to or aggravated by the pregnancy or its management, but not from accidental or incidental causes
Direct deaths	Those resulting from obstetric complications of the pregnant state (that is, pregnancy, labour and puerperium), from interventions, omissions, incorrect treatment, or from a chain of events resulting from any of the above
Indirect deaths	Those resulting from previous existing disease, or disease that developed during pregnancy and which was not due to direct obstetric causes, but was aggravated by the physiological effects of pregnancy
Fortuitous deaths	Death from causes which happen to occur in pregnancy or in the puerperium (such as accidents)
Late deaths	Death occurring between 43 days and one year after delivery or abortion

Maternal deaths per million women aged 15–44 y. This figure assumes that all women of childbearing age are at risk of becoming pregnant. It can be used as a comparison with other causes of death in the same population group.

	All causes of death in women 15–44 y	Maternal deaths/million
1973–75	807.9	9.0 (1.1%) (England & Wales)
1988–90	625.9	4.1 (0.7%) (United Kingdom)
1991–93	605.6	3.8 (0.6%) (United Kingdom)

Maternal deaths per maternities. (Maternities is used rather than births because the number of births will also include multiple births). For the maternal mortality rate: the number of maternities is the sum of live and still births, since other outcomes, e.g. ectopics, terminations, are unreliable.

	Maternities (n)	Direct and indirect deaths	Maternal mortality rate per 100 000 maternities
1973–75	1 921 568	390	20 (England & Wales)
1988–90	2 360 309	238	10 (United Kingdom)
1991–93	2 315 204	228	10 (United Kingdom)

and any other relevant staff concerned with the care of the woman concerned. Anaesthetic assessors review all cases in which an anaesthetist has been involved. A national panel of doctors classifies the cases according to cause of death and identifies avoidable factors. The forms are then destroyed. Collection of forms is almost complete.

About 60 years ago, the maternal mortality rate was approximately 400 per 100 000 deliveries. The maternal mortality rate has halved every 10 years between 1952 and 1984 (Table 2.1). This dramatic reduction was due not so much to socio-economic factors (unlike infant mortality) as to improved maternity care. Similar declines in maternal mortality also occurred in several other countries (with different maternal death rates), and different organizational solutions led to similar results [3]. The initial downturn in maternal mortality can be attributed to the widespread use of antibiotics in the late 1930s (sulphonamides, then penicillin). Subsequent reductions in non-septic deaths can be attributed to improvements in medical management. Blood transfusions and ergometrine were introduced, as well as better management of pre-eclampsia.

Between the *Confidential Enquiries into Maternal Deaths* of 1988–90 [4] and 1991–93 [5], substandard care as the cause of death, irrespective of whether it was the direct or indirect cause, decreased from 49% to 40% of deaths. This is still not an acceptable figure, but it does suggest that the guidance contained in the reports is being heeded. The rate of indirect deaths due to chronic conditions such as diabetes, epilepsy and cardiac disorders should be benefiting from better services, but in the case of epilepsy, eight of the nine women dying from epilepsy in the 1988–90 report [4] had received substandard care, and similar uncertainties of care persisted in the more recent report [5].

Reproductive health changes that may have wider importance are also noted in the *Confidential Enquiries*. There has been an increasing number of multiple pregnancies, a higher age at conception and a continuing rise in the abortion rate (to 1.5% of women of childbearing age). Only 44% of primiparous women were under 25 years of age. Death rates per million maternities are 10 times higher in women above 35 years of age than in women of 25–29 years. The number of primiparous women delivering at the age of 35 years and over is continually increasing, and represented 22% of women in 1991–93 [5]. In particular, the number of women who die from hypertensive disorders increases with age.

Hypertensive disorders of pregnancy and thromboembolism are one of the two main direct causes of maternal death in the United Kingdom (Table 2.2), and most cases are associated with substandard care. Improvements in care of both have been suggested (Table 2.3). It was identified in the report that the risk features of pulmonary embolism had not been recognized. These features are previous thromboembolism, obesity, immobilization, operative delivery and increasing maternal age. There is a need to consider that pain in the leg, chest or dyspnoea in an otherwise healthy pregnant woman is caused by thrombosis or pulmonary embolism until proved otherwise. Accurate diagnosis and full anticoagulation therapy is essential.

Obstetric haemorrhage has been a recurring cause of death that can be prevented. The main causes of bleeding are placenta praevia, placental abruption, postpartum haemorrhage and coagulation failure. Placenta praevia is particularly likely to cause haemorrhage when associated with a uterine scar, and the mother should be counselled with appropriate advice and information, particularly with regard to critical care and hysterectomy. In such cases,

Table 2.2 Numbers of direct maternal deaths classified by causation in England and Wales (1973–75, 1988–90) and in the United Kingdom (1988–90, 1991–93).

Causes	1973–75 (E&W)	1988–90 (E&W)	1988–90 (UK)	1991–93 (UK)
Hypertensive disease	34 (15%)	25 (18%)	27 (19%)	20 (16%)
Pulmonary embolism	33 (15%)	23 (17%)	24 (17%)*	30 (27%)†
Haemorrhage	21 (9%)	21 (15%)	22 (15%)	15 (12%)
Ectopic pregnancy	19 (8%)	15 (11%)	15 (10%)	9 (7%)
Amniotic fluid embolism	14 (6%)	10 (7%)	11 (8%)	10 (8%)
Abortion	27 (12%)	7 (5%)	9 (6%)	8 (6%)
Sepsis (excluding abortion)	19 (8%)	6 (4%)	7 (5%)	9 (7%)
Anaesthesia	27 (12%)	3 (2%)	4 (3%)	8 (6%)
Total‡	227	136	145	129

* 33 in total from thromboembolism.
† 35 in total from thromboembolism.
‡ Other causes are included in the total figure.

Table 2.3 Appropriate management of hypertensive disorders.

Early use of standardized antihypertensive regimes.
Adequate monitoring of blood pressure and proteinuria antenatally and postnatally
   (if necessary starting at 24 weeks' gestation, because the majority of deaths occurred before 32 weeks).
The availability of an eclampsia protocol with referral to regional centres to provide special expertise in the management of eclampsia.
Avoidance of ergometrine in hypertensive disease.
Epidural analgesia should not be relied upon as an antihypertensive method.
Syllabus for training paramedics in the management of obstetric emergencies.

the anaesthetist must be careful not to obtund the sympathetic nervous system, because the normal vasoconstrictive response may be life-saving.

A hysterectomy may be the final outcome. Haemorrhage is a more common cause of death in the older pregnant woman, and age has become an important risk factor. Haemorrhage can also complicate ectopic pregnancy, amniotic fluid embolism and genital trauma. Guidelines for the management of massive obstetric haemorrhage can be found in Section 23.1, p. 419. In brief, the following are essential:

- anaesthetic registrar immediately contacted;
- alert haematologist and porters to arrange blood supply (6 units);
- 14 G × 2 cannulae and central venous pressure monitoring;
- remove 20 mL blood for group, cross match, haemoglobin, platelets and coagulation;
- give fluids, colloid or blood through a pressurized, warmed, intravenous infusion;

- monitor electrocardiograph (heart rate), central venous pressure, intra-arterial pressure, blood gases and acid–base, oxygen saturation, urine output.

When a massive blood transfusion is given, operative interventions are required, or coagulation disorders are occurring, transfer to an intensive-care unit is advised. The contribution that haemorrhage makes to maternal mortality is underestimated. In the past 10 years, it has contributed to 12–15% of direct deaths and up to 17% of total maternal deaths. The recognition of massive haemorrhage may be delayed when moderate 'trickling' vaginal bleeding is allowed to continue for a few hours postpartum, or when a small bleed occurs and a deterioration in clotting abnormalities is allowed to continue.

Anaesthesia became the third commonest cause of maternal death in 1972, and this continued for the next 10 years (Fig. 2.1). Most of the deaths were associated with general anaesthesia, but a number of fatalities associated with regional anaesthesia have now occurred, often from inadequate assessment and management of hypovolaemic shock and inappropriate treatment of dysrhythmias. It is difficult to estimate the risk of death for a particular technique of anaesthesia, because the denominator data—that is, the total number and type of anaesthetics administered—are unknown. There has been an increase in the number of Caesarean sections from the early 1970s onwards, and methods of anaesthesia have changed from general anaesthesia to regional nerve block.

The principal causes of death from general anaesthesia have been a failure to intubate the trachea, usually during emergency Caesarean section and

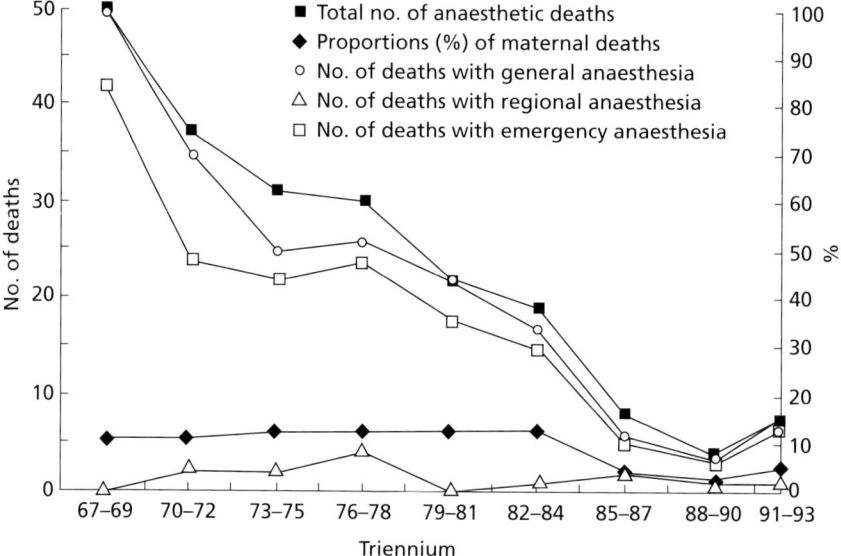

Fig. 2.1 Anaesthesia and maternal death (England and Wales, 1967–84, and United Kingdom, 1985–90).

often in association with undiagnosed oesophageal intubation, and the aspiration of gastric contents. Both causes lead to cerebral hypoxaemia. Airway difficulties can arise not only on induction but also during recovery, and the need for care in this postpartum period is well documented. Good muscle tone and adequate reversal of muscular relaxation are essential to maintain an airway and ventilation. Management of the difficult airway is discussed in Chapter 16, and the protocol for failed intubation is given on p. 313.

Improvements in the quality and safety of anaesthesia have occurred in part as a result of the implementation of the recommendations of the *Confidential Enquiries*. Recent recommendations [4,5] for anaesthetists to improve obstetric anaesthetic care have been:

- adequate consultant involvement and appropriate specialist care, particularly in assessing the severity of illness and in requesting critical care facilities;
- use of appropriate monitoring:
  (i) A carbon dioxide analyser is the best method to diagnose failed intubation during a general anaesthetic. A series of peaks of end-tidal CO_2 concentration corresponding with the first few breaths are confirmatory. This also will detect disconnections or gas leakage.
  (ii) Pulse oximetry is to be used throughout general or regional anaesthesia, into the recovery period and for longer when a patient's condition gives grounds for concern.
- prevention of hypoxaemia and airway obstruction.

The development of acute respiratory distress syndrome should include the administration of histamine H_2-receptor blocking drugs, because despite antacid preparation, aspiration of gastric contents still leads to pulmonary dysfunction, and all measures to avoid or prevent it must be used;

- assistance for the anaesthetist should be provided at all times by an appropriately trained person who maintains competence to practise. Postoperative care is still the responsibility of an anaesthetist, and must only be delegated to a midwife if she is trained in recovery nursing care.

The reporting of late deaths is being continued, because multiple organ support systems are now available and the death of a woman who has an acute complication at delivery may not occur until after six weeks. Forty per cent of direct and indirect maternal deaths were associated with a need for intensive-care unit facilities. Development of acute respiratory distress syndrome mainly followed haemorrhage and sepsis, but hypertensive disorders, aspiration of gastric contents and amniotic fluid emboli were all factors. Additional risks were associated with obesity, cardiac disease and asthma [5].

The two recent reports end with general recommendations. Those of specific relevance to anaesthetists are:

- facilities for high-dependency or intensive care should be available and conveniently sited, and staff should have training in emergency care and resuscitation;

- risks of life-threatening conditions should be explained to a mother. Every effort must be made to improve the quality of information provided and ensure that it is presented appropriately, e.g. with interpreters present;
- diagnosis of thromboembolic disorders should be improved, with close attention being given to the chest symptoms and prophylaxis used;
- appropriate monitoring equipment must be available and training should be provided for its use;
- there should be early consultant anaesthetist involvement, especially in complex deliveries.

2.2 Perinatal mortality

Mortality data relating to the fetus or neonate are presented in three ways.

1 Stillbirths. The stillbirth rate is calculated by the formula: number of babies born dead after 24 weeks × 1000/all births (both live and stillborn). The figure was 5.3 per 1000 in 1992 [6], for babies born after 28 weeks.

2 Neonatal deaths. The rate of neonatal deaths is calculated by the formula: number of babies dying up to 28 days after birth × 1000/number of live births. The figure was 3.9 per 1000 in 1992 [6].

3 Perinatal death rate. This figure groups together all babies whose death may have had some relation to obstetric events, i.e. both stillbirths and early neonatal deaths. The rate is calculated by the formula: stillbirths + neonatal deaths in the first seven days (days 0–6) × 1000/all live births and stillbirths. The figure was 7.6 per 1000 in 1992 [6].

The perinatal mortality rate has more than halved over the past 20 years. Initially, there was a rapid decline, but the rate is now decreasing more slowly.

2.2.1 Interpretation of perinatal death rates

The perinatal mortality rate will not include babies (such as those with lethal congenital abnormalities) who are kept alive in neonatal units until the second or third week of life. Some countries, e.g. Australia, have compromised by including all deaths from days 0–27 in the perinatal morality rates [7]. Artefactual differences in the perinatal mortality rate can occur at the lower limit of registrable stillbirths. At low gestational age, a fetus could be defined as a late spontaneous abortion rather than a stillbirth. The number of cases that could be influenced in this way is substantial [8].

The World Health Organization has recommended the introduction of a weight definition for perinatal morality, such that live or dead infants of > 500 g would be included in national figures and > 1000 g for international comparisons. However, not all infants are weighed at birth, especially if they are severely ill. Some countries, such as Norway, start their registration of births, whether alive or dead, at 16 weeks' gestation—far below the level at which international comparison is to begin—and this method would avoid the criticisms of these statistics.

2.2.2 Causes of perinatal mortality

The three main causes of perinatal mortality in the United Kingdom are hypoxia, low birth weight and congenital abnormalities. Out of 100 babies born, one will die around the time of birth, two will have an abnormality and six will have a birth weight of less than 2500 g. Some mothers are at high risk from these problems:

- the extremes of maternal age (< 20 and > 40 years);
- high parity (more than four babies);
- low socio-economic class;
- some ethnic groups [9] in which perinatal mortality rates are influenced not only by obstetric and midwifery practice, but also by educational, social, nutritional and public health factors.

2.2.3 Methods of improving perinatal death rates

The Department of Health in the United Kingdom has enabled a continuing investigation into perinatal death rates. Its first report, the *Confidential Enquiry into Stillbirths and Deaths in Infancy* [6], made recommendations for improvements in standards of care. Three deficiencies were described throughout the report: failures of communication, lack of training and an absence of clear clinical guidelines.

These identified areas of deficiency are also applicable to obstetric anaesthetic management [10]. Antenatal identification of medical problems that put a mother at risk requires anaesthetic assessment (see Table 1.3), and management during labour or operative delivery in full consultation with senior anaesthetic staff. The antenatal risk factors identified in the report included diabetes, infection, post-term pregnancy and parental behaviour. The recommendation was that professional staff should advise parents that agreed birth plans may need to be modified in the event of a change in clinical findings. Prior discussion with an obstetric anaesthetist is often helpful in this regard.

Peripartum risk factors focused on deficiencies relating in particular to induction of labour, fetal monitoring, lack of staff (especially anaesthetists), and management of emergencies such as shoulder dystocia (large babies, diabetic mothers), haemorrhage and neonatal resuscitation. Recommendations stressed the need for training and practice. Neonatal resuscitation and maternal haemorrhage are both anaesthetic problems, and their management is discussed in Chapters 21 (p. 392) and 23 (p. 420), respectively.

2.2.4 Perinatal bereavement

Attitudes to perinatal death have changed radically in the past 25 years, and current practice is based on the principles recommended by the Stillbirth and Neonatal Death Society [11]. There is an initial problem of how to manage the pain and distress, and there are also secondary, long-term effects of parental mourning [12]. These may even lead to a mother refusing regional analgesia techniques for infant delivery in the future [13], and the patient's next pregnancy should also be considered to be 'at risk' [14].

References

1. Potts M. Safe motherhood. *Lancet* 1990; **i**: 1580.
2. Royston E, Armstrong S, eds. *Preventing Maternal Deaths*. Geneva: World Health Organization, 1989.
3. Loudon I. The transformation of maternal mortality. *Br Med J* 1992; **305**: 1557–60.
4. Department of Health. *Report on Confidential Enquiries into Maternal Deaths in the United Kingdom, 1988–1990*. London: HMSO, 1994.
5. Department of Health. *Report on Confidential Enquiries into Maternal Deaths in the United Kingdom, 1991–1993*. London: HMSO, 1996.
6. Department of Health. *Confidential Enquiry into Stillbirths and Deaths in Infancy: Annual Report for 1 January–31 December 1993*. London: HMSO, 1995.
7. Anon. Perinatal mortality rates: time for change? [editorial]. *Lancet* 1991; **337**: 331.
8. Working Group on the Very Low Birth Weight Infant. European Community collaborative study of outcome of pregnancy between 22 and 28 weeks' gestation. *Lancet* 1990; **336**: 782–4.
9. Lieberman E. Low birth weight: not a black and white issue. *N Engl J Med* 1995; **332**: 117–18.
10. Holdcroft A. The fetus comes of age. *Anaesthesia* 1995; **50**: 925–7.
11. Stillbirth and Neonatal Death Society. *Miscarriage, Stillbirth, Neonatal Death: Guidelines for Professionals*. London: Sands, 1991.
12. Bourne S, Lewis E. Perinatal bereavement: a milestone and some new dangers. *Br Med J* 1991; **302**: 1167–8.
13. Holdcroft A, Parshall AM, Knowles MG, Waite KE, Morgan BM. Factors associated with mothers selecting general anesthesia for lower segment Caesarean section. *J Psychom Obstet Gynecol* 1995; **16**: 167–70.
14. Bourne S, Lewis E. Pregnancy after stillbirth or neonatal death. *Lancet* 1984; **ii**: 31–3.

Section 2
Systematic Physiology and Pathology

3: Cardiovascular System

Pregnancy converts the normal female cardiovascular system into a hyperdynamic, vasodilated, hypervolaemic, hypercoagulable and hypo-osmolar state. The increases in circulating blood volume and cardiac output that occur during pregnancy sustain placental blood flow and function. These changes, together with an enhanced coagulability, provide reserve capacity to compensate for and minimize the effects of the acute blood loss that occurs at delivery. When congenital or acquired cardiac disease is present, the cardiovascular changes of pregnancy make the parturient vulnerable to cardiac failure especially at the end of the second trimester, as well as to dysrhythmias and myocardial ischaemia. The development of hypertension during pregnancy complicates these physiological changes. Parturients with pre-eclampsia generally have a lower cardiac output and higher systemic vascular resistance (SVR) than in normal pregnancy [1], although a combination of high cardiac output and low SVR has been reported [2]. The aetiology of pregnancy-induced hypertensive changes is not fully understood, and symptomatic treatment of identified cardiovascular abnormalities, such as the increase in blood pressure and reduction in circulating blood volume, is common. Treatment of pre-eclampsia is discussed in Chapter 22.

3.1 Blood and body fluids

3.1.1 Blood and blood volume

Blood volume increases by 40–100% through pregnancy. The way in which this change is controlled is described in more detail in the section on renal physiology in Chapter 6. The increase involves two components: the plasma volume and the volume occupied by the cellular blood components, mostly red blood cells (often referred to as the 'red cell mass'). The increase in plasma volume continues until 32–34 weeks' gestation [3]. An earlier view that plasma volume actually decreased during the last eight weeks of pregnancy was based on dye dilution measurements made during the third trimester with patients in the supine position. The aortacaval compression associated with this posture inevitably caused incomplete mixing of dye, and erroneously low plasma volumes were recorded [4]. The plasma volume increase seems to correlate with fetal size or number. Normal singleton pregnancy is associated with an increase in plasma volume of 40–50% [3], but increases of nearly 100% have been recorded in patients with triplet or quadruplet pregnancies [5–7].

The increase in the total volume of circulating red blood cells, or red cell mass, is more variable than the increase in plasma volume. It depends on diet and dietary supplements, as well as the stimulus of pregnancy itself. It is now unusual to see venous haematocrit values much below 32% at term in the parturient who has received regular antenatal care and supplements of iron and folate if her haemoglobin concentration falls below 10 g/dL.

In normal pregnancy, a decrease in haemoglobin concentration to about 12 g/dL occurs. This is a dilutional phenomenon, which is inappropriately referred to as the 'physiological anaemia of pregnancy'. It is not abnormal, nor does it result in any penalty to fetoplacental oxygen availability. The decreasing concentration of haemoglobin obscures the fact that the total quantity of oxygen available to tissues is increased because of an increase in cardiac output.

Optimal diet, together with supplements when necessary, will keep the circulating red cell mass close to non-pregnant values. Maintaining antenatal haemoglobin levels > 12 g/dL has the added benefit that blood transfusion will be less frequently required if operative intervention is needed or postpartum haemorrhage occurs. This is an important consideration, because of the risks of complications such as transmission of infection. The more subtle effects of blood transfusion on the recipient's immune defence mechanisms may in future also come to be considered important factors weighing against administration of homologous blood.

Sickle-cell disorders. The inheritance of haemoglobin S is autosomal, and homozygous women now reach childbearing age. Haemoglobin electrophoresis is required for all parturients with a family background that could indicate genetic transmission, since skin colour is no guide to its presence. Electrophoresis will determine the type and amount of haemoglobin. Haemoglobin can be in combinations of AS, SS and SC with variable amounts of fetal haemoglobin. Haemoglobin C becomes crystallized at low oxygen tensions, but does not deform the red blood cells. Although the SC combination may clinically appear less severe, thrombotic episodes are common. The SS combination has usually been identified in infancy or childhood, and the individual followed up by a haematologist. Varying degrees of anaemia and chronic manifestations of vascular occlusion may be present. During pregnancy, routine maintenance of haemoglobin A at more than 70% of the total haemoglobin concentration can be achieved by exchange blood transfusions. Central nervous system symptoms may present in sickle-cell disorders because of an intracranial sickling crisis. This has to be distinguished from eclampsia in pregnancy.

If anaesthesia is required for pain relief in labour of delivery, adequate oxygenation and avoidance of hypotension and hypothermia is mandatory in the preoperative and postoperative periods in order to avoid sickling of red blood cells. Pregnant women at risk of complications from sickled cells in the tissues include those on bed rest because of circulatory stasis.

Epidural analgesia for labour and delivery is a preferred option, even in sickle-cell crisis [8], because it provides pain relief, vasodilation, and a reduction in endogenous catecholamines, which exacerbate vasoconstriction. Adequate fluids must be infused and inferior venacaval occlusion avoided. Oxygenation may be compromised by shivering, so that monitoring of oxygen saturation and administration of an adequate inspired oxygen is necessary. The use of adrenaline in local anaesthetic solutions is to be avoided because of its vasoconstrictor and acidic properties, and if opioids are used in a regional nerve block, monitoring of respiration is vital.

Thalassaemia. The α- and β-thalassaemias have a reduced production of haemoglobin protein chains. Most patients are asymptomatic, but if the condition is severe, e.g. β-thalassaemia major, anaemia is present. Women are likely to have received multiple blood transfusions, and may suffer from iron overload. In addition, cardiomyopathy and hepatic and pancreatic dysfunction may occur. An anaesthetist will have to assess the heart rhythm and the degree of heart failure and monitor myocardial function. Altered drug pharmacokinetics may result from abnormal liver function. Skeletal deformities may affect the spine and make access to the epidural or intrathecal space difficult.

3.1.2 Coagulation

The increase in the overall coagulability of the blood during pregnancy results from a combination of increased concentrations of coagulation factors I (fibrinogen), VII (antihaemophilic factor), VIII (Stuart–Prower factor) and X (Fig. 3.1) and a decrease in fibrinolytic activity (Fig. 3.2). A substantial rise in the availability of the raw materials needed for successful haemostasis at delivery is thereby achieved, and this also supplies the fivefold increase in the rate of fibrin deposition that occurs during late pregnancy.

The decrease in fibrinolytic activity is possibly due to placental production of inhibitors of fibrinolysis [9]. However, the low level of plasminogen activator measured during normal pregnancy may simply be due to excessive binding of the activator to the increased amount of fibrin present. The increased deposition of fibrin is almost certainly matched by an increased consumption of fibrinolytic factors, and during Caesarean section the deposition of fibrin and subsequent fibrinolysis results in raised levels of fibrin degradation products (FDPs) [10]. The large area of injury and the powerful nature of the coagulation factors available locally and in the circulation can—and occasionally do—stimulate a more widespread coagulation process outside the area of the uterus. This is usually prevented by the fine control exerted by naturally occurring anticoagulant factors. Antithrombin III (At III) and protein C, together with the latter's cofactors, thrombomodulin and protein S, are the main controllers of the coagulation process. Antithrombin III is an inhibitor of

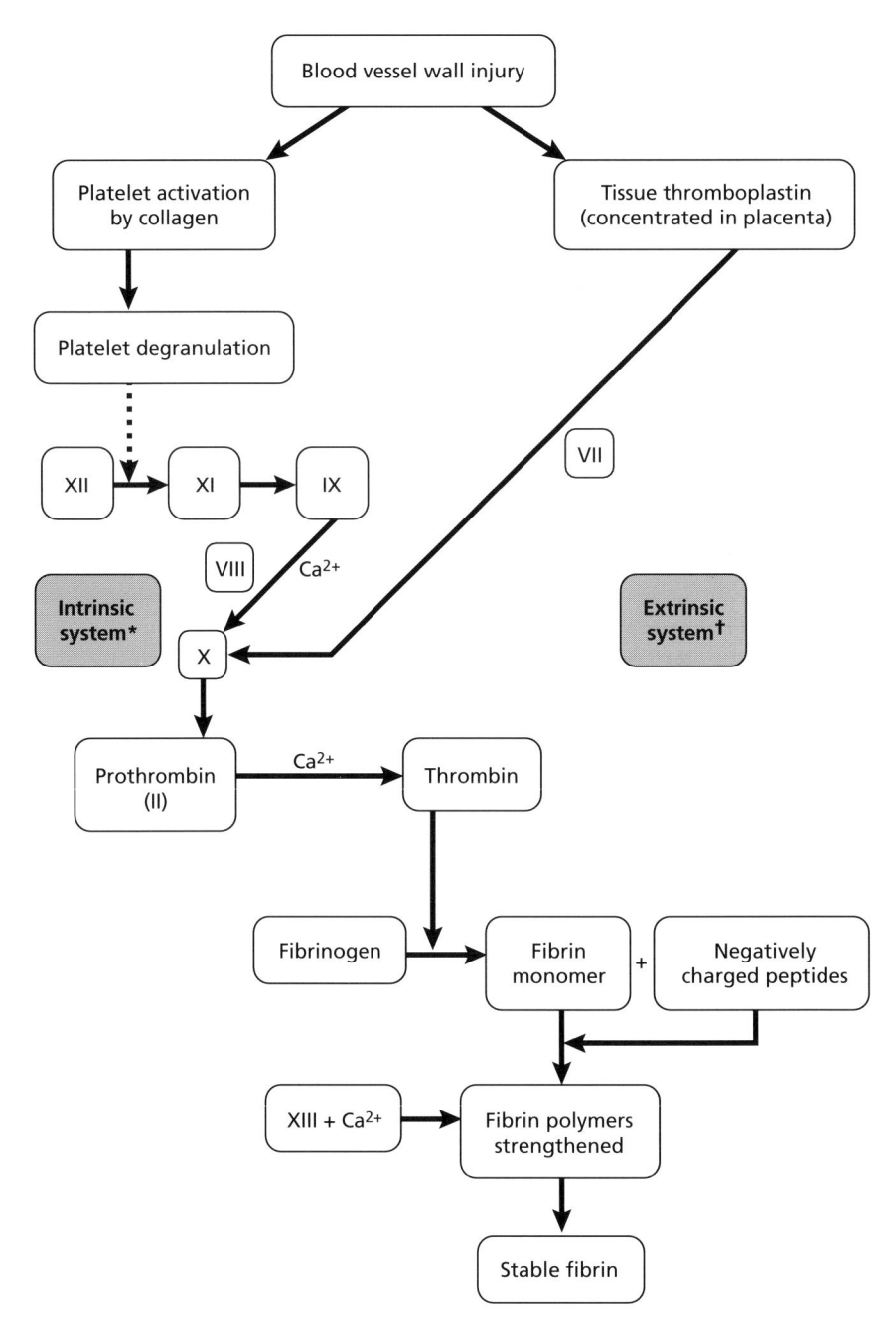

Fig. 3.1 Coagulation of the blood. * Activated partial thromboplastin time (APTT) measures the activity of the intrinsic pathway; † prothrombin time (PT) measures the activity of the extrinsic pathway. The thrombin time measures the activity of the final common pathway (Factor X onwards).

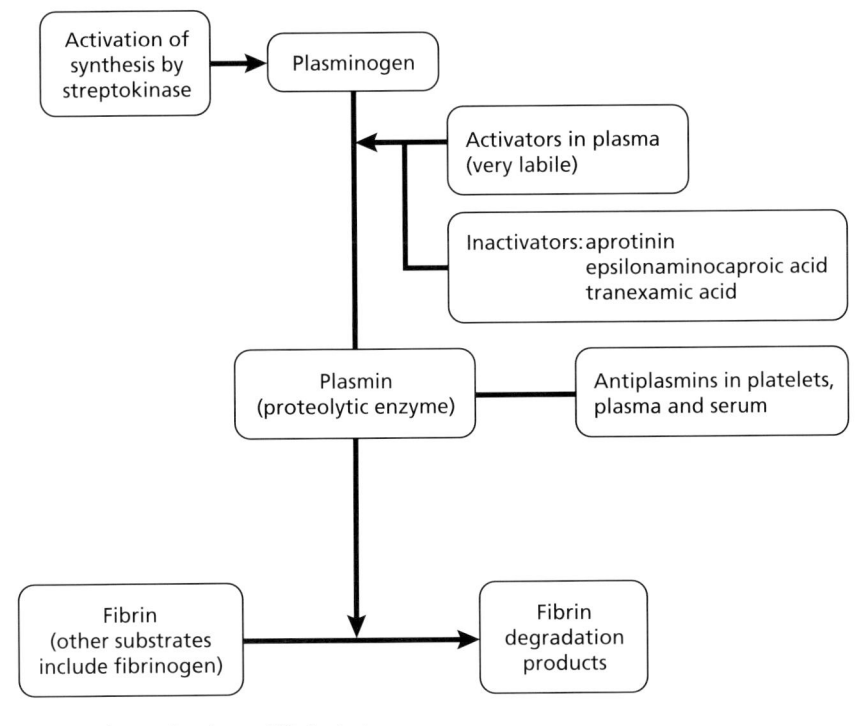

```
                ┌─────────────┐
┌────────────┐  │             │
│Activation of│─▶│ Plasminogen │
│synthesis by │  │             │
│streptokinase│  └─────────────┘
└────────────┘         │
                       ▼
              ┌──────────────────────┐
              │ Activators in plasma │
              │    (very labile)     │
              └──────────────────────┘
              ┌──────────────────────────┐
              │ Inactivators: aprotinin  │
              │    epsilonaminocaproic   │
              │    acid tranexamic acid  │
              └──────────────────────────┘

        ┌──────────────┐      ┌──────────────────────┐
        │   Plasmin    │──────│Antiplasmins in       │
        │(proteolytic  │      │platelets, plasma and │
        │  enzyme)     │      │serum                 │
        └──────────────┘      └──────────────────────┘

   ┌──────────────┐         ┌──────────────┐
   │    Fibrin    │────────▶│    Fibrin    │
   │(other        │         │  degradation │
   │ substrates   │         │   products   │
   │ include      │         │              │
   │ fibrinogen)  │         │              │
   └──────────────┘         └──────────────┘
```

Fig. 3.2 The mechanisms of fibrinolysis.

thrombin, Factor Xa and possibly IXa, XIa and XIIa. Increasing levels of oestrogen during pregnancy may therefore contribute to increasing coagulability by reducing levels of At III. Support for the hypothesis that oestrogen causes a decrease in At III comes from studies of women taking oral contraceptives of two types. Oral contraceptives cause a small decrease in At III levels and are also associated with a slight increase in venous thrombosis problems. The decrease in At III levels has not been seen in women taking progestogen-only oral contraceptives [11], so the decrease in the At III level is likely to be an effect of oestrogen. The anticoagulant factor, protein C, is a vitamin K dependent protein synthesized in the liver. It inactivates Factors V and VIII, and must itself be activated by protein S, another vitamin K dependent glycoprotein, and a cofactor named thrombomodulin derived from endothelial cells. Patients suffering from protein C deficiency will be at increased risk of venous thrombosis, and are therefore maintained on anticoagulant therapy through pregnancy.

In addition to the naturally occurring anticoagulants, the coagulation process is controlled by a fibrinolytic system that comprises plasminogen and plasmin, together with their activators and inhibitors. Plasmin is a proteolytic enzyme that digests fibrin and fibrinogen. It is derived from its inactive precursor, plasminogen, by the action of tissue activators. The uterus is especially rich in activators, which are mainly concentrated around blood vessels, especially veins.

The rise in fibrinogen levels and the inhibition of fibrinolysis are probably the largest of the coagulation changes that take place during pregnancy. However, enhanced coagulability is not the sole mechanism responsible for the limitation of uterine bleeding. Well-maintained contraction of the uterus itself and its exposed maternal blood vessels is the basis of the prevention of postpartum haemorrhage. Uterine contraction is adversely affected by fibrin degradation products, so any further increase in these can exacerbate blood loss by relaxing the uterus. A vicious circle of increasing blood loss, coagulation, fibrinolysis and further release of FDPs can result, and may be difficult to control. Disseminated intravascular coagulopathy (DIC) is a life-threatening development of this sequence of events (see Chapter 23). Even in the presence of well-maintained uterine contraction, the reserve pool of coagulation factors that develops through pregnancy is needed to seal the large raw area left after placental separation.

3.1.3 Platelets

Although the platelet count during normal pregnancy has been extensively studied for the last 25 years, the results vary widely. Earlier studies were carried out on small numbers of parturients, and the counts were performed manually. A study of 2066 women [12] showed significant decreases in platelet counts during the last eight weeks of pregnancy. However, the counts recorded were still within the normal non-pregnant range. Platelet size was increased, which would seem to indicate a preponderance of younger platelets. This shift in the profile of platelet size supported the hypothesis of a chronic intravascular coagulation process during normal pregnancy [13]. Further confirmation of the small decrease in platelet numbers has been obtained from a prospective study of 2263 healthy women [14]. In the latter study, 8.3% of the women exhibited a mild thrombocytopenia at term, the authors using platelet counts of $97–150 \times 10^{-9}$ per litre as their range for mild thrombocytopenia. Significant increases in the number of aggregated platelets have also been recorded [15,16], and would seem to confirm the presence of low-grade disseminated intravascular coagulation as part of normal pregnancy.

3.1.4 Haemostasis and coagulation processes at delivery

More parturients die as a direct result of haemorrhage than from any other single cause of death in the United Kingdom. In the triennium 1988–90 at least 49 women died from haemorrhage, and in 1991–93 the figure was 29 (approximately one-third of all direct deaths). Successful haemostasis is therefore literally life-saving. The size of the physiological challenge to the body's haemostatic mechanisms is daunting. The placental site at term

Table 3.1 Platelet factors released at placental separation.

Thromboxane
Fibrinogen
Factor V
Factor VIII
Serotonin
Adenosine diphosphate
β-Thromboglobulin
Calcium

occupies an area of some 300–350 cm² and receives a continuous blood flow of 500 mL/min. Atonic uterine contraction reduces the size of the bleeding site and blood flow to it through a tourniquet-like effect on uterine vessels. It is an essential part of a rapid and finely controlled response to injury. Most of the coagulation factors involved in haemostasis are carried in the blood as an inert form. They are activated by extrinsic factors released by tissue injury, and by intrinsic factors released from blood vessel endothelial cells and platelets. Following tissue injury or blood vessel injury, platelets accumulate at the site of damage. Once they are adherent at the site of injury, the platelets release a mixture of vasoactive and coagulation factors. These platelet factors include thromboxane, β-thromboglobulin, fibrinogen, Factor V, Factor VIII, serotonin (5-hydroxytryptamine) and calcium. Adenosine diphosphate is also released, and stimulates further aggregation of platelets around the damaged tissue. Serotonin helps with this process, and in addition produces local vasoconstriction (Table 3.1).

Circulating inert coagulation factors are activated at the site, and the coagulation cascade is initiated. Fibrin is formed, and together with platelet contractile proteins it produces a firm, retracted clot. The haemostatic process at the placental site involves both the intrinsic and extrinsic limbs of the coagulation cascade. The intrinsic pathway is initiated by the action of collagen on Factor XII, and is a contact system that is relatively slow to produce fibrin. However, the placenta is very rich in tissue factors, which bypass this contact intrinsic system and produce fibrin within about 12 seconds of being added to blood at the placental site. Fibrin polymer is formed by the action of thrombin on fibrinogen, and the polymer is strengthened by fibrin-stabilizing factor (Factor XIII), which links adjacent areas of the fibrin polymer and produces a strong and insoluble clot.

3.1.5 Plasma proteins and extracellular fluid

In normal pregnancy, the plasma protein concentration decreases during the first three to four months of gestation, and reaches a plateau at approximately 10 g/L below non-pregnant levels. The total amount of circulating albumin probably increases during pregnancy, but the increase in plasma volume is proportionately greater, so albumin concentration decreases. It does so most

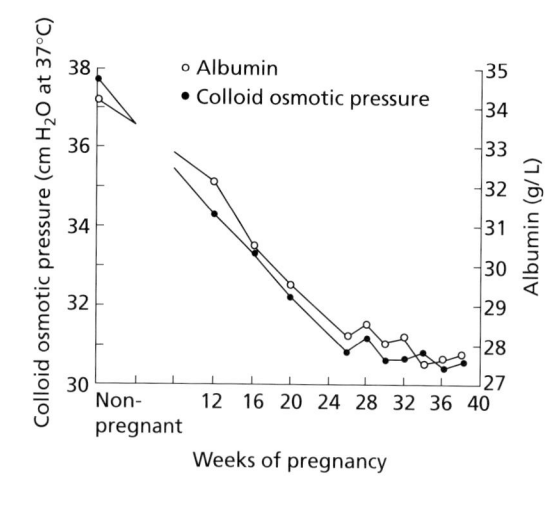

Fig. 3.3 Decreases in plasma albumin and colloid osmotic pressure during non-pregnant and pregnant state (from [17] by kind permission.

rapidly in the first trimester, and by late pregnancy is about 30–35 g/L. Albumin is one of the smaller proteins, and is a major osmotic factor. Plasma colloid osmotic pressure decreases almost linearly with the reduction in albumin concentration (Fig. 3.3) [17]. The association has been well demonstrated by Robertson in a number of publications [18,19], showing that a decrease in albumin concentration of approximately 7 g/L is associated with a decrease in colloid osmotic pressure of approximately 7 cm H_2O. The changes in albumin concentration and colloid osmotic pressure are accompanied by an increase in extravascular water. The extracellular fluid volume increases through pregnancy by 1–2 L. It may increase by as much as 5 L if marked oedema is present.

Oedema is a natural accompaniment to pregnancy, and gravitational oedema is seen commonly. A water load drunk by a parturient in a standing position appears as an increased leg volume of 500–600 mL [20]. When she lies down, diuresis occurs, and this recumbent diuresis is one of the causes of pregnancy-related nocturia.

Increases in lower limb volumes do not account for all the accumulated fluid, and the remaining fluid is distributed to other tissues. The underlying principles of these changes are defined by Starling's equation:

$$F = L_p \times A[(P_c - P_i) - r(COP_p - COP_i)]$$

where:
L_p = membrane hydraulic conductivity per unit area;
A = exchanging surface area;
P_c = capillary hydrostatic pressure;
P_i = interstitial hydrostatic pressure;
COP_p = colloid osmotic pressure of plasma;
COP_i = colloid osmotic pressure of interstitial fluid; and
r = capillary reflection coefficient for plasma proteins.

A number of the factors in this equation, other than the decrease in colloid osmotic pressure, change during pregnancy [21]. Interstitial colloid osmotic pressure (COP$_i$) decreases, and interstitial hydrostatic pressure (P$_i$) tends to rise. These two changes tend to minimize the effect of the decreased plasma colloid osmotic pressure. The increasing extracellular fluid volume of pregnancy is therefore more likely to be due to a rise in capillary pressure, although increasing capillary permeability may also be a contributing factor [22].

The Starling equation relates to oedema arising not only from the systemic but also from the pulmonary circulation. This is of more importance to anaesthetists, because there seems to be a tendency for pregnant women to produce pulmonary oedema easily. Non-cardiogenic pulmonary oedema seems to occur in non-pregnant subjects when colloid osmotic pressure in the pulmonary circulation decreases below 13–16 mmHg [23,24]. The colloid osmotic pressure can decrease to approximately 16 mmHg during and following labour [25,26]. This can occur whether the women deliver vaginally or abdominally, under both epidural and general anaesthesia. The change seems to be greater in those patients given large quantities of crystalloid intravenously during labour. In normal pregnancy, it should be assumed that there is little margin of safety when administering intravenous fluids, and the risk of producing pulmonary oedema should be constantly borne in mind with the pregnant patient. Large volumes of crystalloid solutions, especially 5% dextrose, can and do cause pulmonary oedema. It is surprising that the liberal usage of such solutions, combined with oxytocin (Syntocinon), which has an antidiuretic effect, does not produce the symptoms and signs of excess lung water more frequently.

In protein-losing diseases associated with pregnancy, such as pre-eclampsia, the plasma albumin concentration can reach concentrations as low as 20 g/L. This will cause a significant additional alteration in the balance of circulatory hydrostatic vs. osmotic pressure. Pulmonary oedema fluid will form with relatively small increases in pulmonary capillary pressures. These changes are of importance to the anaesthetist, because both general and regional anaesthesia can themselves cause changes in pulmonary and systemic blood pressures, and the latter may involve administration of significant volumes of intravenous crystalloid. Measurement of albumin concentration is an important investigation that can influence the choice and conduct of anaesthesia. The increased risk of pulmonary oedema with hypoalbuminaemia probably continues until the physiological postpartum diuresis becomes established. However, this diuresis can be delayed for as long as 24–48 hours, during which time an increase in pulmonary interstitial water or frank oedema can develop. When pulmonary oedema occurs, a brisk diuresis should be sought with a loop diuretic in moderate to high doses i.v., e.g. frusemide 40–80 mg. Diuretics should be given to any parturient with the signs of increased lung water, such as cough, increased respiratory effort, wheeze, crepitations on auscultation and falling oxygen saturation on pulse oximetry. Securing an early diuresis may prevent the need for intermittent positive pressure ventilation in an intensive-care unit and the concomitant increased risk of acute respiratory distress syndrome.

3.2 Cardiac function

The human circulatory system consists of a relatively high-resistance systemic circulation and a low-resistance pulmonary circulation. Heart rate, stroke volume and therefore cardiac output increase throughout pregnancy, and an additional low-resistance circulatory system opens in the uteroplacental unit, which at term receives 10–20% of the cardiac output. This second low-resistance system has similarities to an arteriovenous shunt, and may have an antinatriuretic effect, helping to conserve sodium [27].

3.2.1 Arterial blood pressure

The systolic arterial blood pressure during pregnancy decreases slightly, but a much larger decrease in diastolic pressure occurs in mid-pregnancy, rising back to non-pregnant levels at term. This effect increases the pulse pressure, and the peripheral resistance is considerably below normal in mid-pregnancy. These changes are widely recognized as normal. However, there is a large disparity between the actual blood pressures measured, due to observer bias and methodological variability (Fig. 3.4).

The measurement of diastolic blood pressure is open to errors. Indirect measurement using a mercury sphygmomanometer has focused on the Korotkoff sound phases. Phase IV occurs when the sounds muffle, and is poorly reproducible [28], and phase V when the sounds disappear. Intra-arterial diastolic blood pressure is closer to phase V, and is routinely used outside pregnancy. In comparison with direct measurements, sphygmomanometry has been shown to overestimate both the systolic and Korotkoff V diastolic pressure by about 7 and 12 mmHg, respectively [29]. It has been asserted that phase V may never occur, but this is very rare, and may be a technical error. Other technical difficulties include the selection of the correct size of cuff (Table 3.2), posture and observer error. The arbitrary choice of 90 mmHg for the diastolic pressure at which hypertension is diagnosed is based on it being more than two standard deviations from the mean throughout gestation in epidemiological studies [30]. In individual women, variations will exist between those who are mildly hypertensive prior to conception and those with markedly lower diastolic pressures, and these differences should be interpreted in the appropriate context.

In women with hypertensive disease, the use of direct arterial pressure measurements or automated blood pressure-measuring machines such as the Dinamap introduces further confounding factors into the assessment. It has

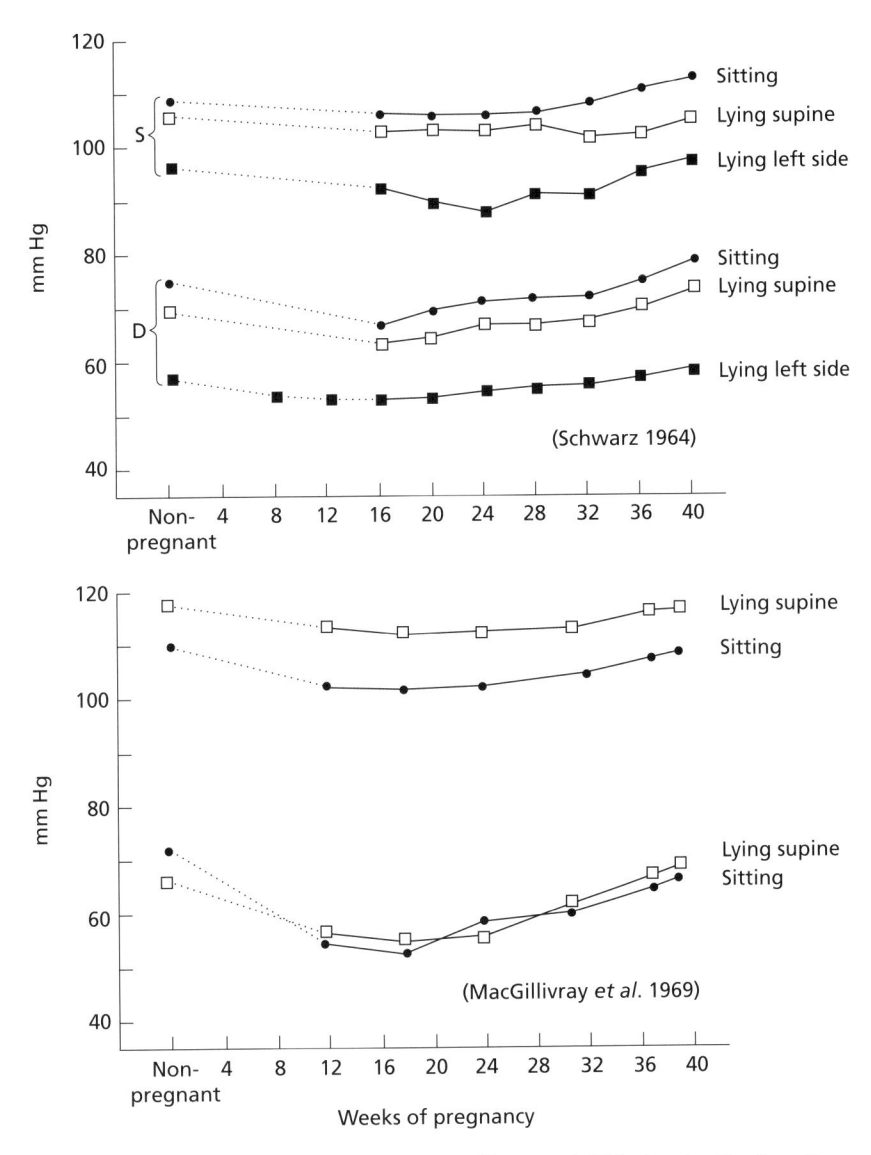

Fig. 3.4 Two studies, by Schwarz [69] and MacGillivray *et al.* [70], showing the disparity between results from different investigators studying the effects of posture. Reproduced with permission from [71].

been shown [31] that the Dinamap underestimates diastolic blood pressures when compared with midwife-read sphygmomanometer readings by approximately 10 mmHg. Such a difference may delay the introduction of therapy unless appropriate corrective factors are applied when considering blood pressure results from automated blood pressure recordings in the hypertensive pregnant patient.

Table 3.2 Factors contributing to variables in blood pressure measurement.

Position of patient
Cuff:
  Cuff type
  Regular (12 × 23 cm)
  Large (15 × 33 cm)
  Thigh (18 × 36 cm)
Speed of cuff deflation
Korotkoff phase
Manual vs. automatic
Direct vs. indirect

Cuff type	*Arm circumference*
Regular (12 × 23 cm)	< 33 cm
Large (15 × 33 cm)	33–41 cm
Thigh (18 × 36 cm)	> 41 cm

3.2.2 Cardiac output

Pregnancy-related increase in cardiac output results from an increase in both heart rate and stroke volume. Sex hormones and prostaglandins generate these effects. Oestrogen is known to increase cardiac output [32,33], but alone is probably not sufficient to account for the recorded increases. It is now believed that vasodilation and a decrease in systemic vascular resistance during pregnancy is another potent influence on cardiac output. Prostaglandins may have a vital role to play in this aspect of cardiovascular changes [34,35]. The most recent and reliable method of accurately measuring cardiac output using non-invasive techniques is the combination of pulsed and continuous-wave Doppler techniques. Using this method, a cardiac output at rest of 7 L/min has been recorded immediately before and then 24 hours after labour [36]. Similar studies have recorded a cardiac output of 7.5 L/min at 38 weeks' gestation, decreasing to about 5.4 L/min in the puerperium [37]. Heart rate and stroke volume both contribute to produce the change in cardiac output, but the change in stroke volume has been claimed to be quite small, and is said by some not to occur [38].

If this is true, the increase in cardiac output is more heart rate-dependent than previously believed. The balance of cardiac output, blood volume and peripheral resistance is such that blood pressure does not change during pregnancy. Whether or not this balance reflects an underfilled or overfilled system remains a matter of debate [39,40]. The cause of the vasodilation and fall in peripheral resistance that occur during pregnancy is equally poorly understood. Both progesterone and oestrogen do have vasodilator actions, but it seems likely that another circulating humoral factor is involved. Studies in the 1950s using ganglion blockade during pregnancy [41] suggested that vasomotor tone is more dependent on sympathetic control in the pregnant as opposed to the non-pregnant patient. Whether a humoral dilator substance is produced from the vascular endothelium, and whether it involves relaxin and nitric oxide pathways remains hypothetical, but is being investigated. However, the dependence on sympathetic tone for maintenance of blood pressure is certainly a major factor in the parturient's susceptibility to the sympathetic block that accompanies both subarachnoid and epidural anaesthesia.

3.2.3 Central venous pressure

Measurements made with the patient in a lateral decubitus position show that central venous pressure (CVP) is well maintained throughout pregnancy.

Changes in central venous pressure during labour depend on the presence or absence of pain. The extremely high central venous pressures reported during 'pushing' are principally due to the very high intrathoracic pressures generated during a Valsalva manoeuvre. They do not reflect the state of the circulating blood volume, nor do they give an accurate impression of venous return.

3.2.4 Aortocaval compression

The enlarging uterofetal mass occupies a position anterior to the abdominal aorta and vena cava. If a parturient adopts the supine position, the uterine mass will press on these vessels. The effect of pressure on the abdominal vena cava is to reduce venous return from the lower part of the body to the heart. In approximately 10% of parturients, systemic hypotension results, and will continue in patients with poor collateral (azygous) venous pathways until the vena caval compression is relieved. This syndrome is referred to as the 'supine hypotensive syndrome'. The history and mechanisms of the syndrome have been the subject of a recent review [42]. The clinical significance and consequences of the pressure of the gravid uterus on the vena cava and aorta when a pregnant woman lies in the supine position were not fully appreciated until 1972. This lack of appreciation and consideration of the effects of caval compression is surprising, because the basic information had been known since the 1930s. Supine hypotension in late pregnancy was described in the Swedish literature in 1932 [43]. In 1937 Ferris and Wilkins [44] recorded, in supine subjects, femoral venous pressure increases during pregnancy that were not matched by increases in right atrial pressure. They observed that there are no valves between these two points of measurement, and suggested that the discrepancy was due to venous obstruction, either caused by the uterofetal mass or high-pressure venous drainage from the uterus itself. Confirmation of the mechanical obstruction followed in 1943 [45], when studies during Caesarean section showed that delivery of the fetus coincided with a sudden decrease in femoral vein pressures. Unfortunately, the relationship between caval obstruction, decreased venous return, decreased cardiac output, hypotension and decreased placental perfusion in late pregnancy was still not fully appreciated. The interaction between supine hypotension and subarachnoid anaesthesia certainly was not realized, and the risk of catastrophic hypotension was one of the factors that led to the view, in the United

Kingdom at least, that spinal anaesthesia was contraindicated for Caesarean section (see Chapter 15). Some 20 years elapsed before the next significant results appeared in the literature. In the 1960s, Scott and his colleagues [46–48] confirmed McLennan's findings and showed that, in late pregnancy and the supine position, the vena cava was completely flattened for the length of the uterus. Venous pressures below the flattening were higher than those above it, and in women with poor collateral venous pathways, the obstruction was accompanied by decreases in right atrial pressure, cardiac output and systemic blood pressure. Finally, the 1972 report by Crawford *et al.* 1972 [49] drew attention to the necessity of the left lateral tilt position for the term pregnant patient, to prevent vena cava compression, maternal hypotension and diminished placental blood flow during Caesarean section.

Vena cava compression is often accompanied by aortic compression [50]. The proportion of parturients affected varies with the posture adopted, the maturity of the pregnancy, uterine contractions and the methods used by investigators. Approximately 40% of parturients probably have some degree of aortic compression during labour [51,52]. Most will have only mild compression of the aorta, with little detectable clinical effect other than some narrowing of the pulse pressure and slightly lower overall systemic pressure in the lower limbs. Approximately 8% of parturients will have severe aortic compression, which becomes worse during uterine contractions and lessens as labour progresses. The latter effect is associated with increasing cervical dilatation and descent of the fetal head. The occipitoposterior position seems to be associated with an increased risk—whether because of slower fetal descent through the pelvis or simply increased intrapelvic and abdominal pressure effects is not clear. A 15° left lateral tilt does not seem to prevent aortic compression, and most patients in Kinsella's series [51] needed a 34° lateral tilt or even full lateral positioning before signs of the aortic compression were abolished.

The great variability in the incidence and severity of both aortic and caval compression is widely recognized, and not surprising given the individual variation in the anatomical shape, size and position of the gravid uterus and great vessels in the posterior wall of the abdomen. There seems to be no position that will guarantee freedom from the problem of aortocaval compression, but the full left lateral and prone positions seem to be only rarely and unusually associated with aortocaval compression. The upright sitting position also seems safe. However, few parturients remain upright when seated—most preferring, and sometimes being encouraged, to lean back at approximately 45°. Reclining at 45° has quite clearly been associated with the symptoms of aortocaval compression [53,54], and is not significantly better than the supine position in some parturients.

Care must be taken to detect aortocaval compression during epidural insertion. Flexing the patient may result in pressure from the thighs pushing the uterus posteriorly onto the vessels of the posterior abdominal wall.

Aortocaval compression during labour is largely a recent problem. It is closely associated with the desire on the part of accoucheurs to manage the patient in the supine position. This desire often overrides maternal choice, and is difficult to understand because labour and delivery can perfectly well be managed with the parturient in the left lateral position as the preferred option.

The severity of aortocaval compression and the associated hypotension is not always matched by symptoms in the parturient [55,56]. The symptoms themselves vary widely from individual to individual, some patients complaining of faintness or nausea with a systolic blood pressure of 95 mmHg, whereas others are symptom-free with systolic blood pressures of 65 mmHg. If the aortocaval compression is not detected in the latter circumstances, fetal distress may occur as the first sign of the problem. The distress is caused by fetal hypoxia, due to reduced placental perfusion from maternal hypotension or direct aortic pressure above the origin of the uterine arteries.

Clinically, these postural factors are of great significance, because unrelieved aortocaval compression can cause maternal or fetal death [57,58]. Maternal or fetal changes can be serious enough to precipitate a demand for immediate delivery, with all the attendant risks of emergency treatment. However, the problem is often best and most rapidly dealt with by appropriate maternal postural change, usually into the full left lateral position, administration of oxygen and, if necessary, intravenous fluid therapy. It is now clear that when urgent Caesarean section is to be performed for fetal distress, the patient should adopt a left lateral tilt, oxytocin infusion should be discontinued and the lateral position should be maintained at all times during transport to theatre. Mothers should ideally travel to theatre in the full left lateral position, breathing as high an inspired oxygen concentration (F_{IO_2}) as possible to minimize or reverse any residual fetal hypoxia. The blood pressure changes are perhaps the most obvious effects of aortocaval compression. However, it must be remembered that in occasional patients, the caval and aortic obstructions are at a level that can affect renal blood flow. The full effects of these factors have only relatively recently been recognized when considering fluctuations in the glomerular filtration rate and electrolyte balance.

3.2.5 Cardiac function changes in labour

The changes in cardiac function that take place during labour depend on many factors. If pain relief is not used or is inadequate, further increases in heart rate, stroke volume and cardiac output are produced. These changes are normal sympathetic responses to pain, and during labour the pain of each contraction will be coupled with intermittent autotransfusions of up to 500 mL of blood from the uteroplacental vasculature. Bearing down during second stage—effectively a Valsalva manoeuvre—can reduce right heart filling and may briefly decrease cardiac output.

Effective pain relief with regional anaesthesia/analgesia prevents much of the sympathetic autonomic response. In patients with good pain relief, heart rate and cardiac output remain similar to the values recorded before the onset of labour. Venodilation by epidural or subarachnoid block may reduce venous return. In doing so, it may cause a bradycardia, probably as a consequence of a negative effect on the Bainbridge/stretch receptor reflex mechanism in the right atrium. This response is known as the Bezold–Jarisch reflex, and adequate intravenous fluid preload together with the uterine autotransfusion already mentioned will reduce the chance of the change in most patients. This potential reflex bradycardia should be borne in mind, however, as one possible cardiovascular consequence of epidural or subarachnoid anaesthesia. The use of ephedrine in this situation is particularly valuable, because its mixed α- and β-adrenergic effect will tend to produce chronotropic as well as inotropic effects. One may wonder whether this fortuitous combination of effects is the reason for the drug's apparently unique place in the treatment of hypotension in pregnant patients, both supporting the systemic blood pressure and returning placental blood flow to normal.

3.3 Cardiovascular disease and pregnancy

Most of the physiological cardiovascular changes are well developed before the end of the first trimester and complete by the end of the second trimester. Hence, patients with little or no cardiac reserve may suffer decompensation and cardiac failure by the end of the second trimester. Patients with stenotic valvular lesions and those with a right-to-left shunt are at particular risk at this time. In the third trimester, obstruction of the inferior vena cava and an increased risk of thromboembolism complicate earlier changes.

3.3.1 Prevalence

The incidence of cardiac disease in parturients in the United Kingdom varies greatly, with a 10-fold variation of approximately 0.4–4.0% being quoted by some authors [59]. In the United Kingdom, both acquired and congenital heart disease are relatively infrequent complications of pregnancy but with the decrease in rheumatic heart disease, congenital heart disease is becoming more common than acquired. The number of maternal deaths from cardiac disease has not decreased in the last 20 years [60]. The most recent report [61] found that two influences are probably responsible for producing an increase in the number of patients at risk. Successful cardiac surgery has extended the survival of women with both congenital and acquired valvular heart disease into childbearing age. Even when residual signs and symptoms of heart disease continue, women are often reluctant to forgo one or more pregnancies even when so advised. Changes in culture have also had an influence. The average age of conception and delivery has increased and obstetric services are caring for an older population, with an increased proportion of smokers. These older parturients, with a longer exposure to smoking, have a greater risk of suffering from ischaemic heart disease. Rheumatic heart disease is still a major problem in many developing countries, and it is common among immigrants. In more developed countries, rheumatic mitral stenosis may be missed, as it is no longer common. Women with regurgitant valve disease can tolerate pregnancy even when the leak is severe, but in rheumatic heart disease there is always a risk of atrial fibrillation, with sudden pulmonary oedema. Congenital heart disease ranges from simple defects to complex malformations. The success of cardiac surgery in infancy has resulted in an increase in the number of women of childbearing age with congenital heart disease.

3.3.2 Risk assessment

The number of 'cardiae' deaths in the United Kingdom is small, but risk management lessons can be learned from the fatalities reported. Pulmonary hypertension is a major complicating feature in a considerable proportion of fatalities. Previous episodes of endocarditis or myocardial infarction are also important risk factors [62]. A significant feature of substandard care relates to the lack of proper assessment. Any patient with a history of heart disease, or showing signs or symptoms suggestive of heart disease, should be thoroughly assessed at the earliest possible stage of pregnancy. Both cardiologists and obstetric anaesthetists should be involved alongside obstetricians in the subsequent management, and detailed assessments should be made at appropriate intervals in order to identify changes in the disease severity.

Early referral of patients with heart disease for an anaesthesia consultation may involve the obstetric anaesthetist in the initial cardiovascular assessment of the patient and planning of further investigations. A detailed medical history should be taken, with careful attention to previous cardiorespiratory problems and their treatment. Some quantification of exercise tolerance and grading of dyspnoea are both essential. The assessment should include an initial grading using the New York State Heart Association classification system:
Class I: no limitation during ordinary physical activity;
Class II: symptoms with ordinary physical activity;
Class III: symptoms provoked easily;
Class IV: breathless at rest.
Using this classification system provides a general description of the functional severity of the heart disease, and when it is used sequentially during pregnancy a change to III or IV gives warning of increasing severity of heart disease or decompensation of a previously functionally normal patient. Patients may present with symptoms of dyspnoea, syncope or ischaemia. Repeated assessments are necessary, because the physiological changes of pregnancy add to the demands made on cardiac reserves. In addition, the increasing concentration of oestrogen and progesterone tend to cause some valvular dilation

Table 3.3 Echocardiographic variables in normal patients during early and late pregnancy (mean ± SD) [64].

	Gestation (weeks)	
	24–28	32–36
Mitral valve area (cm²)	3.69 (0.48)	4.31 (0.67)
Left atrium (cm)	2.95 (0.29)	3.25 (0.22)
Left ventricle (cm)	4.93 (0.37)	5.06 (0.44)
Cardiac output (L/min)	4.06 (0.54)	5.39 (1.01)
Systolic volume (mL)	72.39 (27.25)	93.83 (29.16)
End systolic volume (mL)	29.70 (8.13)	34.26 (10.25)
End diastolic volume (mL)	116.39 (25.73)	130.35 (35.27)
Ejection fraction	0.74 (0.04)	0.76 (0.04)
Aorta (cm)	2.85 (0.19)	3.06 (0.21)

within the heart and, in damaged valves, can predispose to increased regurgitation. These physiological changes can alter the normal values of heart chamber pressures used by cardiologists to assess severity.

Ideally, investigations should be undertaken prior to conception, but the initial referral to an obstetric anaesthetist commonly occurs during pregnancy. The following investigations should be carried out if they have not already been performed. Joint consultations between anaesthesia, obstetrics and cardiology departments should follow as soon as results are available.

1 Haemoglobin estimation.
2 Electrocardiography: 12-lead electrocardiography (ECG). Then, if required:
   (i) a 24-h Holter monitoring tape if dysrhythmias are occurring;
   (ii) an exercise ECG to detect ischaemic disease.
3 A chest radiograph to assess cardiac size and outline, pulmonary vasculature and lung fields. Even in pregnant women, serial investigations from baseline may be necessary with fetal screening [63].
4 Echocardiography can provide much of the information needed to allow the severity of the abnormalities to be assessed. Some reference values have been reported in normal patients during early and late pregnancy, and they are shown in Table 3.3 [64].

Then, where appropriate: invasive measurement of cardiac pressures and flows, e.g. cardiac output, pulmonary artery pressure, pulmonary wedge pressure, central venous and right atrial pressure, pressure gradients across valves.

Transoesophageal echocardiography (TOE) may be useful if transthoracic echocardiography does not provide sufficient information. It is difficult to perform without anaesthetizing the patient, but TOE can also be a useful method for intraoperative or intensive-care unit assessment in difficult cases requiring critical care [65].

3.3.3 Anaesthesia for the parturient with cardiac disease

General considerations

It is usually the mother rather than the fetus who is at risk during anaesthesia. The fetus will be at risk if the mother is hypoxic or placental blood flow is reduced, or both. Conditions that require careful management can be divided into myocardial disorders and major vessel disorders. Recently, women with aortic aneurysms have presented with chest pain. A chest radiograph is vital in the diagnosis. Parturients with coarctation of the aorta have a high blood pressure in the proximal segment, and surges during the stress of labour or intubation can increase the risk of cerebral haemorrhage. Women with the Marfan syndrome may have both cardiac and aortic pathology.

In normal pregnancy, the resting heart rate increases by up to 20 beats/min. Any further increase suggests a failure to increase stroke volume in the absence of non-cardiac causes, e.g. infection. Tachycardia is well tolerated in regurgitant valve disease, but can lead to a marked rise in left atrial pressure in mitral or aortic stenosis, or in severe cases of hypertrophic cardiomyopathy. Tachycardia must be avoided where filling time and diastolic coronary perfusion time are critical to maintain cardiac output. Any stimulus that increases heart rate should be prevented. Ephedrine, with β-sympathomimetic effects, is therefore an inappropriate vasoconstrictor, and methoxamine or phenylephrine should be used in preference. Women with valve prosthesis who are in sinus rhythm usually have ample cardiovascular reserve, and anticoagulation may not be required. In patients with mechanical prostheses, the management of anticoagulation control has to be discussed with the specialist cardiologist [66]. The need to maintain anticoagulation may pre-empt the decision as to whether general or regional anaesthesia can be employed. Accelerated deterioration of bioprosthesis may precipitate emergency replacement. Homografts are more durable than xenografts. Prophylactic antibiotic cover is not needed for normal delivery, except in patients who have had previous infective endocarditis and patients with artificial heart valves.

Determinants of anaesthetic technique include the severity of the cardiac disorder, anticoagulation status, and the method of delivery. Epidural analgesia is indicated in labour to minimize catecholamine release, and the addition of epidural or intrathecal opioids strengthens analgesia and reduces motor and sympathetic blockade by local anaesthetics [67]. The loss of resistance to saline technique should be performed so that any paradoxical air embolus can be avoided in septal defects. Fluid loading for regional nerve block and the use of vasopressors may require cautious management. General anaesthesia allows more invasive monitoring and is particularly indicated in severe cardiac disorders. A decision should be made preoperatively about when to convert a regional nerve block to general anaesthesia, so that appropriate monitoring can be selected.

Table 3.4 Routes of insertion of central venous pressure catheters and associated complications.

Antecubital vein (drum cartridge catheter)
Malposition, e.g. migrates into the jugular vein
Perforation of the vein or cardiac structures

External jugular vein using a short cannula (access to this vein is often difficult)
Haematoma
Poor-quality tracing (position-dependent)
Prevents some movements of the neck

Internal jugular vein. This route is associated with some life-threatening complications, and should only be used if indicated and with suitable experience
Haematoma
Puncture of structures, e.g. pleura: pneumothorax; myocardium: tamponade; thoracic duct (left side): chylothorax
Dysrhythmias

Monitoring for the cardiac patient

During labour or operative delivery, ECG monitoring with leads II and CM5 to detect ischaemia is essential. An indwelling central venous and arterial catheter will allow assessment of pressure within the great veins or right atrium. The choice of routes for insertion of central venous pressure catheters and their complications are listed in Table 3.4. This pressure assesses volume status, circulatory capacity and right heart function. For other aspects of cardiac function, an in-dwelling arterial catheter will measure systemic arterial pressure and allow pressure measurements and blood gas and acid–base status to be monitored. Indirect measures of cardiac output may provide serial assessments from thoracic impedance electrodes, or during general anaesthesia from an oesophageal Doppler probe. A trained operator may aid the diagnosis of a ruptured aortic aneurysm with transoesophageal echocardiography. Direct monitoring of cardiac output and pulmonary capillary wedge pressure should be discussed with the cardiologist in the absence of clear indications such as a change to Grade IV in the New York Heart Classification. A pulmonary artery catheter is associated with increased morbidity, and its use requires evaluation [68].

Specific conditions

The cardiac disorders that pose a serious threat to a woman's life are pulmonary hypertension and severe mitral and aortic stenosis. Operative delivery at term is the usual option in order to avoid the stress of labour.

Mitral stenosis. Increases in preload can be reduced by diuretics if pulmonary congestion occurs. Beta-adrenergic blocking drugs can provide time for left atrial emptying and lower left atrial pressure, increasing stroke volume and reducing the reflex tendency to increase the heart rate. Digoxin is the treatment for atrial fibrillation.

Aortic stenosis. Aortic stenosis may be congenital, in association with a bicuspid valve, or acquired after rheumatic fever, for example. The size of the valve opening varies from 2.5 to 3.5 cm. A valve that has an opening of less than 1 cm will increase left ventricular end-diastolic pressure. If valve replacement is needed, the baby should be delivered before aortic valve replacement.

If a woman has asymptomatic aortic stenosis, she will have a reduced cardiovascular reserve, but normal delivery can be anticipated if she is monitored during labour and has no signs or symptoms of cardiovascular dysfunction, such as ischaemia. If the aortic stenosis is symptomatic, an increase in morbidity and mortality of both the mother and the fetus is to be expected. There may be a pre-existing left ventricular hypertrophy with ischaemia and—if the condition is congenital—an associated left bundle branch block. Labour and blood loss will be hazardous because of the fixed output through the valve, where only an increase in heart rate can increase the cardiac output. Left ventricular failure can result if too high pressures are generated in the left ventricle, and cerebral and myocardial ischaemia if the coronary circulation is compromised by a reduction of blood through the valve.

Management involves planning delivery with risk assessment for the stress of labour and the maintenance of an adequate blood volume. It is important not to allow the development of bradycardia, a reduction in venous return, or a tachycardia of over 140 beats/min, in order to maintain filling pressures in the left ventricle. Vasopressors, such as ephedrine if a bradycardia occurs or the addition of methoxamine if tachycardia is present, should be used to maintain adequate pressures.

Hypertrophic cardiomyopathy. The main risks in hypertrophic cardiomyopathy are from myocardial depression, especially from general anaesthetic agents, and tachycardia. An increase in venous return or increased systemic vascular resistance may also reduce stroke volume if myocardial function is severely disturbed. Treatment of these conditions follows that for congestive cardiac failure.

Aortic coarctation. Antihypertensive medication will be prescribed for women with uncorrected aortic coarctation. There is a small risk of aortic dissection.

Ischaemic heart disease in pregnancy. Ischaemic heart disease is becoming one of the major causes of maternal cardiac deaths, and is associated with smoking, diabetes, obesity and hypercholesterolaemia. It has also become a well-recognized sequel to cocaine use.

Pulmonary hypertension. Primary pulmonary hypertension usually affects younger women, and any increases in pulmonary vascular resistance, e.g.

mild hypoxaemia, hypercarbia and acidosis can lead to death. The contractile state of the right ventricle is important to maintain pulmonary blood flow. During anaesthesia, high central blood volumes with good venous return are needed, together with 100% oxygen in order to supply adequate oxygen to the pulmonary capillaries and avoid hypoxic vasoconstriction. Epoprostenol (prostacyclin) decreases pulmonary resistance, and can be used by infusion.

Intracardiac shunts. These may be acyanotic or cyanotic. Congenital cyanotic heart disease presents special risks to the fetus and has a high morbidity in the mother. Women with pulmonary hypertension and cyanosis, e.g. Eisenmenger syndrome, have a 40–50% morbidity, usually soon after delivery.
- Atrial septal defect. This may be an isolated lesion in association with pulmonary artery stenosis. It is a low-pressure shunt. Supraventricular dysrhythmias may be associated with it.
- Eisenmenger syndrome includes pulmonary hypertension and intracardiac or aortopulmonary shunts, which may be right-to-left or bidirectional and may be associated with peripheral cyanosis. Sudden death can occur at any time in the 7–10 days postpartum. The systemic vascular resistance (SVR) decreases in pregnancy, and a right-to-left shunt therefore increases. The SVR should be maintained by α-adrenergic agonists, e.g. methoxamine and phenylephrine. An increase in pulmonary vascular resistance is detrimental, and a 100% inspired oxygen concentration is necessary to avoid pulmonary vasoconstriction. The patient may be heparinized because of polycythaemia, which may increase after delivery with the attendant risk of pulmonary embolism.

The mortality depends on the severity of the syndrome. The presence of cyanosis or continuing pulmonary hypertension is an indicator of high risk. The mortality associated with spontaneous vaginal delivery is 30%, and after Caesarean section it is 50%. Sudden postpartum death occurs because of pulmonary emboli, hypotension and increased pulmonary vascular resistance. Intensive-care unit management may be preventive, but it is rarely available for the period of risk.

Dysrhythmias. Paroxysmal tachycardia recurs more frequently during pregnancy. Direct current cardioversion can be carried out when necessary without disturbing the fetus, and implantable defibrillators are in use.

Special care facilities for the obstetric cardiac patient

Anaesthetic intervention is not only required for the parturient in labour and for operative delivery, but also in the postoperative management of the obstetric cardiac patient. Monitoring should be continued in a high-dependency unit for up to a week after delivery, particularly for those patients with a high risk of morbidity and mortality. The risk of thromboembolism is increased particularly in cyanotic heart disease, with polycythaemia and sudden deterioration of cardiac function.

References

1. Visser W, Wallenburg HCS. Central hemodynamic observations in untreated pre-eclamptic patients. *Hypertension* 1992; **17**: 1072–7.
2. Easterling TR, Benedetti FJ, Carlson KC *et al.* The effect of maternal hemo-dynamics on fetal growth in hypertensive pregnancies. *Am J Obstet Gynecol* 1991; **165**: 902–6.
3. Pirani BBK, Campbell DM, McGillivray I. Plasma volume in normal first pregnancy. *J Obstet Gynaecol Br Commonw* 1973; **80**: 884–7.
4. Chessley LC, Duffus GM. Posture and apparent plasma volume in late pregnancy. *J Obstet Gynaecol Br Commonw* 1971; **78**: 406–12.
5. Fullerton WT, Hytten FE, Klopper AE, McKay E. A case of quadruplet pregnancy. *J Obstet Gynaecol Br Commonw* 1965; **72**: 791–6.
6. Rovinski JJ, Jaffin H. Cardiovascular hemodynamics in pregnancy, 1: blood and plasma volumes in multiple pregnancy. *Am J Obstet Gynecol* 1965; **93**: 1–13.
7. Rovinchi JJ, Jaffin H. Cardiovascular hemodynamics in pregnancy, 2: cardiac output and left ventricular work in multiple pregnancy. *Am J Obstet Gynecol* 1966; **95**: 781.
8. Finer P, Blair J, Rowe P. Epidural analgesia in the management of labour pain and sickle cell crisis: a case report. *Anesthesiology* 1988; **68**: 799–80.
9. Uszinki M, Abildgard U. Separation and characterisation of 2 fibrinolytic inhibitors from human placenta. *Thromb Diath Hemorrhagica* 1971; **25**: 580–9.
10. Hahn L. Fibrinogen—fibrin degradation products in uterine and peripheral blood during Caesarean section. *Acta Obstet Gynaecol Scand* 1974; **53 (S28)**: 1–7.
11. Conard J, Cazenave B, Samama M, *et al.* At III content and antithrombin activity in oestrogen-progestogen and progestogen-only treated women. *Thromb Res* 1980; **18**: 675–81.
12. Fay RA, Hughes AO, Baron NT. Platelets in pregnancy: hyperdestruction in pregnancy. *Obstet Gynecol* 1983; **61**: 238–40.
13. McKay DG. Chronic intravascular coagulation in normal pregnancy and pre-eclampsia. *Contrib Nephrol* 1981; **25**: 108–19.
14. Burrows RF, Kelton JG. Incidentally detected thrombocytopenia in healthy mothers and their infants. *N Engl J Med* 1988; **319**: 142.
15. O'Brien WF, Saba HI, Knuppel RA, Scerbo JC, Cohen GR. Alterations in platelet concentration and aggregation in normal pregnancy and pre-eclampsia. *Am J Obstet Gynecol* 1986; **155**: 486.
16. Lewis PJ, Boylan P, Friedman LA, Hensman CN, Downing I. Prostacyclin in pregnancy. *Br Med J* 1980; **280**: 1581–2.
17. Hytten FE, Lind T. Diagnostic Indices in Pregnancy. *Documenta Geigy* 1973; 43.
18. Robertson EG. The natural history of oedema during pregnancy. *J Obstet Gynaecol Br Commonw* 1971; **78**: 520–9.
19. Robertson EG. Oedema in normal pregnancy. *J Reprod Fertil* 1969; **9** (Suppl): 27–36.
20. Theobold GW, Lundborg RA. Changes in limb volume and in venous infusion pressures caused by pregnancy. *J Obstet Gynaecol Br Commonw* 1963; **70**: 408.
21. Øian P, Maltau JM, Noddeland H, Fadnes HO. Oedema-preventing mechanisms in subcutaneous tissue of normal pregnant women. *Br J Obstet Gynaecol* 1985; **92**: 113–19.
22. Hunyor SN, McEniery PT, Roberts KA *et al.* Capillary permeability in normal and hypertensive human pregnancy. *Clin Exp Pharmacol Physiol* 1983; **10**: 345–50.

23 Stein L, Beraud JJ, Morisette M et al. Pulmonary edema during volume infusion. *Circulation* 1975; **52**: 483–9.
24 Rackow EC, Fein IA, Leppo J. Colloid osmotic pressure as a prognostic indicator of pulmonary edema and mortality in the critically ill. *Chest* 1977; **72**: 709–13.
25 Cotton DB, Gonik B, Spillman T, Dorman KF. Intrapartum to postpartum changes in colloid osmotic pressure. *Am J Obstet Gynecol* 1984; **149**: 174–7.
26 Gonik B, Cotton DB, Spillman T, Abouleish E, Zavica F. Peripartum colloid osmotic pressure changes: effects of controlled fluid management. *Am J Obstet Gynecol* 1985; **151**: 812–15.
27 Lindheimer MD, Katy AI. Normal and abnormal pregnancy. In: Arieff AI, Defronzo R, eds. *Fluid Electrolyte and Acid–Base Disorders.* Edinburgh: Churchill Livingstone, 1985: 1041.
28 Shennon A, Gupta G, Hallagan A, Taylor DJ, de Sweit M. Lack of reproducibility in pregnancy of Korotkoff phase IV as measured by mercury sphygmomanometer. *Lancet* 1996; **347**: 139–42.
29 Ginsburg J, Duncan S. Direct and indirect blood pressure measurements in pregnancy. *J Obstet Gynaecol Br Commonw* 1969; **76**: 705–10.
30 Rubin P. Measuring diastolic blood pressure in pregnancy using the fifth Korotkoff sound. *Br Med J* 1996; **313**: 4–5.
31 Hassan MA, Thomas T, Prys-Roberts C. A comparison of automatic measurement in the labour ward. *Br J Anaesth* 1993; **70**: 141–4.
32 Walters WA, Lim YL. Haemodynamic changes in women taking oral contraceptives. *J Obstet Gynaecol Br Commonw* 1970; **77**: 1007–12.
33 Lehtovirta P. Haemodynamic effects of combined oestrogen–progestogen oral contraceptives. *J Obstet Gynaecol Br Commonw* 1974; **81**: 517–25.
34 Phippard AF, Horvath JS, Glynn EM et al. Circulatory adaptation to pregnancy: serial studies of haemodynamics, blood volume, renin and aldosterone in the baboon (*Papio hamadryas*). *J Hypertension* 1986; **4**: 773–9.
35 Broughton Pipkin F, Morrison R, O'Brien PM. The effect of prostaglandin E1 upon the pressor and hormonal response to exogenous angiotensin II in human pregnancy. *Clin Sci* 1987; **72**: 351–7.
36 Robson SC, Dunlop W, Boys RJ, Hunter S. Cardiac output during labour. *Br Med J Clin Res Ed* 1987; **295**: 1169–72.
37 Robson SC, Hunter S, Moore M, Dunlop W. Haemodynamic changes during the puerperium: a Doppler and M-mode echocardiographic study. *Br J Obstet Gynaecol* 1987; **94**: 1028–39.
38 Mashini IS, Albazzaz SJ, Fadel HE. Serial noninvasive evaluation of cardiovascular hemodynamics during pregnancy. *Am J Obstet Gynecol* 1987; **156**: 1208–13.
39 Schrier RW, Durr JA. Pregnancy: an overfill or underfill state. *Am J Kidney Dis* 1987; **19**: 284–9.
40 Schrier RW. Pathogenesis of sodium and water retention in high output and low output cardiac failure, nephrotic syndrome, cirrhosis, and pregnancy. *N Engl J Med* 1988; **319**: 1127–34.
41 Assali NS, Vergon JM, Tadda Y, Garber ST. Studies on autonomic blockade, 6: the mechanisms regulating the hemodynamic changes in the pregnant woman and their relation to the hypertension of toxemia of pregnancy. *Am J Obstet Gynecol* 1952; **63**: 978.
42 Kinsella SM, Lohmann G. Supine hypotensive syndrome. *Obstet Gynecol* 1994; **83**: 774–88.
43 Ahlthorp G. Ett fall ar hjartinsufficiens vid rygglage hos gravid kvinna [A case of cardiac insufficiency in the dorsal position in a pregnant woman]. *Svenska Lak-Tidnarig* 1932; **29**: 1378–88.

44 Ferris EB, Wilkins RW. The clinical value of comparative measurements of the pressure in the femoral and cubital veins. *Am Heart J* 1937; **13**: 431.
45 McLennan CE. Antecubital and femoral venous pressure in normal and toxemic pregnancy. *Am J Obstet Gynecol* 1943; **45**: 568.
46 Scott DB, Kerr MG. Inferior vena caval pressure in late pregnancy. *J Obstet Gynaecol Br Commonw* 1963; **70**: 1044.
47 Kerr MG, Scott DB, Samuel E. Studies of the inferior vena cava in late pregnancy. *Br Med J* 1964; **i**: 532–33.
48 Lees MM, Scott DB, Kerr MG, Taylor SH. The circulatory effects of recumbent postural change in late pregnancy. *Clin Sci* 1967; **32**: 453–65.
49 Crawford JS, Burton M, Davies P. Time and lateral tilt at Caesarean section. *Br J Anaesth* 1972; **44**: 477–84.
50 Abitbol MM. Aortic compression and uterine blood flow during pregnancy. *Obstet Gynecol* 1977; **50**: 562–70.
51 Kinsella SM, Whitwam JG, Spencer JAD. Aortic compression by the uterus: identification with the Finapres digital arterial pressure instrument. *Br J Obstet Gynaecol* 1990; **97**: 700–5.
52 Goodlin RC. Importance of the lateral position during labour. *Obstet Gynecol* 1971; **37**: 698–701.
53 Wright L. Postural hypotension in late pregnancy: the supine hypotensive syndrome. *Br Med J* 1962; **i**: 760–2.
54 Sluder HM. The supine hypotensive syndrome of pregnancy. *N Engl J Med* 1956; **19**: 420–2.
55 Oxorn H. Postural hypotension in pregnancy. *Can Med Soc J* 1960; **83**: 436–7.
56 Cato J, Tinaker T. Shock due to supine hypotensive syndrome. *Sanfujinka No Jissai* 1967; **16**: 118–23.
57 Courtney L. Supine hypotensive syndrome during Caesarean section. *Br Med J* 1970; **1**: 797–8.
58 Ricodeau F, Pontier R, Gouin F, Valet C, François G. Le choc postural: deux observations [postural shock: two case histories]. *Anesth Analg Reanim* 1972; **29**: 233–9.
59 Busch RL. Cardiac disease. In: Ostheimer GW, ed. *Manual of Obstetric Anaesthesia*, 2nd edn. Edinburgh: Churchill Livingstone, 1992: 276–91.
60 Department of Health. *Report on Confidential Enquiries into Maternal Deaths in the United Kingdom, 1988–1990.* London: HMSO, 1994.
61 Hibberd BM, Department of Health. *Report on Confidential Enquiries into Maternal Deaths in the United Kingdom, 1991–1993.* London: HMSO, 1996.
62 Department of Health. *Report on Confidential Enquiries into Maternal Deaths in the United Kingdom, 1985–1987.* London: HMSO, 1991.
63 Robers G, Sarton H, Field S. *Making the Best Use of a Department of Clinical Radiology: Guidelines for Doctors*, 2nd edn. London: Royal College of Radiologists, 1993.
64 Carvalho JCA. Cardiac disease. In: Van Zundert A, Ostheimer GW, eds. *Pain Relief and Anesthesia in Obstetrics.* Edinburgh: Churchill Livingstone, 1996: 547–57.
65 Townend JN, Hutton P. Transoesophageal echocardiography in anaesthesia and intensive care. *Br J Anaesth* 1996; **77**: 137–9.
66 Prendergast BD, Banning AP, Hall RJC. Valvular heart disease: recommendations for investigation and management. *J R Coll Physicians Lond* 1996; **30**: 309–15.
67 Sharma SK, Gambling DR, Gajraj NM, Sidawi EJ. Anaesthetic management of a parturient with mixed mitral valve disease and in controlled atrial fibrillation. *Int J Obstet Anesth* 1994; **3**: 157–62.
68 Soni N. Swan song for the Swan–Ganz catheter. *Br Med J* 1996; **313**: 763–4.

69 Schwarz R. Das Verhalten des Kreislaufs in der normalen Schwangerschaft, 1: Der arterielle Blutdruck [The behaviour of the blood circulation in normal pregnancy, 1: the arterial blood pressure]. *Arch Gynäkol* 1964; **199**: 549–70.

70 MacGillivray I, Rose GA, Rowe B. Blood pressure survey in pregnancy. *Clin Sci* 1969; **37**: 395–407.

71 De Sweit M. The Cardiovascular System. In: Chamberlain G, Broughton Pipkin, F, eds. *Clinical Physiology in Obstetrics*, 3rd edn. Oxford: Blackwell Science, 1998: 33–70.

4: Respiratory System

A third of maternal deaths are associated with acute respiratory problems [1]. Acute respiratory distress syndrome alone accounted for 44 deaths in the *Report on Confidential Enquiries into Maternal Deaths for the United Kingdom* between the years 1988 and 1990. Treatment of these patients requires the application of normal maternal values for their period of gestation, in order to allow adequate gas exchange for the fetus.

Studies of respiratory function in pregnancy have been conducted under varying conditions. The position of the mother during the assessment of respiratory function is one such variable. Many physiological studies are performed with the patient sitting rather than supine, yet during anaesthesia the mother is rarely sitting. Whether the mother is placed in a standing, sitting, supine or left lateral position will affect the values of lung volumes, capacities and flows to varying degrees relative to the stage of pregnancy and the physical characteristics of the mother.

The functional respiratory changes of normal pregnancy are produced by the interaction of endocrinological factors with anatomical alterations in the airways, thoracic cage, respiratory muscles and cardiovascular system. The mother must provide for respiratory exchange both in her own lungs and at the placental site. Extra demands for gas exchange occur, because there is an increase in tissue mass, fetal requirements and an increase in cardiac and respiratory work. Oxygen consumption is increased by 20–30%. Any abnormality in maternal cardiorespiratory function will have profound consequences for the fetus.

4.1 Anatomy

4.1.1 Upper airway

The mucosa of the respiratory tract becomes engorged, and nasal stuffiness is a presenting symptom of pregnancy. It is thought to be caused by an increase in oestrogens. The proposed mechanism for these changes is that oestrogens increase the hyaluronic acid component of interstitial tissues and thus increase tissue hydration and oedema. Capillaries become congested, and hyperplastic and mucous glands hypersecrete under the influence of this hormone [2]. The changes are most severe during the third trimester, and are made worse by allergies, upper respiratory tract infections and pre-eclampsia.

The upper airway becomes compromised by the nasal pharyngeal and laryngeal mucosa becoming oedematous and friable, so that minimal trauma

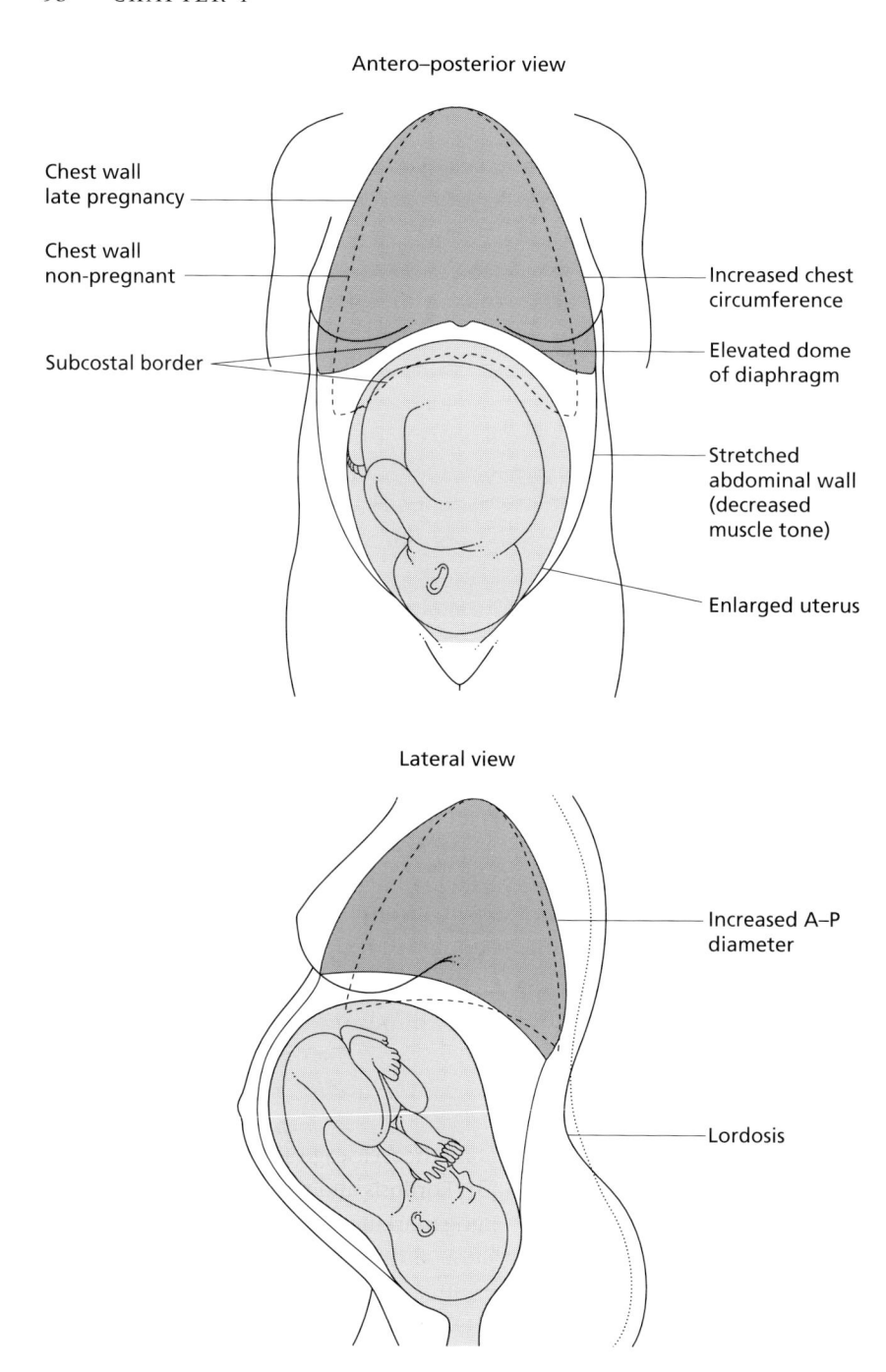

Fig. 4.1 Changes in the thoracic cage in late pregnancy. The dotted lines indicate the non-pregnant state.

can produce complications such as epistaxis and laryngeal oedema [3]. Excessive weight gain in pregnancy may deposit fat in anatomical locations around the airway, both in the pharyngeal structures and in the breasts, shoulders and neck, so that access to the airway is impeded from without and within.

Mouth breathing may make the mother less tolerant of a face mask, either for analgesia in labour or for preoxygenation. Mouthpieces may be preferred for self-administration of analgesic gases or oxygen. Nasogastric tubes may precipitate epistaxis, and smaller-diameter endotracheal tubes, e.g. cuffed 6.0 mm, should be available for intubation [4].

4.1.2 Thoracic cage

The thoracic cage changes in shape during pregnancy, partly as a result of the enlarging uterus, and partly through relaxation of the ligamentous attachments of the ribs. The rib cage moves upwards and laterally. There is an increase in both anteroposterior and transverse diameters of the rib cage, so that chest circumference increases by 5–7 cm. The subcostal angle broadens from an acute to an obtuse angle, and there is a tendency for it not to return to normal. The reduction in length from the apex to the base of the lungs reduces the negative pressure that can be generated, especially at the bases. This can lead to atelectasis and closure of small airways.

The cephalad displacement of the rib margin elevates the peripheral insertion of the diaphragm. The central dome is also elevated because of the changing abdominal contents. However, the abdominal muscles have less tone, and tend to counteract this diaphragmatic movement. The resultant changes are shown in Fig. 4.1. Diaphragmatic elevation of 4 cm occurs with increased excursion of the muscle, so that breathing becomes more diaphragmatic than abdominal [5].

Respiratory muscle function is not changed in pregnancy or one month postpartum [6], but muscle strength may be reduced for up to 24 hours after normal vaginal delivery, and this may be hazardous in situations in which an adequate cough reflex is required [7].

The anatomical changes in the bony thoracic cage alter the normal appearance on radiological examination [8]. Lordosis and rotation displace the apex of the heart upwards and laterally. Lung markings are increased, partly because more alveoli are collapsed on expiration and partly because of increased filling of pulmonary blood vessels. These appearances can simulate those of mild congestive cardiac failure.

4.1.3 Lung volumes

The diaphragmatic elevation acts as a restrictive effect on the residual volume and expiratory reserve volume, reducing both, so that the functional residual capacity decreases by 10–25% in the third trimester [9]. These changes

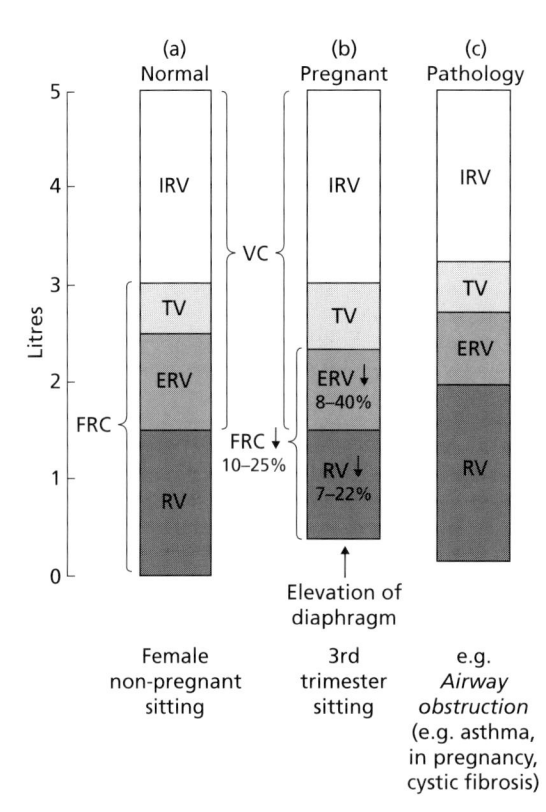

Fig. 4.2 Lung volume changes in women: (a) non-pregnant, (b) in late pregnancy, (c) in obstructive airway disease in pregnancy. ERV: expiratory reserve volume; FRC: functional residual capacity; IRV: inspiratory reserve volume; RV: residual volume; TV: tidal volume; VC: vital capacity.

are increased by obesity [10] and posture, e.g. the supine, lithotomy and Trendelenburg positions. The widening of the rib cage allows good inspiratory activity, and the vital capacity is maintained [11]. Any decrease in vital capacity will be abnormal, and can be an early indication of respiratory or cardiac disorders (Fig. 4.2).

Tidal volume increases markedly from 450–500 mL up to 600–700 mL, a 40% increase at times. It is a major factor in maintaining an increased minute ventilation during pregnancy, because the respiratory rate does not change.

Changes in airway calibre have been described, particularly in the bronchioles. An increase in physiological dead space secondary to dilatation of the smaller bronchioles occurs in pregnancy [12]. Bronchiolar collapse contributes to airway closure, and an increase in closing volume has been described during normal tidal volumes, especially in women with hypertensive disorders who have an abnormal capillary blood flow [13].

4.2 Pulmonary dynamics

4.2.1 Pulmonary mechanics

The forced vital capacity, forced expiratory volume in one second (FEV_1) and lung compliance are not appreciably altered during pregnancy [14–16]. Chest

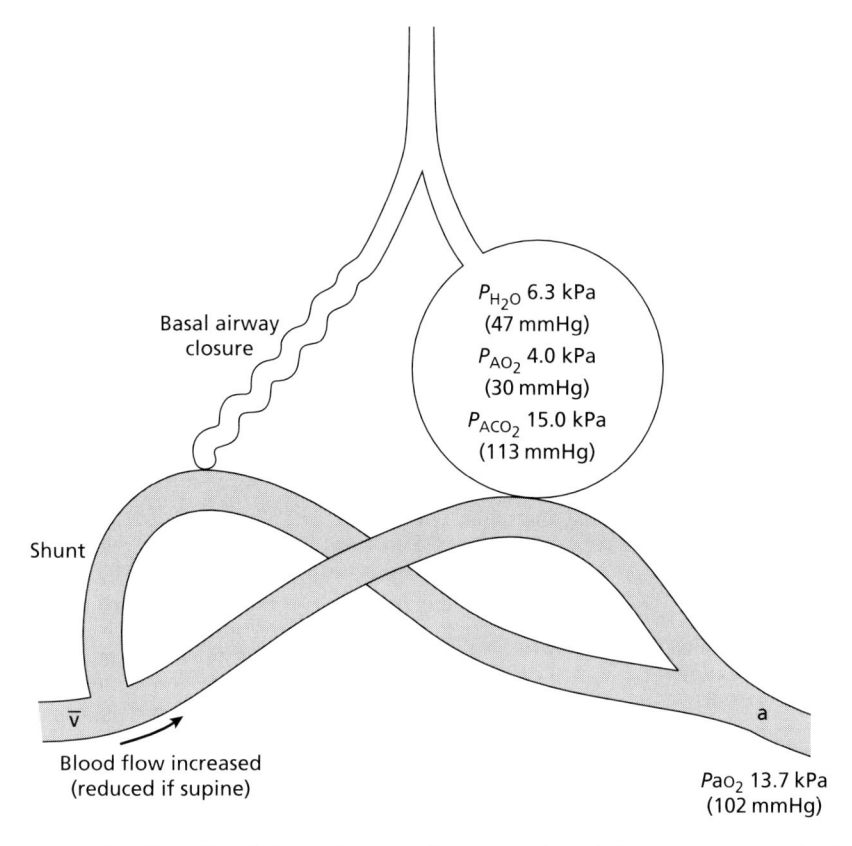

Fig. 4.3 The effect of basal airway closure and increasing shunt in late pregnancy; v, mixed venous and a, arterial blood.

wall compliance is reduced in late pregnancy, but once delivery has been achieved, it improves [17].

Airway resistance is altered both by factors that increase it (such as the reduction in resting lung volume) and those that decrease it (such as hormonal relaxation of bronchial smooth muscle), as well as by increased compliance secondary to hyperventilation [18], so that no significant change occurs.

Figure 4.3 illustrates the potential factors in late pregnancy that can increase ventilation/perfusion abnormalities. Throughout pregnancy there is no change in the alveolar–arterial difference in partial pressure of oxygen (P_{AO_2}–Pa_{O_2}), or in the percentage shunt from normal values, provided that the supine position is avoided [19,20]. A mild degree of anaemia can increase the alveolar–arterial oxygen tension difference for any given degree of physiological shunt. A decrease in cardiac output as a result of inferior vena caval occlusion will tend to reduce the mixed venous oxygenation and reduce arterial oxygen tension. Pathological changes, such as an increase in lung water, may reduce the diffusing capacity and decrease lung compliance.

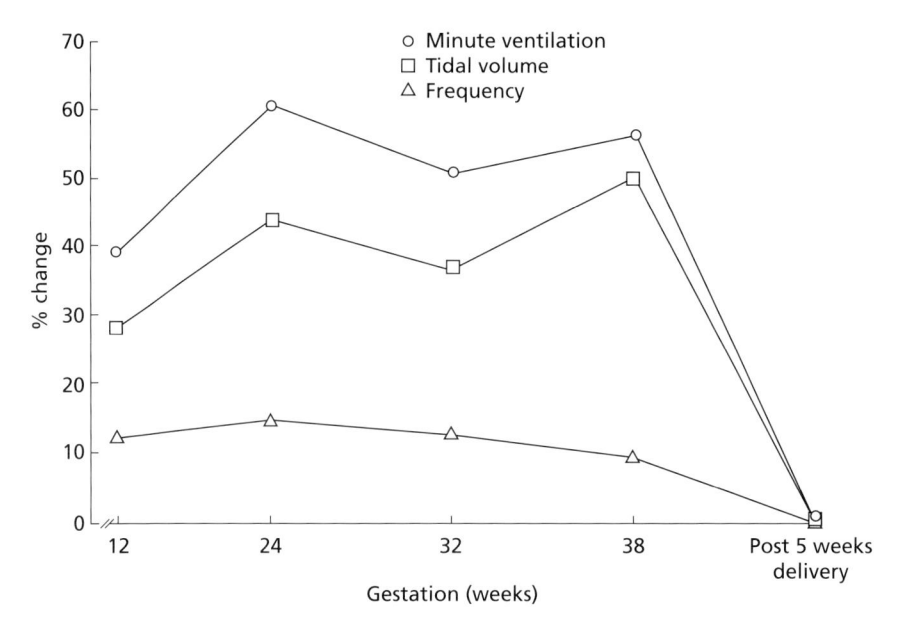

Fig. 4.4 Changes in ventilation during pregnancy [19].

4.2.2 Ventilation

There is an increase in minute ventilation early in pregnancy [21], which is not paralleled by a similar change in oxygen requirements and appears to be an effect of progesterone on the respiratory centre. Subsequent increases in progesterone have no further effect on respiration. Minute ventilation gradually increases in the second and third trimesters, paralleling increases in tidal volume rather than any real change in respiratory frequency (Fig. 4.4) [19].

There is no change in dead space, because the anatomical changes in the thoracic cage shorten airway length, while at the same time there is an increase in the cross-sectional area because bronchial smooth muscle relaxes. Hyperventilation will therefore reduce alveolar and hence arterial carbon dioxide tension. This respiratory alkalosis is compensated for by renal excretion of bicarbonate, so that pH is normalized [22]. The serum bicarbonate decreases to 18–21 mmol/L. The decrease in alveolar CO_2 tension will fractionally increase the alveolar oxygen, by their relationship through the alveolar air equation. An increase in alveolar ventilation will increase the work of breathing, but only marginally.

Many of the respiratory function tests in pregnancy are measured with the mother at rest. However, women exercise, and during labour this is an important stress. The oxygen reserve in the functional residual capacity is decreased and oxygen consumption is increased, so that exercise, if not properly compensated for, could reduce tissue and fetal oxygenation. The respiratory rate response is unchanged during exercise in pregnancy, so that the increase in minute ventilation during exercise is maintained. In the exercising pregnant woman, venous blood returns from the distended overfilled leg veins, so that cardiac output initially increases faster than in the non-pregnant state [23].

4.2.3 Pulmonary circulation

The pulmonary circulation is a low-pressure system that can accommodate increased flow without an increase in pressure. It is controlled by a number of vasoactive mechanisms. The pulmonary endothelium produces both constrictive and relaxing factors, but vasomotor tone is also modulated by neurogenic influences; for example, acetylcholine lowers vascular tone by the arginine–nitric oxide pathway. The capillary endothelium also metabolizes hormones, e.g. oestrogens. The pulmonary capillary network can also act as a filter to trap emboli from thrombi or particles from amniotic fluid.

Flow through the pulmonary circulation will increase as a result of the increase in cardiac output associated with pregnancy. This may improve ventilation/perfusion inequalities, especially in the upper lobes. Pulmonary blood flow will decrease in maternal hypotension, e.g. inferior vena caval occlusion, haemorrhage or sympathetic block and hypoxaemia will develop. Pulmonary vascular resistance increases in pain, stress, hypoxia, intubation, active pushing and mechanical ventilation. When pulmonary capillary pressure is increased and there is a reduction in colloid osmotic pressure, fluid exchange between the capillaries and other lung tissues as governed by Starling's forces (see p. 38) is altered, and there is a tendency to pulmonary oedema [24]. An increase in lung water can reduce the capacity for diffusion of gases across the alveoli to the capillaries.

4.3 Alterations in physiology

4.3.1 Labour

Oxygen consumption increases from the resting state at term (about 30% above non-pregnant volumes) to more than double during labour at 500–750 mL/min, primarily as a result of an increase in the work of breathing [25,26]. Hyperventilation is a response to pain, or can be actively produced as part of childbirth methods. High values of minute ventilation, close to maximum breathing capacity have been recorded [27]. Alkalaemia is secondary to this ventilatory response, and may be partially compensated for by the metabolic tendency towards acidosis. These effects can induce uterine artery vasoconstriction, leading to decreased placental perfusion [28].

The hypocarbia associated with painful contractions may induce apnoea between contractions, leading to hypoxaemia [29], and is more frequent in the second stage when no analgesia is used [30]. This increase in hypoxaemia towards delivery may result from muscle splinting, maternal exhaustion and

Table 4.1 Breathing patterns associated with sleep disorders.

Characteristics
Sleep apnoea
Obstructive
10 apnoeic episodes/h sleep.
Respiratory efforts are made.
Central
Apnoea with no respiratory effect
Mixed
Both obstructive and central effects
Periodic breathing
Tidal volume waxes and wanes
Alveolar hypoventilation
Associated with obesity

Valsalva manoeuvres, which halt respiration and reduce venous return. Effective epidural analgesia markedly diminishes the increase in minute ventilation, which indicates that it is in part caused by the pain of labour [31].

4.3.2 Smoking

The effects of smoking on pulmonary physiology in pregnancy mainly relate to small airways disease, and its severity is directly related to the amount of exposure. The bronchodilatory effect of pregnancy is not sufficient to overcome the deleterious effect on small airway resistance [32].

Fetal oxygen supply is reduced, and consequently fetal growth retardation occurs. Smoking up to 20 cigarettes per day reduces birth weight by 200 g [33]. This may be the result of carbon monoxide inhalation and the additional increase in maternal oxygen consumption from the stimulant effects of nicotine. If a mother stops smoking before the sixteenth week of pregnancy, this weight loss does not occur. Nicotine itself can have adverse effects, so nicotine patches are not recommended in pregnancy to aid cessation of smoking.

4.3.3 Sleep disorders (Table 4.1)

During the first trimester, daytime sleepiness is often noted as a presenting symptom of pregnancy. In the last trimester, the weight gain in pregnancy may contribute to upper airway obstruction during sleep. Nasal obstruction is present during pregnancy, as well as a tendency to hypoxia due to the reduction in functional residual capacity. The mother is protected from some of these effects (Table 4.2) by spending less time sleeping supine, where obstructive sleep apnoea is most common, by a reduction in rapid eye movement (REM) sleep, because her nights are disturbed by discomfort, e.g. urinary

Table 4.2 Potential effects of pregnancy on sleep disorders.

Protective effects
Increased ventilatory drive from progesterone
Less time sleeping supine
Decreased rapid eye movement sleep

Detrimental effects
Weight gain
Nasal obstruction
Thoracic cage alterations

frequency, backache, heartburn, etc., and there is the background ventilatory drive from progesterone [34].

There are several reports of sleep apnoea during pregnancy [35–37] and of fetal heart rate changes related to apnoeic episodes, with intrauterine growth retardation. If hypoxaemia is occurring during sleep, oxygen supplements should be given. Continuous positive airway pressure via the nasal route has been used successfully during pregnancy. Sleep apnoea sufferers are sensitive to opioid drugs. If opioids are used in labour, great care must be taken to detect any early signs of respiratory depression.

When anaesthesia is needed, regional techniques without opioids are the methods of choice. If general anaesthesia is needed, difficulties should be anticipated and recovery from anaesthesia should be managed in a high-dependency unit or intensive-care setting. The additional risks that should be considered are a lack of venous access, intubation difficulties (awake fibre-optic intubation may be needed), problems on arousal and respiratory depression postoperatively.

4.4 Applied physiology

4.4.1 Asthma

Asthma is a chronic inflammation of the airways, with bronchial hyperreactivity and exacerbations of reversible airway obstruction. This is the most common medical respiratory disorder in pregnancy, affecting more than 1% of pregnancies. With good educational, environmental and pharmacological support, the outcome of pregnancy should match that in non-asthmatics [38]. Poor asthma control in pregnancy can lead to increased maternal and fetal complications, such as pre-eclampsia, complicated labours, low birth weight infants and neonatal mortality. No increased incidence of congenital malformation has been found [39]. If the asthma is severe—that is, if wheezing occurs daily—there is an increased incidence of premature rupture of the membranes and labour [40]. Steroids are indicated in severe exacerbations, and can precipitate diabetes. In an acute attack, maternal hypoxaemia causes fetal hypoxia. Sympathetic responses will lead to uterine vasoconstriction.

Hyperventilation will occur, further lowering the arterial Pa_{CO_2}, increasing uterine arterial vasoconstriction and shifting the oxygen dissociation curve to the left, thereby compromising the fetus. Gas trapping will increase intrathoracic pressure and reduce venous return. It is important that asthmatics who become pregnant are jointly assessed by obstetricians and respiratory physicians, so that the correct choice of therapy is made. Fear of fetal drug effects, especially teratogenicity, is a major problem in the treatment of asthma in pregnancy [38]. Effective therapy and the avoidance of status asthmaticus are associated with good fetal outcome, so it is necessary to optimize respiratory care.

Pathophysiology

A mild, tonic constriction exists in all human airways. It is maintained largely by efferent vagal activity, and can be abolished by antimuscarinics such as atropine. Baseline airway size can significantly influence the bronchoconstrictive response, because changes in airflow resistance are related inversely to the fourth power of the airway radius. Any decrease in an already constricted bronchus will produce a greater degree of airway obstruction than the same decrease in a more dilated airway. Airway size is the result of bronchial smooth-muscle tone, mucosal oedema, inflammation and airway secretions, and it is occasionally affected by pressure effects from outside the bronchi (e.g. tumours).

Hyperactivity of the smooth muscle occurs not only in severe asthma but also in mild forms of the disease and in normal subjects after viral infection and exposure to pollutants. Damage to airway mucosa may be the major factor that produces this sensitivity. Loss or dysfunction of the epithelium may result in the loss of substances, e.g. neuropeptides, which degrade constricting substances [41].

A prospective study of 16 asthmatic women initially assessed before pregnancy recorded stable peak expiratory flow (PEF) rates throughout pregnancy and an improvement in observed bronchial responsiveness in the second trimester [42]. An increase in cortisol and progesterone would be expected to decrease bronchomotor tone and airway resistance. Serum concentrations of these hormones did not parallel these observed changes in bronchial responsiveness, because hormone concentrations were maximal in the third trimester.

Deterioration of asthma in pregnancy is not well tolerated by mothers. Decreases in pulmonary reserve, coupled with changes in airway resistance and compliance, increase the work of breathing and recruit accessory muscles, thereby increasing oxygen consumption. Prevention of symptom exacerbation is therefore important. Other causes of dyspnoea should be excluded by objective measures of large airway calibre. The FEV_1 and PEF correlate reliably, and the PEF meter is portable and can be used twice daily by a mother throughout pregnancy to monitor therapy. Allergies and smoking should be avoided. Immunoglobulin E-mediated triggering factors should be excluded so that medication can be reduced. Animals, dust mites and fungal spores are common antigens. Asthma is generated as an inflammatory disorder by the immunoglobulin E (IgE) molecules binding to receptors on mast-cell membranes. This binding initiates the release of mediators, which—in addition to contracting bronchial smooth muscle—increase vascular and mucosal permeability and increase mucus production. Cell damage exposes sensory receptors situated beneath the epithelium, and local reflex or vagally mediated responses develop.

Variations in the prevalence of asthma suggest that environmental rather than genetic factors are operating, and the most important risk factors for death from asthma are being poor and black [43]. Studies comparing different ethnic groups have to take into account factors such as smoking, less medication, higher serum IgE levels, less education and more pregnancies [44]. Few studies have controlled for these important confounding variables. Genetic susceptibility factors are probably of most importance during the inductive stages of the disease, not in acute exacerbations in adult life.

Fetal effects. The fetus, unlike the mother, operates on the steep portion of its oxygen dissociation curve. Decreases in maternal Pao_2 below 8 kPa (60 mmHg) result in a rapid and profoundly decreased fetal oxygen content. Before labour, this can only be detected by abnormalities in the fetal heart rate.

Asthma
Aspiration pneumonitis
Pulmonary oedema
Large airway obstruction
   In lumen, e.g. foreign body
   Outside lumen, e.g. thyroid gland enlargement
Anaphylactic reaction
Amniotic fluid embolus
Left heart failure
Mitral stenosis
Pneumothorax
Pulmonary emboli

Associated specifically with general anaesthesia
Aspiration
Inadequate neuromuscular block
Endotracheal tube
   Kink
   Obstruction
   Endobronchial intubation
   Cuff overinflation

Table 4.3 Differential diagnosis of wheezing.

Table 4.4 Severity of asthma.

Mild	Infrequent cough and wheezing (1 or 2 times a week)
	Good exercise tolerance (not vigorous exercise)
Moderate	More symptomatic
	Occasional severe exacerbations (A & E three times a year)
Severe	Daily wheezing
	Severe exacerbations (more than three times a year)
	Poor exercise tolerance

Indicators of severe asthma (on acute admission) [47]
Recent history of status asthmaticus
Use of corticosteroids
Previous prolonged hospitalization
Endotracheal intubation required in previous admission
Arterial blood gas analysis: values in pregnancy
  $Paco_2$ > 4.7 kPa (35 mmHg)
  pH < 7.35
  Pao_2 in early pregnancy < 13.3–14.7 kPa (100–110 mmHg)
  Pao_2 at term < 12.0–13.3 kPa (90–100 mmHg)

Clinical assessment

Differential diagnosis of wheezing. A parturient who develops wheezing may or may not have a history of asthma. Even if the patient is asthmatic, it is necessary to consider other causes for her symptoms, especially since the physiological effects of pregnancy combined with obstetric and anaesthetic complications can produce airway narrowing [45]. These are summarized in Table 4.3.

Management guidelines for acute and chronic asthma

Asthma is a chronic process characterized by acute exacerbations. It has been classified as mild, moderate or severe, without specific consideration of pregnancy [46]. It is important to be able to identify indicators of a potentially fatal acute asthmatic attack in a pregnant woman. These are outlined in Table 4.4 [47].

Chronic asthma. The currently recommended guidelines [48] describe five steps after provoking factors (e.g. smoking, animals, dust mite) have been reduced when possible:
Step 1: occasional use of relief bronchodilators (short-acting $β_2$-agonists).
Step 2: regular inhaled anti-inflammatory agents (e.g. beclomethasone or cromoglycate) plus bronchodilators (Step 1) as necessary.
Step 3: high-dose inhaled steroids plus bronchodilators (step 1), *or* long-acting $β_2$-agonists.

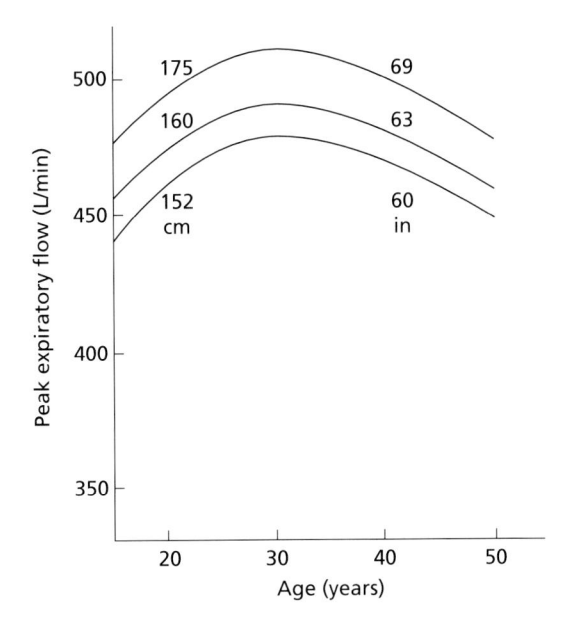

Fig. 4.5 The peak expiratory flow rate variations in normal non-pregnant women of childbearing age [48].

Step 4: high-dose inhaled steroids, bronchodilators and other agents, e.g. anticholinergic agents. Theophylline should be used with caution in pregnancy, and blood levels should be monitored closely (therapeutic range of theophylline 10–20 µg/mL).
Step 5: addition of oral steroids.

Patients will start treatment at the step most appropriate to the initial severity, with step-down after periods of stability. A short course of oral steroids may be needed at any time and at any step. Control is monitored by peak flow rates (Fig. 4.5). The aim of therapy is to achieve a flow rate of ≥ 80% of the predicted or best value. Small diurnal variations usually occur, which are exaggerated in asthma, with excessive decreases in the early morning.

Many pregnant women are managed with inhaled β-agonists and inhaled corticosteroids. Teratogenic effects have not been associated with the use of these [38,49]. Steroid use in pregnancy may induce hyperglycaemia, and blood and urinary glucose should be monitored. For respiratory tract infections in pregnancy, the penicillins, cephalosporins and erythromycin are appropriate. Fetal effects of other antibiotics should be considered before use [50].

Acute asthma. The severity of an acute exacerbation of asthma is often underestimated because of failure to make objective measurements. There may be no signs or subjective distress. Life-threatening features include exhaustion, hypotension, a silent chest and a reduction in peak expiratory flow to less than 33% of normal or best.

Treatment aims to:
- correct hypoxia;
- relieve bronchospasm;
- achieve adequate ventilation;
- optimize uteroplacental function;
- prevent early relapse.

Immediate treatment. Management guidelines for asthma have been approved nationally [48]. These include:
- oxygen must be used at the highest concentration available, with the woman sitting. Carbon dioxide retention is not aggravated by oxygen therapy in asthma;
- high dose of inhaled β-agonists. This can be either 5 mg salbutamol or 10 mg terbutaline via an oxygen-driven nebulizer;
- establish intravenous access, for rehydration and drug administration;
- high doses of systemic steroids must be given early, because they take time to have an effect. Intravenous hydrocortisone 200 mg or prednisolone tablets (30–60 mg), or both may be used;
- no sedatives;
- chest radiograph to exclude pneumothorax. The abdomen and fetus must be shielded;
- if life-threatening features are present: add ipratropium 0.5 mg to the nebulized β-agonist. Also, consider giving a parenteral β-agonist, with the rate of infusion adjusted according to the response of the peak expiratory flow and heart rate;
- in pregnancy, try to avoid aminophylline, because it has not been demonstrated to provide additional benefit over standard treatment [41]. Its action as a phosphodiesterase inhibitor has been disputed in the therapeutic dose range, and bronchodilation may be the result of catecholamine release. Theophylline crosses the placenta. It can cause transient nervousness (irritability) and tachycardia in the neonate;
- monitor the fetal heart rate continuously.

Monitoring of treatment. The electrocardiogram, oxygen saturation and heart rate should be monitored continuously. The peak expiratory flow (PEF) is measured every 15–30 min after starting treatment. Serial measurements of forced expiratory volume in one second (FEV_1) are an alternative to the PEF.

Further measurements of blood gas tensions will be required if the patient was initially hypoxic and (i) the oxygen saturation after immediate treatment has not improved more than 5%; or (ii) if the initial Pa_{CO_2} was normal or increased; or (iii) if the patient's condition deteriorates. Reference to normal blood gas values in pregnancy should be made (Table 4.4). The Pa_{CO_2} in pregnancy is expected to be 4 kPa (30 mmHg), so any value above 4.7 kPa (35 mmHg) is abnormal.

A sputum sample should be obtained if possible, and appropriate antibiotics should be given if bacterial infection is present.

Intensive care

Women with life-threatening factors require intensive monitoring. Not all patients admitted to the intensive care unit need ventilation. Those who have worsening hypoxia or hypercapnia, drowsiness or unconsciousness and those who have had a respiratory arrest require intermittent positive pressure ventilation. Successful perinatal outcomes of pregnancy have been achieved in such circumstances [51].

Prolonged respiratory time constants occur in asthma because of gas trapping. It is usual to ventilate with a long expiratory pause, which can be achieved by a low respiratory frequency, e.g. seven to eight breaths per minute. Successful treatment using high-frequency oscillatory ventilation has been reported in a parturient suffering from a combination of asthma and atypical pneumonia [52]. This method was used because the respiration failure was refractory to conventional intermittent positive-pressure ventilation (IPPV).

Labour and delivery

The severity of asthma may influence the timing and method of delivery. Elective Caesarean section may have to be postponed if the woman is unable to lie supine without shortness of breath. The effect of drugs on asthma and labour, as well as drug interactions with the treatments used, have to be considered. Prostaglandin $F_{2\alpha}$ should not be used to induce labour, and non-steroidal analgesic drugs are to be avoided. Narcotic analgesics which liberate histamine may also be contraindicated. Uterine contractility may be reduced by β-adrenergic agonists, but the latter drugs may have to be continued in order to maintain asthma control. Drugs that sensitize the myocardium, e.g. halothane, are potential dysrhythmics if adrenergic agonists are used. However, halothane has been used as a bronchodilator. When steroid therapy is being given orally, its use during labour and delivery should be continued by a parenteral preparation. There is a rare potential risk of fetal adrenal insufficiency following maternal steroid therapy.

Exacerbating airway responsiveness (e.g. through irritants, cold air, exercise) should be avoided. The mother may be aware of this, but not all the hospital staff may be so well informed. Some aerosols used in hospitals may be irritants. Hyperventilation should be minimized. This is best achieved by adequate pain relief and decreasing stress and anxiety. The mother should also be encouraged to drink small volumes of water-based fluids to maintain her hydration. Throughout labour and delivery, the fetus should be monitored by cardiotocography.

Delivery is unlikely to be complicated by asthma. Although minute ventilation can increase dramatically, high levels of catecholamines or cortisol may protect the parturient at this time.

All types of analgesia have been successfully used to relieve the pain of labour in asthmatics. Active wheezing would contraindicate drugs with histamine-releasing and sedatives effects, e.g. pethidine. Since an asthmatic mother should be considered to be a patient more at risk of obstetric complications, a prophylactic antacid regimen (see Chapter 5, p. 92) should be followed during labour in case emergency delivery is required.

Anaesthesia for Caesarean section

Elective surgery will require a patient who is medically stable and in whom treatment for asthma has been optimized. Lung function assessment will require PEF rate or FEV_1 monitoring. Patients taking steroids should receive parenteral hydrocortisone instead.

General anaesthesia. The prevalence of gastro-oesophageal reflux in asthmatic patients is three times higher than non-asthmatics [53], so pulmonary aspiration of gastric contents is a greater risk in such patients. Maternal gastric acid secretion can be decreased by the preoperative administration of H_2-receptor blocking drugs. The action of these drugs enhances the bronchoconstriction response to histamine. Cimetidine is more likely to have this effect than ranitidine [54]. Both intubation and extubation must be conducted with all precautions to avoid this complication. Endotracheal intubation itself may precipitate bronchospasm, especially if anaesthesia is inadequate to prevent reflex responses. Extubation must be performed with the patient awake, with an adequate cough reflex and in a position to avoid tracheal soiling.

The choice of anaesthetic drugs should avoid those known to release histamine, such as the neuromuscular relaxants *d*-tubocurarine and atracurium. Vecuronium is the non-depolarizing neuromuscular agent of choice for Caesarean section. There is a need to ensure adequate reversal of muscle relaxants. Although neostigmine may increase airway secretions and can precipitate bronchospasm, inadequate reversal of neuromuscular blockade can result in respiratory distress and itself stimulate bronchospasm. The muscarinic effects of neostigmine can be prevented by adequate doses of glycopyrrolate or atropine. Inhalational agents can prevent or reverse antigen-induced bronchoconstriction [55]. Enflurane or isoflurane may be preferred to halothane, which can sensitize the heart to dysrhythmias. Halothane should be avoided in patients receiving sympathomimetics. Ketamine has been reported in the treatment of asthma, but it is not usually the first choice of induction agent [56]. It probably exerts its effects by centrally stimulating increased catecholamines, and when administered with aminophylline it lowers the seizure threshold [57].

Intraoperative ventilation should be adjusted to minimize peak inspiratory pressure and allow time for expiration, thereby preventing air trapping and increased intrathoracic pressure. The differential diagnosis of wheezing must be considered intraoperatively (Table 4.3) and treated according to causation. Coughing is impaired, and mucus plugging of bronchi has to be prevented.

The use of smooth-muscle relaxant drugs to achieve bronchodilation may have effects on uterine tone. Blood loss may potentially be larger than normal.

Regional anaesthesia. Although regional anaesthesia is the method of choice for operative delivery of asthmatic women, because it avoids intubation with its irritant effects and potential for aspiration of gastric contents, it is not without its own problems. The mother has to lie supine with a pelvic tilt. This may not be comfortable for her, especially if she has gastro-oesophageal reflux. The regional block itself will reach dermatome T4, and can have effects on motor and sympathetic function. Unopposed parasympathetic tone to the bronchi may cause bronchoconstriction. Intercostal muscles may be paralysed in a high spinal block and lead to loss of expiratory muscle power and inadequate respiratory gas exchange [58]. Bupivacaine is the drug of choice, because it has a wider sensorimotor block differential than does lidocaine.

4.4.2 Cystic fibrosis

Cystic fibrosis is characterized by widespread dysfunction of exocrine glands, principally in the lungs and pancreas. Aggressive respiratory therapy has dramatically improved the survival of patients with cystic fibrosis into the third decade of life. This may increase further in future with advances in therapy. Nebulized human recombinant deoxyribonuclease (DNase) has been used to reduce the viscosity of secretions [59], and has been found effective in improving lung function over 24 weeks. The major features are malabsorption due to pancreatic insufficiency, chronic suppurative lung disease with bronchiectasis and failure to thrive.

The disorder is usually autosomal recessive, occurring with an incidence of one in 3000. The physiological dysfunction is a defect in chloride transport in the epithelial cells of the respiratory, hepatopancreatobiliary, gastrointestinal and reproductive tracts. The decreased Cl^- transport is accompanied by decreased transport of sodium and water, resulting in dehydrated, viscous secretions. It renders a man infertile because of spermatic cord obstruction and azoospermia, but females are fertile, and genetic counselling should be available to potential parents. The outcome of pregnancy relates to the severity of pulmonary and pancreatic dysfunction [60]. There is a better outcome if pancreatic function is normal, but that may represent a mild form of the disorder. The nutritional requirements of pregnancy may be greater than normal, because of increased cardiorespiratory work and catabolism from chronic infection, and may exceed supply because of malabsorption. Regular monitoring of weight is required, and 85–90% of the ideal weight for height is satisfactory (Table 4.5). Pancreatic enzyme supplements and multivitamin supplementation to prevent deficiency of fat-soluble vitamins are standard

Table 4.5 Management of cystic fibrosis.

Daily
Postural drainage, physiotherapy and exercise
Bronchodilators (plus steroids, if necessary)
Antibiotics
Vitamins
Pancreatic enzymes

Periodic
Team review at regional centre
Weight
Lung function
Sputum culture

therapies. Studies are in progress to develop a gene transfer system to correct the defective gene by targeting the respiratory epithelial cells. An optimal system of delivery resulting in long-term gene expression is required.

Progressive lung damage in cystic fibrosis is due to a combination of chronic infection and a host inflammatory response [61]. Despite frequent use of antibiotics, fetal malformations have not been noted. Experience with the penicillins, and to a lesser extent the cephalosporins, has demonstrated these agents to be safe during pregnancy. It is to be expected that a quarter to one-third of women with cystic fibrosis will require hospitalization during their pregnancy for intravenous antibiotics and intensive chest physiotherapy.

When lung function is compromised—for example, when the forced vital capacity is 50% below that predicted—the overall stability of the patient's disease would be the predictor of whether or not a mother would tolerate pregnancy. Women with cor pulmonale, hypoxaemia and severe airflow obstruction would be at high risk of maternal and fetal complications [62]. Patients with severe impairment of lung function ($FEV_1 < 60\%$ predicted) deliver prematurely, and themselves suffer increased loss of lung function and mortality [63]. Heart and lung transplantation may provide adequate cardiorespiratory reserve for pregnancy, but the increased risk of organ rejections and fetal exposure to potentially teratogenic drugs limits this option [64].

Multidisciplinary care is required for the pregnant woman with cystic fibrosis. She will require an obstetrician, dietician, respiratory physician and physiotherapist. Pancreatic function should be evaluated for diabetes and malabsorption. A quarter of the women will be diabetic prior to pregnancy [65]. Malabsorption of fat will predispose to vitamin K deficiency. The prothrombin time should be checked periodically, and water-soluble parenteral vitamin K should be administered if required. Anticipation and treatment of complications (Table 4.6) will minimize the risks associated with pregnancy.

Careful assessment of cardiorespiratory reserve is necessary at term, before and during labour. It is at this time that a compromised patient will develop right-sided heart failure. This complication will require aggressive diuresis and

Table 4.6 Complications of cystic fibrosis.

Respiratory
Infection
Nasal polyps
Deterioration during and after pregnancy
Pneumothorax
Haemoptysis

Cardiovascular
Cor pulmonale

Gastrointestinal
Cirrhosis, portal hypertension
Cholecystitis

Other
Diabetes mellitus
Salt loss (sweating in labour)
Arthropathy

Fetal
Intrauterine growth retardation
Prematurity

---

oxygen to reduce pulmonary vasoconstriction. Fluid and electrolyte management in labour requires careful attention, because excessive salt loss is associated with sweating.

The anaesthetist should be involved at an early stage in the management of labour and delivery, and should have an up-to-date functional assessment of the pulmonary, circulatory, nutritional and hepatic systems. Close monitoring will be required, and this is best in the high-dependency area of a labour ward. If cardiorespiratory function is not stable, invasive arterial and venous monitoring should be started. Adequate pain relief in labour can most effectively be provided with epidural analgesia. Motor block should be minimized so that respiratory muscle function and power is maintained.

General anaesthesia should be avoided, if possible, because of the potential risks from respiratory complications. If it is required, the anaesthetist should be careful not to use anticholinergic agents, because of their tendency to promote drying and inspissation of airway secretions. The woman may require intensive-care facilities and additional nutritional support [66,67].

4.4.3 Acute respiratory failure

Tissue oxygenation requires the delivery of an adequate quantity of available oxygen. The oxygen content of blood is changed in pregnancy by a reduction in haemoglobin concentration and an alteration in the position of the oxygen dissociation curve. Cardiac output increases in pregnancy, offsetting the

Table 4.7 Causes of acute respiratory failure in pregnancy.

Specific to pregnancy
   Amniotic fluid embolism
   β-Adrenergic tocolytic therapy (manifest as pulmonary oedema with volume overload)

General
Intrapulmonary
   Acute respiratory distress syndrome (ARDS)
   Aspiration of gastric contents
   Embolism
   Severe asthma
   Pneumonia
   Anaphylaxis
   Pneumothorax (second stage of labour)

Extrapulmonary
   Airway difficulties
   Central nervous system (drug depression, pathology)
   Muscle disorders (suxamethonium apnoea, myasthenia gravis)

reduction in oxygen content. Abnormalities of lung function may reduce tissue oxygenation and affect organ survival. Physiological mechanisms that result in inadequate pulmonary oxygen uptake include ventilation/perfusion mismatch, shunting, hypovolaemia, low $P\text{AO}_2$ (by reduced inspired oxygen concentrations) and diffusion abnormalities. A low $P\text{aO}_2$ and widened alveolar–arterial oxygen tension difference are associated with ventilation/perfusion mismatch and shunting. Alveolar hypoventilation also increases the arterial CO_2 from normal pregnant values.

The causes of acute respiratory failure in pregnancy are listed in Table 4.7. These patients will receive treatment in intensive-care units, and present a unique challenge to intensive-care specialists, because baseline pulmonary and cardiovascular values will be different from the non-pregnant patient and there is a necessity to provide adequate respiratory, cardiovascular and nutritional support for both mother and fetus. The potential effects on the fetus, not only of the mother's condition but also of the therapeutic interventions, e.g. medications and radiological procedures, must be considered.

Acute respiratory failure from pulmonary and amniotic fluid embolism accounts for 24% of maternal deaths in the United Kingdom [68]. Other obstetric complications, e.g. haemorrhage and pre-eclampsia, are associated with acute respiratory distress syndrome (ARDS), which has a high mortality when associated with multiorgan system failure. Mortality is a well-defined end point, but the morbidity presented by acute respiratory failure is difficult to assess. One report [69] on obstetric patients admitted to a medical intensive-care unit (ICU) showed that they were younger than the usual ICU population and had a higher mortality. Respiratory failure was the most common cause of admission, but ARDS was present in all maternal deaths in the series. Infant mortality was 35%. Most other studies of ICU care are post-surgical. A further report of obstetric patients admitted to a surgical intensive-care unit after Caesarean section showed a high incidence of anaesthetic respiratory complications following difficult intubation, aspiration and drug-related respiratory depression [70]. A 10-year retrospective review of ICU admissions at an obstetric hospital (61 435 deliveries) identified 16 anaesthetic complications requiring respiratory support. These included anaphylaxis, high regional block, suxamethonium apnoea and failure of tracheal intubation [71].

Pneumothorax

Spontaneous pneumothorax and pneumomediastinum occur most commonly in the second stage of labour [72]. Symptoms include chest or shoulder pain, dyspnoea and subcutaneous emphysema. Chest drainage will be required if air occupies more than a quarter of a hemithorax as seen on a chest radiograph. Subcutaneous emphysema can reduce venous return by a direct pressure effect. Absorption of the air in the tissues will occur more quickly if 100% oxygen is breathed. Nitrous oxide is contraindicated in this situation, in which air is trapped in a confined tissue space, because it will diffuse into the gas and expand its volume, with detrimental effects.

Embolism

Amniotic fluid embolism is discussed in Chapter 23.

Venous air embolism has been described during normal labour, delivery of patients with placenta praevia and criminal abortions. Presumably, subplacental venous sinuses are the site of air entry. Neck vein cannulation with poor technique and patient positioning, especially if the patient is generating large negative thoracic pressures by deep inspiration, can also be complicated by air embolism. Sudden profound hypotension is the most common presentation, followed by respiratory arrest. Electrocardiographic changes of ischaemia and right heart strain may be present. Turbulence in the heart may induce platelet damage, fibrin formation and microemboli. These obstruct the pulmonary arteries and capillaries. If air embolism is suspected, 100% oxygen must be continued. Nitrous oxide should be discontinued, because it has a very low solubility and by diffusing into the air bubbles tends to increase their size in the pulmonary vasculature.

Thromboembolism. The most important intervention to reduce the mortality caused by pulmonary embolism is to prevent venous thrombosis (see Chapter 23).

Acute respiratory distress syndrome

Definition. There is a spectrum of acute lung injury, and when it is severe, it has been termed 'acute respiratory distress syndrome' (ARDS). The presenting signs and symptoms of ARDS are acute non-specific dyspnoea and tachycardia. It is a syndrome of acute onset, with hypoxaemia and a large arterial-inspired oxygen gradient $Pao_2/Fio_2 \leq 26.6$ kPa (200 mmHg), regardless of positive end-expiratory pressure (PEEP), excluding heart failure with a mean airway pressure (Paw) ≤ 18 mmHg and with bilateral infiltrates on the posteroanterior (frontal) chest radiograph. The definitive radiological pattern appears 12–24 hours after the onset of clinical symptoms. Acute lung injury differs only in showing an oxygenation gradient of $Pao_2/Fio_2 \leq 40$ kPa (300 mmHg) [73]. Patients with hypoxaemia and pulmonary infiltrations caused by volume overload or heart failure, or both, do not have acute lung injury ARDS. However, ARDS may coexist with or follow heart failure or volume overload.

ARDS in pregnancy. Patients with pre-eclampsia seem to be at particular risk in these circumstances. Acute lung injury (and ARDS, if severe) is often associated with direct injury such as aspiration, pneumonia or indirect injury, e.g. sepsis. ARDS in parturients is also associated with haemorrhage or hypotension, and a significant number (41%) of women who develop ARDS have hypertensive disorders of pregnancy [68]. When aspiration, pneumonia and cardiogenic oedema were excluded, the causation of ARDS in these women was not clear, and further study was suggested. It is recommended that particular care should be taken to prevent aspiration or pulmonary oedema in women at risk of ARDS, and that these women should receive high dependency care for at least 24 hours after delivery.

Physiological monitoring. Pregnant women will have cardiac output changes that reflect their period of gestation, or stage of labour, but central pressures will not differ significantly from those in non-pregnant women except immediately after delivery, when there is an acute increase in circulating blood volume from the contracted uterus. When hypotension and oliguria fail to respond to moderate hydration, pulmonary artery catheterization is usually indicated in addition to central venous pressure measurement to monitor filling pressures, cardiac output and systemic vascular resistance [74]. Pulmonary artery catheterization is also indicated in the situation in which ventilation of the lungs is required for oxygenation and adequate oxygen tensions can only be achieved by the addition of a positive end-expiratory pressure of 15 mmHg or above [75]. Methods of assessing the degree of pulmonary oedema using pulmonary pressure–volume loops may lack information on the normal physiological changes in pregnancy.

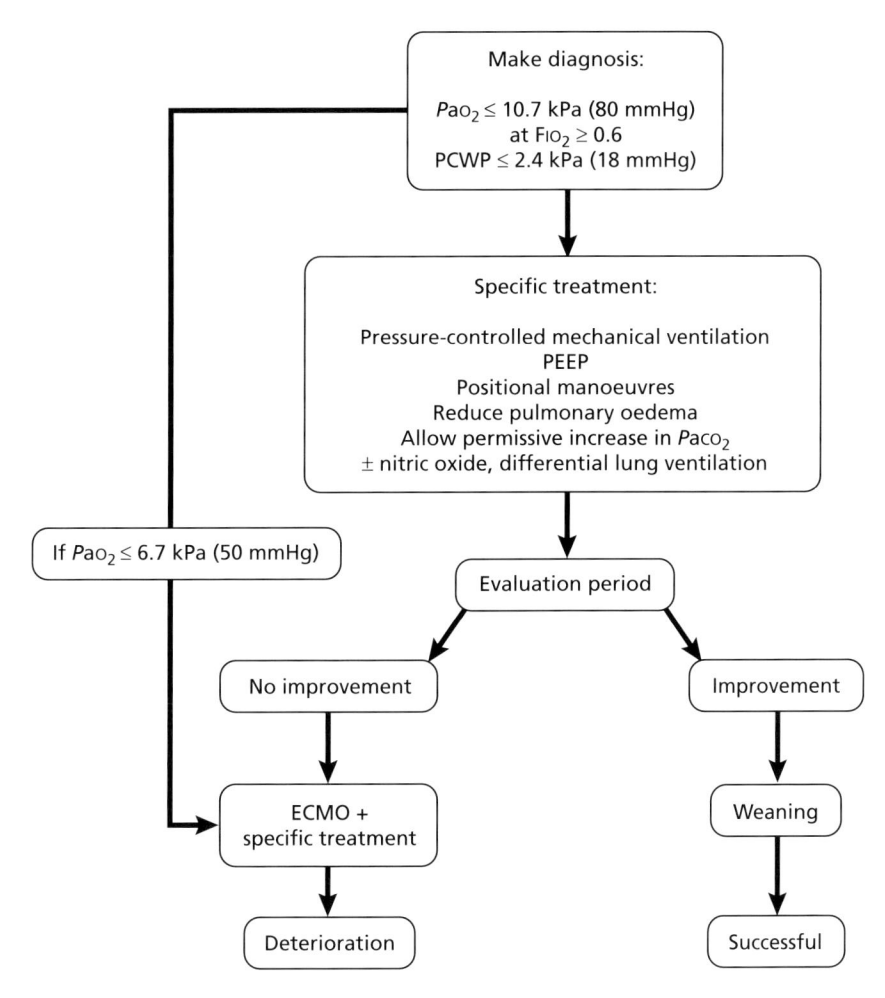

Fig. 4.6 Flow chart for the treatment of acute respiratory distress syndrome (ARDS) [77].

Management of ARDS. Management of ARDS (Fig. 4.6) will include additional oxygen, PEEP, or continuous positive airways pressure (CPAP), mechanical ventilation (if required to maintain oxygenation), avoidance of fluid overload and delivery of care within an ICU. The form of ventilatory support that applies large tidal volumes at low frequency can contribute to the progression of the disease, as well as a high inspired fractional oxygen concentration. The ventilatory manoeuvres required to prevent alveolar collapse and airway closure are a specialized area of intensive care, and have been recently reviewed [76]. The new approach to ventilation attempts to protect the lung from mechanical barotrauma, prevent oxygen toxicity, recruit alveoli in the infiltrated, atelectatic and consolidated lung, and reduce the anatomical and alveolar dead spaces. Additional pharmacological or technical interventions, e.g. steroids, nitric oxide inhalation and extracorporeal membrane oxygena-

Table 4.8 Complications of acute respiratory distress syndrome.

System	Complication	Prevention
Pulmonary	Barotrauma	Avoid high inflation pressures and tidal volumes
	Fibrosis	Aggressive initial therapy
	Emboli	Prevent deep vein thrombosis on i.v. catheters
	Pneumothorax	Careful insertion of pulmonary artery catheter
	Airway occlusion	Good nursing care, attention to cuff
	Pneumonia	Monitor colonization, culture and sensitivity
Gastrointestinal	Ileus, gastric distension	Check medications
	Haemorrhage	Check coagulation, correct hypotension, acidosis
Cardiovascular	Pulmonary hypertension	Relieve hypoxaemia, consider pulmonary artery catheter, vasodilators
	Dysrhythmias	Avoid acidosis, alkalosis, hypoxaemia
	Bacteraemias	Remove infected catheters
Renal	Sepsis	Treat infections aggressively
	Acute renal failure	Maintain fluid balance, avoid nephrotoxic drugs, relieve any obstruction
Metabolic	Malnutrition	Enteral nutrition
	Hyperpyrexia	Reduce body temperature

tion (ECMO) are not considered to be standard methods, and require evaluation. The prognosis for ARDS as determined on ICU admissions is based on the aetiology, its severity, the patient's physiological reserve and other disease processes, especially those that affect the immune system. Once treatment and support have been given, these factors may change.

Complications. Patients with ARDS develop complications (Table 4.8) that can further increase morbidity and mortality. These may be iatrogenic, such as invasive monitoring or drug therapy, or secondary to the primary disorder, such as sepsis [77]. Tissue oxygenation, which is dependent on adequate oxygen delivery and extraction, is critical, and significant reductions will impair organ function and survival. Mixed venous oxygen saturation is often used to measure this. After initial resuscitation and stabilization, the most common causes of reduced tissue oxygenation are either interventions (e.g. occurring with ventilation or medication) or patient-related. The latter include rapid progress of the underlying disease, or the onset of a new pathological event [78]. Pneumothorax and atelectasis occur relatively frequently in mechanically ventilated patients, and abnormalities of oxygenation have been correlated with the quantity of non-inflated lung tissue on computed tomography (CT) scan analysis of patients with moderate to severe ARDS [79]. In pregnant women, tissue oxygen consumption is increased, and it remains above normal levels even after delivery when the majority of women are managed in the ICU. This additional burden on a failing respiratory system could potentially increase multiorgan failure in this disorder.

Pulmonary oedema

Changes in the pressures generated in pregnancy, both within and outside the pulmonary capillaries, are described in Chapter 3. The capillary hydrostatic pressure is the most important factor in determining clinical pulmonary oedema formation [80]. Small increases in capillary hydrostatic pressure cause functional disturbances when capillary permeability is abnormal, e.g. in ARDS and anaphylaxis. However, clinical measurement of pulmonary capillary hydrostatic pressure cannot be made, and conventional measures of preload, such as central venous pressure and pulmonary artery occlusion pressure, are rarely available in pregnant women unless they are critically ill. In acute pulmonary oedema precipitated by excessive intravenous fluid administration, high-concentration oxygen therapy and intravenous diuretics are the immediate treatments. Positive airways pressure will be required if these measures fail to relieve the acute respiratory failure. This can be delivered by securing the airway with tracheal intubation and ventilation, or by face mask [81]. A study of 45 parturient women who developed pulmonary oedema demonstrated unexpected cardiac dysfunction with echocardiography in 47%. This indicates that echocardiography should be considered in evaluation of pulmonary oedema [82].

Pulmonary oedema and anaesthesia. The combination of a tachycardia (iatrogenically produced, such as from tocolysis with salbutamol, or endogenously produced), a preload of intravenous fluid (dextrose water, crystalloid) and a regional nerve block complicated by hypotension is the scenario for morbidity and mortality. The treatment of hypotension is likely to be administration of more fluid and a vasoconstrictor such as ephedrine. In the presence of a tachycardia (sinus or dysrhythmia) of about 140 beats/min and an increase in preload (fluid) and afterload (vasoconstriction), acute pulmonary oedema can be precipitated. The initial response to hypotension should be to check the woman's position so as to avoid inferior vena caval occlusion, which may not be reversed by fluid or vasoconstrictors. A more logical approach would be to determine the heart rhythm by electrocardiography, and reduce the rate if necessary so that adequate atrial filling can be achieved.

Another scenario can occur after general anaesthesia, again where a fluid load has been given and a vasoconstrictor such as ergometrine. The peripheral vasodilator effects of the anaesthetic agents can redistribute the fluid load, but when the patient wakens, the unopposed action of ergometrine is manifest as dyspnoea, hypoxia and pink frothy sputum, diagnostic of pulmonary oedema. This situation can also arise after acid aspiration, and often leads to ARDS.

It may be difficult to differentiate between the causes of these signs and symptoms.

References

1. Hollingsworth HM, Irwin RS. Acute respiratory failure in pregnancy. *Clin Chest Med* 1992; **13**: 723–40.
2. Toppazada H, Michaels L, Toppazada M *et al.* The human respiratory nasal mucosa in pregnancy: an electroimmunoscopic and histochemical study. *J Laryngol Otol* 1982; **96**: 613–26.
3. Fishburne JI. Physiology and disease of the respiratory system in pregnancy. *J Reprod Med* 1979; **22**: 177–89.
4. Camann WR, Ostheimer GW. Physiological adaptations during pregnancy. *Int Anesthesiol Clin* 1990; **28**: 2–10.
5. Gilroy RJ, Mangura BT, Lavietes MH. Ribcage and abdominal volume displacements during breathing in pregnancy. *Am Rev Resp Dis* 1988; **137**: 668–72.
6. Contreras G, Gutiérrez M, Beroiza T *et al.* Ventilatory drive and respiratory muscle function in pregnancy. *Am Rev Respir Dis* 1991; **144**: 837–41.
7. Gupta A, Johnson A, Johansson A, Berg G, Lennmarken C. Maternal respiratory function following normal vaginal delivery. *Int J Obstet Anesth* 1993; **2**: 129–33.
8. Turner AF. The chest radiograph in pregnancy. *Clin Obstet Gynecol* 1975; **18**: 65–74.
9. Cugell DW, Frank NR, Gaensler EA *et al.* Pulmonary function in pregnancy, 1: serial observations in normal women. *Am Rev Tuberc* 1953; **67**: 568–97.
10. Eng M, Butler J, Bonica JJ. Respiratory function in pregnant obese women. *Am J Obstet Gynecol* 1975; **123**: 241–5.
11. Knuttgen HG, Emerson K. Physiological response to pregnancy at rest and during exercise. *J Appl Physiol* 1974; **36**: 549–53.
12. Pernoll ML, Metcalfe J, Kovach PA, Watchel R, Dunham MJ. Ventilation during rest and exercise in pregnancy and postpartum. *Resp Physiol* 1975; **25**: 295–310.
13. Bevan DR, Holdcroft A, Loh L *et al.* Closing volume and pregnancy. *Br Med J* 1974; **i**: 13–15.
14. Milne JA, Mills RJ, Howie AD, Pack AI. Large airways function during normal pregnancy. *Br J Obstet Gynaecol* 1977; **84**: 448–51.
15. Sims CD, Chamberlain GVP, De Sweit M. Lung function tests in bronchial asthma during and after pregnancy. *Br J Obstet Gynaecol* 1976; **83**: 434–7.
16. Gee JBL, Packer BS, Millen JE, Robin ED. Pulmonary mechanics during pregnancy. *J Clin Invest* 1967; **46**: 945–52.
17. Farman JV, Thorpe ME. Compliance changes during Caesarean section. *Br J Anaesth* 1969; **41**: 999–1001.
18. Elkus R, Popovich J. Respiratory physiology in pregnancy. *Clin Chest Med* 1992; **13**: 555–65.
19. Templeton A, Kelman GR. Maternal blood gases, (P_{AO_2}–Pa_{O_2}), physiological shunt and V_D/V_T in normal pregnancy. *Br J Anaesth* 1976; **48**: 1001–4.
20. Awe RJ, Nicotra MB, Newson TD, Viles R. Arterial oxygenation and alveolar–arterial gradients in term pregnancy. *Obstet Gynecol* 1979; **53**: 182–5.
21. Alaily AB, Carrol KB. Pulmonary ventilation in pregnancy. *Br J Obstet Gynaecol* 1978; **85**: 518–24.
22. Prowse CM, Gaenster EA. Respiratory and acid–base changes during pregnancy. *Anesthesiology* 1965; **26**: 381–92.
23. Edwards MJ, Metcalfe J, Dunham MJ, Paul MS. Accelerated respiratory response to moderate exercise in late pregnancy. *Respir Physiol* 1981; **45**: 229–41.

24 Cope DK, Gimbert F, Downey JM, Taylor AE. Pulmonary capillary pressure: a review. *Crit Care Med* 1992; **20**: 1043–56.
25 Reid DHS. Respiratory changes in labour. *Lancet* 1966; **i**: 784–5.
26 Novy MJ, Edwards MJ. Respiratory problems in pregnancy. *Am J Obstet Gynecol* 1967; **99**: 1024–45.
27 Sangoul F, Fox GS, Houle GL. Effect of regional anesthesia on maternal oxygen consumption during the first stage of labor. *Am J Obstet Gynecol* 1975; **121**: 1080–3.
28 Moya F, Morishima HO, Shnider SM, James LS. Influence of maternal hyperventilation on the newborn infant. *Am J Obstet Gynecol* 1965; **90**: 76–84.
29 Huch R. Maternal hyperventilation and the fetus. *J Perinat Med* 1986; **14**: 3–17.
30 Griffin RP, Reynolds F. Maternal hypoxaemia during labour and delivery: the influence of analgesia and effect on neonatal outcome. *Anaesthesia* 1995; **50**: 151–6.
31 Fisher A, Prys-Roberts C. Maternal pulmonary gas exchange: a study during normal labour and extradural blockade. *Anaesthesia* 1968; **23**: 350–6.
32 Das TK, Moutquin JM, Parent JG. Effect of cigarette smoking on maternal airway function during pregnancy. *Am J Obstet Gynecol* 1991; **165**: 675–9.
33 Werler MM, Pober BR, Holmes LB. Smoking and pregnancy. *Teratology* 1985; **32**: 473–81.
34 Yannone ME, McCurdy JR, Coldfien A. Plasma progesterone levels in normal pregnancy, labor and the puerperium. *Am J Obstet Gynecol* 1988; **101**: 1058–61.
35 Bourne T, Ogilvy AJ, Vickers R. Nocturnal hypoxaemia in late pregnancy. *Br J Anaesth* 1995; **75**: 678–82.
36 Feinsilver SH, Hertz G. Respiration during sleep in pregnancy. *Clin Chest Med* 1992; **13**: 637–44.
37 Conti M, Izzo W, Muggiasca ML, Tiengo M. Sleep apnoea syndrome in pregnancy: a case report. *Eur J Anesthesiol* 1988; **5**: 151–4.
38 Barron WM, Leff AR. Asthma in pregnancy. *Am Rev Resp Dis* 1993; **147**: 510–11.
39 Clark SL, National Asthma Education Program Working Group on Asthma and Pregnancy, National Institutes of Health, National Heart, Lung and Blood Institute. Asthma in pregnancy. *Obstet Gynecol* 1993; **82**: 1036–40.
40 Doucette JT, Bracken MB. Possible role of asthma in the risk of premature labour and delivery. *Epidemiology* 1993; **4**: 143–50.
41 Gal TJ. Bronchial hyperresponsiveness and anesthesia: physiologic and therapeutic perspectives. *Anesth Analg* 1994; **78**: 559–73.
42 Juniper EF, Daniel EE, Roberts RS *et al.* Improvement in airway responsiveness and asthma severity during pregnancy: a prospective study. *Am Rev Respir Dis* 1989; **140**: 924–31.
43 Du Bois RM. Respiratory medicine. *Br Med J* 1995; **310**: 1594–7.
44 Sherman CB, Tollerud DJ, Heffner LJ, Speizer FE, Weiss ST. Airway responsiveness in young black and white women. *Am Rev Respir Dis* 1993; **148**: 98–102.
45 Mettam IM, Reddy TR, Evans FE. Life-threatening acute respiratory distress in late pregnancy. *Br J Anaesthesia* 1992; **69**: 420–1.
46 Sheffer AL. Guidelines for the diagnosis and management of asthma (National Heart, Lung and Blood Institute, National Asthma Education Programme Expert Panel report). *J Allergy Clin Immunol* 1991; **88**: 425–534.
47 Hernandez E, Angell CS, Johnson JWG. Asthma in pregnancy: current concepts. *Obstet Gynecol* 1980; **55**: 739–43.
48 Woodhead M. Guidelines on the management of asthma, 1992. *Thorax* 1993; **48**: 51–4.
49 Schatz M. Asthma during pregnancy: interrelationships and management. *Ann Allergy* 1992; **68**: 123–33.
50 Greenberger PA. Asthma in pregnancy. *Clin Chest Med* 1992; **13**: 597–605.

51 Gruteke P, Askari A, Chatterjee TK, Chopra MP, Nwokolo F. Artificial ventilatory management in a severe, pregnant asthmatic: a case report. *Br J Clin Pract* 1992; **46**: 63–4.

52 Raphael JH, Bexton MD. Combined high frequency ventilation in the management of respiratory failure in late pregnancy. *Anaesthesia* 1993; **48**: 596–8.

53 Nelson HS. Worsening asthma: is reflux oesophagitis to blame? *J Rev Resp Dis* 1990; **11**: 827–44.

54 Koga Y, Iwatsuki N, Hashimoto Y. Direct effects of H_2-receptor antagonists on airway smooth muscle and on responses mediated by H_1- and H_2-receptors. *Anesthesiology* 1987; **66**: 181–5.

55 Hirshman CA, Edelstein G, Peetz S, Wayne R, Downes H. Mechanisms of action of inhalation anesthesia on airways. *Anesthesiology* 1982; **57**: 107–11.

56 Hirshman CA, Downes H, Barood A, Bergman NA. Ketamine block of bronchospasm in experimental canine asthma. *Br J Anaesth* 1979; **51**: 713–18.

57 Hirshman CA, Krieger W, Littlejohn G, Lee R, Julien R. Ketamine–aminophylline-induced decrease in seizure threshold. *Anesthesiology* 1982; **56**: 464–7.

58 Freund FG, Bonica JJ, Ward RJ, Akametsu TJ, Kennedy WF. Ventilatory reserve and level of motor block during high spinal and epidural anaesthesia. *Anesthesiology* 1967; **28**: 834–7.

59 Fuchs HL, Borowitz DS, Christiansen DH *et al.* Effect of aerolysed recombinant human DNase on exacerbations of respiratory symptoms and on pulmonary function in patients with cystic fibrosis (Pulmozyme Study Group). *N Engl J Med* 1994; **331**: 637–42.

60 Cohen LF, di Sant' Agnese PA, Friedlander J. Cystic fibrosis and pregnancy: a national survey. *Lancet* 1980; **ii**: 842–4.

61 Colten HR. Airway inflammation in cystic fibrosis. *N Engl J Med* 1995; **332**: 886–7.

62 Kotloff RM, FitzSimmons SC, Fiel SB. Fertility and pregnancy in patients with cystic fibrosis. *Clin Chest Med* 1992; **13**: 623–35.

63 Edenborough FP, Stableforth DE, Webb AK, MacKenzie WE, Smith DL. Outcome of pregnancy in women with cystic fibrosis. *Thorax* 1995; **50**: 170–4.

64 Edenborough FP, Stableforth DE, MacKenzie WE. Pregnancy in women with cystic fibrosis: outcomes for mother and baby have much improved. *Br Med J* 1995; **311**: 822–3.

65 Webb AK, David TJ. Clinical management of children and adults with cystic fibrosis. *Br Med J* 1994; **308**: 459–62.

66 Butler JA, Esmond GM, Mickelsons C, Empey DW, Restrick LJ. Pregnancy assisted by nasal intermittent positive pressure ventilation in a patient with cystic fibrosis. *J R Soc Med* 1997; **90**: 220–3.

67 Bose D, Yentis SM, Fauvel NJ. Caesarean section in a parturient with respiratory failure caused by cystic fibrosis. *Anaesthesia* 1997; **52**: 576–85.

68 Department of Health. *Report on Confidential Enquiries into Maternal Deaths in the United Kingdom, 1988–1990.* London: HMSO, 1994.

69 Collop NA, Sahn SA. Critical illness in pregnancy: an analysis of 20 patients admitted to a medical intensive care unit. *Chest* 1993; **103**: 1548–52.

70 Ng TI, Lim E, Tweed WA, Arulkumaran S. Obstetric admissions to the intensive care unit: a retrospective review. *Ann Acad Med* 1992; **21**: 804–6.

71 Stephens ID. ICU admissions from an obstetrical hospital. *Can J Anaesth* 1991; **38**: 677–81.

72 Karson EM, Saltzman D, Davis MR. Pneumomediastinum in pregnancy: two case reports and a review of the literature, pathophysiology and management. *Obstet Gynecol* 1984; **64**: 39S.

73 Bernard GR, Artigas A, Brigham KL *et al.* The Consensus Committee Report of the American–European Consensus Conference on ARDS: definitions, mechanisms, relevant outcomes and clinical trial co-ordination. *Intensive Care Med* 1994; **20**: 225–32.

74 Hollingsworth HM, Irwin RS. Acute respiratory failure in pregnancy. *Clin Chest Med* 1992; **13**: 723–40.
75 Nolan TE, Wakefield ML, Devoe LD. Intensive hemodynamic monitoring in obstetrics: a critical review of its indications, benefits, complications and alternatives. *Chest* 1992; **101**: 1429–33.
76 Kewandowski K, Falke KJ. Acute respiratory distress syndrome. *Baillière's Clin Anaesthesiol* 1996; **10**: 181–214.
77 Pingelton SK. Complications of acute respiratory failure. *Am Rev Resp Dis* 1988; **137**: 1463–96.
78 Glauser FL, Polatty RC, Sessler CN. Worsening oxygenation in the mechanically ventilated patients: causes, mechanisms and early detection. *Am Rev Resp Dis* 1988; **138**: 458–65.
79 Gattinoni L, Pesenti A, Bombino M *et al.* Relationships between lung computed tomographic density, gas exchange, and PEEP in acute respiratory failure. *Anesthesiology* 1988; **69**: 824–32.
80 Allen SJ, Drake RE, Williams JP, Laine GA, Gabel JC. Recent advances in pulmonary edema. *Crit Care Med* 1987; **15**: 963–70.
81 Bersten AD, Holt AW, Vedig AF, Skowronski GA, Baggoley CJ. Treatment of severe cardiogenic pulmonary edema with continuous positive airway pressure delivered by face mask. *N Engl J Med* 1991; **325**: 1825–30.
82 Mabie WC, Hackmann BB, Sibai BM. Pulmonary edema associated with pregnancy: echocardiographic insights and implications for treatment. *Obstet Gynecol* 1993; **81**: 227–34.

5: Gastrointestinal System

Changes occur throughout the gastrointestinal tract during pregnancy. The alterations in gastric motility and secretions, together with changes in the oesophagus and gastro-oesophageal junction, are of principal interest to the anaesthetist because they increase the incidence of reflux of gastric acid into the oesophagus and regurgitation of acid subsequently in the pharynx, with the attendant risk of pulmonary aspiration.

The perioperative risk of aspiration of gastric contents is not restricted to the pregnant woman. It is, potentially, a problem in any patient with a full stomach who becomes, or is rendered, unconscious. However, the pregnancy-related changes of gastric and lower oesophageal sphincter function increase the risk, especially during labour.

5.1 Gastric function

Gastrointestinal motility in the non-pregnant individual is a complex, cyclical activity. In the fasting state, the stomach exhibits a cycle of activity in three phases: a quiescent period, a period of irregular contractions and short periods of intense contractions [1,2]. The rhythm of activity of the fasting stomach may follow a slow undulation of the activity of the sodium–potassium pump in smooth muscle membranes. The slow waves of electrical change that make up this basic rhythm do not in themselves cause muscle contractions. Contractions are dependent on spike potentials developing in the resting membrane of the smooth muscle of the gut. The spike potentials seem to appear when the peaks of the slow waves rise above −40 mV. These action potentials are produced by a rapid influx of calcium ions into the gastrointestinal smooth muscle cells via calcium–sodium channels. These channels have a very slow response time, being much slower to open and close than the rapid sodium channels that are responsible for action potentials in nerve cells. The slow opening and closing of these channels allows the movement of large amounts of calcium ions into the interior muscle fibres, and this build-up of calcium is important during contraction of intestinal smooth muscle. Motility within the gastrointestinal tract is largely dependent on internal reflexes, which are controlled by the myenteric neuronal plexus and a number of hormones. Most of the hormones that affect the motility of parts of the gastrointestinal tract also control gastrointestinal secretion. Cholecystokinin is secreted by the mucosa of the jejunum when fatty substances are present in the jejunal lumen. It inhibits gastric motility and slows the emptying of food from the stomach. Secretin is secreted by the mucosa of the duodenum in response to acid entering the duodenal lumen. It also has an inhibitory effect on the motility of most of the gastrointestinal tract. Gastric inhibitory peptide is secreted by the mucosa of the small intestine. Secretion of this peptide is stimulated by the presence of fats and carbohydrates, and it has a depressant effect on the motor activity of the stomach. During pregnancy, hormonal changes in oestrogens and progestogens, together with a reduction in circulating motilin, alter both the patterns of motility and secretion of acid by the stomach.

Ingestion of small volumes of water does not seem to disturb or change the sequence of contractions, so the rate of passage of the fluids through the stomach will be largely dependent on the phase of motility existing at the moment of ingestion. Large volumes of fluid are processed differently. Ingestion of a large volume of liquid will convert the existing pattern of fasting gastric motility into a more active phase, so gastric emptying rates increase as the volume of ingested fluid increases. The nature of the ingested material is also of significance. The underlying physiological control of gastric activity seems to be aimed at achieving a rate of stomach emptying that is regulated in order to deliver calories to the duodenum at a constant rate. The greater the energy density of the food ingested and the larger the energy content of the duodenum, the slower will be the rate of gastric emptying. Food characteristics that slow gastric emptying are high osmolarity, high fat content and acidity [3–5]. In contrast, the presence of partially digested protein or other secretagogues seems to increase gastric motility and the rate of emptying of the stomach.

5.2 Gastric motility during parturition

A hypomotile state exists in pregnancy and especially labour, and has been confirmed by a number of investigations. The variability during parturition of the onset and degree of decreased gastric emptying rates is still not clear. What is clear is that the onset of labour impairs gastric emptying significantly, and the administration of epidural opioids—even in very dilute concentrations via the epidural space [6]—will further decrease the emptying rate. Most anaesthetists recognize the dangers of aspiration of stomach content and have worked to reduce them. The danger is now less obvious, but still remains. However, midwifery pressure groups in particular are now advocating a more permissive attitude towards eating in labour.

In the 1950s, radiological studies of gastric emptying were performed using barium meals taken during labour [7,8]. Both studies showed that gastric emptying was much reduced during labour and, as expected from the results in non-pregnant patients, the administration of pethidine caused retention of up to 20% of the test meal for at least five hours. Several methods have been used to study gastric emptying rates in pregnancy: radiology, paracetamol absorption, ultrasound and scintigraphic assessments.

The use of radiographic investigations is now ethically unacceptable, and more recent methods of assessment include paracetamol absorption and ultrasound scanning. Paracetamol absorption as a measure of gastric emptying, acceptable for fluids, may not be as reliable when the transit time of solid material is measured [9,10]. Presumably, liquids will carry paracetamol from the stomach into the duodenum easily, while solid material is retained in the stomach for further processing. These limitations of the paracetamol absorption method must be taken into account when interpreting the findings that pregnancy is associated with a delay in gastric emptying that begins at 12 weeks [11]. Paracetamol absorption may be more reliable when used to compare two groups of patients who are differentiated by a single variable. Such studies have shown that the administration of opioids during labour, either systemically or via the epidural space, delays gastric emptying [6,12,13].

More recently, ultrasound scanning techniques have compared gastric emptying rates in healthy volunteers, parturients at term but not in labour, and parturients in active labour [14]. Gastric emptying was complete by four hours after a standardized meal in both non-pregnant and pregnant volunteers. However, during labour, food was present in the stomach for many hours after ingestion. Two-thirds of women in labour who had eaten solids at any time from eight to 24 hours previously had detectable residual food in their stomachs. These ultrasound findings were consistent with vomitus produced by four patients following their ultrasound examination, and with gastric contents aspirated via a large-bore gastric tube in three patients undergoing Caesarean delivery under general anaesthesia. Similar results were obtained in another study [15] using ultrasound assessment of the stomach and comparing parturients in labour who had been allowed a light, standardized low-fat diet with those allowed only water by mouth. Those women who were allowed to eat had significantly greater gastric antral cross-sectional areas, were more likely to vomit, and when they did produced significantly greater volumes of vomitus. Eating, during or within four hours of the onset of labour, will therefore increase the volume of gastric contents for many hours. These findings confirm the earlier work of Roberts and Shirley [16] and indicate that eating in labour is an unsafe practice, which increases the risk of aspiration during anaesthesia [15].

There are categories of women in whom restrictions of fluid may also be necessary. These are women with severe pre-eclampsia, those whose fetus has significant cardiotocographic abnormalities and those in whom there is a high risk for instrumental delivery. It is the recommendation of the *Report on Confidential Enquiries into Maternal Deaths in the UK, 1988–1990* [17] that 'H_2-receptor blocking drugs should be administered to all patients who may require anaesthesia and to patients with pre-eclampsia.' This encompasses a substantial number of at-risk women, as listed in Table 5.1.

There have been few studies of the postpartum period, and they have reported rather conflicting results. Recently, a delay in postpartum gastric

Table 5.1 High-risk pregnancies.

Any hypertensive disorder
Diabetes
Gestation < 36 weeks
Intrauterine growth retardation
Oligohydramnios
Meconium
Abnormal admission cardiotocogram
Antepartum haemorrhage
Multiple pregnancy
Breech
Oxytocin infusion
Previous Caesarean section
Any other case identified as high risk by the medical staff on admission

emptying has been reported during the first two hours postpartum, but not beyond 18 hours after delivery [18].

After normal delivery, a recent preliminary study using scintigraphic and ultrasound assessment showed that the rate of gastric emptying for solids returned to normal within 18 hours after delivery [19]. It would seem, therefore, that gastric emptying returns to normal by 24 hours after delivery in most parturients. Again, it must be assumed if systemic or spinal opioids are used that gastric emptying will be delayed, and suitable antacid preparations should be made for anaesthesia in the puerperium.

5.3 Gastric secretions

Studies of the effects of pregnancy on gastric secretion indicate that the rate of gastric secretion is reduced during pregnancy. Measurements have been made following stimuli such as histamine stimulation, saline test meals and water test meals. The reduction seems to be greatest in the first and second trimester [20]. Peptic ulceration is rare in pregnancy, and remission of symptoms in proven peptic ulcer sufferers has been reported [21]; but whether this indicates reduced gastric secretory activity in the stomach or increased secretion of gastric mucus [22] is not known.

There is now general agreement that gastric secretion returns to normal or slightly above normal in the third trimester. The combination of normal or increased secretory function, reduced motility, and an incompetent lower oesophageal sphincter produces, in the third trimester, a woman who is at high risk of having a large intragastric volume of acid material which is easily refluxed and, given the right circumstances, regurgitated and aspirated. The secretory function returns to normal in the postpartum period, but exactly when this occurs probably varies from individual to individual.

5.4 Oesophageal sphincters

Pregnancy affects the two oesophageal sphincters—the lower oesophageal sphincter (LOS) and the upper (UOS). The upper sphincter prevents regurgitation of gastric contents from the oesophagus into the pharynx. Regurgitation of acid into the pharynx is recognized as the symptom of 'water brash', which is also common in patients with hiatus hernia. The LOS is responsible for preventing the reflux of gastric contents from the stomach into the oesophagus, and neuronal control is mediated via the vagus nerve. Gastric reflux passing through the LOS into the oesophagus may cause symptoms of retrosternal burning pain or 'heartburn', which is common in pregnancy. However, oesophageal reflux can occur without symptoms [23–25].

Intra-abdominal pressure changes across the LOS in the awake subject—for example, during a Valsalva manoeuvre or when adopting the lithotomy position—seem to produce only few episodes of reflux [23]. Reflux can occur following brief episodes of relaxation of the LOS. The phenomenon is referred to as 'spike refluxing', and is probably a normal physiological event. Spikes are neuronally mediated and may be due to gastric distension [26]. Reflux spikes are usually followed by a brief period of secondary oesophageal peristalsis, which removes acid from the lower oesophagus.

The high incidence of reflux during pregnancy probably occurs because of high concentrations of plasma progesterone. Oral contraceptives containing progesterone have been shown to reduce the lower oesophageal sphincter pressure [26]. Whether the progesterone affects the muscle of the LOS or its neuronal control seems to be unclear. Vagal blockade, as well as general anaesthesia, will affect control of the LOS [27]. Once general anaesthesia is established, any increase in the pressure gradient across the sphincter (such as might occur during hiccup or straining during induction of anaesthesia) can be associated with episodes of reflux [28]. When this occurs, the gastric contents will remain in the oesophagus, so that with subsequent relaxation of the upper oesophageal sphincter (UOS) regurgitation can result. These mechanisms are discussed and illustrated in the section on general anaesthesia (Chapter 16).

The UOS consists of the cricopharyngeus muscle and the posterior aspect of the cricoid cartilage. The cricopharyngeus is inserted into the lateral aspects of the cricoid cartilage, so that it acts as a posterior sling around the oesophagus. Contraction of the muscle obliterates the lumen of the oesophagus by pressure against the posterior aspect of the cricoid cartilage. The cricopharyngeus muscle is under both voluntary and involuntary control, and produces sphincteric pressures that vary markedly. Pressures as high as 40 mmHg have been measured in awake subjects [29,30]. During deep sleep, the pressure may decrease to 8 mmHg. The UOS performs the important role of preventing refluxed gastric content from being regurgitated into the pharynx, and it continues to do so during light general anaesthesia when no muscle relaxant has been used [28]. The importance of the UOS in parturients who are about to undergo, or are recovering from, general anaesthesia is therefore considerable. Clinically, it is wise to assume that any parturient presenting for anaesthesia will be suffering from oesophageal reflux, whether or not she has symptoms and whether or not she has fasted. General anaesthesia, or loss of consciousness from whatever cause, will remove the UOS barrier. Prophylactic measures that will reduce the risk of acid gastric content being regurgitated and aspirated should therefore be instituted in all high-risk parturients. H_2-receptor blocking drugs, non-particulate antacids and metoclopramide should be used. Cricoid pressure and rapid-sequence induction with intubation of the trachea are the combined methods of choice for general anaesthesia in the antenatal and peripartum period, and the antacids and H_2-receptor blockers are an essential form of prophylaxis before regional anaesthesia.

5.5 Aspiration prophylaxis

Acid aspiration pneumonitis developing in the pregnant patient is referred to as Mendelson's syndrome. It was first described by Hall in 1940 [31] and in 1946 by Mendelson [32]. In the United Kingdom, its contribution to maternal mortality has been recorded in the triennial reports on *Confidential Enquiries into Maternal Deaths* since the reports began in 1952. In spite of an improvement in our understanding of pregnancy-related changes in gastrointestinal function and strenuous attempts to control the acidity and volume of gastric secretions and their regurgitation into the laryngopharynx, aspiration deaths still occur. In the reports for the period 1988 to 1993 [33,34], four anaesthesia related deaths were caused by aspiration of gastric contents. A further 10 deaths in 1988–90 and an unspecified number in 1991–93 from acute respiratory distress syndrome (ARDS) occurred as a complication of aspiration of gastric contents. The risk of regurgitation and aspiration and the development of chemical pneumonitis will always be greater during pregnancy; for the anaesthetist, obstetrician and midwife, this should be an ever-present concern, and precautions should be taken to avoid it.

Regimens that are widely used to prevent acid aspiration are summarized in Table 5.2.

5.5.1 Antacids

In 1970, 20 years after deaths from acid aspiration began to be recorded, Crawford advocated that antacids should be administered at two-hourly intervals during labour, with a further dose before anaesthesia was induced [35]. Initially, magnesium trisilicate, a particulate antacid, was used routinely in many units, in spite of the fact that non-particulate alternatives had been suggested as early as 1973 [36]. Eventually, in 1980, the poor mixing characteristics of particulate antacids were demonstrated [37]. A year earlier, Gibbs

Table 5.2 Aspiration prophylaxis (Timings are shown in italics).

Drugs used for reduction of gastric acidity and volume of gastric contents
    Antacids, e.g. sodium citrate 30 mL (0.3 M) *less than 30 min before induction*
    Prokinetic drugs, e.g. metoclopramide 10 mg i.v. *before induction or orally 2 h preoperatively*
        (cisapride has no parenteral preparation)
    Direct inhibition of gastric secretion
    —H_2-receptor antagonists, e.g. ranitidine *150 mg orally the evening before and 2 h prior to surgery (i.m. not less than 50 mg 30 min before general anaesthesia)*
    —Proton-pump inhibitors, e.g. omeprazole *orally the evening before and 2 h prior to surgery (not cost-effective)*

Physical methods
    Wide-bore oral tube after a meal *prior to induction*
    Orogastric tube (the nasal mucosa is congested—bleeding may occur) *during anaesthesia, prior to extubation*

Rapid-sequence induction (preoxygenation, cricoid pressure, cuffed endotracheal tube, (trained assistant)

Others
    Suction apparatus
        Wide-bore oropharyngeal sucker; *check prior to induction*
        Negative pressure of −400 mmHg
    Tipping table (head-down if necessary)
    Magill forceps

Postoperatively
    Full muscle tone, adequate ventilation, no airway obstruction
    Position lateral for extubation
    Avoid central nervous system depression

and colleagues had reported that the aspiration of particulate antacids was potentially as damaging as the aspiration of acid solutions [38]. In consequence, 30 mL of sodium citrate 0.3 mol/L recommended by Lahiri *et al.* [36] has become the antacid of choice for the neutralization of residual gastric acidity in the labouring parturient. A number of studies [39–41] have confirmed that sodium citrate mixes rapidly with gastric contents and has a duration of action of approximately 30 minutes, depending on any delay in gastric emptying. However, the efficacy of any antacid is variable, so the use of oral antacids alone is not a reliable method of maintaining an intragastric pH above 3, which is required to prevent chemical pneumonitis. Furthermore, intermittent two-hourly administration of any solution will increase gastric volumes. This is not a desirable outcome. A combination of an H_2-receptor blocker two hours prior to surgery with sodium citrate immediately before induction of anaesthesia is the minimum prophylaxis to prevent acid aspiration. Prophylaxis for extubation, with nasogastric suction and administration of sodium citrate, should be considered if optimal preoperative preparation has not been given.

5.5.2 Reducing gastric secretion

H₂-receptor blocking drugs

The H$_2$-receptor blockers act by inhibiting the effects of the gastrin/acetylcholine stimulus on the H$_2$ receptors of gastric parietal cells, and thereby reducing hydrogen ion output. Both of the commonly available drugs, cimetidine and ranitidine, have been used in parturients [42,43]. Although both drugs are effective in reducing gastric acidity, they cannot influence acid that is already present in the stomach prior to administration, which must be neutralized by a non-particulate antacid. Both H$_2$ blockers, but cimetidine in particular, can cause cardiovascular disturbances with intravenous injection, so only ranitidine can be given by this route, albeit by slow injection. Cimetidine, followed by 30 mL sodium citrate 0.3 molar shortly before induction of anaesthesia was reported to be effective in all of 100 patients studied [44]. The drug must be given as a dose of 200 mg intramuscularly at the time of the decision to undertake Caesarean section. Ranitidine should be given in doses of 150 mg orally or 50 mg intramuscularly or intravenously. The combination of ranitidine and sodium citrate can reduce the gastric volume and pH to clinically acceptable levels [45]. In a randomized double-blind study [46] of 595 women undergoing emergency Caesarean section, 30 mL of sodium citrate 0.3 molar was administered with either intravenous saline as a control or intravenous ranitidine 50 mg. The combination of ranitidine and sodium citrate prevented the risk of acid aspiration syndrome (defined as pH less than 3.5 and volume greater than 25 mL) in all 595 parturients at induction, and reduced the aspiration risk to a very small percentage (0.3%) in gastric samples drawn immediately prior to extubation. The citrate and intravenous saline group had a 3.2% incidence of acid gastric contents at intubation and a 5.6% incidence in samples drawn prior to extubation. The ranitidine in this study was given more than 30 minutes before induction of anaesthesia in order to achieve this effect. It is quite obvious that the differences in the times of onset of action and duration of action of ranitidine and sodium citrate make timing of administration of paramount importance. When used intravenously, the H$_2$-receptor blocker must be given at least 30 minutes prior to induction of anaesthesia, and when used orally it must be given at least two hours before induction. Sodium citrate, on the other hand, has an almost immediate buffering effect on gastric contents, and should be given no more than 20 minutes before induction of anaesthesia. Of the two H$_2$-receptor blocking drugs, ranitidine has the longer half-life, and has less inhibitory side effects on the cytochrome P450 system. The longer duration of action makes ranitidine the drug of choice, because its effect on gastric secretion has the potential to last into the recovery period. It should be used in combination with sodium citrate for all patients undergoing elective and emergency Caesarean section, no matter whether they are receiving a general anaesthetic or a regional technique. Ranitidine should also be used in all high-risk parturients during labour, and especially in moderate and severe pre-eclampsia, when the parturient is at increased risk of receiving one or other form of anaesthesia and also of losing consciousness during an eclamptic fit. During the last decade, the combined use of ranitidine/sodium citrate has become widespread, and it is likely that the number of general anaesthetics given to parturients has declined by no more than 10%. It is salutary to note that since 1984, there have been no aspiration maternal deaths in the United Kingdom in which a properly timed combined H_2-blocker/non-particulate antacid prophylactic regimen was given.

Proton-pump inhibitors

Omeprazole decreases gastric acid secretion by inhibiting H^+/K^+ ATPase, effectively the proton pump of the gastric parietal cell. Omeprazole requires a prokinetic agent to maximize its effects on gastric acid volume, and is inadequate for prophylaxis as a single dose prior to emergency anaesthesia [47]. It is more expensive than either of the H_2-receptor antagonists described, and is not widely used in parturients.

Prokinetic drugs

Metoclopramide increases lower oesophageal barrier tone, reverses delayed gastric emptying and decreases the risk of oesophageal reflux [48]. Intravenous, but not intramuscular, metoclopramide antagonizes the delay in gastric emptying caused by morphine premedication in elective surgery patients [49]. Intravenous metoclopramide given to mothers who had received 50 mg of pethidine has also been shown to increase gastric emptying rates [50]. Metoclopramide 10 mg can be used orally or intravenously in combination with the H_2-receptor blockers and antacids. The drug helps to empty the stomach of acid gastric contents at the time of its administration. When its administration is followed by ranitidine and sodium citrate, their effects are enhanced in the presence of lower gastric volumes. In addition, but rather more slowly, metoclopramide can increase the tone or barrier pressure of the lower oesophageal sphincter [51].

Physical methods

In some circumstances, prophylaxis with the agents discussed above may be considered inappropriate or inadequate, and physical emptying of the stomach may be felt necessary. It is possible, though unpleasant for the parturient, to pass a wide-bore orogastric tube, for instance, to remove a recently ingested and substantial meal as far as possible. The emetic effect of passing the wide-bore tube is probably as great as the subsequent aspiration of stomach contents via the tube. Thankfully, the combination of an urgent need for anaesthesia and surgery in the face of recent ingestion of a full meal will be rare. If physical stomach emptying is needed, it should be remembered that nasogastric tubes are usually ineffective and too small for the removal of solid gastric contents. If the feasibility of physical emptying is doubted, it should be remembered that the method is used effectively in other countries—for example, prior to 44% of emergency Caesarean sections in Norway [52].

Prevention of aspiration of gastric contents postoperatively may also include drainage of the stomach through an orogastric tube passed and aspirated during anaesthesia [53]. This helps to prevent postpartum aspiration of stomach contents.

Anticholinergics

Anticholinergics such as atropine, glycopyrrolate and hyoscine decrease the secretion of gastric acid by blocking the vagally mediated acetylcholine stimulus to the oxyntic glands. Their use in the control of gastric secretions in the parturient is limited, however, because atropine reduces the barrier pressure of the lower oesophageal sphincter and is therefore likely to increase the severity of gastro-oesophageal reflux. It is only now used for its cardiovascular effects in the reversing of any pronounced bradycardia resulting from anaesthetic procedures or surgical traction on viscera.

5.6 Management of aspiration

Mendelson's report of the problem of acid aspiration and the subsequent development of pneumonitis appeared before intermittent positive-pressure ventilation became an integral part of general anaesthesia for parturients. None of Mendelson's patients died from their acid aspiration pneumonitis. Fatalities occurred because of asphyxia due to solid food material lodging in the upper airways. We can but speculate that Mendelson's patients developed a less severe form of aspiration pneumonitis than the one we see today. This difference in severity may have been due to a difference in the spread of the gastric content within the lung. It is quite possible that intermittent positive-pressure ventilation (IPPV) is responsible for widespread dissemination of any tracheal pollutant. This possibility will govern the anaesthetist's first response to any visible signs of tracheal aspiration. Any sign of tracheal soiling, or even profuse pharyngeal secretions, should be dealt with by thorough tracheal and pharyngeal suction once the endotracheal tube is in place and before the institution of IPPV. The immediate suctioning of the upper airway should be followed by gentle IPPV using an inflation pressure and tidal volumes that are as low as is consistent with good patient oxygenation. Fibre-optic bronchoscopy and suction should be carried out as soon as possible in order to identify and remove any remaining debris or foreign material. Lavage of the airways is not recommended, because it seems only to disseminate further the effects of the original aspiration. Symptomatic treatment with bronchodilators and increased inspired oxygen fraction will usually be required. The pH of any suctioned material, whether from the airways or the pharynx, should be measured. If material from the airways is shown to have a low pH, aspiration of gastric contents must be assumed to have occurred. Early postoperative transfer of the patient to an intensive-care unit should take place before the development of the more florid changes, which, once present, will make transfer difficult.

Even when aspiration is not suspected, the unexplained onset of clinical signs such as wheezing and decreased oxygen saturation should alert the anaesthetist to the possibility of aspiration.

These signs may appear during the anaesthetic or shortly thereafter. The patient should not be returned to the postnatal ward at this time. Instead, she should be kept under close surveillance with continuous pulse oximetry, frequent repeated auscultation of the chest and an early chest radiograph. She should be nursed in a high-dependency unit and referred to an intensive-care unit should her condition deteriorate.

Supplementary oxygen and ventilatory support are usually required if aspiration has occurred. The intensive-care management of these patients is difficult, and can be very protracted. They are likely to develop acute respiratory distress syndrome (ARDS), and because many units use high ventilatory pressures, pneumothorax is not uncommon. If inspired oxygen fractions and airway pressures can be kept to modest levels, the patients will do better. It is possible that alternative types of cuirass or negative-pressure rapid-frequency style ventilators may benefit these parturients, but experience is too small to do more than speculate about this at present.

5.7 Gastrointestinal symptoms

5.7.1 Nausea and vomiting

Nausea is a common symptom in early pregnancy. It can be associated with vomiting, particularly on rising in the morning. When these symptoms are severe, hyperemesis gravidarum occurs (see Section 7.2.1). Nausea and vomiting frequently complicate first-trimester and second-trimester terminations or miscarriages. A phenothiazine with antihistamine properties, such as prochlorperazine, may be a useful therapy. Nausea and vomiting are also common in labour, and may be associated with the effects of visceral stimulation from the uterus. They can also complicate regional analgesia for Caesarean section, particularly if hypotension is present. The treatment during operative delivery is intravenous atropine with correction of hypotension.

5.7.2 Constipation

Constipation and exacerbation of haemorrhoids are common complications of pregnancy, and persist into the postpartum period. They are particularly distressing after opioid analgesia, and prophylactic laxatives should be prescribed. During labour, pain from prolapsed or thrombosed haemorrhoids can be troublesome. Paradoxically, this pain can become a greater problem once the pain of labour is relieved. During the latter phase of first-stage labour, it can be difficult to distinguish between the perineal pain from haemorrhoids and that due to labour itself. Extending an epidural nerve block to relieve the former is possible, but leads on to greater perineal motor and sensory effects than would be considered desirable. Confirmation of both the stage and the source of the pain is important, and it may be more appropriate to treat haemorrhoid pain with local applications of proprietary preparations.

References

1. Kelly RA. Motility of the stomach and gastroduodenal junction. In: Johnson CR, ed. *Physiology of the Gastrointestinal Tract*. New York: Raven Press, 1981: 393–410.
2. Code CF, Myelet JA. The interdigestive myoelectric complex of the stomach and small bowel of dogs. *J Physiol* 1975; **246**: 289–309.
3. Hunt JN, MacDonald I, Spurrell WR. The gastric response to pectin meals of high osmotic pressure. *J Physiol* 1951; **15**: 185–95.
4. Hunt JN, MacDonald I. The influence of volume on gastric emptying. *J Physiol* 1954; **226**: 459–74.
5. Hunt JN, Knox MT. The slowing of gastric emptying by *nine* acids. *J Physiol* 1969; **201**: 161–79.
6. Wright PMC, Allen RW, Moore J, Donnelly JP. Gastric emptying during lumbar extradural analgesia in labour: effect of fentanyl supplementation. *Br J Anaesth* 1992; **68**: 248–51.
7. La Salvia LA, Steffen EA. Delayed gastric emptying time in labor. *Am J Obstet Gynecol* 1950; **50**: 1075–88.
8. Crawford JS. Some aspects of obstetric anaesthesia. *Br J Anaesth* 1956; **28**: 201–8.
9. Heading RC, Nimm WS, Prescott LF, Tarthill P. The dependence of paracetamol absorption on the rate of gastric emptying. *Br J Pharmacol* 1973; **47**: 415–21.
10. Petring OU, Adelhoj B, Ibsen M, Poulsen HE. The relationship between gastric emptying of semi-solids and paracetamol absorption. *Br J Clin Pharmacol* 1986; **22**: 659–62.
11. Simpson KH, Stakes AF, Miller M. Pregnancy delays paracetamol absorption and gastric emptying in patients undergoing surgery. *Br J Anaesth* 1988; **60**: 24–7.
12. Nimmo WS, Wilson J, Prescott LF. Narcotic analgesics and delayed gastric emptying during labour. *Lancet* 1975; **i**: 890–3.
13. Holdsworth JD. Relationship between stomach contents and analgesia in labour. *Br J Anaesth* 1978; **50**: 1145–8.
14. Carp H, Jayaram A, Stoll M. Ultrasound examination of the stomach contents of parturients. *Anesth Analg* 1992; **74**: 683–7.
15. Scrutton MJL, Metcalfe GA, Lowy C, Seed PT, O'Sullivan G. Eating in labour. A randomized controlled trial assessing the risks and benefits, *Anaesthesia* 1999; **54**: 329–34.

16 Roberts RB, Shirley MA. Reducing the risk of acid aspiration during Cesarean section. *Anesth Analg* 1974; **53**: 859–68.
17 Department of Health. *Report on Confidential Enquiries into Maternal Deaths in the United Kingdom, 1988–1990.* London: HMSO, 1994.
18 Whitehead EM, Smith M, Dean Y, O'Sullivan G. An evaluation of gastric emptying times in pregnancy and the puerperium. *Anaesthesia* 1993; **48**: 53–7.
19 Scrutton M, Holleron D, Page C, O'Doherty O'Sullivan G. Scintigraphic and ultrasound assessment of postpartum gastric emptying of solids, *Int J Obstet Anes* 1997; **6**: 201.
20 Murray FA, Erskine JP, Fielding J. Gastric secretion in pregnancy. *J Obstet Gynaecol Br Emp* 1957; **64**: 373.
21 Clarke DH. Peptic ulcer in women. *Br Med J* 1953; **i**: 1254.
22 Parbhoo SP, Johnston IDA. Effect of oestrogens and progesterone on gastric secretion in patients with duodenal ulcer. *Gut* 1966; **7**: 612–18.
23 Vanner RG, Goodman NW. Gastro-oesophageal reflux in pregnancy at term and after delivery. *Anaesthesia* 1989; **44**: 808–11.
24 Dent J, Dodds WJ, Friedman RH *et al.* Mechanism of gastroesophageal reflex in recumbent asymptomatic human subjects. *J Clin Invest* 1980; **65**: 256–67.
25 Dodds WJ, Dent J, Hogan WJ *et al.* Mechanisms of gastroesophageal reflux in patients with reflux esophagitis. *N Engl J Med* 1982; **307**: 1547–52.
26 Van Thiel DH, Gavaler JS, Strempel J. Lower esophageal sphincter pressure in women using sequential oral contraceptives. *Gastroenterology* 1976; **71**: 232–5.
27 Martin CJ, Patrikios J, Dent J. Abolition of gas reflux and transient lower esophageal sphincter relaxation by vagal blockade in the dog. *Gastroenterology* 1986; **91**: 890–6.
28 Vanner RG. Gastroesophageal reflux and regurgitation during general anaesthesia for termination of pregnancy. *Int J Obstet Anesth* 1992; **1**: 123–8.
29 Davidson GP, Dent J, Willing J. Monitoring of upper oesophageal sphincter pressure in children. *Gut* 1991; **32**: 607–11.
30 Cook IJ, Dent J, Shannon S, Collins SM. Measurement of upper esophageal sphincter pressure: effects of acute emotional stress. *Gastroenterology* 1987; **93**: 526–32.
31 Hall GC. Aspiration pneumonitis as an obstetric hazard. *JAMA* 1940; **114**: 72.
32 Mendelson CL. Aspiration of stomach contents into lungs during obstetric anesthesia. *Am J Obstet Gynecol* 1946; **53**: 191–205.
33 Department of Health. *Report on Confidential Enquiries into Maternal Deaths in the United Kingdom, 1988–1990.* London: HMSO, 1994.
34 Hibberd BM, Department of Health. *Report on Confidential Enquiries into Maternal Deaths in the United Kingdom, 1991–1993.* London: HMSO, 1996.
35 Crawford JS. The anaesthetist's contribution to maternal mortality. *Br J Anaesth* 1970; **42**: 70–3.
36 Lahiri SK, Thomas TA, Hodgson RMH. Single dose antacid therapy for the prevention of Mendelson's syndrome. *Br J Anaesth* 1973; **45**: 1143–6.
37 Holdsworth JD, Johnson K, Mascall G, Gwyn-Roulston R, Tomlinson PA. Mixing of antacids with stomach contents: another approach to the prevention of the acid aspiration (Mendelson's) syndrome. *Anaesthesia* 1980; **35**: 641–50.
38 Gibbs CB, Schwartz DJ, Win JW, Hood CI, Cluck EJ. Antacid pulmonary aspiration in the dog. *Anesthesiology* 1979; **51**: 380–5.
39 O'Sullivan G, Bullingham RES. The assessment of gastric acidity and antacid effect in pregnant women by a non-invasive radiotelemetry technique. *Br J Obstet Gynaecol* 1984; **91**: 973–8.
40 O'Sullivan G, Bullingham RES. Does twice the volume of antacid have twice the effect in pregnant women at term? *Anesth Analg* 1984; **3**: 752–6.
41 O'Sullivan G, Bullingham RES. Non-invasive assessment by radiotelemetry of antacid effect during labor. *Anesth Analg* 1985; **64**: 95–100.

42 Foulkes E, Jenkins LC. A comparative evaluation of cimetidine and sodium citrate to decrease gastric acidity: effectiveness at the time of induction of anaesthesia. *Can Anaesth Soc J* 1981; **28**: 29–32.
43 McAuley DM, Moore J, McCaughey W, Donnelly DB, Dundee JW. Ranitidine as an antacid before elective Caesarean section. *Anaesthesia* 1983; **38**: 108–14.
44 Thorburn J, Moir DD. Antacid therapy for emergency Caesarean section. *Anaesthesia* 1987; **42**: 352–5.
45 Tordoff SG, Sweeney BP. Acid aspiration prophylaxis in 288 obstetric anaesthetic departments in the United Kingdom. *Anaesthesia* 1990; **45**: 776–80.
46 Route CC, Rocke DA, Gouws E. Intravenous ranitidine reduces the risk of aspiration of gastric contents at emergency Cesarean section. *Anesth Analg* 1993; **76**: 156–61.
47 Orr DA, Bill KM, Gillon RW *et al*. Effects of omeprazole, with and without metoclopramide, in elective obstetric anaesthesia. *Anaesthesia* 1993; **48**: 114–19.
48 Cotton BR, Smith G. Single and combined effects of atropine and metoclopramide on the lower oesophageal sphincter pressure. *Br J Anaesth* 1981; **53**: 869–79.
49 McNeill MJ, Ho ET, Kenny GMC. Effect of i.v. metoclopramide on gastric emptying after opioid premedication. *Br J Anaesth* 1990; **64**: 450–2.
50 Murphy DF, Nally B, Gardener J, Unwin A. Effect of metoclopramide on gastric emptying before elective and emergency Caesarean section. *Br J Anaesth* 1983; **56:** 1113–16.
51 Brock-Utne JG, Dow TGB, Welman S, Dimopoulos GE, Moshal MG. The effect of metoclopramide on the lower oesophageal sphincter in late pregnancy. *Anaesth Intensive Care* 1978; **6**: 26–9.
52 Soreide E, Holst-Larssen H, Steen PA. Acid aspiration syndrome prophylaxis in gynaecological and obstetric patients: a Norwegian survey. *Acta Anaesthesiol Scand* 1994; **38**: 863–8.
53 Department of Health. *Report on Confidential Enquiries into Maternal Deaths in England and Wales, 1982–1984.* London: HMSO, 1989.

6: Renal System

6.1 Renal physiology

6.1.1 Changes in pregnancy

Renal physiology changes during pregnancy just as markedly as that of the cardiovascular or respiratory systems, and overlap of systemic effects occurs, so that the pregnant woman is more vulnerable to acidosis and hypoxaemia. Some of the changes are reflected in altered levels of plasma electrolytes, and an understanding of the different, but essentially normal, values will prevent clinical misinterpretation of the pregnant woman's renal function, especially when organ failure occurs. The physiological changes in the kidney often have superimposed on them the effects of pregnancy-related diseases such as pre-eclampsia. Pre-existing disease with renal involvement also complicates pregnancy. Pre-existing hypertension, chronic renal failure, systemic lupus erythematosus and diabetes are the most obvious examples.

6.1.2 Anatomical changes

The kidney becomes larger and heavier by approximately 20% during pregnancy. Glomerular size increases, but not cell numbers [1]. Much of the increase in kidney size seems to be due to increased vascularity, blood volume, blood flow and water content [2,3].

Dilatation of the calyces, renal pelvis and ureter begins early in the first trimester, and is well established in 90% of parturients by the third trimester. Obstruction and hormonal effects probably combine to produce these changes, which are usually more marked on the right side [3]. The smooth muscle of the ureters hypertrophies, and the frequency and force of ureteric contractions increase [4]. Mechanical obstruction seems to occur at the pelvic brim, where the ureter passes through a thick fibrous sheath that effectively prevents dilatation at this point. Errors may occur in any timed urinary collection for biochemical analysis, because urine may be held back within the increased capacity of the dilated urinary tract. The errors can be minimized by placing the patient in a full lateral position for the last hour of the urine collection [5]. In addition, gross dilatation of the ureter and renal pelvis can give rise to an overdistension syndrome. Sufferers may have only mild loin pain, but some experience severe loin and abdominal pain, radiating to the groins [6,7]. When this problem occurs in the peripartum period, the signs can be very misleading and can lead to unnecessary laparotomy and requests for epidural

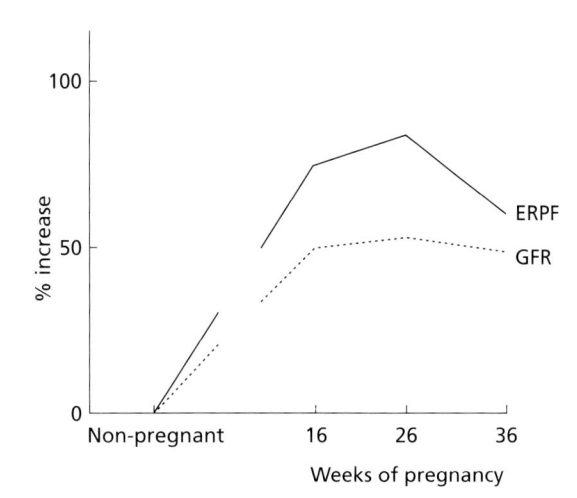

Fig. 6.1 Renal haemodynamic changes during normal pregnancy, showing average values for glomerular filtration rate (GFR) and effective renal plasma flow (ERPF). With permission from [8]

analgesia. Placing the patient in the lateral or knee–chest position may be helpful in this syndrome, but ureteral catheterization, stenting or nephrostomy may be necessary. Ureteral dilatation may continue for up to four months after delivery, and is permanent in approximately 10% of parturients. Urinary stasis can lead to urinary tract infections. The most common organism is *Escherichia coli*, which spreads retrogradely through the dilated system.

6.1.3 Renal blood flow and glomerular filtration rate

There have been conflicting estimates of renal blood flow changes during pregnancy, as there have with many other haemodynamic measurements. Postural and methodological variations have caused some of the differences. The effective renal plasma flow rises by approximately 75% during the first half of pregnancy and then decreases until, at term, it is approximately 50% above non-pregnant values (Fig. 6.1).

The glomerular filtration rate (GFR) is controlled by glomerular plasma flow, glomerular blood pressure, hydrostatic extravascular pressure in Bowman's capsule, the plasma oncotic pressure and the glomerular capillary ultrafiltration coefficient. A 50% increase in GFR mirrors the change in effective renal plasma flow, and is produced by increased intrarenal perfusion and vasodilatation.

Glomerular filtration rate changes can be studied experimentally using inulin clearance, or clinically estimated using creatinine clearance. Inulin clearance increases by 50% in the first trimester of pregnancy, and thereafter remains at that level throughout the second and third trimesters. Creatinine clearance rises by 25% in the first month of pregnancy, and is 45% above pre-pregnant values by nine weeks' gestation [9]. Clearance rates fall thereafter, and reach non-pregnant values by term. They commonly rise slightly for the first few days of the puerperium [10,11]. These normal variations make the diagnosis of renal failure during pregnancy more difficult. A creatinine concentration of 75 mol/L and a urea concentration of 4.5 mmol/L, which are acceptable values in non-pregnant women, are suspect in pregnancy. Serial estimates of creatinine clearance values are needed if reliable assessments are to be made of renal function.

6.1.4 Plasma osmolality and the kidney

Plasma osmolality decreases by approximately 10 mosm/kg H_2O in the first trimester in pregnancy [12], principally because of a reduction in plasma electrolyte and protein concentrations. There is a simultaneous decrease in the osmotic threshold for antidiuretic hormone (arginine vasopressin, AVP) release, so a diuretic response to the established hypo-osmolality is not seen in pregnancy. Thirst is also decreased, and both these effects may be due to circulating human chorionic gonadotropin. Later in pregnancy, the enzyme vasopressinase is secreted by the placenta in large amounts, and at the same time clearance of AVP from the blood increases markedly. The placenta itself seems to be able to destroy AVP, and may account for up to 30% of the increased metabolism of the hormone [13]. The lack of sensitivity to hypo-osmolality may well contribute to the otherwise incomprehensible ease with which the pregnant woman retains water. During pregnancy, water intoxication and various forms of oedema (including pulmonary oedema) can result from the administration of relatively small volumes of electrolyte and protein-free fluids such as 5% dextrose [14].

6.1.5 Electrolyte balance

The interaction between hormonal changes and kidney function during the course of pregnancy is complex. The differences between non-pregnant and pregnant values for some plasma constituents are shown in Appendix 1.

Increased effective renal plasma flow and GFR inevitably lead to increased sodium loss in the resulting filtrate. The decreased serum albumin concentration that accompanies normal pregnancy will also tend to inhibit sodium reabsorption. These factors enhancing sodium loss are balanced by increases in aldosterone, oestrogens and desoxycorticosterone, which cause sodium retention. Paradoxically, desoxycorticosterone is derived from increased levels of progesterone, a natriuretic, by the oestrogen-enhanced activity of 21-hydroxylase. Retention of sodium during pregnancy is therefore particularly reliant on a very effective hormonally controlled reabsorption.

Posture also affects sodium retention. The upright and supine positions are both antinatriuretic. Both positions are associated with increased intraureteral luminal pressures. They are also associated with decreased venous return to the right side of the heart in a substantial proportion of parturients. Hypothetically, at least, the venous pooling that occurs because of vasodilatation in normal pregnancy is enhanced by these two postures, and atrial and arterial volume receptors effectively sense a reduced blood volume and further stimulate sodium retention. The delicate balance of sodium excretion can be affected by anaesthetic agents [15], and particularly the stress response to surgery.

The reduction in maternal Pa_{CO_2} increases the maternal–fetus carbon dioxide concentration gradient without any need for the fetus to develop high circulating levels of carbon dioxide. This fetal advantage is not without its cost, however. The lowered maternal Pa_{CO_2} would cause a respiratory alkalosis, except that it is matched by a loss of plasma bicarbonate by the kidney to maintain normal pH. Bicarbonate values of 18–22 mmol/L are normal in pregnancy. The loss of bicarbonate probably contributes to the reduction of serum sodium. These processes reduce the buffering capacity in pregnancy.

6.1.6 Uric acid and urates

Plasma urate is a product of purine metabolism. Concentrations fall by approximately 25% during the early stages of a normal pregnancy. As pregnancy progresses, the balance of glomerular filtration and tubular reabsorption changes, and plasma levels rise again. Plasma urate levels rise significantly during pre-eclampsia [16], and a urate level of 350 mol/L seems to be the threshold above which perinatal mortality increases. Single isolated estimations are unreliable, because of physiological changes and variability between individuals. Serial measurements should therefore be used in order to assess the severity and progress of pre-eclampsia.

Maternal urate levels also increase when fetal growth retardation is present, but the significance of the measurement is unclear. Serial rising plasma urate levels increase the likelihood of a demand for urgent surgical intervention and delivery. The fact that they are associated with poor fetal condition may also affect the choice of anaesthesia, and alerts the anaesthetist to the possibility of an increased need for fetal resuscitation.

6.2 Renal disease

Renal disease can present acutely as a complication of pre-eclampsia, or chronic renal disease can worsen intrapartum, leading to increased fetal morbidity and mortality.

6.2.1 Acute renal failure

Acute renal failure in pregnancy is the most common cause of all acute renal failure in young women. The causes are listed in Table 6.1, and can be divided into prerenal, renal or postrenal complaints. Particular conditions occur at different times in pregnancy; for example, sepsis can complicate abortion in

Table 6.1 Causes of acute renal failure in pregnancy.

Hypovolaemia
Haemorrhage
  Antepartum
  Postpartum
  Tranfusion reactions
Severe vomiting

Pre-eclampsia

Disseminated intravascular coagulation
Amniotic fluid embolism
Fetal death

Septic shock

Nephrotoxins
Antibiotics
Non-steroidal anti-inflammatory drugs

early pregnancy, whereas haemorrhage and pre-eclampsia occur later in pregnancy. Nephrotoxic effects of non-steroidal anti-inflammatory analgesics occur particularly in pre-eclampsia or hypovolaemic states, because they prevent prostaglandin synthesis in the kidney and lead to renal vasoconstriction. Monitoring of right heart filling pressures can help the control of fluid replacement in prerenal failure after a fluid challenge of 500 mL normal saline given rapidly intravenously.

6.2.2 Chronic renal failure

Fertility declines as renal function diminishes. However, a substantial number of patients with mild or moderate chronic renal insufficiency do conceive, and pregnancy usually has little or no adverse effect in patients with mild chronic renal disease. Some uncommon forms of mild disease are, however, more susceptible to pregnancy-related exacerbations. Those with lupus nephropathy (focal glomerular sclerosis) and membranoproliferative glomerulonephritis have been particularly identified as having a greater risk of renal deterioration during pregnancy [17].

The likelihood of acute or chronic problems supervening and exacerbating renal disease correlates with the severity of preconceptual renal insufficiency. A loss of 75% of functioning nephrons represents a 50% loss of renal functional capacity, and plasma creatinine levels will be unaffected and remain below 125 mol/L. Patients will usually be symptom-free until their GFR falls to 25% of normal.

In patients with moderate renal insufficiency, indicated by plasma creatinine levels of between 125 and 250 mmol/L, serious renal deterioration,

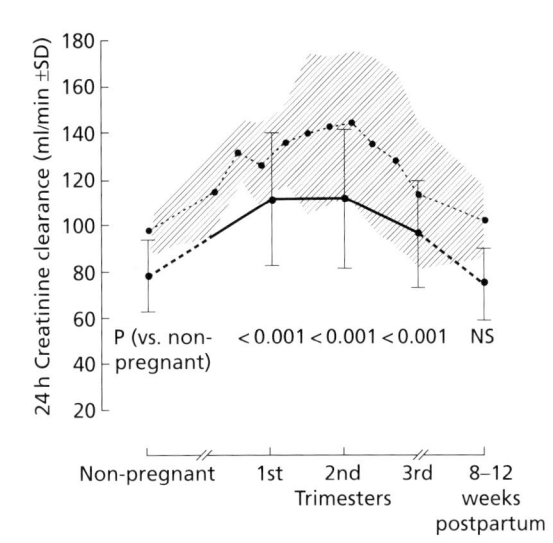

Fig. 6.2 Changes in creatinine clearance during the course of pregnancy in parturients with chronic renal failure (solid line), in comparison with normal healthy patients (shaded area). [18]

uncontrolled hypertension and postdelivery renal problems have been reported [18,19]. About 60% of infants born to women with this degree of renal impairment will be premature and small for gestational age. Fetal mortality has declined to less than 10% with modern intensive care for newborns, but for the mother, loss of renal function persists after delivery in about half of the women [20]. Therefore, all parturients suffering from renal disease, no matter what the severity, should have their renal function assessed at regular intervals throughout their pregnancy. Creatinine clearance and assessment of protein excretion should be used in addition to routine estimations of plasma urea and electrolytes (Fig. 6.2). Any fluid or electrolyte imbalance should be detected as early as possible since a small number of patients will inevitably develop reversible causes of deterioration, such as urinary tract infection or dehydration. Prompt treatment may prevent further renal damage. Frequent and regular assessment of maternal blood pressure is required, because the combination of hypertension with worsening renal function is usually a warning sign of serious impending renal problems. Antihypertensive medication is aggressively employed by renal physicians. There is an increased risk of toxicity if magnesium is administered in the acute situation.

In women with pre-existing severe renal insufficiency (creatinine > 250 mol/L), there is a 50% risk of fetal loss, and the risk–benefit ratio of pregnancy is poor. Such patients should be advised that the priority is to preserve renal function whenever possible and, when appropriate, to undergo renal transplantation prior to conception.

6.2.3 Long-term haemodialysis

Women undergoing long-term haemodialysis are prone to volume overload and severe hypertension, and many of the factors influencing blood volume

Table 6.2 A summary of the limitations of drugs used in anaesthesia for pregnant women with renal impairment of varying degrees.

Drug	Degrees of renal impairment	Comment
Muscle relaxants		
Suxamethonium	Moderate	Risk of hyperkalaemia in acute renal failure with existing high potassium concentration
'Obstetric drugs'		
Ergometrine	Severe	Manufacturer advises avoidance
Magnesium	Moderate	Increased risk of toxicity—reduce dosage and monitor concentration
Ephedrine	Severe	Increased risk of CNS toxicity related to catecholamine release
Analgesics		
Non-steroidal anti-inflammatory drugs	Mild	Causes serious renal deterioration; avoid use
Opioids	Moderate	Reduce dosage
	Severe	Avoid pethidine, dextropropoxyphene and tramadol

CNS, central nervous system.

and acid–base balance are more critical. The anaemia of chronic renal disease is aggravated, and transfusion of blood presents a particular hazard of hyperkalaemia, because potassium excretion and movements of the ion between red cells, plasma and the intracellular compartment are abnormal. Intravenous access and coagulation status should be checked prior to anaesthesia.

6.2.4 Renal transplantation

Patients with a successful transplant who become pregnant may present a number of complications. They suffer a 9% rate of graft rejection, and 50% experience early spontaneous rupture of membranes and preterm labour. Approximately one-third of them become hypertensive. Despite the pelvic location of the transplanted kidney, vaginal delivery is not impeded. However, Caesarean section, if it proves necessary, is often surgically difficult. The choice of general or regional anaesthesia should be made antenatally, after a discussion of potential problems between the woman and her anaesthetist, obstetrician and renal physician.

6.2.5 Anaesthetic management (Table 6.2)

Preservation of the existing renal function is essential by maintaining renal blood flow and preventing any toxic effects of anaesthetic drugs on the kidney, such as non-steroidal anti-inflammatory analgesics and volatile agents that liberate reactive fluoride ions (e.g. enflurane). It is not uncommon for coagulopathies to be associated with renal dysfunction, so a clotting screen is necessary prior to any form of anaesthesia.

General anaesthesia should be avoided if possible, because volatile anaesthetic agents decrease renal blood flow and the glomerular filtration rate. Isoflurane is the preferred agent only because it is least metabolized. Induction of anaesthesia requires careful consideration of:

1 the dose of induction agent, because of pharmacokinetic alterations in drug distribution and excretion;
2 the use of suxamethonium, which may cause hyperkalaemia;
3 the presence of hypertension, which may be exacerbated by intubation and extubation.

Non-depolarizing muscle relaxants may cause a prolonged block, and atracurium is preferred.

Epidural analgesia will reduce catecholamine release during labour, and if anaesthesia is required for Caesarean section, acute fluid loading and use of vasoconstrictors such as ephedrine must be monitored using direct continuous pressure measurements in severe renal failure. The composition of the fluid can be chosen depending on the blood chemistry. Opioids may be added to local anaesthesia solutions, but prolonged effects—especially on respiration—must be sought by appropriate monitoring. The intrathecal route may not provide the desired cardiovascular stability. Maintenance of blood pressure is obviously important, but the balance of fluid preload and sympathomimetic drugs must be carefully judged. When the vasodilating effects of epidural or subarachnoid anaesthesia fade, the excess intravascular volume of fluid may not be excreted quickly enough by a failing kidney, and circulatory overload and pulmonary oedema result. Caution must also be exercised when giving ephedrine, as it is excreted unchanged from the body within 24 hours. Doses may need to be reduced, otherwise they may have a more prolonged effect.

References

1 Sheehan HL, Lynch JB, eds. *Pathology of Toxaemia of Pregnancy*. Edinburgh: Churchill Livingstone, 1973: 44.
2 Cietak KA, Newton JR. Serial quantitative nephrosonography in pregnancy. *Br J Radiol* 1985; **58**: 405.
3 Cietak KA, Newton JR. Serial qualitative nephrosonography in pregnancy. *Br J Radiol* 1985; **58**: 399–404.
4 Marchant DJ. Alterations in anatomy and function of the urinary tract during pregnancy. *Clin Obstet Gynecol* 1978; **21**: 855–61.
5 Fainstat T. Ureteral dilatation in pregnancy: a review. *Obstet Gynecol Surv* 1963; **18**: 845–60.
6 Meyers SJ, Lee RV, Munschauer RW. Dilatation and nontraumatic rupture of the urinary tract during pregnancy: a review. *Obstet Gynecol* 1985; **66**: 809–15.
7 Meares EM. Urologic surgery during pregnancy. *Clin Obstet Gynecol* 1978; **21**: 207–20.

8 Baylis C, Davison J. The Urinary System. In: Hytten F, Chamberlain G, eds. *Clinical Physiology in Obstetrics, 2e*. Oxford: Blackwell Scientific Publications, 1991: 249.
9 Davison JM, Noble MC. Serial changes in 24-hour creatinine clearance during normal menstrual cycles and the first trimester of pregnancy. *Br J Obstet Gynaecol* 1981; **88**: 10–17.
10 Davison JM, Dunlop W, Ezimokhai M. 24-hour creatinine clearance during the third trimester of normal pregnancy. *Br J Obstet Gynaecol* 1980; **87**: 106–9.
11 Dunlop W, Davison JM. Renal haemodynamics and tubular function in human pregnancy. *Baillière's Clin Obstet Gynaecol* 1987; **1**: 769–87.
12 Davison JM, Vallotton MB, Lindheimer MD. Plasma osmolality and urinary concentration and dilution during and after pregnancy: evidence that lateral recumbency inhibits maximal urinary concentrating ability. *Br J Obstet Gynaecol* 1981; **88**: 472–9.
13 Landon MJ, Copas DK, Shiells EA, Davison JM. Degradation of radiolabelled arginine vasopressin (1251-AVP) by the human placenta perfused *in vitro*. *Br J Obstet Gynaecol* 1988; **95**: 488–92.
14 Lauerson NH, Birnbaum SJ. Water intoxication associated with oxytocin administration during saline-induced abortion. *Am J Obstet Gynecol* 1975; **121**: 2–6.
15 Thomsen K, Olesen OV. Effect of anaesthesia and surgery on urine flow and electrolyte excretion in different rat strains. *Renal Physiol* 1981; **4**: 165–72.
16 Redman CW, Beilin LJ, Bonnar J, Wilkinson RH. Plasma urate measurements in predicting fetal death in hypertensive pregnancy. *Lancet* 1976; **26**: 1370–3.
17 Lindheimer MD, Katz AI. Gestation in women with kidney disease: prognosis and management. *Baillière's Clin Obstet Gynaecol* 1994; **8**: 387–404.
18 Hou SH, Grossman SD, Madias NE. Pregnancy in women with renal disease and moderate renal insufficiency. *Am J Med* 1985; **78**: 185–94.
19 Hou S. Peritoneal dialysis and haemodialysis in pregnancy. *Baillière's Clin Obstet Gynaecol* 1987; **1**: 1009–25.
20 Jones DC, Hayslett JP. Outcome of pregnancy in women with moderate or severe renal insufficiency. *N Engl J Med* 1996; **335**: 226–32.

7: Hepatobiliary System

7.1 Physiology

The liver receives none of the increase in cardiac output that accompanies pregnancy, so that the proportion of cardiac output received by the liver decreases from 35% to 29% [1]. There are two systems to supply oxygenated blood to the liver: the well-oxygenated hepatic arterial system and the portal venous system. Normally, hepatic blood flow varies with daily activity, such as digestion. The hepatic artery transmits high pressure and shows some autoregulation, but hypotension can reduce blood flow. The portal venous system has no capacity for autoregulation and does not compensate for hypotension. An increase in intra-abdominal pressure, such as occurs in late pregnancy, may tend to reduce portal venous flow, but there is usually no significant change in total liver blood flow at any stage of pregnancy.

The liver does not change in size or weight during pregnancy, but there are changes in its metabolic substrates and some of the metabolic processes. These can be detected in altered liver function tests and drug handling during pregnancy. Mild hypoalbuminaemia results chiefly from haemodilution. An increase in plasma cholesterol concentration [2] is associated with an increase in biliary cholesterol secretion, and may account for the increased incidence of gallstones in multiparous women. The plasma concentration of bilirubin tends to rise in normal pregnancy because secretion of organic anions is impaired, but levels should not exceed the upper limit of normal.

At term, plasma alkaline phosphatase concentrations are usually twice normal due to increased release of both placental and bone isoenzymes [3]. Elevation of other types of enzyme activity, such as γ-glutamyl transferase, aspartate aminotransferase and alanine aminotransferase, is an indication of hepatocellular damage.

7.2 Hepatic disease (Table 7.1)

The characteristics of four liver diseases which may cause problems demanding anaesthesia or intensive care are shown in Table 7.1. Acute severe liver dysfunction during pregnancy may be coincidental with or exacerbated by pregnancy, or may be specific to pregnancy. The latter disorders include hyperemesis gravidarum, intrahepatic cholestasis of pregnancy, and acute fatty liver of pregnancy. Acute viral hepatitis is the most common cause of jaundice during pregnancy [4], and severe liver dysfunction may result from it. The hypercoagulable state of pregnancy may predispose to thrombosis of

Table 7.1 Characteristics of liver disease in pregnancy [24].

	Viral hepatitis	Intrahepatic cholestasis of pregnancy	Acute fatty liver of pregnancy	HELLP syndrome
Characteristics occur	Any time	2nd–3rd trimester	3rd trimester	2nd–3rd trimester
Incidence in pregnancy	Same as general population	0.1–0.2%	0.008%	0.1% (4–12% in women with pre-eclampsia)
Associated or predisposing factors	Contact with virus	Multiple gestation	First pregnancy	Increased blood pressure Caucasian > 35 y
Clinically	Prodromal symptoms Jaundice	Jaundice (20–60%) Pruritus	Prodromal symptoms Jaundice DIC > 75%	Thrombocytopenia Abdominal pain DIC 20–40%
Plasma bilirubin	Increased (late)	Increased	Increased	Normal
Plasma alkaline phosphatase	No change	Increased	Increased	No change
Aspartate alanine aminotransferase	Greatly increased > 500 U/L	Mainly no change	< 500 U/L	60–150 U/L (increases with infection)

DIC, disseminated intravascular coagulation; HELLP, haemolysis, elevated liver enzymes, and low platelet count.

the hepatic veins, producing abdominal pain, ascites and hepatomegaly, known as the Budd–Chiari syndrome, which is very rare. It can occur acutely postpartum [5], and has a high maternal mortality [6].

Chronic liver disease can be present during pregnancy. Alcoholic cirrhosis can present both the problems of liver cell dysfunction and fetal alcohol syndrome, with congenital abnormalities [7]. Increased fetal loss occurs partly because fetal nutrition is jeopardized by maternal steatorrhoea. Pregnancy can be successful after liver transplantation [8].

Profound changes occur in the circulating levels of sex hormones. Competition for metabolism by liver enzymes occurs. This can affect normal physiological functions such as bilirubin metabolism and drug metabolism. High circulating levels of progesterone, which is mainly bound to albumin, together with a decrease in plasma albumin, may be expected to elevate the unbound concentration of highly bound drugs and enhance toxic or therapeutic actions. Pregnant women can develop spider angiomas and palmar erythema, most likely due to increased circulating oestrogen levels. These conditions do not usually persist after pregnancy, and do not indicate the presence of underlying liver disease.

Table 7.2 Differential diagnosis of pruritis and jaundice (without severe pain, hepatomegaly, splenomegaly or fever). Ultrasound imaging can identify the enlarged gallbladder characteristic of intrahepatic cholestasis. However, a percutaneous biopsy of the liver may be necessary in atypical cases.

Intrahepatic cholestasis of pregnancy
Gallstones
Primary biliary cirrhosis
Sclerosing cholangitis
Viral hepatitis
Autoimmune chronic active hepatitis
Drug hepatotoxicity

7.2.1 Liver disorders specific to pregnancy

Hyperemesis gravidarum

This is defined as intractable vomiting associated with pregnancy, and can lead to dehydration and ketosis serious enough to require hospitalization. It is not rare, and occurs in between one in 100 and one in 1000 pregnancies. Liver involvement may be expected in 50% of patients with hyperemesis gravidarum [9], and is characterized by increased aminotransferase values of 600–1000 U.

The condition has no known aetiology, but has an association with obesity and transient hyperthyroidism. It is more common in nulliparous women and in those with more than one fetus. A successful outcome of pregnancy is to be expected despite the severity of the symptoms.

Intrahepatic cholestasis of pregnancy

Cholestasis of pregnancy is the most common liver disorder peculiar to pregnancy. The differential diagnosis of pruritus and jaundice is shown in Table 7.2. Severe, generalized itching is a classic symptom of the disease in the second or third trimester of pregnancy, often only after the 30th week, and is more common with multiple births. The pruritus associated with cholestasis has been linked to increased availability of opioid receptors in the brain to bind their agonist ligands [10]. Obstructive jaundice follows after a variable period, commonly of two to four weeks, and subclinical steatorrhoea may impair nutrition. Vitamin K dysfunction can account for some cases of uterine or intracranial haemorrhage. The pruritus settles one or two days after delivery, but the jaundice may take several weeks to clear.

It is a mild, self-limiting disease of unknown pathogenesis, although abnormal sex steroid metabolism has been implicated [11,12]. Usually, the plasma bilirubin is less than 100 µmol L^{-1}, and aminotransferases are normal. Total resolution of signs and symptoms occurs spontaneously, and symptomatic treatment of pruritus with cholestyramine along with reassurance are the main therapies. Maternal morbidity can be considerable, with insomnia from itching, anorexia, malaise and epigastric discomfort. The fetal prognosis is not so favourable, as the perinatal mortality rate is increased up to five times. Early referral to an obstetrician is therefore required so that management can be optimized. There have been increased rates of premature labour, intrauterine death and intrapartum hypoxia [13–15].

The condition may return with subsequent oral contraceptive use, i.e. oestrogen therapy or pregnancies [16]. There is a familial tendency, with fathers transmitting susceptibility to their daughters, and the condition has been reported mainly in Scandinavia, South America and China.

Women with severe pruritus that is probably caused by intrahepatic cholestasis of pregnancy, or who have a family history of cholestasis or jaundice exacerbated by oestrogens, require referral to an obstetrician early in pregnancy. Serial measurements of serum concentrations of bile acids, albumin, and alkaline phosphatase should be made. Cholestyramine, which helps to relieve the pruritus, binds bile acids, anionic drugs and fat-soluble vitamins, so treatment with vitamin K should be considered. Substances for relieving itching may only benefit some individual women. In addition to cholestyramine, they include: phenobarbital, charcoal, ultraviolet light, evening primrose oil, intravenous S-adenosyl-L-methionine and epomediol [17].

7.2.2 Disorders associated with pre-eclampsia

Pre-eclampsia is a common multisystem disorder in which liver involvement occurs in a minority of women. Hepatic abnormalities increase in severity with the severity of the pre-eclamptic process. Elevated plasma aminotransferase concentrations occur in 24% of patients with mild hypertension, and this rises to over 80% in those with severe hypertension [18]. However, abnormal liver function tests do not correlate with liver injury. It is necessary to treat this disorder aggressively, primarily with delivery. The mother will complain of epigastric or right upper-quadrant pain, nausea and vomiting when there is hepatic involvement, and the liver is often tender on palpation. The hepatic architecture can be damaged by ischaemia or haemorrhage [19].

Haemorrhage may rupture through the liver capsule into the peritoneal cavity [20]. Hypovolaemic shock is precipitated. The diagnosis can be confirmed by ultrasound, abdominal computed tomography (CT) scanning, or on abdominal paracentesis. Management will include delivery and treatment of any coagulopathy.

HELLP syndrome

The *h*aemolysis, *e*levated *l*iver enzymes and *l*ow *p*latelet count (HELLP) syndrome is probably the extreme end of a continuum of liver involvement in

Table 7.3 Management of HELLP syndrome [25].

Antepartum
Mother
    Correct coagulopathy if present
    Prophylactic anticonvulsant
    Antihypertensives
    Intensive care
    Ultrasound of liver if suspected haematoma

Fetus
    Steroids if immature
    Delivery if mature
    Assess fetal distress

Postpartum
Differential diagnosis:
    Thrombotic thrombocytopenic purpura (elevated von Willebrand factor multimers)
    Haemolytic uraemic syndrome

pre-eclampsia [21]. The haemolysis associated with the syndrome is similar to that observed in acute fatty liver of pregnancy. It is a microangiopathic haemolytic anaemia. Thrombocytopenia can complicate pre-eclampsia without the development of HELLP, but if progression occurs, more serious coagulopathies follow, with disseminated intravascular coagulation in severe cases [22,23]. The main liver enzyme to be elevated is the plasma aminotransferase. Haematological abnormalities may peak after delivery. The differential diagnoses are summarized in Table 7.2. Risk factors for HELLP include pre-eclampsia, maternal age above 25 years, multiparity and white ethnic origin [24]. Perinatal mortality is higher than maternal mortality, and the main treatment is delivery of the fetus. Other treatments are supportive (Table 7.3). This is similar to acute fatty liver of pregnancy, so that liver biopsies to differentiate between them are not usually required.

The presence of HELLP is not an indication for immediate operative delivery. If there is fetal immaturity, steroids should be given to accelerate lung maturity while the fetal and maternal conditions are continuously assessed. Patients in labour should be allowed to deliver vaginally in the absence of obstetric contraindications [25]. The use of regional analgesia is contraindicated because of the risk of bleeding. Before general anaesthesia for Caesarean section, platelet administration should be considered, extra blood should be ordered for transfusion, and wound drainage should be used to avoid haematomas.

If the patient is in shock from liver rupture, an immediate laparotomy is required and also massive blood transfusions with fresh frozen plasma and platelets. Embolization of the appropriate hepatic artery may be an alternative.

HELLP syndrome may develop postpartum, and although hypertension control can be more aggressive, there is an increased risk of pulmonary oedema and acute renal failure. It may be difficult to differentiate this from other causes of postpartum hepatic dysfunction .

Acute fatty liver of pregnancy

Acute fatty liver of pregnancy is a rare complication (one in 13 300 pregnancies), and presents from the 32nd week of gestation in a first pregnancy [26]. The patient complains of a sudden onset of vomiting, abdominal pain, fatigue, headache and fever. These prodromal symptoms rapidly lead to jaundice, coagulopathy and other signs of liver failure. Renal failure follows. Many patients with acute fatty liver of pregnancy have signs of pre-eclampsia, and it has been suggested that these diseases may be related [27,28]. Accurate diagnosis is provided by liver biopsy, which shows centrilobular microvesicular fatty infiltration of the hepatocytes. Fatty infiltration may also be found in the pancreas, brain and kidneys. Biopsy may not be practicable due to severe coagulopathy and the need for urgent delivery. Biochemical abnormalities show mild elevation of the aminotransferases and plasma bilirubin. The peripheral blood film shows marked leucocytosis, microangiopathic haemolysis and thrombocytopenia. An ultrasound examination should exclude other liver conditions, e.g. gallstones, and the Budd–Chiari syndrome. Serological tests will exclude recent infection with hepatic viruses.

Treatment consists of supportive care for the hepatic failure plus urgent delivery of the fetus once the diagnosis is established. There is no specific therapy, and the mechanism of fatty infiltration is unknown. Early delivery and good medical management have helped to improve the mortality rates. Maternal survival rates can reach 90% [11], but it is still a life-threatening condition, both for the mother and the fetus.

References

1 Robson SC, Mutch E, Boys RJ, Woodhouse KW. Apparent liver blood flow during pregnancy: a serial study using indocyanine green clearance. *Br J Obstet Gynaecol* 1990; **97**: 720–4.
2 Svanborg A, Vikrot O. Plasma lipid fraction, including individual phospholipids at various stages of pregnancy. *Acta Med Scand* 1965; **178**: 615–30.
3 Adenii FA, Olatunbosun DA. Origins and significance of the increased plasma alkaline phosphatase during normal pregnancy and pre-eclampsia. *Br J Obstet Gynaecol* 1984; **91**: 857–62.
4 Hammerli UP. Jaundice during pregnancy, with special emphasis on recurrent jaundice during pregnancy and its differential diagnosis. *Acta Med Scand Suppl* 1966; **444**: 1–66.
5 Ilan Y, Oren MD, Shouval D. Postpartum Budd–Chiari syndrome with prolonged hypercoagulable state. *Am J Obstet Gynecol* 1990; **162**: 1164–5.
6 Khuroo MS, Datta DV. Budd–Chiari syndrome following pregnancy: report of 16 cases with roentgenologic, hemodynamic and histologic studies of the hepatic outflow tract. *Am J Med* 1980; **68**: 113–21.

7 Hanson JW, Streissguth AP, Smith DW. The effects of moderate alcohol consumption during pregnancy on fetal growth and morphogenesis. *J Pediatr* 1978; **92**: 457–60.
8 Ville Y, Fernandez H, Samuel D, Bismuth H, Frydman R. Pregnancy in liver transplant recipients: course and outcome in 19 cases. *Am J Obstet Gynecol* 1993; **168**: 196–902.
9 Riely CA. Hepatic disease in pregnancy. *Am J Med* 1994; **96**: 18S–22S.
10 Jones EA, Bergasa NV. The pruritus of cholestasis and the opioid system. *JAMA* 1992; **268**: 3359–62.
11 Lunzer MR. Jaundice in pregnancy. *Baillière's Clin Gastroenterol* 1989; **3**: 467–83.
12 Reyes H, Simon FR. Intrahepatic cholestasis of pregnancy: an oestrogen-related disease. *Semin Liver Dis* 1993; **13**: 289–301.
13 de Sweit M. *Medical Disorders in Obstetric Practice.* Oxford: Blackwell Scientific Publications, 1984.
14 Johnston WG, Basket TF. Obstetric cholestasis: a 14 year review. *Am J Obstet Gynecol* 1979; **133**: 299–301.
15 Reid R, Vey KJ, Rencoret RH *et al.* Complications of obstetric cholestasis. *Br Med J* 1976; **i**: 870–2.
16 Gonzalez MC, Reyes H, Arrese M *et al.* Intrahepatic cholestasis of pregnancy in twin pregnancies. *J Hepatol* 1989; **9**: 84–90.
17 Fagan EA. Intrahepatic cholestasis of pregnancy: timely intervention reduces perinatal mortality. *Br Med J* 1994; **309**: 1243–5.
18 Chesley CC. *Hypertensive Disorders in Pregnancy.* New York: Appleton-Century-Crofts, 1978.
19 Manas KJ, Welsh JD, Rankin RA, Miller DD. Hepatic haemorrhage without rupture in preeclampsia. *N Engl J Med* 1985; **312**: 424–6.
20 Neerhof HG, Zelman W, Sullivan T. Hepatic rupture in pregnancy. *Obstet Gynecol Surv* 1989; **44**: 407–9.
21 Weinstein L. Syndrome of hemolysis, elevated liver enzymes, and low platelet count: a severe consequence of hypertension in pregnancy. *Am J Obstet Gynecol* 1982; **142**: 159–68.
22 Patterson KW, O'Toole DP. HELLP syndrome: a case report with guidelines for diagnosis and management. *Br J Anaesth* 1991; **66**: 513–15.
23 Martin JN, Blake PG, Perry KG *et al.* The natural history of HELLP syndrome: patterns of disease progression and regression. *Am J Obstet Gynecol* 1991; **164**: 1500–13.
24 Sibai BM, Taslimi MM, El-Nazar A *et al.* Maternal perinatal outcome associated with the syndrome of hemolysis, elevated liver enzymes, and low platelets in severe pre-eclampsia/eclampsia. *Am J Obstet Gynecol* 1986; **155**: 501–9.
25 Barton JR, Sibai BM. Care of the pregnancy complicated by HELLP syndrome. *Gastroenterol Clin North Am* 1992; **21**: 937–49.
26 Kaplan MM. Acute fatty liver of pregnancy. *N Engl J Med* 1985; **313**: 367–70.
27 Rolfes DB, Ishak KG. Liver disease in toxemia of pregnancy. *Am J Gastroenterol* 1986; **81**: 1138–44.
28 Reily CA, Latham PS, Romero R, Duffy TP. Acute fatty liver of pregnancy: a reassessment based on observations in nine patients. *Ann Intern Med* 1987; **106**: 703–6.

8: Nervous System

8.1 Physiological changes and anaesthesia

Local anaesthetic requirements for epidural block are reduced in pregnancy. This occurs through a combination of increased sensitivity of nerves to local anaesthetics during pregnancy [1,2] and through engorgement of the epidural veins, decreasing the volume of the epidural space and preventing loss of local anaesthetic solution through the intervertebral foramina [3]. The spread of local anaesthetic solution will therefore be more extensive than in the non-pregnant state. In addition, cephalic spread of solutions may also be enhanced in pregnancy as a result of alterations in body contours. For example, in the horizontal lateral position, a pregnant woman is in a slightly head-down position because of an increase in pelvic width, in contrast to the non-pregnant state, where in the same position a woman would be slightly head-up. Similarly, in the recumbent position, the increased lumbar lordosis associated with pregnancy will allow solutions to migrate cephalad due to gravity.

During pregnancy, the minimum alveolar concentration (MAC) of inhalational anaesthetics is reduced by 25% for halothane and 40% for isoflurane [4]. The mechanism for this reduction in MAC is hormonally mediated. Progesterone, which is a steroid hormone, has been identified as the most likely agent, because of its sedative effects [5].

Baseline pressures in the epidural space are often positive at term, in contrast to negative pressures in the non-pregnant state. As labour progresses, this pressure is increased by an increase in blood flow through the epidural veins during contractions and by an increase in venous pressure generated by pushing in the second stage. Increases of up to 10 cmH$_2$O can occur during contractions, and further reduction in the volume of the epidural space may result. Cerebrospinal fluid pressures can reach 70 cmH$_2$O during bearing-down efforts.

8.2 Neurological symptoms and disorders

The commonest neurological symptoms in pregnancy are headache, convulsions, paraesthesia and muscle weakness. These neurological symptoms have many differential diagnoses. Neurological disorders may be classified into those that are not affected by pregnancy, those exacerbated by pregnancy and those that are precipitated by pregnancy (Table 8.1). Normal pregnancy and labour can cause or exacerbate neurological symptoms, as can obstetric and anaesthetic interventions.

NERVOUS SYSTEM

Table 8.1 Classification of neurological disorders in pregnancy.

Affected by pregnancy	Precipitated by pregnancy	Obstetric and anaesthetic complications
Epilepsy	Carpal tunnel syndrome	Cerebral vein thrombosis
Cerebral tumour	Meralgia paraesthesia (lateral cutaneous nerve of thigh)	Amniotic embolism
Multiple sclerosis		Eclampsia
Migraine	Bell's palsy	
	Lumbospinal nerve root lesions	
Subarachnoid haemorrhage		
Myasthenia gravis		

8.2.1 Headache

The most common request for an obstetric anaesthetic consultation for a headache is after regional nerve blockade. The management of postdural puncture headache is discussed in Chapter 15 (Section 15.8.9) as a complication of epidural and subarachnoid anaesthesia. It is very easy to assume that the performance of dural puncture during regional anaesthesia is responsible for the problem and to overlook other treatable conditions, which are listed in Table 8.2. As with any parturient presenting with headache during pregnancy

Table 8.2 Causes of headache.

Causes	Distinguishing features
Vascular	
e.g. migraine	Usually lasts about 12 h, unilateral visual disturbances, vomiting, photophobia
e.g. hypertension/pre-eclampsia	Increased blood pressure, proteinuria, oedema
Muscle contraction	
Cervical spondylosis	Cervical spine X-ray abnormalities
Trauma (e.g. abnormal position in labour)	Bilateral occipital/neck pain
Depression	Mood disturbance, postpartum period
Meningeal irritation	
Meningitis	Fever, meningism
Subarachnoid haemorrhage	CSF contains blood; neurological disorders
Intracranial pressure	
Raised, e.g. tumour	Optic discs: papilloedema
Lowered, e.g. postdural puncture headache	Continuous bilateral severe frontal and/or occipital pain, which may involve the neck and improves on lying down
Extracranial disorders: metabolic (hypoglycaemia)	Blood glucose estimation

Table 8.3 Investigation of postpartum headache.

History
Previous headaches
Characteristics
 Site
 Quality
 Severity
Associated symptoms
 Visual
 Vomiting
 Photophobia
 Rigors
 Other pains

Physical examination
Position adopted and behaviour
Mental status (alert, depressed, confused)
Temperature
Blood pressure
Heart rate
Neck movements (meningism, muscle spasm)
Sensory function
Motor function
Reflex activity

Investigations
Full blood count, electrolytes, glucose
CT or MRI scan (if neurological lesion suspected)
Cervical spine X-ray (if cervical spondylosis suspected)
Diagnostic lumbar puncture (if subarachnoid haemorrhage suspected)

Follow-up
4-hourly temperature, pulse, blood pressure, respiration
Repeat neurological examination
Neurological opinion

or labour, the postpartum woman must have a careful history and neurological examination recorded, as outlined in Table 8.3. Details of the nature, duration and distribution of the pain are important. Factors that improve or worsen the problem can be diagnostic. The postural nature of postdural puncture headache is almost pathognomonic, and the presence of a pyrexia, neck stiffness and pain on flexion of the head and neck are indicative of meningeal irritation.

If the diagnosis is in any doubt, an urgent neurological opinion and radiological consultation should be obtained, and relevant imaging investigations should be performed. Computed tomography (CT) scanning and magnetic resonance imaging (MRI) will identify or exclude the presence of space-occupying lesions of any type, including neoplasms, abscesses or blood. Full investigations should be expedited in doubtful cases because of the potentially serious consequences of some causes of headache.

When the headache is severe, adequate analgesia must be given. Paracetamol is usually insufficient; it has been tried and has failed to provide relief. Care should be taken in using non-steroidal analgesics, in case further bleeding is precipitated. Adequate hydration is necessary to treat low-pressure headaches, and occasionally caffeine abstinence will cause postpartum headache.

8.2.2 Convulsions

Loss of consciousness occurring for the first time in early pregnancy is most likely to be due to syncope, but may herald the development of epilepsy. In the second half of pregnancy, from about 20 weeks' gestation, an epileptic seizure has to be distinguished from an eclamptic seizure. The causes of convulsions during parturition are summarized in Table 8.4. Initially, the treatment of a convulsion of whatever cause is similar, as outlined below, but thereafter the management diverges according to the cause. The treatment of eclampsia is described in Chapter 22. Symptoms arising from tumours and vascular lesions are rare, but may present at any time during pregnancy.

Table 8.4 Causes of convulsions during parturition.

Eclampsia
Epilepsy
Drug and/or alcohol withdrawal
Brain tumour
Cerebrovascular abnormality
Metabolic disturbances/acute infection

Epilepsy

Idiopathic epilepsy is the most prevalent cause of convulsions during pregnancy. Generalized convulsions can produce hypoxia in the fetus. The frequency of seizures can increase in the first trimester, during labour, or in the puerperium. The increases are often a result of subtherapeutic serum drug levels caused by altered pharmacokinetics. The volume of distribution increases, protein binding is reduced, and an increase in hepatic metabolism and renal excretion occurs. In addition to physiological changes, some women will stop treatment to avoid drug effects on the fetus. Counselling and careful prescribing are necessary, and when therapy is essential, single-drug treatment is preferred [6]. Blood concentrations of the drug should be measured regularly so that the reason for reduced drug concentration can be investigated. Drug regimens should be reassessed after delivery, and doses should be reduced when necessary to avoid toxicity. Combined obstetric and neurological antenatal care is required, with regular monthly reviews.

Table 8.5 Epilepsy and anaesthesia.

Enzyme induction from anticonvulsants
Increased concentration of anaesthetic drug metabolites, e.g. fluoride
Increased clearance of narcotics, barbiturates

Neuromuscular function
Phenytoin has an additive effect with some non-depolarizing muscle relaxants, e.g. *d*-tubocurarine, vecuronium [7]

Seizure threshold
Reduce factors that predispose to seizures—pain, anxiety, hyperventilation, sleep deprivation
Avoid enflurane (high doses), ketamine, methohexital, etomidate
Avoid fluid overload, acid-base disturbance and hypoxia

Local anaesthetics
Anticonvulsant in low doses
Convulsant in high doses

Caesarean section/postpartum
Close monitoring in recovery and postpartum period, since convulsions are more likely during this period [8]
Anticonvulsant dosage requirement decreases

Neonatal
Vitamin K
Congenital abnormalities
Sedation/withdrawal symptoms from antiepileptic drugs

Women should be counselled prior to conception in order to discuss the risks and benefits of treatment, with a view to minimizing the risk of fetal abnormalities while still controlling the seizures. Many congenital abnormalities are minor, but the frequency of congenital malformations in children born to mothers with epilepsy is three times the normal rate, and this is largely the result of anticonvulsant teratogenesis. There is less risk for women taking monotherapy.

At birth, oral prophylactic vitamin K should be given to the neonate if enzyme-inducing anticonvulsants such as carbamazepine, phenytoin, or phenobarbital have been taken, because they can cause a bleeding tendency in neonates. Placental transfer of phenytoin, phenobarbitone, diazepam or primidone occasionally causes neonatal depression. Anticonvulsants will pass to the fetus during breast-feeding, but this should not deter a mother, because only subtherapeutic levels will be achieved.

Epilepsy and labour (Table 8.5). Epileptic women are at risk of drug interactions and fetal effects. Fluid retention may lead to cerebral oedema, which will in turn lower the seizure threshold. Any therapy that can cause fluid retention must therefore be avoided, or used sparingly. Particular problems can occur with oxytocin infusions and the use of 5% dextrose. Alkalosis, e.g. due to hyperventilation, also provokes seizures, and can be avoided in labour by adequate pain relief. An epidural nerve block can reduce factors that predispose to convulsions, e.g. pain, anxiety, hyperventilation and sleep deprivation—and is indicated for pain relief in labour. The choice of local anaesthetic agent depends on clinical requirements rather than any advantage of the agent in seizure control. Administration of anticonvulsant medication during labour and delivery is essential, and should be given by the parenteral route if necessary.

Treatment of epileptic convulsions. This is an obstetric emergency, which will require continuing intensive care if seizures are recurrent. Oxygenation and ventilation, protection of the airway, intravenous access, and maintenance of uterine displacement are routine measures. Immediate treatment includes intravenous diazepam (as Diazemuls, an oil-in-water emulsion) at a dose of 10–20 mg in 2–4 mL at a rate of 0.5 mL/30 s until convulsions stop. A second dose should be given if seizures last longer than or recur after 30–60 minutes. After a bolus injection, unwanted effects such as respiratory depression or hypotension occur in > 10% of women [7], so maternal cardiorespiratory monitoring should be used. Fetal monitoring may detect signs of fetal distress, such as bradycardia and reduced heart rate variability. Long-term anticonvulsant therapy should be started by slow intravenous injection, because diazepam redistributes quickly and seizures can recur 10–20 minutes after its administration. Phenytoin can be administered intravenously over 20 minutes in a loading dose of up to 18 mg/kg. The rate should not exceed 50 mg/min, because rapid infusions can cause cardiac dysrhythmias. Diazepam and phenytoin are not miscible. Treatment also requires any precipitating factor to be corrected, so venous blood samples should be sent for anticonvulsant level, glucose and electrolyte estimation. Arterial blood gases and acid–base status should also be assessed. Both maternal and fetal monitoring should be available continuously.

8.2.3 Vascular disorders

Vascular abnormalities and tumours in the spinal cord, although rare, may present with signs and symptoms during pregnancy, because their vascular supply is increased. They may be asymptomatic until epidural or subarachnoid analgesia is used.

The onset of central cerebrovascular events is often sudden and severe. In life-threatening situations prior to delivery, a successful fetal outcome is possible if Caesarean section is performed within a few minutes after cardiopulmonary resuscitation starts. The performance of a postmortem Caesarean section later than 15 minutes post-arrest is unlikely to produce a satisfactory outcome. In less acute presentations, accurate diagnosis and treatment may be delayed by fetal considerations. If the presentation is postpartum, complications

Table 8.6 Causes of cerebrovascular disorders in pregnancy.

Thrombosis
Arterial. In pregnancy: middle cerebral; postpartum: internal carotid. Risk factors: pre-eclampsia, eclampsia, smoking, sickle-cell disorder, drugs (ergot derivatives, vasopressors)
Venous. Cerebral venous sinus, e.g. sagittal sinus, lateral sinus. NB, venous sinus thrombosis increases intracranial pressure

Emboli (rare)
Risk factors: atrial fibrillation, myocardial infarction
Paradoxical: amniotic fluid

Subarachnoid haemorrhage
Rupture of congenital aneurysm
Arteriovenous malformations
Vasculitis, e.g. systemic lupus erythematosus

Vasospasm
Migraine

Drug-induced
Cocaine
Alcohol

---

such as cerebral vein or venous sinus thrombosis may mimic postdural puncture headache.

Table 8.6 summarizes the aetiology of these vascular disorders. Historically, venous sinus thrombosis was associated with puerperal infection, but the range of predisposing factors now includes blood disorders, abnormalities of blood flow and infiltrative or inflammatory conditions that may promote thrombosis [8]. Thrombosis that occurs in the lower limb veins and cerebral vascular system is a major cause of death in pregnancy [9], and more than one site of thrombosis may occur, e.g. deep-vein thrombosis and internal carotid artery occlusion. A cerebrovascular haemorrhage or ischaemic episode may be aetiologically heterogenous. Any neurological impairment associated with anaesthesia requires systematic evaluation. Where risk factors for a stroke are present, an anaesthetist should take precautions to protect the woman from surges in blood pressure, to reduce the risk of cerebral bleeds and to use antithrombotic therapy as prophylaxis against cerebral thrombosis. This is particularly relevant to the postpartum period, where it was found in a large study that the risks of a stroke were increased in the six weeks after delivery rather than during pregnancy when compared with the incidence in non-pregnant women [10].

Methods of delivery: anaesthetic management

Previous surgery. Women who have had clipping or repair of an intracranial vascular lesion will usually be allowed to labour and deliver vaginally.

Generally, care should be taken to prevent increases in intracranial pressure. This is best achieved using epidural analgesia, which reduces the likelihood of a hypertensive response to pain and can be used to remove the urge to push once the cervix is fully dilated. Although a 10-mL epidural injection may produce an increase in intracranial pressure, this can be prevented by slow injection of small doses and a continuous infusion technique. In the second stage of labour, when intracranial pressure rises with the increase in intrathoracic pressure during active pushing, instrumental forceps or ventouse delivery is indicated, and the analgesia provided by an epidural nerve blockade will help to prevent significant increases in intracranial pressure. The parturient should not be asked to push even then; instead, the obstetrician should time his traction to match uterine contractions.

Caesarean delivery. In disorders in which an increase in intracranial pressure occurs, such as cortical venous sinus thrombosis, measures should be taken to reduce the intracranial pressure. Preoperatively, dexamethasone and furosemide can be used, but mannitol, an osmotic diuretic, is not recommended since water passes from the fetus to the mother [11]. During induction and maintenance of anaesthesia, fluctuations in blood gases and blood pressure should be avoided. This can be achieved by preventing the hypertensive response to intubation and continuously monitoring the oxygen saturation and expired carbon dioxide concentration. Although suxamethonium can increase intracranial pressure, its benefits in allowing rapid intubation may outweigh this risk, especially if preoperative measures are taken to reduce cerebral oedema.

Where Caesarean section is to be followed by craniotomy to correct a vascular abnormality or to remove a tumour, the fetus should be viable. The goals of anaesthetic management are to prevent fluctuations in systemic blood pressure and avoid fetal depression. Preoperatively, the mother is likely to have received barbiturates or benzodiazepines to treat complications such as convulsions and also antihypertensive agents. General anaesthesia is required for this combined procedure, with precautions to obtund the hypertensive response to intubation. Direct arterial pressure monitoring should begin before the induction of anaesthesia.

8.2.4 Hydrocephalus

Hydrocephalic women with cerebrospinal fluid shunts are now surviving to reproductive age. Extracranial shunting catheters allow drainage of fluid at a pressure of between 60 and 80 mmH$_2$O. During pregnancy, and particularly during labour, cerebrospinal fluid pressure increases, but because venous pressure also increases, temporary blockage of flow in a ventriculoatrial shunt can occur. Ventriculoperitoneal shunts can also be blocked by the increase in intra-abdominal pressure. Adequate analgesia and the avoidance of Valsalva manoeuvres (e.g. by preventing pushing with epidural analgesia and a forceps delivery) can minimize these pressure increases. Prophylactic antibiotic therapy should be given during vaginal or abdominal delivery, because bacteraemia may introduce sepsis into a ventriculoperitoneal shunt.

A small group of 18 women with shunts were studied during 21 pregnancies [12]. When symptoms of raised intracranial pressure developed, shunt obstruction had occurred and required surgery. Less common problems were exacerbation of seizures and severe headache. Caesarean section has been recommended for delivery of the neurologically unstable woman with general anaesthesia [13]. Table 8.7 summarizes the anaesthetic management of parturients with an increase in intracranial pressure.

Table 8.7 Anaesthetic management in neurological disease.

Presenting problem	Management
Respiratory function	Assess lung function by test and arterial blood gases. Serial measurements useful to monitor stability
	Avoid respiratory complications, e.g. aspiration of gastric contents, pneumonia
	Consider drug effects: local anaesthetic drugs block intercostal muscles; opioids and sedative drugs depress respiration
	Postoperative care: secure airway, maintain cough/physiotherapy
Bulbar paralysis	Assess risk of aspiration. Secure airway
	Consider awake intubation
Skeletal muscle deterioration	Consider drug effects: suxamethonium-induced hyperkalaemia; variations in sensitivity to muscle relaxants. Titrate dose. Monitor neuromuscular function
Ability to move	Assess and preserve skin integrity. Avoid pressure sores/ulceration
Smooth muscle	
Bladder	Assess function. Avoid over-distension
Gastrointestinal tract	Take precautions to prevent aspiration of stomach contents
Skeleton	Assess respiratory dysfunction and access to the vertebral canal
Families, e.g. dystrophia myotonica	Check family history. Avoid triggers
Intracranial pressure increase	Identify causes: tumours (benign, malignant); haemorrhage; venous sinus obstruction
	Avoid regional nerve block
	Use general anaesthesia
	Avoid hypertension during intubation
	Prevent increases in venous pressure (e.g. coughing)
	Hyperventilate (a pregnant woman is normally hyperventilating) using inhalational agent, e.g. isoflurane
	Postoperative recovery care should be planned, to:
	Avoid sedation (and prevent hypercarbia etc.)
	Monitor Glasgow coma scale

8.3 Motor and sensory function

The anaesthetic management of women with abnormal motor function in skeletal, cardiac or smooth muscle is summarized in Table 8.7. Each case must be individually assessed, and the appropriate management chosen. For example, a denervated or degenerating muscle is especially sensitive to suxamethonium, and muscles leak potassium. This can cause cardiac dysrhythmias, leading to cardiac arrest. Neuromuscular disease, such as dystrophies and multiple sclerosis, can also respond in this way. Skeletal muscle weakness from any chronic cause is not usually associated with or accompanied by impairment of uterine contractility. However, weakness of the abdominal or perineal muscles may reduce a parturient's expulsive power, and second-stage assistance may be required.

8.3.1 Spinal cord injury

The problems and management of women with chronic spinal cord injury are summarized in Table 8.8. During pregnancy, most women are able to continue with their normal bladder management, but in late pregnancy, an indwelling catheter may have to be sited if bladder drainage is obstructed by the fetus. Chronic traumatic paraplegia is associated with urinary tract infections and anaemia, and these may be further exacerbated by pregnancy. Antenatal anaesthetic assessment should include not only haematological and neurological deficiencies, but also respiratory function, such as the peak

Table 8.8 Problems and management in chronic spinal cord injury.

Problems
  Poor respiratory reserve
  Sympathetic nerve paralysis
  Lack of sympathetic reflexes to respond to haemorrhage
  Impaired thermoregulation
  Urinary tract infections

Management
Anaesthetic assessment
  Document sensory and motor deficiencies
  Pulmonary function
  Renal function

General anaesthesia
  Avoid depolarizing muscle relaxant (regional anaesthesia is indicated for Caesarean
    section)
  Hyperkalaemia can develop
  Deep anaesthesia prevents autonomic hyperreflexia—light anaesthesia may not
    (NB, inhalational agents may increase blood loss if used at high concentrations)

expiratory flow rate and any alterations in renal function, particularly secondary to chronic urinary tract infections. Potential improvements in organ function should be sought prior to delivery, for example by suitable antibiotic therapy.

Labour may be precipitated, especially when damage above the lower thoracic segments has occurred, because contractions will be painless. Sympathetic nerve paralysis will block normal responses to haemorrhage, and cardiovascular monitoring at the time of labour is essential. Thermoregulation is also impaired, and hyperthermia can occur, since regulation of heat loss by sweating is disturbed. In labour, close observation and maintenance of normal maternal temperature are both needed in order to prevent hyperthermia and subsequent fetal distress.

Labour can be complicated by autonomic hyperreflexia, which is induced by uterine activity. This is a sudden reflex sympathetic discharge below the level of cord damage, resulting in generalized vasoconstriction and hypertension with a throbbing headache, sweating and bradycardia. Fetal tachycardia has been reported to occur during such episodes [14]. The clinical picture is similar to that of pre-eclampsia, and it must be distinguished from this condition. It occurs if the lesion is above T7 [15] and is the result of unopposed or unmodified transmission of impulses via cutaneous or visceral afferent nerves, which are free from spinal inhibitory controls [16].

The excessive responses can be relieved by subarachnoid or epidural block. Sometimes, however, additional antihypertensive measures may be needed, although vasodilator agents themselves can produce symptoms mimicking those of autonomic hyperreflexia, such as headache and palpitations. Epidurally administered local anaesthesia interrupts nociceptive transmission from the viscera, whereas fentanyl alone does not [17]. Epidural analgesia may prevent the complications of hypertension, such as unconsciousness, convulsions and cerebral haemorrhage. However, the dosage of local anaesthetic used must be carefully titrated to prevent excessive spread of analgesia and hypotension. It will usually be necessary to site an epidural catheter before labour in anticipation of autonomic hyperreflexia, and to maintain a nerve block into the postpartum period until precipitating factors are minimized [18]. When epidural or subarachnoid analgesia is contraindicated and general anaesthesia has to be given, the stimulations that can occur during light anaesthesia may also precipitate autonomic hyperreflexia.

8.3.2 Acute lumbar disc prolapse

Acute lumbar disc herniation is rare, although women may have pre-existing chronic lumbar disc abnormalities. Herniations most commonly present at the L5–S1 level, but it is a central disc herniation that is hazardous, because it can cause the cauda equina syndrome with saddle anaesthesia, loss of bladder control, stress urinary incontinence, extreme constipation, difficult defaecation and rectal incontinence. Women who present antenatally with a history of chronic lumbar disc symptoms should be examined by a combination of orthopaedic, obstetric, physiotherapeutic and anaesthetic specialists, and magnetic resonance imaging is required if the lesion has not been imaged (see backache, Chapter 24). If a chronic problem is present without an acute exacerbation, the mother should receive antenatal advice on the best positions to adopt for labour and delivery, and about the risks associated with epidural or subarachnoid anaesthesia. Where subarachnoid surgery has been pe formed, epidural insertion is more likely to result in dural puncture, due to adhesions with the dura or loss of normal tissue resistance. Epidural analgesia may also be patchy in these women, and they should be advised of this before an epidural is sited. For Caesarean delivery, subarachnoid anaesthesia is usually easier to perform, has more predictable results and is the regional technique of choice.

8.3.3 Multiple sclerosis

This is a remitting, patchy demyelinating disease of the central nervous system with a female predominance and a very variable prevalence of usually less than one in 1000 of the population, depending on geographical location and age. Random demyelinations produce acute symptoms that clear after several weeks, and immunosuppressant therapy, e.g. with steroids, can shorten exacerbations. Residual nervous dysfunction produces disability, but in young women severe disability from multiple sclerosis is rare. Baclofen can be used to treat muscle spasticity.

Pregnancy does not seem to have any significant effect on the disease, but relapse can occur in the puerperium. Relapses may be caused by infections, fatigue, or stress, and rest is helpful. Regional nerve block by the epidural or subarachnoid route is not contraindicated [19–21], but the mother should be aware that loss of sensory and motor function with local anaesthetics is transient [22] and disease relapse may occur at any time, including immediately postpartum. Bladder control is often affected in multiple sclerosis, and this problem may be exacerbated by epidural analgesia. Adequate bladder emptying at regular intervals is particularly important in women with multiple sclerosis in order to prevent bladder distention and the risk of future dysfunction. Epidural analgesia may help to relieve muscle spasticity, but may also make muscle weakness worse.

Prior to any anaesthetic intervention, a full neurological examination is required, and assessment of any respiratory impairment. Women who are receiving steroids for therapy require additional parenteral doses. The blood–brain barrier is impaired in these women, and a toxic response to local anaesthetics may occur at lower than expected doses [23]. Dilute solutions of local anaesthetics, e.g. < 0.1% bupivacaine, should be used for maintenance of epidural analgesia rather than concentrations of 0.5% or 0.25%. The long-term effects of epidural or subarachnoid opioids for labour or delivery have not been described.

If general anaesthesia is required, particular care should be taken to avoid pulmonary complications and any increase in body temperature, which can exacerbate the disease. The choice of neuromuscular blocking agent for intubation may be limited, because suxamethonium is to be avoided in women with severe muscular involvement. The alternative is an awake intubation, which may prevent problems of aspiration and be more easily achieved if muscle weakness is present.

8.3.4 Myasthenia gravis

This is an autoimmune disease, with antibodies to the subunit acetylcholine receptor being present in 90% of women [24]. Thymic hyperplasia can occur. It is a rare disorder (one in 20 000 adults), but more common in women of childbearing age than older years. Muscle fatigue is the prime symptom, typically starting asymmetrically in the extraocular muscles, the bulbar muscles (affecting speech and swallowing) and then spreading to the arms, legs and trunk. The anticholinesterase group of drugs provides symptomatic improvement. Pyridostigmine is the preferred treatment, as it has a longer action than neostigmine. Thymectomy may relieve the symptoms, and immunosuppressive drugs such as steroids are sometimes used.

Table 8.9 Anaesthetic assessment in myasthenia gravis.

Respiratory function: spirometry (vital capacity) and peak flow rate
Bulbar weakness: swallowing difficulties may affect nutrition
Treatment: anticholinesterase drugs, steroids
Electrocardiogram

Anaesthetic care (Table 8.9)

Pregnancy has a varied effect on myasthenia gravis, but the majority of changes occur during the first trimester [25]. These women should be seen and assessed by the relevant anaesthetist early in pregnancy, and there should be continuing consultations at a frequency dependent on the severity of the condition. Sufferers usually understand the disease, and especially how it affects them, better than a medical practitioner. They are often used to monitoring their peak flow rate at home. Any worsening of the result should be reported to the anaesthetist concerned, and the woman's condition should be reviewed. The woman should be directly consulted when decisions on the management of the pregnancy, labour, delivery and postpartum care are being discussed or made. In the majority of cases, delivery would be expected to be normal, except that skeletal muscle weakness and fatigue may develop during the second stage, and assistance with delivery may be required.

A number of drugs, particularly those used in anaesthesia [26], can be hazardous.
- Magnesium sulphate: magnesium inhibits the release of acetylcholine and causes neuromuscular block.
- Narcotics/sedatives (including general anaesthetic drugs): respiratory depression may be precipitated.
- Aminoglycoside antibiotics (e.g. gentamycin) exacerbate symptoms.
- Neuromuscular blocking drugs:
  the action of suxamethonium is prolonged
  there is sensitivity to non-depolarizing relaxants, so they should be used in small doses and with caution.

Atracurium is recommended by the authors because of its pharmacokinetic profile.

Myasthenic and cholinergic crisis

A myasthenic crisis begins with increasing muscle weakness, difficulty in swallowing and talking, and develops into respiratory failure. Intravenous edrophonium 2–10 mg will reduce symptoms. Edrophonium is a quaternary ammonium compound that does not cross the placenta.

A cholinergic crisis is caused by drug overdosage and muscarinic symptoms can predominate, e.g. abdominal cramp, that may be similar to labour pains and diarrhoea. An edrophonium test (2 mg i.v.) will confirm the diagnosis and does not produce bradycardia.

Labour and delivery

Medication is best given parenterally during labour, because enteral absorption may be delayed. Adequate rest should be encouraged before and after delivery, and respiratory muscle strength can be tested by serial peak expiratory flow rates. Neonatal myasthenia can develop due to the passage of maternal antireceptor antibodies.

Regional nerve block can be used [27,28]. Care should be taken to avoid a high intercostal block in order to retain adequate respiratory function. Ester-type anaesthetics are best avoided, because anticholinesterases may prevent them from being metabolized.

8.3.5 Dystrophia myotonica

Myotonia describes the state of delayed relaxation following contraction. This develops because of an abnormal re-entry of calcium through malfunctioning ion channels in the sarcoplasmic reticulum [29]. There may be a decrease in muscle power and an increase in myotonia in the last trimester of pregnancy. The smooth muscle of the uterus may be affected, and uterine inertia may develop and second-stage delay [30]. If the mother has the autosomal dominant form, which is the most common of the myotonic dystrophies, the fetus is likely to be affected *in utero*, and polyhydramnios may develop due to depression of fetal swallowing activity.

Smooth muscle in the gut is also affected, and so there is an increased risk of regurgitation and aspiration of gastric contents at induction of anaesthesia or extubation of the trachea. There is an extreme sensitivity to inhalational agents and intravenous analgesics, so that central nervous system depression is increased [31]. Administration of suxamethonium to myotonics causes masseter spasm [32], so awake intubation may be a necessary first step in general anaesthesia.

Epidural or subarachnoid anaesthesia is preferred. Shivering may precipitate a myotonic crisis, so efforts to prevent it must be taken. Warming the woman, maintaining hydration with parenteral fluids and parenteral administration of small, incremental doses of an opioid have been advocated [33,34]. Epidural opioids should probably be avoided because of the risk of respiratory depression [35]. An acute myotonic crisis can be treated with quinine 300–600 mg i.v., dantrolene or large doses of steroids. Muscle relaxants and regional blocks are ineffective.

Postoperative care includes prevention of shivering and adequate analgesia. Respiratory function should be monitored so that respiratory depression is detected and treated promptly.

8.3.6 Disturbances of micturition

The anatomy of the bladder is shown in Fig. 8.1. Micturition can be initiated by a local reflex mechanism, and this can occur even after traumatic damage to the spinal cord or multiple sclerosis. Normally, voluntary mechanisms inhibit this reflex and exert control over the hypothalamic and pontine facilitatory centres and the pelvic floor muscles. During labour, pressure on the bladder and urethra can lead to urinary retention. This can be exacerbated by loss of sensation from epidural nerve block. If the detrusor muscle becomes overstretched, it will not function properly postpartum and overflow incontinence will occur. A single episode of bladder overdistension can produce irreversible damage to the detrusor muscle. During delivery, stretching and pressure on the bladder and its sphincters and nerves in the pelvic floor can lead to an autonomous bladder with dribbling incontinence as there is reduced sensation, particularly of bladder fullness.

Newly occurring stress incontinence is present in 11% of women postpartum [36], and is associated with a long second stage of labour, large babies and increasing maternal age. In another study, Caesarean section resulted in fewer symptoms [37], and this potential long-term deleterious effect of vaginal delivery on bladder function has led to a demand for Caesarean deliveries.

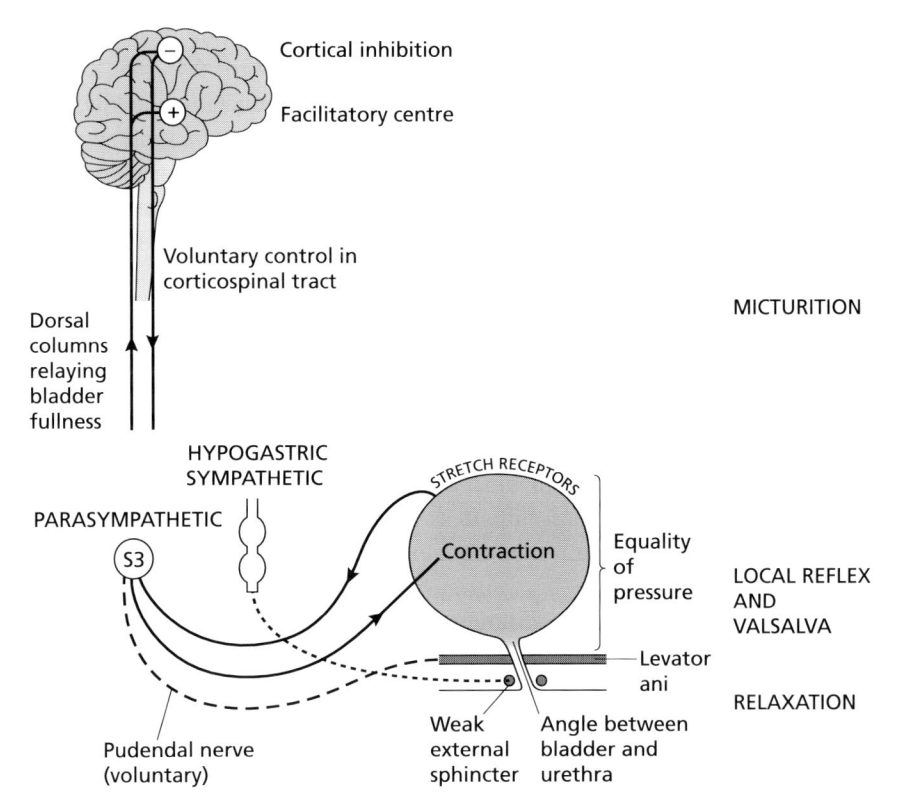

Fig. 8.1 Anatomy of the bladder.

8.4 Local infection: abscesses

Subarachnoid epidural abscess is a rare condition, but rapid recognition is required since swift treatment will limit or prevent nerve damage. The abscess usually represents an underlying spinal traumatic or degenerative condition [38], or bacteraemia. The abscess rarely occurs secondary to epidural injection [39]. In the unlikely event that an abscess follows epidural injection, the presentation of back pain and fever usually occurs up to two weeks afterwards. *Staphylococcus aureus* is the most common bacterial agent [40], and early diagnosis with magnetic resonance imaging and early laminectomy are the most important prognostic factors. Specific antibiotics can be used once the causative organism has been cultured, but since *Staphylococcus aureus* is very common, cephalosporins and metronidazole are appropriate initial treatments.

8.5 Peripheral nerve disorders

Sensory symptoms with numbness on the outer and anterior aspect of the thigh are the largest group of neurological symptoms after childbirth, but they are transient and occur in one in 100 women.

8.5.1 Carpal tunnel syndrome

The median nerve is compressed in the carpal tunnel, and painful symptoms usually develop at night when tissue oedema forms in the area. They can also be reproduced when a blood pressure cuff repeatedly occludes the arterial circulation. If a woman presents with an antenatal history of carpal tunnel syndrome, considerable care should be taken with the frequency of non-invasive blood pressure measurements during anaesthesia. Occasionally, surgical decompression is required in pregnancy, and infiltration local anaesthesia is appropriate.

8.5.2 Meralgia paraesthetica

This rare problem (compression of the lateral cutaneous nerve of the thigh) can either complicate an otherwise normal pregnancy or result from excessive retraction during Caesarean section. The lateral cutaneous nerve of the thigh is compressed as it passes laterally under the inguinal ligament, close to the attachment of the ligament to the ileum [41]. It produces an area of pain and numbness or altered sensation on the anterolateral surface of the thigh. It can be differentiated from compression of the lumbar nerve roots by a lack of motor effects.

Resolution usually occurs within three months of delivery, but if the symptoms are troublesome, infiltration with local anaesthetic solution where the nerve passes below the inguinal ligament can help. Transcutaneous electrical nerve stimulation (TENS) therapy has also been reported to be useful [42].

8.5.3 Root and nerve lesions in the leg

Traumatic nerve damage associated with labour and delivery usually affects the lower extremity. Injury is mainly caused by compression of the lumbosacral trunk by the descending fetus. Nerve roots L4 and L5 cross the pelvic rim (Fig. 8.2) to reach the lumbosacral plexus. They are not covered by the psoas muscle at this point, and are therefore vulnerable to pressure. The obturator nerve, which also crosses the pelvic inlet, may rarely be injured during delivery. Prolonged labour, abnormal maternal anatomy, e.g. in cephalopelvic disproportion such as occurs with a large baby relative to the size of the pelvis—and high forceps delivery may increase the frequency of these pressure effects, as may disorders of the nerves themselves, such as those occurring in diabetes and alcoholism.

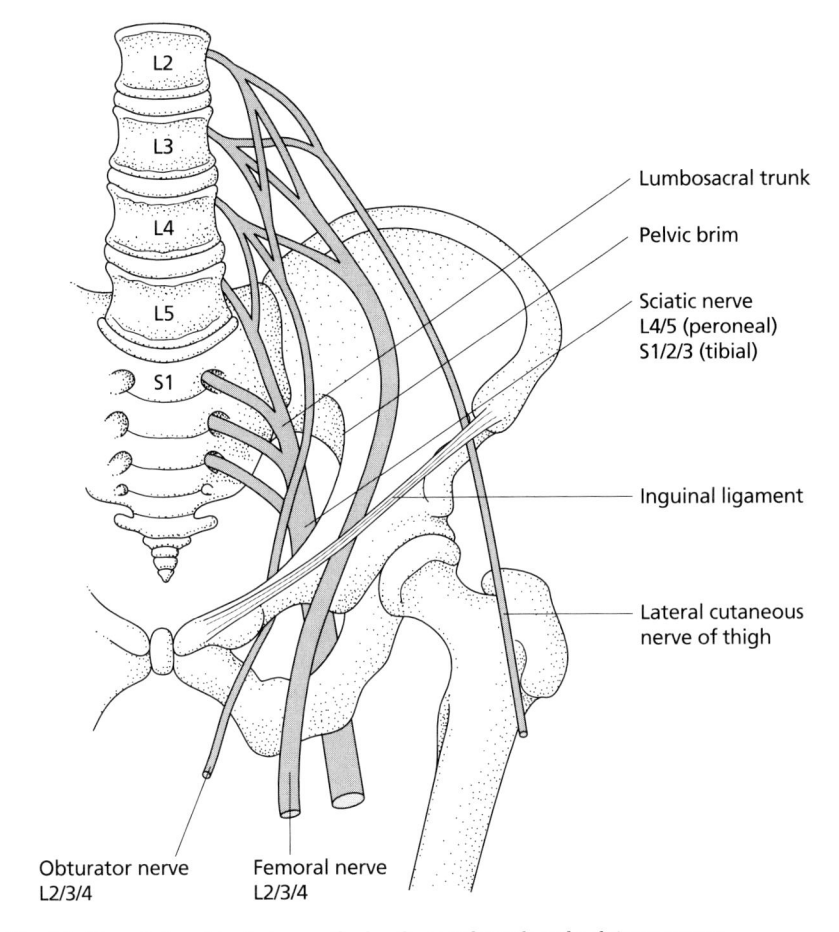

Fig. 8.2 The relationships between the lumbosacral trunk and pelvic structures.

Recognition of nerve lesions

Obturator nerve (L2, L3, L4). Postpartum, the lesion is usually unilateral. Sensation is decreased over the medial aspect of the thigh, and there is an inability to adduct the leg.

Femoral nerve (L2, L3, L4). When the femoral nerve is damaged, there will be decreased sensation on the anteromedial surface of the thigh and leg as far as the medial malleolus. The femoral nerve also supplies the muscles that extend the knee, so the knee jerk will be affected and the woman will have difficulty climbing stairs.

Root lesions of L2, L3 or L4 are very unlikely to be the result of disc disease. The femoral nerve may be injured with retractors during Caesarean section.

Sciatic nerve. The sciatic nerve may be damaged by an incorrectly administered intramuscular injection, as it lies in the buttock. A foot drop is the most commonly seen motor deficit, and this can be associated with compression of the L4–L5 contributions of the lumbosacral trunk as they cross the pelvic brim. The nerve has two divisions: the common peroneal nerve (roots L4, L5), and the tibial nerve (roots S1, S2, S3).

Common peroneal nerve (L4, L5). This nerve is most commonly injured, as it passes superficially over the head of the fibula lateral to the knee joint. Pressure at this point may be exerted in the lithotomy position. Loss of sensation occurs over the anterolateral aspect of the calf and the dorsum of the foot—often just the dorsum of the foot. Foot drop occurs, with loss of inversion, eversion and dorsiflexion. Occasionally, bilateral palsies occur after a prolonged second stage in the squatting position.

Tibial nerve S1, S2, S3. This nerve is rarely injured. However, disc lesions often affect the S1 root, and the ankle can be affected, as well as sensation at the back of the thigh down to the sole of the foot.

8.6 Mood disorders and pregnancy

The parturient woman experiences a time of great hormonal variation during and after pregnancy, often accompanied by stressful family, social and economic consequences that are not always desired. Pregnancy itself frequently generates emotional well-being, but mood instability can occur, and pregnancy is a risk factor for depressive illness. Psychiatric disorder is one of a number of factors underlying failure to attend the antenatal clinic.

Depressive illness usually presents in the first trimester. If it is severe and a woman is suicidal, treatment is required throughout pregnancy. The tricyclic drugs have powerful anticholinergic effects and have toxic effects on the newborn such as jitteriness, hyperexcitability and suckling problems up to 10 days after delivery. Monoamine oxidase inhibitors are not used, due to teratogenicity. Fluoxetine is a selective inhibitor of serotonin uptake, and is the preferred long-term treatment for severe depression in pregnancy. Confounding factors in studies of antidepressants include the depression itself and maternal outcome without treatment; neonatal–maternal adaptations; and the use of other psychoactive drugs in at least one-third of women [43].

References

1 Butterworth JF, Walker FO, Lysak SZ. Pregnancy increases median nerve sensitivity to lidocaine. *Anesthesiology* 1990; **72**: 962–5.
2 Fagraeus L, Urban B, Bromage PL. Spread of epidural analgesia in early pregnancy. *Anesthesiology* 1983; **58**: 184–7.

3 Bromage PL. Continuous lumbar epidural analgesia for obstetrics. *Can Med Assoc J* 1961; **85**: 1136–40.
4 Palahnuik RJ, Shnider SM, Eger EIII. Pregnancy decreases the requirements for inhaled anaesthetic agents. *Anesthesiology* 1974; **41**: 82–3.
5 Merryman W. Progesterone 'anesthesia' in human subjects. *J Clin Endocrinol Metab* 1954; **14**: 1567–9.
6 Brodie MJ. Management of epilepsy during pregnancy and lactation. *Lancet* 1990; **336**: 426–7.
7 Cleland PG. Management of pre-existing disorders in pregnancy. *Epilepsy Prescr J* 1996; **36**: 102–9.
8 Enevoldson TP, Russell RW. Cerebral venous thrombosis: new causes for an old syndrome? *Q J Med* 1990; **77**: 1255–75.
9 Department of Health. *Report on Confidential Enquiries into Maternal Deaths in the United Kingdom, 1988–1990.* London: HMSO, 1994.
10 Kittner SJ, Stern BJ, Feeser BR *et al.* Pregnancy and the risk of stroke. *N Engl J Med* 1996; **335**: 768–74.
11 Bruns PD, Linder RO, Drose VE, Battaglia F. The placental transfer of water from fetus to mother following the intravenous infusion of hypertonic mannitol to the maternal rabbit. *Am J Obstet Gynecol* 1963; **86**: 160–6.
12 Wisoff JH, Kratzert KJ, Handwerker SM, Young BK, Epstein F. Pregnancy in women with cerebrosubarachnoid fluid shunts: report of a series and review of the literature. *Neurosurgery* 1991; **29**: 827–3.
13 Gar MJ, Grubb RL, Strickler RC. Maternal hydrocephalus and pregnancy. *Obstet Gynecol* 1983; **63**: 296–315.
14 Young BK, Katz M, Klein S. Pregnancy after spinal cord injury: altered maternal and fetal response to labour. *Obstet Gynecol* 1983; **62**: 59–63.
15 Ciliberti BJ, Goldfein J, Rovenstine EA. Hypertension during anaesthesia in women with spinal cord injury. *Anaesthesia* 1953; **15**: 273–9.
16 Stirt JA, Marco A, Conklin KA. Obstetric anesthesia for a quadriplegic woman with autonomic hyperreflexia. *Anesthesiology* 1979; **51**: 560–2.
17 Abouleish EI, Hanley ES, Palmer SM. Can epidural fentanyl control autonomic hyperreflexia in a quadreplegic parturient? *Anesth Analg* 1989; **68**: 523–6.
18 Kobayashi A, Mizobe T, Tojo H, Hashimoto S. Autonomic hyperreflexia during labour. *Can J Anaesth* 1995; **42**: 1134–6.
19 Schapira K, Poskanzer DC, Newell DJ, Miller H. Marriage, pregnancy and multiple sclerosis. *Brain* 1966; **89**: 419–28.
20 Bernardi S, Grass MG, Bertollini R, Orzi F, Feischi C. The influence of pregnancy on relapses in multiple sclerosis: a cohort study. *Acta Neurol Scand* 1991; **84**: 403–6.
21 Roullet E, Verdier-Taillefer MH, Amarenco P *et al.* Pregnancy and multiple sclerosis: a longitudinal study of 125 remittent women. *J Neurol Neurosurg Psychiatry* 1993; **56**: 1062–5.
22 Warren TM, Datta S, Ostheimer GW. Lumbar epidural anesthesia in a woman with multiple sclerosis. *Anesth Analg* 1982; **61**: 1022–3.
23 Eickhoff K, Wikstrom J, Poser S, Bauer H. Protein profile of cerebrospinal fluid in multiple sclerosis, with special reference to the function of the blood–brain barrier. *J Neurol* 1977; **214**: 207–15.
24 Lindstrom JM, Seybold ME, Lennon VA, Whittingham S, Duane DD. Antibody to acetylcholine receptor in myasthenia gravis: prevalence, clinical correlates, and diagnostic value. *Neurology* 1976; **26**: 1054–9.
25 Plauche WE. Myasthenia gravis in pregnancy. *Am J Obstet Gynecol* 1964; **88**: 404–6.
26 Baraka A. Anaesthesia and myasthenia gravis. *Can J Anaesth* 1992; **39**: 476–86.

27 Coaldrake LA, Livingstone PA. Myasthenia gravis in pregnancy. *Anaesth Intensive Care* 1983; **11**: 254–7.
28 Rolbin SH, Levinson G, Snider SM, Wright RG. Anesthetic considerations for myasthenia gravis and pregnancy. *Anesth Analg* 1978; **57**: 441–50.
29 Ptacek LJ, Johnson KJ, Griggs RC. Genetics and physiology of the myotonia disorders. *N Engl J Med* 1993; **328**: 482–9.
30 Hopkins A, Wray S. The effect of pregnancy on dystrophic myotonica. *Neurology* 1967; **17**: 166–8.
31 Speedy H. Exaggerated physiological responses to propofol in myotonic dystrophy. *Br J Anaesth* 1990; **64**: 110–12.
32 Mitchell MM, Ali HH, Savarese JJ. Myotonia and neuromuscular blocking agents. *Anesthesiology* 1978; **49**: 44–8.
33 Matthews NC, Corser G. Epidural fentanyl for shaking in obstetrics. *Anaesthesia* 1988; **43**: 783–5.
34 Sevarino FB, Johnson MD, Lema MJ *et al.* The effect of epidural sufentanil on shivering and body temperature in the parturient. *Anesth Analg* 1989; **68**: 530–3.
35 Russell SH, Hirsch NP. Anaesthesia and myotonica. *Br J Anaesth* 1994; **72**: 210–16.
36 MacArthur C, Lewis M, Knox EG. Health after childbirth. *Br J Obstet Gynaecol* 1991; **98**: 1193–5.
37 Snooks SJ, Swash M, Mathers SG, Henry MM. Effect of vaginal delivery on the pelvic floor: a 5-year follow up. *Br J Surg* 1990; **77**: 1358–60.
38 Ericsson M, Algers G, Schliamser SE. Subarachnoid epidural abscess in adults: review and report of iatrogenic cases. *Scand J Infect Dis* 1990; **22**: 249–57.
39 Mamourian AC, Dickman CA, Drayer BP, Sonntag VKH. Subarachnoid epidural abscess: three cases following subarachnoid epidural injections demonstrated with magnetic resonance imaging. *Anesthesiology* 1993; **78**: 204–7.
40 Ngan Kee WD, Jones MR, Thomas P, Worth RJ. Epidural abscess complicating epidural anaesthesia for Caesarean section. *Br J Anaesth* 1992; **69**: 647–52.
41 Rhodes P. Meralgia paraesthesia in pregnancy. *Lancet* 1957; **ii**: 831.
42 Fisher AP, Hanna M. Transcutaneous electrical nerve stimulation in meralgia paraesthetica of pregnancy. *Br J Obstet Gynaecol* 1987; **94**: 603–5.
43 Robert E. Treating depression in pregnancy. *N Engl J Med* 1996; **335**: 1056–8.

9: Metabolism and its Disorders in Pregnancy

During pregnancy, the changing energy requirements of maternal, placental and fetal tissues have to be met. Energy in the form of adenosine triphosphate (ATP) is generated, predominantly by the breakdown of either carbohydrates or fat (Fig. 9.1). The relative contribution of these substrates is dependent on their availability and on factors influencing enzyme activity. These can be influenced by the pregnant state itself, or by pathological disorders. The changes in energy requirements during pregnancy can be divided into those associated with the development of fat stores in the second trimester, and those connected with fetal growth requirements in the third trimester (Fig. 9.2).

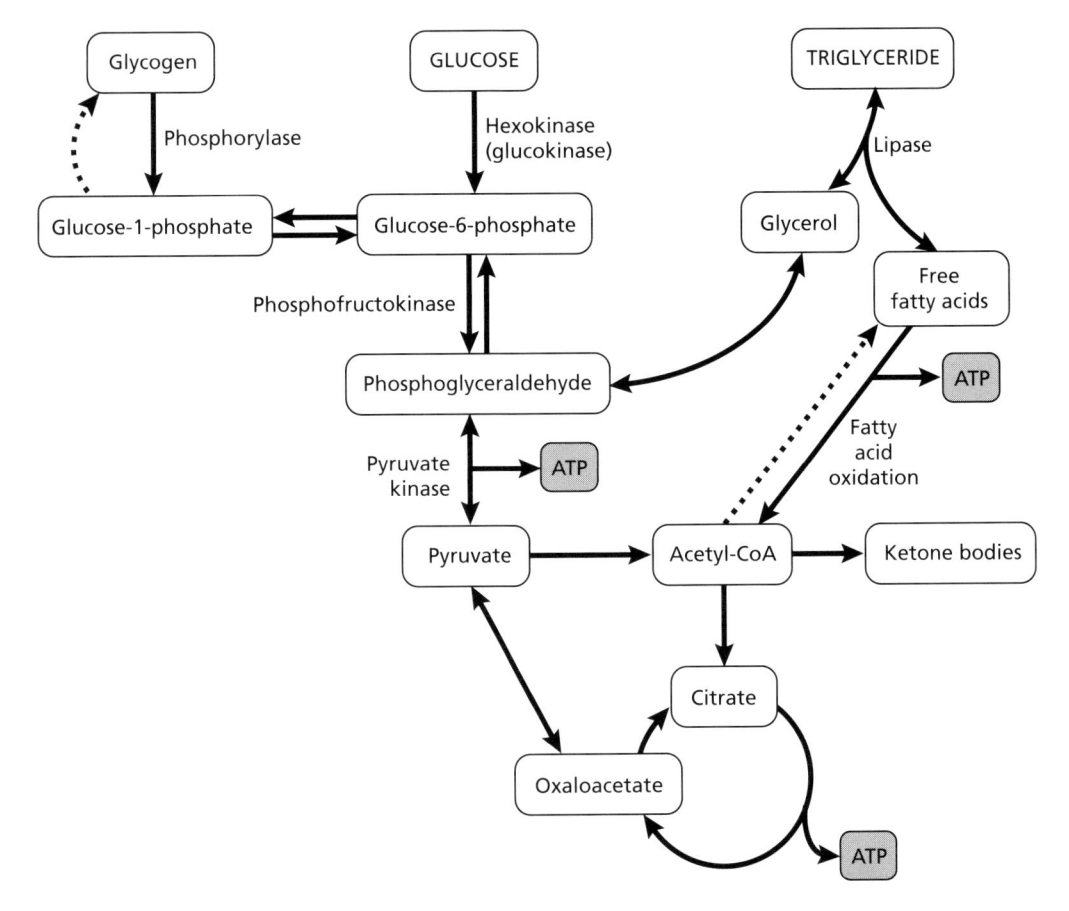

Fig. 9.1 The main pathways of energy production, as adenosine triphosphate (ATP), from carbohydrate and fat sources.

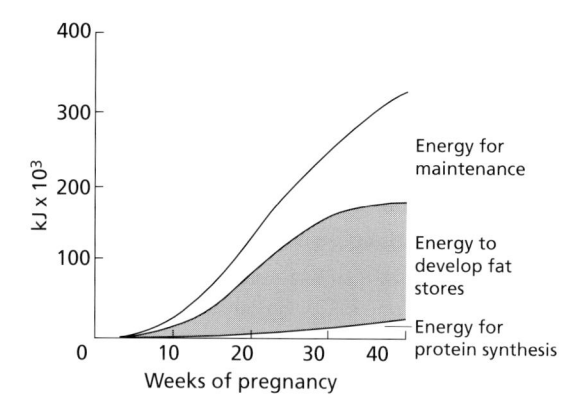

Fig. 9.2 The cumulative energy cost of pregnancy and its components. (Adapted with permission from [66].)

Table 9.1 Nutrients in blood.

Changes in pregnancy		Comments
Proteins		
Albumin	*Plasma concentration decreases early in pregnancy* (total protein mirrors changes)	Colloid osmotic pressure decreases (the risk of pulmonary oedema increases)
		Carrier protein function may be altered (no specific problems occur, probably because the total circulating amount is normal)
Globulins	*Small rise*	This is the result of complex changes, e.g. immunoglobulins, specific pregnancy proteins
Lipids	*A considerable increase in most plasma lipids*	Diet has no effect
Cholesterol		Low levels in mid-pregnancy are consistent with storage
Free fatty acids		Increasing levels in the last trimester are associated with lipolysis
Lipoproteins		Increase in high-density lipoproteins

9.1 Nutrition

The daily energy requirements are increased during the last trimester of pregnancy by 0.8 MJ/day (200 kcal/day) [1]. This value may be lower in some ethnic groups such as Asian women, when glucose intolerance is present. A carbohydrate intake of 200 g/day should provide just under half of the daily energy requirement. Daily energy requirements cannot be provided by 5% glucose. This contains 50 g of glucose per litre, which is only 840 kJ (200 kcal). The dietary protein requirement in pregnancy is about 1 g/kg/day, and it increases by 5 g/day during lactation. Daily mineral requirements are 15 mg of iron, 100 µg of folic acid and 800 mg of calcium [1]. The changes in nutrients in the blood in pregnancy are described in Table 9.1.

9.2 Carbohydrates

Glucose is the basic substance for energy production in the cell, and it is broken down by glycolysis to pyruvate. It is phosphorylated to form glucose-6-phosphate, a reaction catalysed by hexokinase. There is an additional enzyme in the liver called glucokinase that has a greater specificity for glucose, and which—unlike hexokinase—is increased by insulin and decreased in diabetes. Glycogen is the storage form of glucose. Storage occurs mainly in the liver and skeletal muscle. Phosphofructokinase is the enzyme that adds energy into the glycolytic pathway. Interconversions between carbohydrates, fats and protein include the conversion of glycerol to an intermediate in the glycolytic pathway. Glucose can be converted to fats through acetyl-CoA, but the conversion of pyruvate to acetyl-CoA is irreversible, so that there is very little conversion of fats to carbohydrate. Glycolysis to pyruvate occurs outside the mitochondria. Pyruvate then enters the mitochondria, and is oxidized to release energy in the citric acid cycle. Lactate is produced under anaerobic conditions.

9.2.1 Alterations in carbohydrate metabolism in pregnancy

The pregnant state is associated with hormones that have diabetogenic properties (such as human placental lactogen, progesterone, prolactin and cortisol), with a reduced activity in the liver of the enzymes glucokinase and phosphofructokinase [2] and peripheral insulin resistance, predominantly in muscle tissue. Normal pregnant women counteract this by augmenting insulin secretion [3].

Women with gestational diabetes do not have the capacity to increase insulin secretion, so that glucose accumulates. Fat and protein metabolism are accelerated, and consequently protein depletion can occur. Ketone bodies form, and the plasma level of free fatty acids increases. This augments maternal–fetal fat transfer. Increased fatty acid oxidation may reduce pyruvate kinase activity in both the mother and fetus [4]. The altered glycogen metabolism in fetal lungs may be associated with decreased synthesis of surfactant and with an increased incidence of respiratory distress in the newborn of diabetic mothers [5].The reduction in pyruvate kinase can result in a reduction in blood pyruvate. This can alter the ratio of lactate/pyruvate, but does not signify the presence of lactic acidosis [6].

Glucose

Circulating glucose (Fig. 9.3) is obtained from dietary sources, the hydrolysis of glycogen stored in the liver (glycogenolysis), and the production of glucose from non-carbohydrate sources (gluconeogenesis). The liver can remove glucose from the blood to store it as glycogen or it can raise blood glucose levels by glycogenolysis, depending on whether or not the mother has taken food.

140   CHAPTER 9

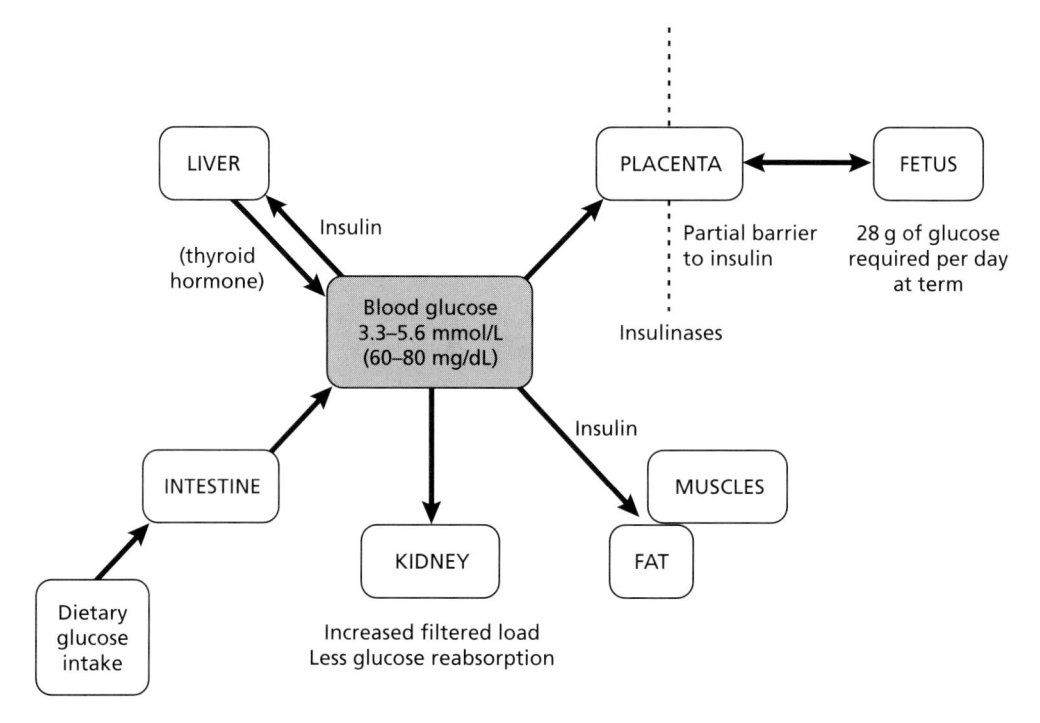

Fig. 9.3 Maintenance of blood glucose level.

Expanded maternal blood volume
Placental transfer of glucose
Altered hormonal balance

Table 9.2 Causes of decreased fasting blood glucose level in pregnancy.

The activity of the liver in maintaining normal levels of glucose is influenced by various hormones, principally insulin, which also reduces blood glucose levels by stimulating an increase in peripheral glucose uptake and utilization (Table 9.2). Blood glucose levels are increased by growth hormone, glucocorticoids, glucagon, catecholamines and thyroid hormones.

Glucose is lost from the circulation in pregnancy via the kidneys because of a low renal threshold, and through the placenta by facilitated diffusion. Placental metabolism accounts for 60% of the glucose taken up from the maternal circulation. Transplacental transfer of glucose is dependent on maternal plasma concentration, and so is highest after a meal. Utilization of glucose by the fetus continues while a mother fasts. Maternal fasting venous glucose concentration decreases by 10–15% in the last trimester of pregnancy compared with the non-pregnant state; average values are 3.7 mmol/L (68 mg/dL) and 4.4 mmol/L (80 mg/dL), respectively [7]. This decrease occurs despite an increase in systemic glucose production, and could be the result of increased distribution space [8].

Glucose is freely filtered by the glomeruli in the kidney, but is almost all reabsorbed in the proximal tubules. The renal threshold is the plasma level at which glucose first appears in the urine in more than the usual minute amounts. It is 10 mmol/L (180 mg/dL). Pregnancy-induced glycosuria in rats is due to the decrease in reabsorption from the distal portions of the nephron [9]. Glycosuria of pregnancy could be the result of an increase in filtered load from the increase in glomerular filtration rate, or a change in tubular reabsorption, or a combination of the two. Glucose reabsorption is less complete in pregnancy [10] and depends on many factors, including pregnancy hormones. However, the filtered load is probably the most important factor.

The demands of the growing fetus and increased maternal metabolism necessitate the availability of more glucose, and hence insulin secretion, to maintain intracellular availability. Resistance to peripheral insulin activity develops during pregnancy, especially in the third trimester. Hormonal factors have been implicated. Human placental lactogen is produced by the syncytiotrophoblast of the placenta, and the size and structure of the molecule are similar to that of growth hormone, an insulin antagonist. Oestrogen and progestogen also progressively increase, and may contribute to insulin resistance effects. Whole-body insulin resistance is increased to about three times that observed in the non-pregnant state. This increase is mainly caused by cellular, post-insulin receptor events generated by one or more of the pregnancy hormones and free cortisol [3]. After the placenta is delivered, insulin resistance decreases very rapidly. Consequently, close attention must be directed to insulin requirements in the diabetic parturient following delivery.

An adequate reserve of beta cell pancreatic mass is necessary to meet the increased insulin requirements, particularly during the last trimester of pregnancy. If this functional beta cell mass is not available, gestational diabetes will emerge. The onset of gestational diabetes parallels the progression of insulin resistance that develops in the second half of pregnancy. Additional demands for insulin secretion may be caused by stress such as surgery, infection or steroid treatment, and may unmask subclinical gestational diabetes.

Detection of hyperglycaemia

When plasma glucose is elevated over a period of time, small amounts of haemoglobin are non-enzymatically glycosylated to form haemoglobin A_{1c} (HbA_{1c}), with a glucose molecule attached to the terminal valine in each beta chain. Glycosylated haemoglobin is a poor transporter of oxygen [11]. HbA_{1c} can be measured, and its concentration reflects glycaemic control during the prior four weeks (or more). A glycosylated haemoglobin value of 8% corresponds to an average daily blood glucose concentration of about 11 mmol/L (200 mg/dL) [12]. The normal amount is below 6%. Albumin is also glycosylated, but has a more rapid turnover and is therefore not such a useful marker of hyperglycaemia.

Insulin and blood glucose control

The placenta has always been considered to be a barrier to insulin, but glucose passively crosses from the mother to the fetus. Passage of insulin as an antibody-bound complex from mother to fetus has been demonstrated in diabetic patients [13]. Maternal insulin exerts an effect on both maternal and fetal energy sources. Fetal glucose levels reflect maternal levels, but may lag behind them if maternal insulin therapy is given as boluses. If maternal hyperglycaemia is present throughout pregnancy, the fetus will be exposed to it, and this may result in beta cell hyperplasia in the fetus and hyperinsulinaemia. This response may outlast the stimulus, and such a fetus when delivered is at risk of hypoglycaemia. Fetal hyperinsulinaemia can also result in increased birth weight, with problems of shoulder dystocia complicating delivery.

There is a transition in the fetus from intrauterine dependence on maternal glucose to extrauterine activation of catabolic processes and the mobilization and utilization of endogenous fuel sources. The surges of glycogen and epinephrine at birth, coupled with a decrease in insulin secretion, develop patterns of receptor changes and enzyme activity such as phosphorylase activation [14].

Metabolism in labour

Muscular activity in the uterus or skeletal muscles as a consequence of pain, respiratory activity and shivering increases metabolic requirements dramatically. Tissue demands for oxygen may not be met because of reduced blood flow if dehydration is present. Anaerobic metabolism will then occur, with increased blood lactate levels, in an effort to produce adequate energy. Thus, acidosis predominates over the respiratory alkalosis. Situations that aggravate these acid–base disorders include vomiting, hypothermia and haemorrhage.

Metabolism is also affected by hormones that interfere with glucose utilization, such as catecholamines and cortisol. All of these increase in labour, particularly when pain relief is inadequate [15,16].

9.3 Disorders of metabolism

9.3.1 Diabetes

Pregnancy is characterized by several factors tending to lead to glucose intolerance, mainly the secretion of diabetogenic hormones and increasing insulin resistance. Pregnancy can be viewed as a physiological stress on the beta cells, and glucose tolerance will depend on the adequacy of maternal beta cell reserves (Fig. 9.4). The frequency of gestational diabetes within a population reflects that of impaired glucose tolerance and the development of non-insulin-dependent diabetes in older women. When a glucose load is given to a patient,

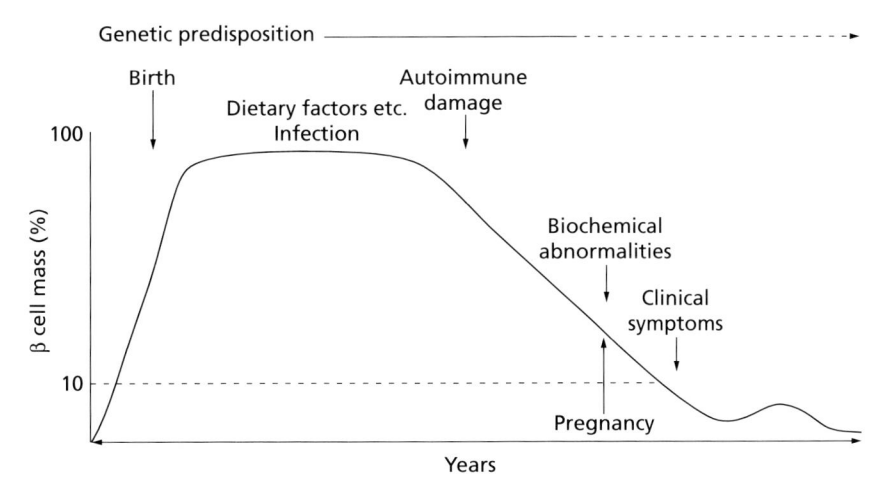

Fig. 9.4 The gradual changes in beta cell mass that can develop in gestational diabetes or insulin-dependent diabetes.

the blood glucose response is an indirect measure of pancreatic function. The distribution curve of blood glucose values in a population shows no separate population with higher than 'normal' levels [17]. The definition of diabetes is therefore arbitrary. The gestational nature of a patient's diabetes can theoretically only be confirmed retrospectively when responses to a glucose load have returned to normal. Deterioration of glucose tolerance following gestational diabetes is associated with factors related to insulin sensitivity, e.g. obesity, ethnic group and a positive family history of non-insulin-dependent diabetes (Table 9.3).

Glucose tolerance test

The glucose load, its route and the method of glucose analysis are variable. The oral route of administration is preferred. Amounts of 100 g (USA), 75 g (WHO) and 50 g (Europe, Australasia) have been advocated [18]. Arterial, venous and capillary sampling have all been used. Plasma levels of glucose measured by the glucose oxidase or hexokinase methods are higher than whole-blood measurements using the Somogyi–Neilsen method, because the latter also measures non-glucose-reducing substances. Individual hospitals and laboratories have their own limits of normality, and although international standardization may not be possible, individual criteria will not vary greatly. Screening of patients with glycosuria with an oral glucose tolerance test and plasma or serum sampling for gestational diabetes usually occurs at 28 weeks of pregnancy. Earlier screening is likely to miss a small percentage of cases. A short, 50-g, one-hour glucose challenge test with a cut-off point of 7.8 mmol/L (140 mg/dL) is followed, if positive, by a 100-g oral glucose tolerance test. The cut-off points for venous plasma or serum samples are:

Table 9.3 Risk factors for the development of diabetes in pregnancy.

Family history of diabetes
Previous gestational diabetes
Obesity
Previous large baby
Poor obstetric history
Age

Table 9.4 Characteristics of gestational diabetes.

Complicates 2–3% of pregnancies
Babies no longer have an increased risk of congenital abnormalities if the diabetes is well controlled
At risk of large fetus
10–20% of gestational diabetics develop non-insulin-dependent diabetes later
70% develop non-insulin-dependent diabetes if obese
Diabetic complications such as ketoacidosis and vascular problems are now rare
Commoner in Asian-born than Caucasian women

- fasting, 5.8 mmol/L (105 mg/dL);
- one hour, 10.5 mmol/L (190 mg/dL);
- two hours, 9.2 mmol/L (165 mg/dL);
- three hours, 8.1 mmol/L (145 mg/dL).

diabetes is the most common medical disorder in pregnancy. The two-hour serum diagnostic level for diabetes mellitus is more than 11.1 mmol/L (200 mg/dL). A figure of 8–11 mmol/L indicates some impairment of glucose tolerance. Of the 2–3% of pregnancies that are complicated by diabetes (Table 9.4), more than 90% have this impairment of glucose tolerance. In a large multicentre study on glucose tolerance in normal pregnancy [19], more than 10% of women had two-hour glucose concentrations of more than 8 mmol/L after an oral 75 g glucose tolerance test. It is unlikely that such a high percentage of women have a disordered carbohydrate metabolism.

Complications of diabetes

Maternal. Maternal complications are more common if diabetes is present before 24 weeks' gestation [20]. The disease itself can be associated with considerable variability in blood sugar and ketoacidosis, and with organ-specific problems related to vascular disturbances in the renal circulation (Table 9.5), cardiovascular circulation and retinal circulation. These may exacerbate the hypertensive disorders of pregnancy [21]. Renal function may deteriorate further after associated secondary infection in the renal tract. Obstetric complications (Table 9.6) [22] include pre-eclampsia, polyhydramnios and preterm delivery.

Table 9.5 Problems associated with diabetic nephropathy.

Abnormal renal function affects drug excretion
Proteinuria
Hypertension
Coexistent retinopathy
Pre-eclampsia is more common, further increasing protein loss and affecting blood pressure control

Table 9.6 Incidence of obstetric complications associated with diabetic nephropathy.

Pre-eclampsia	40%
Intrauterine growth retardation	18%
Fetal distress	24%
Anaemia	42%
Polyhydramnios	27%
Preterm delivery	
< 37 weeks	56%
< 32 weeks	23%
Perinatal mortality	3%

Fetal. The fetal complications associated with diabetes that have been described include major congenital abnormalities, intrauterine fetal distress, macrosomia and birth trauma. These have been reduced to normal levels because of improved maternal blood glucose control (especially at the time of organogenesis), ultrasound and early delivery by Caesarean section [23]. Neonatal complications associated with uncontrolled diabetes include respiratory distress syndrome, hypoglycaemia, hyperglycaemia and hyperbilirubinaemia.

Management of diabetes

Historical. The management of diabetes in pregnancy has changed in the past few years, and differs considerably from when the condition was initially recognized. Before the availability of insulin in 1923, there were reports of non-insulin-dependent gestational diabetes. Fetal hypoglycaemia was recognized as a complication, and associated congenital malformations were reported. Once insulin became available, early delivery was advocated to avoid the trauma of a large baby, but that policy led to fetal deaths due to prematurity and respiratory distress syndrome. In the 1970s, a policy of metabolic normalization and continued fetal surveillance was initiated. This continued more rigorously into the 1980s, with meticulous control of maternal glucose levels and antepartum fetal biophysical profiles such as ultrasonography, fetal movements, heart rate changes, and hormonal and amniotic fluid phospholipid changes, as well as Doppler studies [24].

It was found that if euglycaemia was achieved before conception and main-tained throughout pregnancy, congenital malformations could be

Table 9.7 Signs of diabetic ketoacidosis. NB, this is an acute emergency with a high risk of fetal mortality.

Vomiting
Thirst
Polyuria
Weakness
Hyperventilation
Altered mental state
Hypotension and tachycardia
Fruity odour on breath

Biochemistry
Plasma glucose variable, above 11 mmol/L (200 mg/dL)
Bicarbonate ≤ 15 mmol/L
Arterial pH ≤ 7.30
Positive serum ketones

prevented [25], and morbidity and mortality could be reduced to non-diabetic levels.

Combined specialist care. Pregnant women known to be diabetic, and those who are screened and found to have an abnormal glucose tolerance test, should be referred to a combined obstetric and endocrine clinic in which the obstetric and medical diabetic management teams work in consultation. Such teams will produce management guidelines.

Diet alone is often sufficient to control gestational diabetes. The daily amount of carbohydrate in the diet is adjusted to the size of the patient, so that slim women would have 160 g of carbohydrate, whereas obese women would have 120 g. A 10–12 kg weight gain in pregnancy would be expected.

Frequent daily capillary blood glucose estimates, e.g. with glucose oxidase strips and portable reflectance colorimeter [26], with weekly verification of venous blood glucose measurements in the laboratory, are required [27]. The aim is to achieve preprandial levels of less than 5.0 mmol/L and postprandial levels less than 7.0 mmol/L, i.e. within normal concentrations of 4–6 mmol/L. If this is not achieved by diet, insulin is administered twice daily as a mixture of short-acting and intermediate-acting insulin preparations. The patient's compliance with these requirements is checked by monthly measurements of HbA_{1c}, which should be below 7%. If compliance or blood glucose control is inadequate, in-patient admission may be required. The combined clinics also check for signs of fetal or placental abnormalities and diabetic complications, and routinely test the urine for infection.

Renal tract infection is a common cause of difficulties with blood glucose control. Diabetic ketoacidosis may be precipitated by infections, or may be the presenting problem in newly diagnosed diabetes. A lower presenting blood glucose level is likely to occur in pregnant women. Table 9.7 lists the signs of diabetic ketoacidosis. It is an acute emergency, and is diagnosed by positive serum ketones, an arterial blood pH ≤ 7.30 and/or a serum bicarbonate

Table 9.8 Sliding scale for insulin infusions during vaginal delivery in diabetic parturients.

Capillary blood glucose level (mmol/L)	Insulin dosage
0–4	None
4.5–9.0	2 U/h
9.5–13.0	3 U/h
13.5–17.0	4 U/h

⩽ 15 mmol/L. Admission to hospital and intensive combined care are required to prevent morbidity and mortality. Intravenous fluid and electrolyte management and insulin administration should be started immediately. The most serious complication is the onset of cerebral oedema, with headaches and deterioration in the level of consciousness. The pathophysiology of the condition is poorly understood [28].

Diabetes and labour

Metabolic problems. Both hyperglycaemia and starvation can increase the production of ketones. The resulting ketoacidosis compounds the normal acidosis that occurs in labour. Close monitoring of blood sugar levels is therefore important, and appropriate insulin dosage should be controlled with a sliding scale. The increase in catecholamines that occurs in labour will increase the production of ketones and lactate. Epidural analgesia is positively indicated in this situation to avoid the catecholamine surge. It will also help to prevent fetal hyperglycaemia with consequent neonatal hypoglycaemia.

Intrapartum management of diabetes. Local guidelines should be available in each obstetric unit. The following outline of management is that followed at Hammersmith Hospital, London.

1 *Vaginal delivery.* Labour is often induced between 38 and 40 weeks' gestation in order to avoid complications such as cephalopelvic disproportion or placental insufficiency. Earlier intervention may be required, depending on the type and severity of the complications. The woman fasts overnight before artificial rupture of the membranes early in the morning. Her usual morning dose of insulin is withheld in case fetal distress necessitates urgent delivery. At induction of labour, an infusion of 500 mL of 5% dextrose and 10 mmol KCl is commenced at 100 mL/h. This will provide 5 g of glucose per hour, and is the minimum requirement. A separate infusion of 50 units of insulin (Actrapid) in 50 mL 0.9% NaCl is started if the capillary blood glucose (NB, the mother is fasting) is more than 4.5 mmol/L. The infusion is given according to a sliding scale (Table 9.8). The capillary blood glucose level is measured every hour, and the sliding scale is adjusted as required. The aim is to keep the level between 4 and 5 mmol/L. Every four hours, the venous blood glucose and urea and electrolytes are measured by the laboratory.

2 *Caesarean section.* After overnight fasting, the venous blood glucose level and urea and electrolytes are measured by the laboratory. The dextrose and insulin infusions are started as described above for vaginal delivery, and capillary blood glucose is measured half-hourly. A blood glucose level of 4–5 mmol/L (70–90 mg/dL) should be maintained. The insulin infusion is commenced at 1 mL/h, and the operation is scheduled for early to mid-morning. Insulin requirements after delivery will reduce rapidly, and may be nothing for the first 24 hours postpartum. Hypoglycaemia should be treated with 5–10 g glucose intravenously.

Postpartum management. Treatment with insulin should stop after delivery if diabetes has been first diagnosed in pregnancy, i.e. it is gestational diabetes. If the woman is a known diabetic, the requirements for insulin will be reduced within 24 hours of delivery.

Hypoglycaemia

1 Maternal. Although a lower fasting blood glucose is usual in the third trimester, the hypoglycaemic threshold for symptoms does not change. Rigorous insulin therapy in diabetes can precipitate hypoglycaemia, with the potential to cause maternal coma and fetal death. The urgent administration of 20 g of glucose intravenously is a life-saving treatment. Patients with the haemolysis, elevated liver enzymes and low platelet count (HELLP) syndrome present a similar picture, because of fulminant liver failure. Other rare conditions, such as insulinoma, will need to be excluded from the differential diagnosis.

2 Fetal. In healthy parturients, the administration of more than 20 g glucose intravenously per hour can precipitate neonatal hypoglycaemia.

Table 9.9 Antenatal assessment for anaesthesia in a diabetic mother.

Maternal
Control of diabetes
Previous obstetric and anaesthetic history
Vascular complications
   Hypertension
   Retinopathy
   Coronary artery disease
   Nephropathy
   Fetal intrauterine growth retardation
Obesity
Neuropathy (including the autonomic nervous system)
Ripening of cervix

Fetal
Gestation (prematurity)
Estimated weight
Degree of fetal distress

Diabetes and anaesthetic management

1 Antenatal assessment (Table 9.9). Diabetes is a multisystem disorder. It can be associated with obesity, hypertension, myocardial ischaemia, renal failure, and neuropathies of the peripheral or autonomic nerves. The severity of these complications has to be defined, and any anaesthetic technique must be tailored to minimize further disturbances to both the mother and the fetus. Antenatal anaesthetic consultations should therefore be organized for any diabetic parturient with poor diabetic control or signs of involvement of any of these systems in their disease.

Anaesthetic complications that can be anticipated, and for which management plans can be formulated, are:
- metabolic, e.g. ketoacidosis from dehydration and unstable diabetes, or associated with catecholamine release;
- cardiovascular instability due to hypertensive disorders or autonomic neuropathy;
- pharmacokinetic, e.g. as a result of renal failure reducing drug excretion;
- technical, e.g. airway obstruction in obesity;
- fetal resuscitation.

If β-sympathomimetic drugs are given to arrest premature labour or corticosteroids are given to the mother to induce fetal lung maturation, hyperglycaemia and ketoacidosis can result, and can lead to a substantial increase in insulin requirements.

2 Intrapartum care (Table 9.10). An anaesthetist should expect a vaginal delivery to be attempted if there is a cephalic presentation, the fetus has an estimated weight of less than 3500 g, and the woman is either multiparous or primiparous and less than 30 years of age [29]. In patients with diabetic retinopathy, straining should be avoided at delivery. A Caesarean section will be the preferred method of delivery if there is fetal distress, macrosomia (above 4000 g), an unripened cervix and instability in diabetic control. Neonatal resuscitation should be expected following any type of delivery, and care should be taken to avoid, or identify and treat, hypoglycaemia and hyperbilirubinaemia in the neonate.

(i) *Vaginal delivery.* The diabetic parturient is more likely to experience complications that may affect the course of labour. Fetal distress is more common because of reduced placental blood flow, and HbA_{1c} decreases oxygen carriage. Continuous fetal monitoring by scalp electrode or cardiotocography and monitoring of acidosis by fetal scalp sampling is essential. The mother will not be able to have a normal oral intake, so acidosis occurs more frequently unless adequate fluid is administered and glucose control is achieved [30]. Dehydration must be avoided. Excess water loss can occur with hyperventilation or excessive sweating. If the mother becomes acidotic, ketones can cross the placenta and affect fetal acid–base status.

Table 9.10 General requirements for maternal diabetic anaesthetic care.

Action	Comment
Reassess insulin requirements immediately after delivery	Insulin resistance is reduced after delivery
Avoid hypoglycaemia	Monitor blood glucose closely after delivery
	It may interfere with uterine action
	It may be undiagnosed during general anaesthesia and lead to cerebral dysfunction
	It can cause fits
	It can lead to unconsciousness, lack of airway control and aspiration of stomach contents
Avoid hyperglycaemia	It may increase the risk of fetal distress
	Neonatal hyperglycaemia is associated with it
	Ketoacidosis may result
Avoid dehydration	Maintain a good urine output
Prevent infection	Sterility in all procedures, e.g. urethal catheterization, epidural cannulation
Good pain control	Avoid catecholamine release
Two separate intravenous cannulae	This allows one for the insulin and glucose infusion and one for rapid access
Prevent hypotension	It may lead to further tissue acidosis
	Use non-glucose-containing fluids and ephedrine if hypotension occurs
	Use spinal anaesthesia with caution; it is associated with a higher incidence of hypotension than epidural or general anaesthesia
	It may further compromise an already distressed fetus

- During labour, adequate pain control is needed to reduce catecholamine release and metabolic acidosis. This can best be provided by epidural analgesia, which modifies the normal metabolic responses in labour [30,31]. An epidural block may also be indicated, because during the second stage of labour, good perineal relaxation is required for delivery of a large baby. It is also helpful to have functioning epidural analgesia in labour if there is a high risk of vaginal or abdominal operative delivery.

(ii) *Caesarean section.* Anaesthesia for Caesarean section in a diabetic mother may be planned as an elective procedure. Diabetic management will proceed as outlined above (pp. 147–8). There would be a preference for epidural or spinal analgesia in order to avoid intubation difficulties in an obese diabetic woman, and because it is associated with normal acid–base status in both mother and neonate when glucose and insulin infusions are used [6].

- The presence or absence of a diabetic neuropathy should be confirmed with a Valsalva manoeuvre before instituting anaesthesia. More aggressive support of systemic blood pressure may be needed in the presence of a neuropathy.
- General anaesthesia may be indicated for emergency Caesarean section because of complications of the diabetic state, e.g. abruptio placenta, which can produce hypovolaemia, fetal distress and coagulopathy.

9.3.2 Thyroid function

The basal metabolic rate in pregnancy is increased, but not as a result of a change in thyroid status. Hypothalamic and pituitary regulation maintain normal levels of thyroid-stimulating hormone. Although the total concentrations of the thyroid hormones triiodothyronine (T_3) and thyroxine (T_4) in the blood are increased due to oestrogens increasing the binding capacity of thyroxine-binding globulin, the levels of free thyroxine and triiodothyronine are normal. This is in contrast with thyrotoxicosis, in which both free T_3 and free T_4 levels are raised. Renal clearance of iodine increases, as does the iodine turnover by the thyroid gland.

Transient thyroid dysfunction can occur up to six months after delivery in 5% of parturients [32]. Hypothyroidism is more common than hyperthyroidism, and may cause symptoms of tiredness and depression. The state of immune suppression that occurs during pregnancy ameliorates autoimmune thyroid disease, but exacerbations of the disease follow delivery [33].

The placenta produces factors that play a role in regulating maternal thyroid function [34]. It also acts as a barrier to thyroid-stimulating hormone, produced by both the mother and the fetus, but other thyroid hormones pass through in variable amounts. Untreated hypothyroidism or hyperthyroidism in the mother is associated with fetal loss.

Anaesthetic problems associated with disorders of thyroid function

Enlarged thyroid gland. In areas of endemic goitre where there is iodine intake deficiency, the enlarged thyroid gland can cause airway obstruction. It may not be clinically apparent if the goitre is retrosternal. Respiratory obstruction from an enlarged thyroid gland is usually long-standing, and symptoms can include dysphagia as well as dyspnoea. Haemorrhage into a nodule can occur at any time and cause acute respiratory obstruction requiring tracheal intubation. The true cause of this emergency may not be immediately obvious in the last trimester of pregnancy [35].

The neonatal effects of treating iodine deficiency in the mother are the development of an enlarged thyroid gland, which may cause hyperextension of the head, with difficulty in vaginal delivery and respiratory obstruction.

Hyperthyroidism [36]

Women who develop thyrotoxicosis during pregnancy, or have pre-existing disease, will be treated with carbimazole or propylthiouracil. Both of these drugs cross the placenta, and there is a risk of fetal hypothyroidism occurring unless dosages are minimized. Thyrotoxicosis often improves spontaneously during pregnancy, so a small maintenance dose is required, and by the third trimester, antithyroid drugs may be withdrawn completely. If drugs are withdrawn, close observation of the woman is required, and treatment should be restarted if thyrotoxicosis recurs. If the mother requires to breast-feed, the lowest dose needed to treat the woman should be used.

If satisfactory control of thyrotoxicosis is not achieved with these drugs, partial thyroidectomy can be performed in the second trimester, or in the postpartum period if possible. If thyroid surgery is urgently needed, the anaesthetist should have immediately available the means to treat airway problems and thyroid crises in the perioperative period. Postoperative complications that should be anticipated are airway difficulties (laryngeal oedema, recurrent laryngeal nerve palsy and pressure on the trachea from a concealed haematoma) and thyroid storm [37]. The latter problem may be precipitated not only by surgery, but also by the stress of labour or infection. It is characterized by a high metabolic rate, tachycardia, an increase in body temperature (leading to a fluid loss from sweating) and cardiovascular collapse. Immediate oxygen (to meet tissue requirements), cooling, hydration and antibiotics are required, and aggressive therapy with antithyroid drugs, intravenous steroids (to block the conversion of T_4 to T_3) and β-adrenergic blocking drugs.

Prevention of these complications is necessary if emergency surgery is planned and the woman is not euthyroid. Catecholamine release must be avoided, so sedation is helpful, and sympathomimetics and vasopressors should be used with extreme caution. Airway assessment and tracheal intubation are mandatory. Anticholinergic drugs, which may cause tachycardia and reduce heat loss, should be avoided. Postoperative monitoring, especially of the airway and cardiovascular system, is required for at least 24 hours.

Rarely, neonatal thyrotoxicosis can occur. This may be indicated by fetal tachycardia. When there is this risk, an endocrinologist should assist in supervising the pregnancy.

Hypothyroidism [38]

Hypothyroidism should be treated with daily thyroxine to restore normal function. However, the features of hypothyroidism can be masked by pregnancy. Hypotension and bradycardia may not be present, but the pregnancy-related increases in cardiac output and heart rate may be less than normal. The electrocardiogram will show low-voltage complexes, which will aid diagnosis.

Table 9.11 Obstetric anaesthetic agents that may trigger porphyria.	Barbiturates Hydralazine Nifedipine Cimetidine Enflurane

Drug dosages may need to be reduced, although intravenous induction of anaesthesia will be slower than normal. Congestive cardiac failure is easily precipitated, and hypotension may be resistant to treatment with vasopressors.

The rate of drug metabolism is reduced, so that respiratory depression from narcotic, sedative and inhalational agents occurs. A nerve stimulator must be used to avoid overdosage by muscle relaxants. A regional anaesthetic technique is therefore useful, provided that hypotension is prevented. Ephedrine can be titrated to achieve this.

Adequate care in recovery is necessary. Body temperature, adequacy of ventilation, fluid balance and cardiovascular stability must all be closely monitored.

9.3.3 Acute intermittent porphyria

This is a rare, inherited disorder with an episodic nature. Exacerbations of the disease can be triggered by pregnancy or by one of a number of anaesthetic agents, listed in Table 9.11 [39]. The successful use of 0.5% hyperbaric bupivacaine for emergency Caesarean section in a patient with known acute intermittent porphyria has been described [40].

9.3.4 Plasma cholinesterase

There are several variants of plasma cholinesterase that hydrolyse acetylcholine esters. Their function is not fully understood, but they all have a catalytically important serine amino acid in the active centre, similar to acetylcholinesterase. Both plasma cholinesterase and acetylcholinesterase are heterogenous proteins. They have separate genes that encode them, and these genes are structurally related [41,42]. Acetylcholinesterase is present wherever acetylcholine is the neurotransmitter, so it is present in the junctional clefts of muscles and ganglia, but it is also present in red blood cells. It breaks down acetylcholine to choline and acetate. Plasma cholinesterase is less specific, and it is found in the liver (where it is synthesized), plasma and pancreas. Plasma cholinesterase concentration depends on genetic factors, liver disease and functional impairment by drugs (e.g. oestrogens, anabolic steroids), malnutrition or infection, and dilution in plasma. Its enzyme activity can be reversibly inhibited by cholinergic drugs, e.g. neostigmine and ecothiopate, or irreversibly by organophosphorus compounds. A significant

Table 9.12 Plasma cholinesterase and pregnancy.

Rapid decline in activity in first trimester
Low levels of activity in second and third trimester
Lowest levels of activity in the first postpartum week

Clinical guidance
The reduction in plasma cholinesterase levels may not reflect the clinical risks of a prolonged effect of suxamethonium
Women with abnormal genes may be more sensitive to suxamethonium when pregnant than when not pregnant

---

reduction in its concentration or activity can affect the duration of action and toxicity of drugs that are metabolized by the enzyme. These are neuromuscular relaxants such as suxamethonium and the newer non-depolarizing agents such as mivacurium, and the ester local anaesthetic drugs, such as procaine and cocaine. The latter drug, if abused, is also metabolized by placental esterases.

Effects of pregnancy (Table 9.12)

Cholinesterase activities have been measured in blood sent for routine grouping at all stages of pregnancy in 941 women [43]. Activity started to decrease in the first four to eight weeks, and continued to decrease to 20 weeks' gestation. The number of women with activity in the range that could result in a prolonged neuromuscular block from suxamethonium increased from 1% at four to eight weeks of pregnancy to 8% from 20 weeks onwards. Cholinesterase activity was depressed for up to a week after delivery, with 12% of women being at risk of sensitivity to suxamethonium in the postpartum period. The majority of these women were phenotypically normal. The pattern of activity in the postpartum period has been examined in more detail [44]. Women with normal genotype were studied from delivery to five weeks postpartum. The mean level of cholinesterase activity was depressed by 30% at delivery and by 40% in the first week postpartum. Concentrations then increased, and reached non-pregnant values by five weeks postpartum. A few women took longer to reach non-pregnant levels.

These effects cannot be explained simply by the change in circulating blood volume that occurs during pregnancy, because a diuresis occurs postpartum and the plasma volume is lost. This would produce an increase rather than a decline in plasma cholinesterase activity postpartum. Plasma volume changes may therefore not be relevant to plasma cholinesterase activity changes.

The changes parallel changes in albumin concentration, and can be produced by oestrogen–progestogen contraceptives [45]. These hormones are thought to cause their effects by increasing membrane permeability. If molecular dimensions are considered, this could explain the decrease in serum albumin (molecular weight 69 kDa) but not the decrease in plasma cholinesterase (300 kDa). It is postulated that a reduction in protein synthesis occurs in response to oestrogen. Hormonal control may switch biosynthesis from cholinesterase to increase plasma fibrinogen, which increases rapidly and has an active role in blood clotting after delivery [46].

Assay methods may affect the levels of measured plasma cholinesterase activity. Monoclonal antibodies have enabled the development of an enzyme-linked immunosorbent assay. These assays are more sensitive and accurate, and they confirm the low activity of cholinesterase in the second trimester [47].

Relevance to anaesthesia

Clinically, high doses of suxamethonium given by infusion have not led to a high incidence of prolonged paralysis, so changes in plasma cholinesterase activity may not relate to the duration of suxamethonium apnoea. The normal reduction in cholinesterase activity in pregnancy may therefore bring more women into the range of cholinesterase activity often associated with, but not diagnostic of, suxamethonium apnoea. Women who were genotypically normal but had a reduction in plasma cholinesterase activity of 60–80% were found to have a duration of apnoea after suxamethonium (in a dose of 1 mg/kg intravenously) of 22 minutes [48]. Women with atypical genes who were studied in pregnancy [44] had more significant reductions in cholinesterase activity compared with normal genes. Women with pre-eclampsia are reported to have reduced levels of plasma cholinesterase activity [49].

The use of metoclopramide in women undergoing postpartum tubal ligation has been observed to prolong suxamethonium-induced neuromuscular block in a dose-related manner. Metoclopramide in doses of 10 and 20 mg increased the mean duration of neuromuscular block by 23% and 56%, respectively. An *in vitro* study demonstrated that metoclopramide produced a potent non-competitive dose-dependent inhibition of plasma cholinesterase [50].

9.3.5 Malignant hyperthermia

This is a rare disorder that may be associated with diseases of the musculoskeletal system, such as Duchenne muscular dystrophy and some of the myotonic dystrophies. The underlying problem is an abnormality in sarcoplasmic reticulum function. Total cellular calcium content is greater than normal, because of an imbalance between release and uptake from the sarcoplasmic reticulum. The result is prolonged high concentrations of calcium surrounding the contractile proteins that maintain contractile activity. This sustained contracture produces high concentrations of potassium and hydrogen ions, giving rise to hyperkalaemia and acidosis. Similar reactions may occur during drug abuse with cocaine and drug therapy for psychotic conditions, which can induce the malignant neuroleptic-like syndrome.

Anaesthetic management

Prophylaxis
- Avoid trigger agents: volatile anaesthetic agents, suxamethonium, ketamine. Suxamethonium is mainly used in obstetrics to prevent aspiration of gastric contents during a rapid-sequence induction, and difficult intubation is more common in pregnancy, so that the presence of masseter spasm may be overlooked.
- Use a regional technique.
- Monitor with oxygen saturation, capnography and temperature measurement.
- Use an anaesthetic machine that is not contaminated by volatile anaesthetic agents.
- Dantrolene (caution: uterine hypotonia and fetal transfer). The preoperative prophylactic dose is 2–4 mg/kg i.v. over 15 minutes.

Treatment
1 Dantrolene: intravenous bolus with repeated injections.
2 100% oxygen and ventilation.
3 Cooling.
4 Correction of acid–base and electrolyte balance.
5 Maintenance of renal function.

The most commonly encountered trigger agents in anaesthesia are volatile inhalational anaesthetics and suxamethonium. Both are integral parts of general anaesthesia in obstetrics, but must be avoided in women with a predisposition to malignant hyperthermia. Operative obstetric procedures in such women are best carried out under regional anaesthesia whenever possible. Forward planning during the antenatal period will avoid the sudden emergency need for general anaesthesia in most cases. When general anaesthesia cannot be avoided and an awake intubation would be difficult, alternative relaxant strategies must be used for endotracheal intubation, and the small increase in the risk of aspiration must be accepted. The contraindication to volatile anaesthetic agents demands an alternative strategy for the maintenance of unconsciousness. Intravenous agents such as barbiturates and benzodiazepines can be used, as can most opioids. Propofol also seems to be a safe agent.

It is essential to discuss and explain the problem with malignant hyperthermia to any susceptible woman, so that she understands clearly the reasoning behind advice that may otherwise be unacceptable to her.

Table 9.13 Risks of obesity.

General
Respiratory failure
Aspiration
Cardiovascular failure
Pulmonary embolism
Infection
Hepatic dysfunction and fatty infiltration
Renal dysfunction

Obstetric
Gestational diabetes
Hypertension
Operative difficulty, e.g. at Caesarean section: increased blood loss, increased operating time, wound infection
Twins
Older
Increased mortality

9.3.6 Obesity

Measures of obesity

The ideal weight for a person can be calculated from the formula:

Ideal weight (kg) = height (cm) − 100

This is called the Broca index. An increase in weight of less than 20% of the ideal weight can be defined as 'overweight'. A weight in excess of 20% more than the ideal weight is 'obese', and 'morbid obesity' is present when the ideal weight is doubled.

The body mass index (Quetelet index) correlates with body fat. It is the body weight (in kg) divided by the square of the height (in m). The normal value of the BMI is 20–26 kg/m². Values above 29 represent obesity, and are more than two standard deviations above the population mean [51,52].

Physiology and pharmacology

Obesity is an excess of body fat. About 20–25% of female body weight is fat, and this proportion tends to increase with age and parity [53]. Obesity is associated with physiological and anatomical changes, and altered pharmacokinetics. When pregnant, obese women have a higher incidence of medical problems [54,55], including cardiovascular disease (such as hypertension and coronary artery disease), gallbladder disease and diabetes (Table 9.13) [56].

The triennial reports on *Confidential Enquiries into Maternal Deaths* do not classify obesity as a cause of death, but have, for many years, identified it as risk factor. It was also present in the majority of deaths from pulmonary embolism in the 1988–90 report [57].

Physiological changes associated with obesity

Obesity adds a further mechanical burden of excess fat during pregnancy, particularly related to cardiorespiratory function and metabolism. The magnitude of the combined changes in any one person has to be assessed on an individual basis.

1 Respiratory.
- Upper airway. There is a continuation from obesity into airway obstruction with sleep apnoea, and at an extreme, 'Pickwickian' syndrome.
- Pulmonary changes. Chest wall compliance is reduced by the increase in abdominal fat and the development of a thoracic kyphosis. This can increase the work of breathing by 30% [58]. A restrictive pattern of breathing will be obtained on spirometry. The inspiratory reserve volume is decreased. This will reduce functional residual capacity (FRC), and hypoxaemia can occur, especially when the woman is recumbent, as a result of closing capacity equalling FRC and encroaching on normal tidal volume gas exchange. Ventilation/perfusion abnormalities and pulmonary arteriovenous shunting increase [59,60].

2 Cardiovascular. The increase in body mass is associated with an increase in cardiac output and blood volume. Normally, this meets the tissue requirements for oxygen supply. However, when oxygen consumption is increased in labour, there may not be adequate oxygen delivery to match tissue oxygen requirements.

3 Gastrointestinal tract. Obese pregnant women in labour are more likely to continue to eat, and this contributes to an increase in gastric volume [61].

Pharmacological effects associated with obesity

The increase in circulating blood volume increases the volume of distribution of drugs, and may make drug elimination time longer [62]. This should be considered if intravenous induction agents are used. The reduction in functional residual capacity will speed equilibration of anaesthetic vapours in the alveoli with inspired concentrations. Tissue concentration—particularly in the brain and uterus—may also be more rapid, but increased distribution volumes and tissue depots may negate this effect. Theoretically, the more fat-soluble volatile anaesthetic agents would be deposited in adipose tissue. This additional uptake will have to be metabolized or mobilized during the recovery period. Both the chest and the abdominal tissues will be heavier and more bulky. The abdominal stiffness may be interpreted as a lack of muscle relaxation if neuromuscular monitoring of non-depolarizing agents is not used.

Resumption of spontaneous ventilation of the lungs postoperatively will be adversely affected, and respiratory inadequacy may follow. Inappropriate dosage with muscle relaxant can complicate this scenario. Careful choice of short-acting muscle relaxant and frequent monitoring of its effects should help to prevent postoperative muscle weakness and respiratory difficulties.

Anaesthesia in the obese parturient

The increased incidence of malpresentations and other obstetric complications associated with obesity should alert the labour ward anaesthetist to the potential need for emergency anaesthesia. Preparation for this eventuality should be started so that appropriate investigations and equipment are available prior to any anaesthetic technique being required. Obese patients (defined as > 90 kg or BMI > 30 kg/m²) should be seen by an obstetric anaesthetist in the antenatal period, when any investigation of respiratory function or airway difficulty can be undertaken. They should also be seen on admission for delivery in order to identify any changed circumstances and to arrange control of gastric contents with ranitidine, sodium citrate and metoclopramide. Intravenous access should be secured at an early stage, as it is difficult to achieve in many obese parturients.

Preliminary clinical assessment in the labour suite of all women with a BMI > 30 kg/m² is also necessary in order to re-examine the airway, intravenous and lumbar spinal access, and clinical signs and symptoms such as shortness of breath and heartburn. Apart from a full blood count and blood grouping, blood profile for renal and hepatic function is a useful baseline. Lung function can initially be assessed clinically and a vitalograph can be obtained if necessary. Pulse oximetry and, if necessary, blood gases on air would confirm hypoxaemia. A baseline may be difficult to obtain during labour due to ventilatory disturbances, and antenatal or pre-induction figures are therefore useful. An electrocardiogram is also necessary. If venous access is difficult, consideration should be given to the siting of a central venous pressure line, which may also assist in assessing hydration during parturition.

Table 9.14 summarizes the anaesthetic problems in the obese patient. Women whose weight was more than 136.4 kg were studied postoperatively for anaesthetic and obstetric outcome. A retrospective matching control group was selected for each of the 117 patients. Caesarean section was three times more common in the obese women, epidural analgesia was associated with placement failure, and difficult tracheal intubation occurred in one-third of the general anaesthetics [63]. A multivariate analysis of risk factors associated with difficult intubation in obstetrics identified obesity as a significant factor, and it had a strong association with a short neck. The probability of experiencing a difficult intubation with no other factors involved, e.g. a receding mandible or protruding maxillary incisors, was less than 20%, but when combined with other factors, this probability increased to over 50% [64].

Table 9.14 Anaesthetic problems in the obese patient.

Technical
Airway management
Monitoring: mother, e.g. blood pressure (consider measuring direct intra-arterial pressure); fetus (thick abdominal wall)
Insertion of cannulae, catheters (need long needles for epidural/spinal block)
Physical size: moving into position; choice of equipment

Pathophysiological
Gastric contents (increased volume, more acid)
Aortocaval compression (lateral displacement of the uterus is difficult)
Lung function deteriorates in the recumbent (lateral) or Trendelenburg (with wedge) positions
Pathological risk factors: prevention if possible

General anaesthesia. General anaesthesia is associated with risks from failed intubation, difficulties in airway management, gastric aspiration from a larger volume, more acidic stomach contents and hypoxaemia. Management of the difficult airway is described in Chapter 16. The obese pregnant patient will desaturate more rapidly after preoxygenation if ventilation is not achieved, due to an increase in oxygen consumption and a decreased functional residual capacity. If ventilation is achieved, tidal volumes should be increased to compensate for the decreased compliance and, if necessary, positive end-expiratory pressure. Care should be taken not to reduce cardiac output with these manoeuvres, especially if the mother is hypovolaemic.

Regional anaesthesia. If the choice between general anaesthesia and regional anaesthesia has to be made, the advantages of regional anaesthesia usually outweigh its disadvantages. Both epidural and spinal anaesthesia require location of the correct needle position. Choice of technique may be limited by the length of the needles available. A 16-gauge Tuohy needle of 15 cm may be used. Smaller-gauge spinal needles may have to be supported during insertion by shorter introducers.

The expected surgical operating time should be considered. An obese patient often has longer surgical operation times than normal-sized patients, and spinal anaesthesia without an epidural catheter may not last long enough. A spinal anaesthetic followed by a small dose of local anaesthetic drug epidurally when the nerve block wanes should avoid a total spinal block and may be the preferred technique, especially if difficulty in intubation has been assessed preoperatively.

Maternal position, both for siting the regional nerve block and for its maintenance, should be considered. It is helpful to locate the midline with the mother sitting upright. If she flexes, the increased abdominal mass may cause caval occlusion. Once the block is sited, it may not be comfortable for the woman to be positioned in the left lateral position for surgery, because thoracic kyphosis is often present and the position of her spinal column often causes considerable interindividual variability in block height [65].

The combined spinal–epidural technique, with the advantages of spinal anaesthesia but with the reinforcement of an epidural block for prolonged surgery, is indicated in the obese patient. Hypotension must be assessed, and intra-arterial monitoring sited prior to the nerve block. Intravenous access must also be secured so that fluids or vasopressors, or both, can be given effectively.

Postpartum. After surgery, the immediate postoperative recovery period is critical in obese patients. If endotracheal intubation has been used to maintain anaesthesia, the tracheal tube should be kept in position until the mother is fully awake. The mother should always be nursed on her side, preferably with her head down, so that aspiration is prevented postoperatively. Return of adequate neuromuscular function should be measured and documented, because there may be residual effects of neuromuscular blocking drugs, central sedation, or a reduced respiratory reserve. Respiratory failure should be prevented. An inspired oxygen concentration of 40% or more should be administered for at least 24 hours postoperatively, and through the second postoperative night. Good muscle tone in the patient's legs is also required to act as a muscle pump and prevent venous stasis, which may lead to thromboembolism. Prophylaxis against deep vein thrombosis must be used. Ambulation requires adequate pain relief. Intramuscular injections of opioid drugs may not reach the muscles and can be deposited subcutaneously. This can lead to unrecognized prolonged effects. Opioids can also compound respiratory depression. If a regional technique cannot be used, patient-controlled analgesia by incremental intravenous bolus may be adequate. The expectation of respiratory dysfunction for longer than the normal recovery period requires the mother to be nursed in a monitored area, e.g. a high-dependency area, for at least 24 hours.

Analgesia for labour. The increased risk of obstetric complications in the obese patient and the need to reduce the respiratory and cardiac changes in labour would indicate the necessity for epidural analgesia in labour. This would enable adequate pain relief for all stages of labour and instrumental delivery if required. Monitoring of maternal oxygen saturation, pulse and blood pressure, as well as direct fetal monitoring, should be available continuously if possible. The mother is best positioned sitting upright, to allow adequate diaphragmatic excursion, and there should be minimal motor block to avoid venous stasis and intercostal nerve paralysis. Additional inspired oxygen may be required. If the mother refuses epidural block, analgesia can be given in the form of Entonox, but between contractions oxygen should also be supplied.

References

1 Committee on Medical Aspects of Food Policy. *Dietary Reference Values for Food Energy and Nutrients for the United Kingdom: Report of the Panel on Dietary Reference Values of the Committee on Medical Aspects of Food Policy.* London: HMSO, 1991. (Reports of health and social subjects, 41.)
2 Anderson O, Kuhl C. Adiposite insulin receptor binding and lipogenesis at term in normal pregnancy. *Eur J Clin Invest* 1988; **18**: 575–81.
3 Kuhl C. Aetiology of gestational diabetes. *Clin Obstet Gynaecol* 1991; **5**: 279–92.
4 Diamant YZ, Kissilevitz R, Shafir E. Changes in activity of enzymes related to glycolysis, gluconeogensis and lipogenesis in placentae from diabetic women. *Placenta* 1984; **5**: 55–60.
5 Singh M, Feigelson M. Effects of maternal diabetes on the development of carbohydrating enzymes, glycogen deposition and surface active phospholipid levels in the fetal rat lung. *Biol Neonate* 1990; **43**: 33–42.
6 Ramanathan S, Khoo P, Arismendy J. Perioperative maternal and neonatal acid–base status and glucose metabolism in patients with insulin dependent diabetes mellitus. *Anesth Analg* 1991; **73**: 105–11.
7 Lind T, Billewicz WZ, Brown G. A serial study of changes occurring in the oral glucose tolerance test during pregnancy. *J Obstet Gynaecol Br Commonw* 1973; **80**: 1033–9.
8 Persson B, Hanson U. Hypoglycaemia in pregnancy. *Clin Endocrinol Metab* 1993; **7**: 731–9.
9 Bishop JHV, Green R. Glucose handling by distal portions of the nephron during pregnancy in the rat. *J Physiol* 1983; **336**: 131–42.
10 Davison JM, Hytten F. The effect of pregnancy on the renal handling of glucose. *J Obstet Gynaecol Br Commonw* 1975; **8**: 374–81.
11 Madsen H, Ditzel J. Changes in red blood cell oxygen transport in diabetic pregnancy. *Am J Obstet Gynecol* 1982; **143**: 421–4.
12 Viberti GC. A glycemic threshold for diabetic complications? *N Engl J Med* 1995; **332**: 1293–4.
13 Menon RK, Cohen RM, Sperling MA *et al.* Transplacental passage of insulin in pregnant women with insulin-dependent diabetes mellitus. *N Engl J Med* 1990; **323**: 309–15.
14 Menon RK, Sperling MA. Carbohydrate metabolism. *Semin Perinatol* 1988; **12**: 157–62.
15 Lederman RP, McCann DS, Work B. Endogenous plasma epinephrine and norepinephrine in the last trimester of pregnancy and labor. *Am J Obstet Gynecol* 1977; **129**: 5–8.
16 Maltau JM, Eielsen OV, Stokke KT. Effect of stress during labor on the concentration of cortisol and estriol in maternal plasma. *Am J Obstet Gynecol* 1979; **134**: 681–4.
17 Pearson DWM. Inheritance and development of diabetes mellitus. *Clin Obstet Gynecol* 1991; **5**: 257–75.
18 Coustan DR. Screening and diagnosis of gestational diabetes. *Clin Obstet Gynaecol* 1991; **5**: 293–313.
19 Lind T, Phillips PR. Influence of pregnancy on the 75-g OGTT: a prospective multicentre study. *Diabetes* 1991; **40**: 8–13.
20 Berkowitz GS, Roman SH, Lapinski RH, Alvarez M. Maternal characteristics, neonatal outcome, and the time of diagnosis of gestational diabetes. *Am J Obstet Gynecol* 1992; **167**: 976–82.
21 Peterson CM, Jovanovic-Peterson L, Mills JL *et al.* The Diabetes in Early Pregnancy Study: changes in cholesterol, triglycerides, body weight and blood pressure. *Am J Obstet Gynecol* 1992; **166**: 513–8.
22 Coombs CA, Kitzmiller JL. Diabetic nephropathy and pregnancy. *Clin Obstet* 1991; **34**: 505–15.

23 Mimouni F, Miodovnik M, Rosenn B, Khoury J, Siddiqi TA. Birth trauma in insulin dependent diabetic pregnancies. *Am J Perinatol* 1992; **9**: 205–8.
24 Landon MB, Gabbe SG. Fetal surveillance in the pregnancy complicated by diabetes mellitus. *Clin Obstet Gynecol* 1991; **34**: 535–43.
25 Fuhrmann K, Reiher H, Semonler K *et al*. Prevention of congenital malformations in infants of insulin-dependent diabetic mothers. *Diabetes Care* 1983; **6**: 219–23.
26 Coustan DR. Recent advances in the management of diabetic pregnant women. *Clin Perinatol* 1980; **7**: 299–311.
27 Carr S, Coustan DR, Martelly P, Brosco F, Rotondo L. Precision of reflectance meters in screening for gestational diabetes. *Obstet Gynecol* 1989; **73**: 727–31.
28 Lebovitz HE. Diabetic ketoacidosis. *Lancet* 1995; **345**: 767–72.
29 Chamberlain G. Medical problems in pregnancy, 1. *Br Med J* 1991; **302**: 1262–6.
30 Pearson JF. The effects of continuous lumbar epidural block on maternal and fetal acid–base balance during labour and delivery. In: Doughty A, ed. *Proceedings of the Symposium on Epidural Analgesia in Obstetrics, Kingston Hospital, Kingston upon Thames, 18 March 1971*. London: Lewis, 1972: 26.
31 Shnider SM, Abboud T, Artal R. Maternal endogenous catecholamine decrease during labor after epidural anesthesia. *Am J Obstet Gynecol* 1983; **147**: 13–15.
32 Toft AD. Thyroxine therapy. *N Engl J Med* 1994; **331**: 174–80.
33 Chiovato L, Lapi P, Fiore E, Tonacchera M, Pinchera A. Thyroid autoimmunity and female gender. *J Endocrinol Invest* 1993; **16**: 384–91.
34 Glinoer D. Maternal thyroid function in pregnancy. *J Endocrinol Invest* 1993; **16**: 374–8.
35 Shaha A, Alfonso A, Jaffe BM. Acute airway distress due to thyroid pathology. *Surgery* 1987; **102**: 1068–74.
36 Stehling LC. Anesthetic management of the patient with hyperthyroidism. *Anesthesiology* 1974; **41**: 585–95.
37 Pugh S, Lalwani K, Awal A. Thyroid storm as a cause of loss of consciousness following anaesthesia for emergency Caesarean section. *Anaesthesia* 1994; **49**: 35–7.
38 Murkin JM. Anesthesia and hypothyroidism: a review of thyroxine physiology, pharmacology and anesthetic implications. *Anesth Analg* 1982; **61**: 371–83.
39 Harrison GG, Meissner PN, Hift RJ. Anaesthesia in porphyric patients. *Anaesthesia* 1993; **48**: 417–21.
40 McNeill MJ, Bennet A. Use of regional anaesthesia in a patient with acute porphyria. *Br J Anaesth* 1990; **64**: 371–3.
41 Pantuck EJ. Plasma cholinesterase: gene and variations. *Anesth Analg* 1993; **77**: 380–6.
42 Gnatt A, Ginzberg D, Lieman-Hurwitz J *et al*. Human acetylcholinesterase and butyrylcholinesterase are encoded by two distinct genes. *Cell Mol Neurobiol* 1991; **11**: 91–104.
43 Evants RT, Wroe JM. Plasma cholinesterase changes during pregnancy. *Anaesthesia* 1980; **35**: 651–4.
44 Robson N, Robertson I, Whittaker M. Plasma cholinesterase changes during the puerperium. *Anaesthesia* 1986; **41**: 243–9.
45 Whittaker M, Charlier AR, Ramaswamy S. Changes in plasma cholinesterase isoenzymes due to oral contraceptives. *J Reprod Fertil* 1971; **26**: 373–5.
46 Whittaker M, Jones JW, Braven J. Immunological studies of plasma cholinesterase during pregnancy and the puerperium. *Clin Chim Acta* 1991; **199**: 223–30.
47 Hangaard J, Whittaker M, Loft AGR, Norgaard-Pedersen B. Quantification and phenotyping of serum cholinesterase by enzyme antigen immunoassay: methodological aspects and clinical applicability. *Scand J Clin Lab Invest* 1991; **51**: 349–58.
48 Viby-Mogensen J. Correlation of succcinylcholine duration of action with plasma cholinesterase activity in subjects with genotypically normal enzyme. *Anesthesiology* 1980; **53**: 517–20.

49 Kamban JR, Perry SM, Entman S, Smith BE. Effect of magnesium on plasma cholinesterase activity. *Am J Obstet Gynecol* 1988; **159**: 309–11.

50 Kao YJ, Tellez J, Turnder DR. Dose-dependent effect of metoclopramide on cholinesterases and suxamethonium metabolism. *Br J Anaesth* 1990; **65**: 220–4.

51 Keys A, Fidanza F, Karvonen MJ, Kimura N, Taylor HL. Indices of relative weight and obesity. *J Chronic Dis* 1972; **25**: 329–43.

52 Smith DE, Lewis CE, Caveny JL *et al.* Longitudinal changes in adiposity associated with pregnancy: the CARDIA Study. *JAMA* 1994; **271**: 1747–51.

53 King JC. New National Academy of Sciences guidelines for nutrition during pregnancy. *Diabetes* 1991; **40** (Suppl 2): 151.

54 Maeder EC, Barno A, Mecklenburg F. Obesity: a maternal high-risk factor. *Obstet Gynecol* 1975; **45**: 669–71.

55 Wolfe HM, Zador IE, Gross TL, Martier SS, Sokol RJ. The clinical utility of maternal body mass index in pregnancy. *Am J Obstet Gynecol* 1991; **164**: 1306–10.

56 Johnson SR, Kolberg BH, Varner MW. Maternal obesity and pregnancy. *Surg Gynecol Obstet* 1987; **164**: 431–7.

57 Department of Health. *Report on Confidential Enquiries into Maternal Deaths in the United Kingdom, 1988–1990.* London: HMSO, 1994.

58 Sharp JT, Henry JP, Sweany SK, Meadows WR, Pietras RJ. The total work of breathing in normal and obese men. *J Clin Invest* 1964; **43**: 728–39.

59 Eng M, Butler J, Bonica JJ. Respiratory function in pregnant obese women. *Am J Obstet Gynecol* 1975; **123**: 241–5.

60 Templeton A, Kelman GR. Maternal blood gases, (P_{AO_2}–Pa_{O_2}), physiological shunt and V_D/V_T in normal pregnancy. *Br J Anaesth* 1976; **48**: 1001–4.

61 Roberts BR, Shirley MA. Reducing the risk of acid aspiration during Cesarean section. *Anesth Analg Curr Res* 1974; **53**: 859–68.

62 Jung D, Mayersohn M, Perrier D, Calkins J, Saunders R. Thiopental disposition in lean and obese patients undergoing surgery. *Anesthesiology* 1982; **56**: 269–74.

63 Hood DD, Dewan DM. Anesthetic and obstetric outcome in morbidly obese parturients. *Anesthesiology* 1993; **79**: 1210–18.

64 Rocke DA, Murray WB, Rout CC, Gouws E. Relative risk analysis of factors associated with difficult intubation in obstetric anesthesia. *Anesthesiology* 1992; **77**: 67–73.

65 Pitkänen MT. Body mass and spread of spinal anesthesia with bupivacaine. *Anesth Analg* 1987; **66**: 127–31.

66 Campbell-Brown M, Hytten FE. Nutrition. In: Chamberlain G, Broughton Pipkin, F, eds. *Clinical Physiology in Obstetrics,* 3nd edn. Oxford: Blackwell Science, 1998: 165–191.

10: Immunity and Infection

The immune system has two interactive parts (Fig. 10.1): the innate system and the adaptive system. The innate system recognizes foreign material indiscriminately, and is not enhanced by repeated exposure. It has two types of cells, natural killer cells and phagocytes (e.g. macrophages, monocytes, mast cells, eosinophils, platelets and neutrophils). Their effects are augmented by soluble factors. These are: complement, cytokines, lysozymes, interferons and acute-phase proteins. The adaptive system recognizes and memorizes the specificity of antigens. The cells and factors of the two systems interact, and a variety of physical methods are used to produce the immune response, e.g. opsonization by C-reactive protein (CRP), immunoglobulin G (IgG) and complement, which assist phagocytosis.

Human leucocyte antigens (HLA), from the major histocompatibility complex (MHC) region on the short arm of chromosome 6, are expressed on the cell surface. They are of two types: class 1 antigens (A, B or C), which are expressed on almost every cell of the body and are key factors in defining 'self'; and class II antigens, with more restricted expression. They are expressed on cells involved in the immune response. The MHC region also contains genes encoding cytokines, e.g. tumour necrosis factor (TNF).

Cytokines are short-acting soluble factors that generate an efficient immune response by affecting cell migration and function so that close cellular contact occurs. Cytokines produced by and released from lymphocytes are called lymphokines. Gene cloning (using recombinant DNA technology) has enabled the identification of pure factors. These are termed 'interleukins', and act as signals between cells of the immune system. Interleukin-1 (IL-1) is secreted by activated macrophages as an initial reaction, and drives the elaboration of the inflammatory cytokines. Interleukin-6 (IL-6) produces the hepatic acute-phase response [1], T- and B-cell activation, and prostaglandin production, and interleukin-8 (IL-8) attracts neutrophils to the inflammatory site.

Cytokines help to recruit and activate other inflammatory cells, thus perpetuating the immune response. Recognition of these antigens has been made possible by the use of monoclonal antibodies (MAB). International agreement has grouped MABs according to their reactions with specific antigens. The groups are termed 'clusters of differentiation' (CD). Techniques are now available to isolate the genes encoding the CDs, and their functional properties are being studied. The CD4 antigen functions as a receptor on the T lymphocyte for the human immunodeficiency virus (HIV).

B cells produce and secrete all antibodies, and mature to form plasma cells. They can switch gene expression from immunoglobulin M (IgM) to IgG

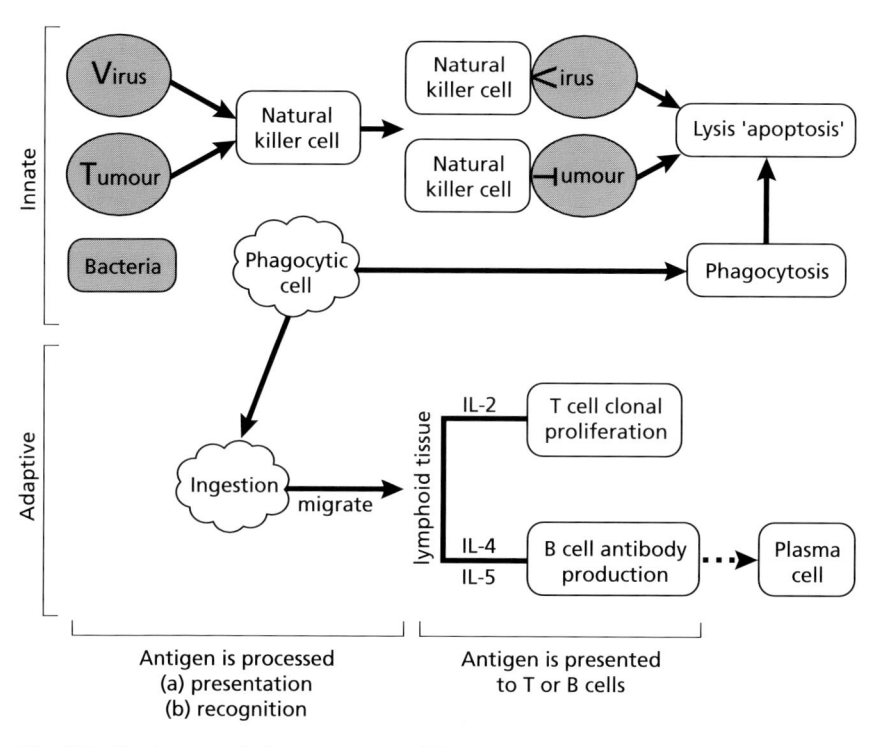

Fig. 10.1 The innate and adaptive systems of the immune response.

Table 10.1 Properties of antibodies.

	IgG	IgA	IgM	IgD	IgE
Molecular KDa weight	150 000	160 000 Smallest Immunoglobulin	900 000 Large molecule Poor tissue penetration	180 000	190 000
Placental transfer	Yes (active process)	No	No	No	No
Complement activation	Yes	No	Yes	No	No
Serum half-life (days)	28	4–5	4–5	2–8	1–5
Effects	Generates secondary immune response	Surface mucosal antigen	Neutralization, e.g. tetanus toxin Early primary immune response	Activation of β-lymphocytes	Type I reactions (IgE is produced by plasma cells, but attaches to receptors on mast cells and basophils)

(Table 10.1). This maturation fits the kinetics of the antibody response, which primarily produces IgM and then secondarily IgG.

10.1 Immunity

10.1.1 Regulation

Production of cytokines is tightly regulated by a variety of mediators, including steroid hormones, prostaglandins and other cytokines. Glucocorticoids have a direct effect on lymphokine production by the genes in the T cells by interference with transcription factors [2]. Sex steroids affect immune function, but their mechanism has not been elucidated. Glucocorticoids are released on stimulation of the immune system via a neuroendocrine immune network. Their physiological role is not just immunosuppressive but also immunomodulatory. A peripheral neuroimmune link exists with endogenous opioids. Opioid receptors are up-regulated during inflammation, and help to attenuate pain from inflammation [3].

Prostaglandin E_2 is an immunomodulator. It inhibits the proliferation and differentiation of macrophage precursors, T and B cells, and also inhibits macrophage production of IL-1 and TNF and expression of class II MHC molecules. It affects the production of antigen, but not T-cell proliferation. Leukotriene B_4 (LTB_4) is another modulator. It is a lipoxygenase product secreted by activated macrophages and neutrophils. It enhances the innate system and stimulates interleukin-2 (IL-2) production.

Sepsis is a cause of morbidity and mortality in obstetrics (see pp. 176–7 and Chapter 2, p. 23). Time-related events occur in the regulation of the immune response that have diagnostic clinical significance. IL-1 and TNF release occurs in minutes, peaks quickly and disappears relatively rapidly [4]. The IL-6 levels gradually rise, and are then sustained at high serum concentrations for several hours. Finally, IL-8 is released and sustained for up to 24 hours.

These inflammatory cytokines provoke increased synthesis of 'acute-phase proteins' in the liver. CRP has a half-life of a few hours, and serum levels reflect rapid changes in inflammation. This is in contrast to fibrinogen, another acute-phase protein (measured in the erythrocyte sedimentation rate), in which changes are much slower.

Regulatory effects can produce acute and chronic clinical disorders. Recognition of antigen by antibodies can cause incidental tissue damage as well as the intended destruction of the antigen. Reactions resulting in tissue damage are called 'hypersensitivity reactions'. They are not confined to single types (previously, types I–IV were described), but usually involve a mixture of mechanisms. For example, anaphylaxis clinically describes a group of symptoms that can be produced by several mechanisms; overproduction of antibodies may account for the strong association of specific MHC antigens

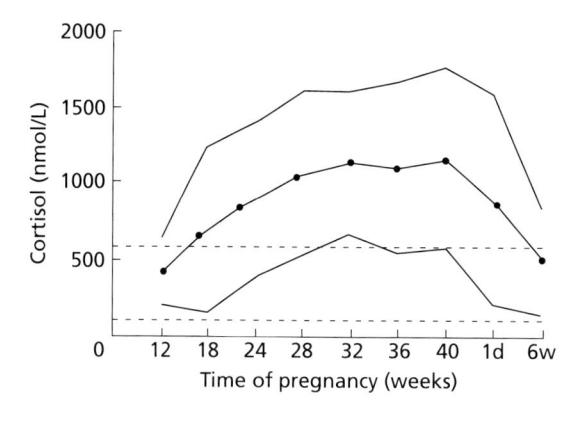

Fig. 10.2 Gestational changes in cortisol production as mean ± standard deviation showing the reference range as dotted lines. (Reprinted with permission from [54].)

with particular diseases, e.g. systemic lupus erythematosus (SLE) and myasthenia gravis (see Chapter 8). It appears that the normal host defence mechanism becomes hostile, but the mechanisms that produce a variety of abnormal immunological clinical states have yet to be defined.

10.1.2 Pregnancy and the immune system

There is little clinical evidence that the pregnant woman is significantly immunocompromised, despite *in vitro* evidence to the contrary. Pregnancy does not affect antibody response, but the effect on cell-mediated immunity and immune system regulation is less clear. Increases in endogenous corticosteroids (Fig. 10.2) suppress lymphocyte function; oestrogen, prolactin and other sex hormones can regulate cytokine production [5]. Pregnancy-specific proteins such as alpha-fetoprotein suppress *in vitro* lymphocyte function. Serum complement levels are often increased due to an increase in synthesis, and fibrinogen concentrations increase markedly.

Fetomaternal immune relationships

Normal. Reproduction involves the introduction of genetically alien spermatozoal cells and seminal plasma proteins. Activation of immunological processes would lead to their destruction. Very rarely, acute hypersensitivity reactions can occur to the seminal plasma proteins, but the usual lack of response has not yet been explained.

A conceptus has antigens that the maternal immune systems should recognize and react against. It does not do this, so the fetus becomes an allogenic graft. There is never any continuity of the intravascular compartment between mother and fetus. The trophoblast is the only fetal tissue to have direct contact with the maternal cells. It is of embryonic origin, and must avoid maternal rejection. The trophoblast is both a barrier and a pathway for the exchange of substances between the mother and fetus. Most of these exchanges occur on the surface of the chorionic villi. Immunohistological studies have provided evidence for the absence of HLA antigens A, band C [6] on the syncytiotrophoblast. The phenomenon of syncytiotrophoblast embolization to the lungs, which leads to a local response, has no known significance. Suppression of specific maternal immune responses to fetal antigens has little supportive evidence. Some non-specific factors may be immunosuppressive. Corticosteroids, progesterone, oestrogen and placental hormones may cause local immunosuppression. Pregnancy-associated plasma proteins, including human placental lactogen, are immunosuppressive *in vitro*, but their role *in vivo* is not known.

There are, however, antigens that have the potential to stimulate maternal immune responses, and there are antibodies that cross into the fetus. Anti-HLA antibodies are detectable in some pregnancies. Fetal leucocytes may leak into the maternal circulation and stimulate their production. Haemorrhage at delivery augments this, and there is an increase in detectable anti-HLA antibody postpartum. Transmission of maternal antibodies into the fetus occurs in two ways: antenatally by transfer across the placenta, and then from breast milk. IgG is actively transferred *in utero*, and the fetal serum level rapidly increases at 26–34 weeks' gestation. Immunoglobulin A (IgA), which protects the gut against enteric infections, is transferred in human breast milk. The neonate replaces maternal antibodies by its own production of immunoglobulins during the first three months of life, and this is complete by one year.

Disorders
- *Isoantibodies.* Access of fetal erythrocytes, leucocytes and platelets to the maternal circulation at the time of haemorrhage or termination of pregnancy can elicit maternal IgG by isoimmunization. Rhesus haemolytic disease is the most severe form of this condition, where maternal antibodies produced by earlier or previous immunological challenges against the Rh(D) antigen of fetal erythrocytes bind to the red cells and cause them to lyse.
- *Autoantibodies.* Autoimmune disease in pregnancy sometimes produces maternal IgG autoantibodies that cross the placenta. They may bind to fetal cellular receptors in thyrotoxicosis and myasthenia gravis, or form circulating immune complexes in SLE, or activate compliment and effector cells in autoimmune haemolytic anaemia. The effects are usually transient, reflecting the catabolism of maternal immunoglobulins, and disappear in the fetus within three months of age.
- *Fetal immune system.* The fetal immune system is able to respond to infection from approximately 12 weeks' gestation. The response includes fetal synthesis of immunoglobulins, particularly IgM and IgG. Maternal vaccination may also enhance fetal antibody response. Theoretically, inactivated vaccines do not put the fetus at risk of infection or teratogenicity.

The main placental transfer of IgG occurs after 32 weeks' gestation, and premature infants are susceptible to infection, since this transfer has not occurred. The half-life of IgG is three weeks, so the period of three weeks to six months after birth is a phase of relative immunoglobulin deficiency.

10.1.3. Clinical disorders

Immunodeficiency

Immunodeficiency may be the result of congenital or acquired disease, and may even be due to therapy for malignancy, or immune suppression for transplant viability. There may be deficiencies in various parts of the immune system, e.g. cellular, humoral and factors.

The protective role of the complement system is illustrated by congenital deficiencies. A C1 esterase inhibition deficiency with an incidence of one in 50 000, as a result of new mutations, is of particular anaesthetic and obstetric importance because acute recurrent mucosal or skin oedema can occur. Vaginal delivery may be impeded by perineal oedema. Recurrent abdominal pain may occur at any time, and should be included in the differential diagnosis of obstetric complications. Regional anaesthesia is to be preferred to general anaesthesia for operative delivery, as laryngopharyngeal oedema may complicate airway manoeuvres. Treatment in pregnancy and labour is with C1 esterase inhibitor [7].

Human immunodeficiency virus (HIV) binds to the CD4 molecule and integrates into the host cell. The host can be any cell expressing the CD4 receptor, such as the T cell, macrophage, monocyte and some cells in the central nervous system. Infected cells malfunction, and a decline in CD4-expressing T cells can be measured. This is an important monitor of progression towards acquired immune deficiency syndrome (AIDS).

Tissue transplantation and immunosuppression

It is the T lymphocyte that develops an immune response to transplanted tissue. These cells can be killed by a purine antimetabolite such as azathioprine, but the patient becomes susceptible to infections and cancer. Glucocorticoids inhibit the production of IL-2 and therefore T cell proliferation, but have side effects. T cells can be suppressed by antibodies such as antilymphocyte globulin. Division of activated T cells is prevented by cyclosporin A.

Interactions can occur between immunosuppressive therapy and anaesthesia. Cyclosporin A decreases levels of cytochrome P450 and hence decreases the rate of drug metabolism, and potentially can prolong the action of barbiturates and opioids [8,9]. Prolonged neuromuscular blockade has also been described following the use of non-depolarizing muscle relaxants in patients taking cyclosporin [10] and azathioprine [11].

Hypersensitivity reactions

Gell and Coombs described four hypersensitivity reactions against extrinsic and intrinsic antigens: types I, II and III are mediated mainly by antibodies, and type IV has cell-mediated immunity. This classification is no longer clinically useful, as it does not take into account the possible aetiological factors. Prophylaxis and treatment have therefore not yet been fully clarified, since the different types overlap. Their basic characteristics are as follows.

- *Type I* are rapid reactions in which an antigen interacts with immunoglobulin E (IgE) bound to tissue mast cells or basophils. IgG-mediated reactions can also occur.
- *Type II* reactions are initiated by antibody reacting with antigens that are part of the cell membrane. The consequences of this depend on further immune interactions. IgG and IgM can be involved. This type of reaction includes autoimmune diseases, e.g. myasthenia gravis, and reactions against blood, such as mismatched transfusions. Not all autoimmune diseases follow a type II reaction.
- *Type III* reactions result from the presence of immune complexes in the circulation or in the tissues. They can accumulate in large amounts.
- *Type IV* reactions are initiated by T cells, which react with antigen and release lymphokines. Lymphokines then attract other cells. This reaction takes days, compared with the type I, II and III reactions, which occur within minutes or hours. The factors that can cause this reaction to become pathological may include the nature of the antigen, e.g. it may not be degradable. On laboratory examination, type IV reactions may have type II reactions present as well.

Initiation and detection of IgE activity. The acute type I IgE responses are usually directed against antigens entering at epithelial surfaces. Multiparous women will have had multiple exposures to antigens (drugs or agents) used in labour. There may be a family history of type I allergic reactions (such as atopy, or anaphylaxis), but a genetic basis is not yet determined. Mast cells liberate their granules and release histamine, heparin, leucotrienes (arachidonic acid metabolites) and other mediators of acute inflammation. Anaphylactoid reactions are accompanied by the same mediators, but are not initiated by IgE activity. Hypersensitivity reactions from IgE activity are usually identified both by the production of immunological factors and by skin testing [12]. IgE can be detected by radioimmunoassay techniques, particularly the specialized radioallergosorbent test (RAST) or the enzyme-linked immunosorbent assay (ELISA) for quantitative measures without the use of isotopes. A normal IgE level does not exclude a type I reaction, either because it is consumed in such reactions or because the particular IgE responsible for the clinical reaction makes only a small contribution to the total IgE level. Complement assays are not diagnostic. The tryptase level is a marker of mast cell degranulation. Skin testing, preferably with the prick test [13] may help to distinguish the agent

Table 10.2 Clinical signs of acute anaphylactic (IgE-mediated) or anaphylactoid (non-IgE-mediated) reaction.

System	Sign	Differential diagnosis
Cardiovascular	Hypotension	Total spinal
		Sympathetic blockade caused by regional nerve block
		Haemorrhage
		Drug overdosage (e.g. local anaesthetic)
		Myocardial infarction
	Cardiac arrhythmias	
Respiratory	Bronchospasm	Asthma
	Acute respiratory failure (tachypnoea, cyanosis)	Pulmonary embolism
		Amniotic fluid embolism
		Aspiration of stomach contents
	Laryngeal oedema	
	Pulmonary oedema	Acute heart failure
Skin	Itching	Epidural opioids
	Weals	Angioedema
	Flushing	Vasodilation
Gastrointestinal	Abdominal pain	Obstetric complications
	Diarrhoea	Infection

causing the reaction, particularly with anaesthetic agents where more than one drug has usually been administered. A negative test, however, does not guarantee a negative response to a systemic challenge.

Specific IgE antibodies to thiopental, suxamethonium, non-depolarizing neuromuscular blocking drugs and pethidine have been identified. Antibodies to other potent antigens used in obstetrics, such as latex [14], chlorhexidine and ethylene oxide [15] have also been identified. Neuromuscular blocking drugs account for 70% of the hypersensitivity reactions in anaesthesia, but only 30–40% of such reactions have a history of previous exposure to the drug. Vecuronium has an inherently safe molecule, because the quaternary ammonium group is monovalent. Cross-reactivity occurs between substances with quaternary ammonium groups, which are commonly found in cosmetics, and household chemicals, as well as anaesthetic drugs. A history of hypersensitivity reactions in the home should alert the anaesthetist to the possibility of problems during anaesthesia. Preventive measures for latex allergy have been described [16].

Clinical anaphylactic and anaphylactoid reactions. When an anaphylactic or anaphylactoid reaction occurs during pregnancy, cutaneous, systemic or life-threatening reactions can occur. The main associated clinical signs of severe systematic reactions are bronchospasm, flushing, hypotension and tachycardia (Table 10.2). These clinical signs may be mimicked during magnesium administration for the treatment of pre-eclampsia. Fetal distress will commonly be induced by the rapid onset of hypoxaemia and poor placental blood flow, and can be further aggravated by aortocaval compression. The relative hypovolaemia from vasodilation that accompanies the reaction may be confused with side effects of regional anaesthesia, because autonomic blockade can contribute to the speed and severity of the circulatory failure. The combination of a failed epidural and anaphylaxis during induction of general anaesthesia is potentially fatal [17], and reactions that were refractory to treatment have been described in the presence of a drug-induced beta blockade [18]. The differential diagnosis of these cardiovascular changes together with acute respiratory distress in a parturient woman includes aspiration of gastric contents, drug overdosage, myocardial infarction, acute heart failure, thromboembolism and amniotic fluid embolism.

- *Reactions associated with oxytocin* (Syntocinon). Hypersensitivity reactions to oxytocin have occurred during epidural and spinal anaesthesia after delivery of the fetus [19–21]. Oxytocin often has additives in solution, and one patient reacted to the chlorbutol used in the oxytocin preparation. The reaction led to a laparotomy to exclude intra-abdominal haemorrhage, and presented difficulties in tracheal tube placement because the larynx was oedematous, further exposing the patient to risks. All the patients reacting to oxytocin initially received oxygen, crystalloids or ephedrine. Bronchodilators were also used in two of the women, and steroids and epinephrine (adrenaline) in separate patients.

- *Reactions associated with antibiotics.* Obstetric patients are routinely given antibiotics and antacid prophylaxis prior to or during Caesarean section. At this stage in pregnancy, any hypersensitivity reaction can affect the fetus if hypotension and hypoxia occur for a critical period of time. A hypotensive reaction to ampicillin resulted in a severely acidotic fetus with long-term central neurological deficits [22].

- *Reactions associated with ranitidine.* Reactions to ranitidine, given orally or intravenously prior to Caesarean section, have presented with dyspnoea [23–25]. Oxygen, chlorphenamine and hydrocortisone were the main therapies. Epinephrine was not used in the case of a woman in labour, because the fetus was bradycardic and assumed to be already distressed. The ranitidine had been administered for prophylaxis because the woman was considered to have a high risk of operative delivery. Another woman who had a reaction to ranitidine started to labour, and spinal anaesthesia was chosen in order to avoid a difficult intubation from laryngeal oedema. Although it was seven hours after the reaction, severe hypotension occurred during the operation. This was probably the result of a sympathetic block plus the relative hypovolaemia from circulatory and tissue effects of the reaction.

- *Reactions associated with local anaesthetics.* Allergic reactions to amide local anaesthetics are very rare [26]. The reactions that are most frequently observed result from relative overdose, intravascular injection, or the effect of other agents in the solution, such as vasopressors or preservatives.

Table 10.3 Treatment of anaphylaxis in pregnancy.

Immediate
Stop giving drug/using agent
Summon help urgently/start cardiopulmonary resuscitation if necessary
Lateral tilt or lift uterus up to prevent inferior vena cava occlusion
Maintain airway, supply 100% oxygen, ensure adequate ventilation
Establish i.v. access with a large bore cannula (central venous cannula if necessary)
Give ephedrine 30 mg i.v.
Start rapid volume expansion with crystalloid solution
Consider delivery if fetus is *in utero*

Then
Epinephrine (50–100 µg boluses) if ephedrine does not restore blood pressure in 1–2 mins
Treat bronchospasm with salbutamol i.v. (250 µg loading dose followed by 5–20 µg/min as infusion). NB, *causes uterine relaxation and may increase bleeding*
Antihistamine: chlorphenamine 10–20 mg i.v. slowly (crosses the placenta, and can cause neonatal depression)
Steroids: hydrocortisone 100 mg i.v.
Take blood for arterial blood gases, electrolytes, clotting screen, haematocrit and investigation of case
Intensive-care unit admission

Patient follow-up
Skin prick tests
Immunological tests
Report reaction to Committee on Safety of Medicine via Yellow Card system (pharmacy will have them)
Document results in patient's notes
Inform the patient, verbally and in writing
Inform the patient's general practitioner in writing
Patient wears warning device

General treatment. Table 10.3 summarizes the treatment of a suspected anaphylactic reaction. Inferior vena caval occlusion must be swiftly avoided by uterine displacement. Additional oxygen must be administered through a patent airway [27], and ventilation with 100% oxygen must be instituted if hypoxia is not corrected quickly. Epinephrine is the drug of choice in non-pregnant women [12]. There are reservations concerning its use in obstetrics due to its adverse effects on placental perfusion, leading to fetal compromise [28]. Ephedrine has been used effectively and may be less arrhythmogenic [29], but in the clinical scenario of severe hypotension and bronchospasm, epinephrine is the drug of choice even with a fetus *in utero*, provided that it is given in small intravenous bolus doses (50–100 µg, i.e. 0.5–1.0 mL of 1 : 10 000 epinephrine) until a circulatory or bronchopulmonary response is obtained.

Type I reactions may be treated by antagonizing type I pathways and limiting tissue damage. Methods used to antagonize type I pathways, such as inhaled sodium cromoglycate and parenteral steroids, are not sufficiently fast-acting to be used as first-line therapy. Once a reaction has occurred, these methods can only be used to prevent further damage.

Protocols for rapid treatment of anaphylaxis have been written for non-pregnant patients [12], and the principles underlying them apply also when treating the parturient. The severity of clinical symptoms differs between organ systems, and their times of onset and the response to treatment are variable, but immediate management is designed to maintain tissue oxygenation. Secondary management treats symptoms. Tissue oxygenation should be achieved by adequate ventilation with oxygen, and normalization of venous return (preventing inferior vena cava occlusion) with intravascular volume expansion (not dextran in pregnancy [30]) and a vasopressor.

The changes associated with hypersensitivity reactions can produce fetal hypoxia by various mechanisms. Blood flow to the uterus may be affected, microemboli of immune complexes may cause placental insufficiency, and immunological function in the fetus may be disturbed. When the fetus is *in utero*, treatment of maternal hypersensitivity reactions may have to be modified. If the reaction is mild, premature fetal delivery may be postponed. However, most case reports describe reactions at delivery with varying fetal effects after the administration of either ephedrine or epinephrine. Epinephrine is the standard drug in anaphylaxis, because it has both α-adrenergic and β-adrenergic effects. It can cause both vasoconstriction and bronchodilation. Its deleterious effects on placental flow may be mitigated by judicious use of titrated doses.

Autoimmunity

Certain combinations of MHC class II molecules and autoantigens can result in overproduction of antibodies. This can account for some of the strong association of diseases with particular regions of the MHC on chromosome 6. Systemic lupus erythematosus differs in its loci from rheumatoid arthritis, myasthenia gravis, thyrotoxicosis (Graves disease) and Goodpasture's syndrome.

Women with diseases unrelated to pregnancy may become pregnant and physiological changes associated with pregnancy may significantly modify the disease, or the fetus can be affected by the disease or by therapeutic measures intended to suppress the maternal disease. These effects on mother and fetus are summarized in Table 10.4.

Systemic lupus erythematosus (SLE). SLE is predominantly a disease of young women. One in five patients first presents during pregnancy. The fetal survival rate with active disease is only 64% [31], whereas if the disease is quiescent the rate increases to 83%. Renal involvement is a major risk factor for fetal mortality. Careful monitoring of blood pressure and serum creatinine and urea levels is required. Renal disease and hypertension compromise the utero-placental circulation, and regular fetal assessment is also required.

Table 10.4 Autoimmune diseases and their major pregnancy complications.

Disease	Maternal complications	Fetal complications
Systemic lupus erythematosus	Hypertension Steroid therapy Worsening renal function Thrombosis (treated with low-dose aspirin) Thrombocytopenia (*differential diagnosis: pre-eclampsia*)	Stillbirth Prematurity Intrauterine growth retardation Neonatal lupus (congenital heart block)
Rheumatoid arthritis	Remission during pregnancy Positioning the patient may be difficult Relapse in the puerperium	Effects of immunosuppressive agents
Myasthenia gravis	Unpredictable	Transient myasthenia in 10% of infants
Idiopathic thrombocytopenia	Haemorrhage in labour Relapse may occur during pregnancy	Neonatal thrombocytopenia

The anaesthetist is not only concerned with renal function in this condition, but also with haematological disorders, since anaemia occurs in more than 70% of the women and is accompanied by thrombocytopenia, which can lead to bleeding disorders. Immunosuppressive therapy with azathioprine in addition to oral steroids is recommended for these complications [32]. Cardiopulmonary features of SLE should also be assessed by an anaesthetist. Pericardial disease is the most common complication. Lung function tests show a greater degree of respiratory tract involvement than is evident clinically. Neurological lesions may also be present, and although convulsions are rare, they may mimic eclampsia. Depression and anxiety are also common. The anaesthetist must also be aware that cross-matching problems may arise due to abnormal antibodies in the patient's serum.

Anaesthetic care should focus on a full evaluation of all systems, minimizing renal dysfunction, choosing drugs and techniques compatible with the patient's renal, cardiac and respiratory disease, and prescribing parenteral steroid cover if the parturient is being maintained with oral steroids. Women with the disease should be delivered where intensive-care facilities for the fetus are available.

Sepsis

There is evidence that pregnancy may increase susceptibility to the effects of endotoxin [33], and the pregnant woman should be considered to be a compromised bacterial host. Endotoxin produces maternal pyrexia, which can limit maternal–fetal temperature exchange and cause the release of compounds such as cytokines. It can also activate the complement system and clotting cascade. Vasoactive compounds are also released that increase vascular permeability and vasodilation.

The number of woman dying from genital tract sepsis, excluding abortion, in the past 10 years has not declined. Prophylactic antibiotics are now recommended [34] for Caesarean section. Diabetic women and those receiving steroid therapy may be more at risk of sepsis, and diagnosis of early infection is difficult in these women as the white blood cell count is normally elevated (10 000–15 000 cells/mm³) in pregnancy.

Women are at risk antenatally, as well as at delivery, from bacterial infection. Bacteraemia is commonly associated with renal tract infection, chorioamnionitis, abortion and listeriosis. The principles of antibiotic therapy have to be applied rigorously in order to prevent generalized sepsis and septic shock (see Section 24.2.3, p. 433]. For example, renal tract infections require antibiotic drugs that are concentrated in the renal system, and retained products of conception have to be removed before broad-spectrum antibiotics can be used to treat endometritis. Blood and vaginal cultures are essential, and antibiotics should be prescribed according to the organism's sensitivity.

Pyrexia

The physiological changes associated with fever in pregnancy can be detrimental to the fetus. Uterine activity increases, and premature labour can result. Fever and pain associated with uterine contractions increase ventilation, further reducing carbon dioxide tension. Alkalaemia shifts the oxyhaemoglobin dissociation curve to the left, decreasing oxygen transport. Oxygen consumption increases in fever, and the basal metabolic rate is increased by 14% for each degree Celsius rise in body temperature. Heart rate and cardiac output will also be increased above pregnant values. Catecholamines released by the hyperthermic process generate these cardiovascular changes and decrease uterine blood flow. Lactic acidosis may result from an inadequate tissue oxygen supply.

Uterine blood flow maintains the fetal–maternal temperature difference of about 0.5°C by heat exchange. When maternal temperature increases, the fetal temperature also increases, because there is a limited reserve capacity in the heat exchange system, and fetal distress occurs. Fetal tachycardia is observed initially, and then heart rate irregularities. An emergency Caesarean section may be required.

The anaesthetist confronted by a septic pyrexial patient must first assess maternal tissue oxygenation and cardiovascular function. The choice of techniques in the presence of infection is discussed in Section 15.2.3, p. 229 and Section 15.8.8, p. 274. Pain relief may limit some of the cardiovascular changes, and active cooling should be considered, as well as providing additional oxygen by mask. Peripheral vasodilation is associated with sepsis, and active peripheral cooling should be undertaken urgently to minimize fetal risks. Adequate intravenous fluids should be provided with central venous pressure control, and urinary output should be measured. An arterial catheter is useful for monitoring acid–base changes and arterial blood pressure.

10.2 Specific infections

Although neither viral or other infections (e.g. tuberculosis) seem to be more common in pregnancy, nor are localized infections more likely to become generalized, the course and outcome of infections occurring in pregnancy may be altered by physiological changes; for example, the pulmonary complications of measles and varicella tend to be more severe [35], may affect the fetus, and also present a risk to attending personnel.

Maternal viral infections can affect the fetus directly by viraemic placental transmission or by ascending genital infection. Rubella virus, cytomegalovirus, varicella-zoster virus, human immunodeficiency viruses and occasionally hepatitis B virus cross the placenta. Systemic effects of infections, such as fever and septicaemia with hypoxia and tissue acidosis, are detrimental to the fetus. Viral infections present a greater risk than bacterial infections, since there are no direct treatments. Vaccination can be used as a protective measure, e.g. hepatitis B vaccination [36], but it is not available for some viral diseases, and protection against transmission therefore has to be provided.

Anaesthetic risk factors for the patient include the potential introduction of infection, either to the central nervous system during a regional nerve block, or—when general anaesthesia is used—into the respiratory tract. Viruses that may affect the mother and have serious consequences for the child include rubella, cytomegalovirus, herpes simplex, hepatitis B, papilloma and HIV. When *in utero* infection of the fetus has occurred, fetal distress may present in labour, and the anaesthetist should be prepared for an emergency Caesarean section or neonatal resuscitation, or both.

The anaesthetist may become involved in the intensive-care management of parturient patients when viral pneumonia necessitates mechanical ventilation. Maternal mortality from this condition is increased in the third trimester [37], and smokers have a higher risk of lung complications following varicella [38]. Intravenous acyclovir would be the treatment of choice in these high-risk groups, despite the theoretical role of fetal damage.

10.2.1 Tuberculosis

Pulmonary tuberculosis is common in areas of poverty, and infection is acquired through the respiratory tract. Among the homeless, drug-resistant forms are increasing [39]. Factors such as decreased immunity due to disease (HIV infection) play a major role in the pathogenesis, especially in parts of the developing world. In pregnancy, tuberculous endometriosis and mastitis can increase the likelihood of transmission to the fetus or neonate, respectively.

Patients may be asymptomatic or have a cough, sputum production, weight loss and night sweats. The differential diagnosis will include other causes of pneumonia, pulmonary embolism and carcinoma. The diagnosis of active pulmonary tuberculosis can be made by sputum stained for acid-fast bacilli. If active infection is present, the anaesthetist must use disposable equipment and protect non-disposable and non-sterilizable equipment, such as mechanical ventilators, from contamination. There may be septicaemia during active infection, and a regional nerve block may be complicated by meningitis. Transmission of infection to health workers and other patients should be prevented by using isolation facilities for the patient and bacille Calmette–Guérin (BCG) vaccination for all attendants. In treated or inactive disease, there is no need to isolate the infant from the mother as long as she has been on effective chemotherapy for two weeks and her sputum cultures are negative.

10.2.2 Human immunodeficiency virus (HIV)

The human immunodeficiency virus penetrates T cells, and an antibody response gradually develops over a variable time, but it does not eradicate the virus or confer immunity. It indicates active infection. There are three main routes of transmission of the virus:
- intimate physical contact (mainly sexual);
- perinatal transmission;
- exposure to blood or blood products.

The prevalence of HIV infection in antenatal clinic populations in the United Kingdom varies from one in 5000 to one in 16 000, depending on the population studied [40]. During parturition, a number of highly infective fluids are shed, so that the fetus/neonate and obstetric health-care workers are at risk. The fluids most likely to transmit infection are blood, amniotic fluid and vaginal secretions. Cerebrospinal fluid is also able to transmit the virus. Nasal secretions, saliva, sweat, urine and vomitus are not considered to present a significant transmission risk unless they are visibly contaminated with blood [36]. All obstetric patients should therefore be regarded as being in a higher than normal risk category for the disease, and all units must always have guidelines on the use of protective practices.

The primary illness, with 'flu-like' symptoms, is followed by an asymptomatic period that may last several years, during which serum antibodies can confirm that infection has occurred. HIV infection in pregnancy may be recognized by known infection, screening, or the appearance of clinical disease. Pregnancy does not change the natural history of HIV infection. Universal screening is not yet accepted for social and political reasons, and risk assessment is therefore usually based on medical history. A high risk of the infection is associated with intravenous drug use, clinical features of HIV, indiscriminate promiscuous sexual behaviour (e.g. multiple sexual partners), blood transfusion given before HIV screening, and areas of high prevalence, e.g. urban areas. Women with high-risk histories should be offered testing after counselling. Anaesthetists may assume that such high-risk histories have been taken in antenatal clinics, but where patients are transferred to hospitals in emergency or have neglected to attend for antenatal care, these assumptions may not be correct. It will be necessary to adopt precautions (see p. 182) if a woman has not been screened but is identified as being in a high-risk group.

About 28% of the babies of infected mothers become infected *in utero*, and 20% during labour [41,42]. Vertical transmission of HIV can occur from mother to child. There is strong evidence that perinatal transmission can be significantly reduced by the administration of zidovudine [40]. Presumably, transmission is prevented by decreasing maternal viraemia or preventing infection in the fetus. The long-term effects of exposure of the fetus to zidovudine have still to be assessed. Strategies to reduce the infant's exposure to HIV-infected maternal blood and vaginal secretions have included Caesarean section delivery and drug therapies. There is accumulating evidence that Caesarean section is protective [42]. However, data from the European Collaborative Study, with information on maternal status, the type of delivery, and long-term infant follow-up establishing the best method of delivery. The protective effects of any one method have to be balanced against its risks (for the mother with symptomatic disease, or through occupational exposure of the obstetrician) and the costs involved. Attempts to develop a randomized controlled trial of delivery have not been successful [43].

Fetal welfare during labour must be assessed only by non-invasive methods, because there is a risk to the fetus of transmission of infection if fetal scalp electrode monitoring or sampling of scalp blood is used.

Clinical manifestations of progressive disease are summarized in Table 10.5. A detailed systematic history and examination are required before anaesthesia in order to assess the risks of intervention for an obstetric procedure. The association of HIV with drug abuse may have prevented the mother from seeking antenatal care [44]. Florid complications may therefore be present, but more insidious may be the development of pneumonia. Neurological manifestations must be defined before any anaesthetic intervention, but neurological deficits themselves would not be a contraindication to regional analgesia unless there was an increase in intracranial pressure or an alteration of consciousness.

Regional anaesthesia can be performed without adverse sequelae [45], but it is contraindicated if a coagulopathy is present. The choice of the subarachnoid or epidural route may depend not on the patient's symptoms but on the anaesthetist deciding to avoid cerebrospinal fluid leakage. Since the virus is most likely to be present in cerebrospinal fluid, the introduction of infection there is not considered to be a danger to the mother. In the event of a postdural puncture headache, the risks of an autologous blood patch for the anaesthetist may be avoided by extradural saline infusion or heterologous HIV-negative

Table 10.5 Systemic manifestations of acquired immune deficiency syndrome.

System	Disorders	Anaesthetic problems
Central nervous system	Encephalopathy	Confusion
	Meningitis	
	Toxoplasmosis	Increased intracranial pressure
	Dementia	Poor cooperation
	Peripheral neuropathy	Neurological complications
Respiratory	Bacterial pneumonia (tuberculosis, *Pneumocystis carinii*)	Hypoxia
		Acute respiratory failure
	Fungal pneumonia (aspergillosis)	
Gastrointestinal	Colitis	Dehydration and fluid and electrolyte imbalance
	Oral candidiasis	Difficult airway management (easily traumatized)
Haematological	Anaemia	Tissue hypoxia
	Thrombocytopenia	Coagulation disorders
	Leukopenia	Infection susceptibility
Cardiovascular	Myocarditis	Dysrhythmias, heart failure
Immune	Immunodeficiency	Bacterial sepsis (epidural abscess)
	Diffuse adenopathy	Tonsillar hypertrophy may cause airway obstruction or difficult intubation

blood [46]. In some centres, autologous blood patch is routine, because the mother is assumed to have central nervous system infection.

The choice and dosage of drugs for general anaesthesia will depend on the function of the respiratory and cardiovascular systems and predictable complications. Weight loss is a feature even in pregnancy, and drug dosage should take into account altered pharmacokinetics. Convulsions can complicate HIV infections, and agents such as enflurane and ketamine, which are epileptogenic, should therefore be avoided. The induction of general anaesthesia may be complicated by oral fungal infections, which increase the fragility of the mucous membranes and cause bleeding, and poor mobility of the larynx at intubation.

Prevention of occupational exposure to HIV

Transmission of HIV from patients to heath-care personnel has occurred by blood contact through non-intact skin, mucous membranes, or direct penetration and most commonly follows a needle-stick injury [47]. The risk following needle-stick injury involving contaminated blood is 0.4%, and prophylactic treatment should be sought within one or two hours of exposure. Adoption of strict infection control guidelines is the most effective means of preventing the transmission of infection, because there is no cure for this disease. When a woman is known to be infected with HIV, operating theatre policies will limit staff access to the theatre, staff will wear protective gowns, glasses and gloves, and the theatre will be cleaned after use. Infected patients will therefore require commensurately more theatre time to allow these measures to be taken.

Universal precautions

HIV-infected patients may not always be identified, so blood and body fluids should be considered potentially infective. Professional guidelines for universal precautions have been published by the Association of Anaesthetists of Great Britain and Ireland [36] to protect anaesthetists from viral blood-borne infections. These precautions should be adhered to strictly. The incidence of needle-stick injury can be reduced by the use of blunt, non-pointed needles, such as hollow quills for drawing up drugs, and if a sharp needle has to be used for injection purposes it should be disposed of immediately in marked, tough, disposal bins, and should not be resheathed. Needles should not be handed from one person to another but should be placed in a tray and picked up by the other person. Gloves must be worn for all anaesthetic techniques, and where substantial spillage of blood is likely, e.g. with an intra-arterial line, a plastic apron, mask and eye protection should be worn. Gloves should be changed after induction and any other procedures involving blood or airway secretion contamination. Used gloves should be removed before handling notes, equipment, etc. Any skin abrasions or cuts must be protected by a water-proof dressing. All items used in airway maintenance should be disposed of or sterilized between patient use. Whenever possible, disposable items should be used. An appropriate disposable filter should be placed between the mother and the breathing system. Any blood-contaminated floors or surfaces should be washed with a solution of hypochlorite containing 10 000 p.p.m. available chlorine, and then washed with detergent and water. The same care and precautions must also be followed during resuscitation of a neonate from a high-risk mother.

When blood samples are sent to the laboratory, they should be identified as being infective if the patient is known to have a blood-borne infection. Any incident of exposure must be reported so that postexposure management can start immediately. The hospital's occupational health service would be responsible for this type of care.

10.2.3 Hepatitis B

Infection with hepatitis B virus is a major problem throughout the world. Following infection, an acute illness and/or the carrier state develops. The carrier state occurs in 5–10% of infected adults, and about one in 500 of the adult population in the United Kingdom is a carrier. The long-term consequences of infection include cirrhosis, chronic active hepatitis and primary liver cancer. Hepatitis B virus is more easily transmitted than HIV, and small amounts of blood, vaginal secretions and breast milk can be a source of infection for the fetus, neonate or health personnel.

All pregnant women are screened for hepatitis B viral infection, because transmission can easily occur after contact with very small quantities of blood. It is because of the highly infective nature of the hepatitis B virus that all anaesthetists must know their immune status and have an adequate antibody titre. This will be monitored by an occupational health service.

10.2.4 Hepatitis C

Mother-to-infant transmission is unusual, and although hepatitis C virus RNA has been found in breast milk, infection of infants by breast-feeding has not been reported.

10.2.5 Hepatitis E

This has been reported to cause intrauterine infection and perinatal morbidity and mortality. Infection is faecal–oral, and although chronic disease is lacking, sporadic disease is common and viraemia can be protracted.

10.2.6 Herpes simplex

Herpes simplex virus types 1 and 2 can both cause genital infection and can be transmitted to the neonate through the placenta or at delivery. The incidence is rare in the United Kingdom (less than three per 100 000 live births, in contrast to the United States, where the rate is one in 7500 live births). Herpes simplex virus type 2 may commonly be shed from the genital tract without producing symptoms. Both viruses infect neural and epidermal tissues. The first episode of genital herpes may occur in the peripartum period and result in a large area of infection on the vulva and cervix, infecting the newborn during labour. Transmission to the fetus occurs in 33–50% of primary cases, 3% of symptomatic recurrences and less than 0.01% of asymptomatic shedding [48]. Maternal complications of primary genital infection include aseptic meningitis and superinfection with bacteria or fungi. Neonatal herpes infection may lead to mucocutaneous disease, encephalitis and disseminated disease to major organs such as the liver and lungs.

Acyclovir is the main treatment for herpes simplex infections. It has less effect in recurrent infections. Prophylactic use of the drug, either in patients with severe recurrent genital infection or in those in whom immunosuppressive therapy is being used, can reduce the number of recurrences but does not eradicate the disease. Transmission of the virus to the neonate has been prevented by early identification of mothers with a primary infection and subsequent delivery by Caesarean section [49]. However, placental transmission may occur before delivery, and postnatal transmission may also occur.

Anaesthesia and herpes simplex

It is important to remember that anaesthetists should protect themselves against viral transmission of infection from oral secretions by routinely wearing gloves and eye protection when performing airway manipulations.

Regional techniques—both subarachnoid and epidural block—have been used without difficulties in patients suffering from herpes simplex. Theoretically, however, there is a possibility of introducing the virus into the central nervous system during the placement of a spinal or epidural needle, and this must be considered in the differential diagnosis of postpartum headache or neurological sequelae after regional analgesia. If a herpetic lesion is present near the lumbar region, regional anaesthesia is best avoided. In a retrospective study of 169 patients (delivered by Caesarean section because of primary or secondary infection) who received general anaesthesia or spinal or epidural anaesthesia, no patients with secondary infection had septic or neurological complications related to the anaesthetic. One patient with primary herpes infection who received spinal anaesthesia had a transient postpartum neurological defect [50]. Epidural anaesthesia for Caesarean section in 89 women with recurrent herpes simplex was without complication in an anaesthetic retrospective study [51]. However, the numbers in both studies were small, and the negative findings do not exclude the possibility of the complication.

The use of spinal narcotics has been controversial, because it was suggested that epidural morphine triggered reactivation of herpes simplex virus infection [52]. However, in a study of two groups, one of which received epidural block and the other intramuscular opioids, the groups were found to have a similar positive viral serology and a low incidence of oral viral shedding [53]. Low-dose intrathecal morphine for Caesarean section delivery in a large group of women with herpes in remission was not associated with reactivation of the virus [54]. The trauma caused by scratching in response to itching due to high-dose morphine may, however, initiate clinically apparent lesions, so prompt treatment of pruritus should be given. Pruritus in the area of the trigeminal nerve as a result of epidural morphine may generate scratching and the trauma necessary to reactivate the virus. Further prospective randomized controlled studies are needed, and in the meantime the risk of reactivating the disease should be discussed with the mother prior to pain relief.

References

1 Heinrich PC, Castell JV, Andus T. Interleukin-6 and the acute phase response. *Biochem J* 1990; **265**: 621–36.

2. Dudley DJ. The immune system in health and disease. *Baillière's Clin Obstet Gynaecol* 1992; **6**: 393–416.
3. Stein C. The control of pain in peripheral tissue by opioids. *N Engl J Med* 1995; **332**: 1685–90.
4. Creasey AA, Stevens P, Kenney J *et al.* Endotoxin and cytokine profile in plasma of baboons challenged with lethal and sublethal *Escherichia coli. Circ Shock* 1991; **33**: 84–91.
5. Lahita RG. The effect of sex hormones on the immune system in pregnancy. *Am J Reprod Immunol* 1992; **28**: 136–7.
6. Hunt JS, Hsi BL. Evasive strategies of trophoblast cells: selective expression of membrane antigens. *Am J Reprod Immunol* 1990; **23**: 57–63.
7. Cox M, Holdcroft A. Hereditary angioneurotic oedema: current management in pregnancy. *Anaesthesia* 1995; **50**: 547–9.
8. Cirella VN, Pantuck CB, Lee YJ, Pantuck EJ. Effects of cyclosporine on anesthetic action. *Anesth Analg* 1987; **66**: 703–6.
9. Augustine JA, Zemaitis MA. The effects of cyclosporine (C_sA) on hepatic microsomal drug metabolism in the rat. *Drug Metab Dispos* 1986; **14**: 73–8.
10. Sidi A, Kaplan RF, Davis RF. Prolonged neuromuscular blockade and ventilatory failure after renal transplantation and cyclosporine. *Can J Anaesth* 1990; **37**: 543–8.
11. Gramstad L. Atracurium, vecuronium and pancuronium in end stage renal failure. Dose–response properties and interactions with azathioprine. *Br J Anaesth* 1987; **59**: 995–1003.
12. Association of Anaesthetists of Great Britain and Ireland and the British Society of Allergy and Clinical Immunology. *Suspected Anaphylactic Reactions Associated with Anaesthesia.* London: AAGBI, 1995.
13. Fisher M. Intradermal testing after anaphylactoid reaction to anaesthetic drugs: practical aspects of performance and interpretation. *Anaesth Intensive Care* 1984; **12**: 115–20.
14. Laurent J, Malet R, Smiejan M, Madelenat P, Herman D. Latex hypersensitivity after natural delivery. *Allergy Clin Immunol* 1992; **89**: 779–80.
15. McKinnon RP, Wildsmith JA. Histaminoid reactions in anaesthesia. *Br J Anaesth* 1995; **74**: 217–28.
16. Dakin MJ, Yentis SM. Latex allergy: a strategy for management. *Anaesthesia* 1998; **53**: 774–81.
17. Fisher M. Personal communication. 1995.
18. Hannaway PJ, Hopper JD. Severe anaphylaxis and drug-induced beta blockade. *N Engl J Med* 1983; **308**: 1536.
19. Emmott RS. Recurrent anaphylactoid reaction during Caesarean section. *Anaesthesia* 1994; **45**: 62.
20. Morris WW, Lavies NG, Anderson SK, Southgate HJ. Acute respiratory distress during Caesarean section under spinal anaesthesia: a probable case of anaphylactoid reaction to Syntocinon. *Anaesthesia* 1994; **49**: 41–3.
21. Maycock EJ, Russell WC. Anaphylactoid reaction to Syntocinon. *Anaesth Intensive Care* 1993; **21**: 211–12.
22. Heim K, Alge A, Marth C. Anaphylactic reaction to ampicillin and severe complication in the fetus. *Lancet* 1991; **337**: 859–60.
23. Barry JES, Madan R, Hewitt PB. Anaphylactoid reaction to ranitidine in an obstetric patient. *Anaesthesia* 1992; **47**: 360–1.
24. Powell JA, Maycock EJ. Anaphylactoid reaction to ranitidine in an obstetric patient. *Anaesth Intensive Care* 1993; **21**: 702–3.
25. Greer IA, Fellows K. Anaphylactoid reaction to ranitidine in labour. *Br J Clin Pract* 1990; **44**: 78.
26. Aldrete JA, Johnson DA. Allergy to local anesthetics. *JAMA* 1977; **237**: 1594–5.

27 Klein VR, Harris AP, Abraham RA, Niebyl JR. Fetal distress during a maternal systemic allergic reaction. *Obstet Gynecol* 1984; **64**: 15S–17S.
28 Edmondson WC, Skilton RWH. Anaphylaxis in pregnancy: the right treatment? *Anaesthesia* 1994; **49**: 454–5.
29 Fisher M. Treatment of acute anaphylaxis. *Br Med J* 1995; **311**: 731–3.
30 Berg EM, Fasting S, Sellevold OFM. Serious complications with dextran 70 despite hapten prophylaxis: is it best avoided prior to delivery? *Anaesthesia* 1991; **46**: 1033–5.
31 Hayslett JP. Effect of pregnancy in patients with SLE. *Am J Kidney Dis* 1982; **2**: 223–8.
32 [Editorial.] Systemic lupus erythematosus in pregnancy. *Lancet* 1991; **338**: 87–8.
33 Beller FK, Schmidt EH, Holzegrave W, Hauss J. Septicemia during pregnancy: a study in different species of experimental animals. *Am J Obstet Gynecol* 1985; **151**: 967–75.
34 Department of Health. *Report on Confidential Enquiries into Maternal Deaths in the United Kingdom, 1988–1990.* London: HMSO, 1994.
35 Stirrat GM. Pregnancy and immunity: changes occur, but pregnancy does not result in immunodeficiency. *Br Med J* 1994; **308**: 1385–6.
36 Association of Anaesthetists of Great Britain and Ireland. *HIV and Other Blood-Borne Viruses: Guidance for Anaesthetists.* London: AAGBI, 1992.
37 Smego RA, Asperila MO. Use of acyclovir for varicella pneumonia during pregnancy. *Obstet Gynecol* 1991; **78**: 1112–16.
38 Ellis ME, Neal KR, Webb AK. Is smoking a risk factor for pneumonia in adults with chicken pox? *Br Med J* 1987; **294**: 1002.
39 Fischl MA, Darkos GL, Uttamchandoni RB *et al.* Clinical presentation and outcome of patients with HIV infection and tuberculosis caused by multiple-drug-resistant bacilli. *Ann Intern Med* 1992; **117**: 184–90.
40 Johnson AM. Epidemiology of HIV infection in women. *Baillière's Clin Obstet Gynaecol* 1992; **6**: 13–31.
41 Connor EM, Sperling RS, Gelber R *et al.* Reduction of maternal–infant transmission of human immunodeficiency virus type 1 with zidovudine treatment (Pediatric AIDS Clinical Trials Group Protocol 076 Study Group). *N Engl J Med* 1994; **331**: 1173–80.
42 Peckham C, Gibb D. Mother-to-child transmission of the human immunodeficiency virus. *N Engl J Med* 1995; **333**: 298–302.
43 [Anon.] Caesarean section and risk of transmission of HIV-1 infection (The European Collaborative Study). *Lancet* 1994; **343**: 1464–7.
44 Brettle RP. Pregnancy and its effect on HIV/AIDS. *Clin Obstet Gynecol* 1992; **6**: 125–36.
45 Hughes SC, Dailey PA, Landers D *et al.* Parturients infected with human immunodeficiency virus and regional anesthetic. *Anesthesiology* 1995; **82**: 32–7.
46 Tom DJ, Gulevich SJ, Shapiro HM *et al.* Epidural blood patch in the HIV-positive mother: review of the clinical experience. *Anesthesiology* 1992; **76**: 943–7.
47 Tokars JI, Marcus R, Culver DH *et al.* Surveillance of HIV infection and zidovudine use among health workers after occupational exposure to HIV-infected blood. *Ann Intern Med* 1993; **118**: 913–19.
48 Dwyer DE, Cunningham AL. Herpes simplex virus infection in pregnancy. *Clin Obstet Gynecol* 1993; **7**: 75–105.
49 Randolph AG, Washington AE, Prober CG. Cesarean delivery for women presenting with genital herpes lesion: efficacy, risks, costs. *JAMA* 1993; **270**: 77–82.
50 Bader AM, Camann WR, Datta S. Anesthesia for Cesarean delivery in patients with herpes simplex virus type-2 infection. *Reg Anesth* 1990; **15**: 261–3.
51 Crosby ET, Halpern SH, Rolbin SH. Epidural anaesthesia for Caesarean section in patients with active recurrent genital herpes-simplex infection: a retrospective study. *Can J Anaesth* 1989; **36**: 701–4.

52 Crone LA, Conly JM, Clark KM *et al.* Recurrent herpes simplex virus labialis and the use of epidural morphine in obstetric patients. *Anesth Analg* 1988; **67**: 318–23.
53 Crone LA, Conly JM, Storgard C *et al.* Herpes labialis in patients receiving epidural morphine following Cesarean section. *Anesthesiology* 1990; **73**: 208–13.
54 Abouleish E, Rawal N, Rashad MN. The addition of 0.2 mg subarachnoid morphine to hyperbaric bupivacaine for Cesarean delivery. *Reg Anesth* 1991; **16**: 137–40.
55 Lockitch G. *Handbook of Diagnostic Biochemistry and Hematology in Normal Pregnancy.* Surrey: CRC Press, 1993: 170.

11: Uterine and Placental Function

11.1 Uterine anatomy

The enlarged uterus at term comprises a muscle mass increased by approximately 4 kg and a cavity containing 2 kg of amniotic fluid, the placenta and 3.4 kg of fetus. The enlarging uterine muscle mass provides protection for the fetus and for its interface with maternal circulation at the placental site. The ability of this muscle to contract rhythmically and strongly is under hormonal control, so that spontaneous vaginal delivery can be achieved, while effective haemostasis after delivery depends on tonic, sustained contraction while involution and endometrial repair are completed.

11.2 Placenta

The placenta is localized to an area about a quarter of the space provided by the mucosal lining of the uterus. The epithelium of the uterus is invaded, so that maternal blood comes into direct contact with the syncytiotrophoblast, which covers the fetal capillary villi. The syncytiotrophoblast is largely a syncytium, so that there is minimal chance of intracellular transfer between the maternal and fetal compartments. The villous surface area at term is 11 m², and the actual area for exchange is increased by microvilli.

The uterine arteries, which in the first 10 weeks of pregnancy carry a blood flow of 50 mL/min, provide at term a flow of 500–700 mL/min for the uteroplacental unit (Fig. 11.1). Eighty per cent of uterine blood flow passes through the placenta, and the remainder supplies the myometrium. Blood flow is mainly dependent on systemic blood pressure, but adrenoreceptors are present in uterine arteries. The spiral arterioles have their walls destroyed by trophoblast and become passive channels.

11.3 Placental transport

11.3.1 Oxygen and carbon dioxide

At the intervillous space (Fig. 11.2), carbon dioxide diffuses rapidly from the fetus to the mother. The oxygen affinity of maternal haemoglobin decreases while that of the fetus increases, since the pH of the maternal blood decreases while that of the fetus increases, thus facilitating transfer of oxygen. This is the double Bohr effect (Fig. 11.3). Carbon dioxide enters the maternal blood from dissolved gas or bicarbonate or carbaminohaemoglobin. The transfer of

UTERINE AND PLACENTAL FUNCTION

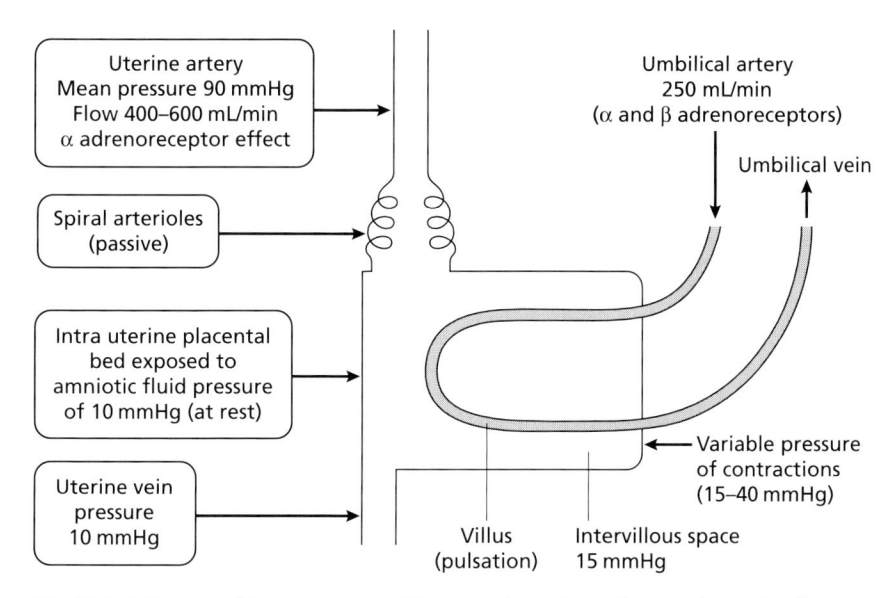

Fig. 11.1 A diagram of the pressures and flow rates in a schematic uteroplacental unit.

Uterine artery
Mean pressure 90 mmHg
Flow 400–600 mL/min
α adrenoreceptor effect

Spiral arterioles (passive)

Intra uterine placental bed exposed to amniotic fluid pressure of 10 mmHg (at rest)

Uterine vein pressure 10 mmHg

Umbilical artery
250 mL/min
(α and β adrenoreceptors)

Umbilical vein

Variable pressure of contractions (15–40 mmHg)

Villus (pulsation)

Intervillous space 15 mmHg

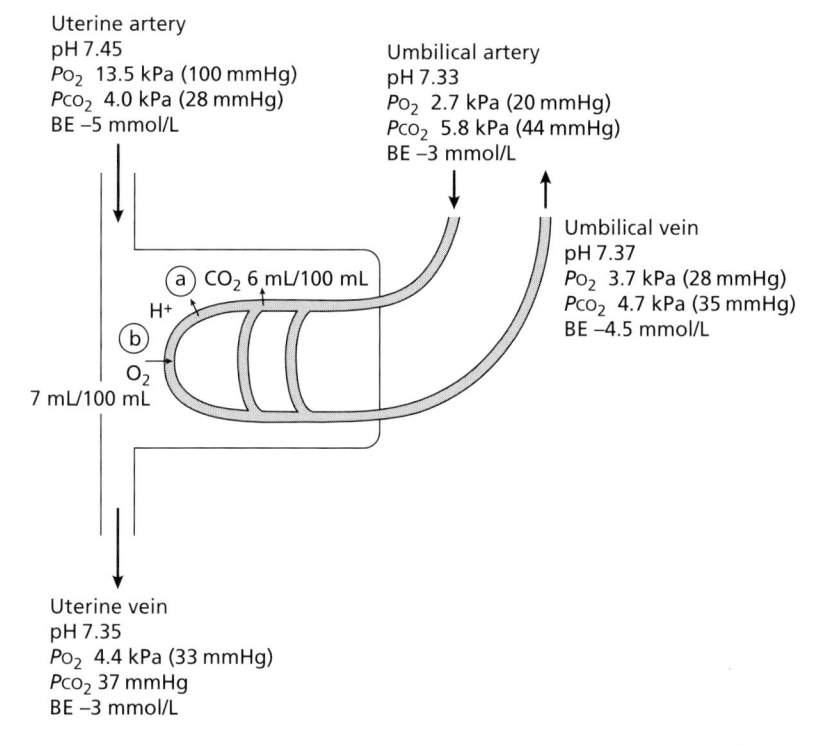

Fig. 11.2 The uteroplacental unit. At (a) the double Bohr effect results from a shift to the right in the maternal oxyhaemoglobin dissociation curve and a shift to the left in the fetal curve, and at (b) Oxygen diffuses and forms oxyhaemoglobin in the fetus. This liberates more carbon dioxide—the double Haldane effect.

Uterine artery
pH 7.45
P_{O_2} 13.5 kPa (100 mmHg)
P_{CO_2} 4.0 kPa (28 mmHg)
BE –5 mmol/L

Umbilical artery
pH 7.33
P_{O_2} 2.7 kPa (20 mmHg)
P_{CO_2} 5.8 kPa (44 mmHg)
BE –3 mmol/L

(a) CO_2 6 mL/100 mL
H+
(b)
O_2
7 mL/100 mL

Umbilical vein
pH 7.37
P_{O_2} 3.7 kPa (28 mmHg)
P_{CO_2} 4.7 kPa (35 mmHg)
BE –4.5 mmol/L

Uterine vein
pH 7.35
P_{O_2} 4.4 kPa (33 mmHg)
P_{CO_2} 37 mmHg
BE –3 mmol/L

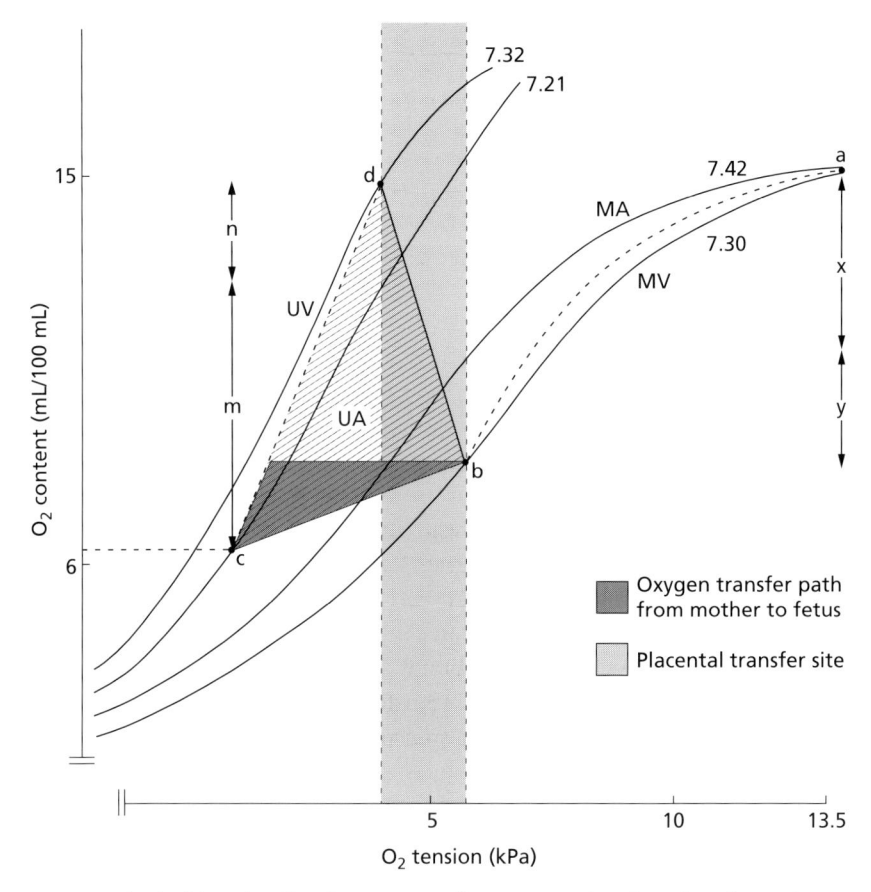

Fig. 11.3 The double Bohr effect diagrammatically represented to show the release of oxygen from maternal blood, its transfer across the placental site and the uptake by fetal blood. MA = maternal artery; MV = maternal vein; UA = umbilical artery; UV = umbilical vein; x = volume of oxygen given up as a result of the pressure gradient; y = additional volume of oxygen generated by the Bohr effect in maternal blood; n = additional volume of oxygen generated by the Bohr effect in fetal blood; m = volume of oxygen received by umbilical blood as a result of the pressure gradient. Points on the curves represent typical samples from (a) the uterine artery, (b) the uterine vein, (c) the umbilical artery and (d) the umbilical vein.

oxygen from mother to fetus leads to the dissociation of carbaminohaemoglobin and facilitates carbon dioxide elimination, as oxyhaemoglobin has less affinity for carbon dioxide than reduced haemoglobin. This is the double Haldane effect.

11.3.2 Plasma contents

The transfer of electrolytes and nutrients is summarized in Table 11.1. Fetal excretion of urea is by passive diffusion. Lipid-soluble unconjugated bilirubin also diffuses for conjugation and excretion by the mother.

Table 11.1 Transfer of electrolytes and nutrients from mother to fetus.

Na+Cl− K+ Ca^{2+} PO$_4$$^{2-}$	Sparse information. Not inert diffusion Active transport
Lactate Glucose	Facilitated diffusion
Amino acids	Active transport except glutamic and aspartic acid
Protein	Impermeable
Free fatty acids	Passive transfer
Cholesterol	Facilitated transfer (saturable)

11.3.3 Drugs

Drugs used for analgesia and anaesthesia pass rapidly from mother to fetus by passive diffusion. This requires no energy. Unlike active transport, it is dependent on a concentration gradient, and is determined by the Fick equation. The physical factors involved are blood flow, concentration gradient, surface area for diffusion, thickness of the membrane and the diffusion constant of the drug. During a contraction, placental transfer depends on the time when the drug was injected. Flow-dependent transport will govern the situation in which a drug is given at the beginning of a contraction, with less drug then passing to the fetus. Appropriate timing of drug administration may minimize neonatal depression.

The concentration gradient depends on the fraction of un-ionized : ionized drug present in plasma. The amount of drug in the un-ionized state depends on the pK_a value for the drug and the pH of fetal (and maternal) blood. Fetal acidosis will therefore enhance the maternofetal transfer of basic drugs such as pethidine, fentanyl and amide-linked local anaesthetics (Table 11.2). Their ionization and retention increases in an acidotic fetus, so their dose should be

Table 11.2 The pK_a of anaesthetic drugs. The relationship between pH and pK_a is:

$$pH = pK_a + \log_{10} \frac{[\text{concentration of nonionized base}]}{[\text{concentration of protonated form}]}$$

This means that for a weak base with a pK_a of 9, a change in pH of the plasma from pH 7 to pH 6 causes a 10-fold reduction in the concentration of non-ionized base.

Drug	pK_a
lidocaine	7.9
bupivacaine	8.1
fentanyl	8.4
pethidine	8.5

reduced to avoid trapping. The diffusion constant for the drug depends on its molecular weight, degree of ionization and lipid solubility.

The lipid solubility of a molecule also plays an important part in placental transfer. Transfer of lipid-insoluble molecules is dependent on microscopic aqueous channels that exist between cellular layers on the villi. Rapid transfer via this route will only occur with molecules < 100 KDa. Lipid-soluble molecules (< 1000 KDa) cross the placenta more rapidly. Whether lipid-soluble or water-soluble, it is only the free or unbound molecules that take part in the placental exchange. Highly protein-bound molecules (such as bupivacaine) do not cross easily from mother to fetus. Many anaesthetic agents in free, unbound form are lipid-soluble, low molecular weight, largely un-ionized compounds, so their transfer is rapid. However, quaternary ammonium compounds such as neuromuscular blocking drugs and neostigmine, which are highly ionized, are unable to cross in significant amounts. There is little evidence that the placental metabolism of drugs plays a major role in determining fetal effects from anaesthetic drugs.

The degree of protein binding can change the total amount of drug transferred to the fetus. Fetal albumin concentrations rise at term to exceed maternal concentrations slightly. Diazepam is bound to albumin and can concentrate in the fetus. In contrast, the concentration of α1-acid glycoprotein, a globulin, rises more slowly, and the fetal concentration at term is less than the maternal one. Basic drugs bound to this protein (e.g. alfentanil, pethidine and local anaesthetics) may not accumulate in the fetus to the amount suggested by ion trapping. Once protein-bound, the drug–protein complex can act as a reservoir and prolong the drug effect. In fact, the albumin concentration in the neonate decreases after birth, so that the free drug concentration of diazepam, for example, can actually increase.

Many studies measure and compare plasma concentrations of free, bound, or total drug present. Simple studies can easily compare the umbilical vein : maternal vein ratios. However, maternal venous concentrations differ markedly from maternal arterial concentrations. It is the arterial concentration that is presented to the placenta for drug transfer. To obtain a more accurate picture, the total mass of drug present in both mother and fetus should be measured, as well as the free fraction. Also the rate of decline; for example, the maternal concentration may vary after a bolus injection, so that fetal/maternal ratios for a drug such as thiopental can vary considerably depending on time relations alone. Other factors, such as tissue distribution, also require consideration [1].

Reference

1 Reynolds F, Knott C. Pharmacokinetics in pregnancy and placental drug transfer. In: Milligan S, ed. *Oxford Reviews of Reproductive Biology,* vol. 2. Oxford: Oxford University Press, 1989: 389–449.

12: Puerperium

12.1 Physiology

The puerperium is commonly thought of as the period of parturition during which most physiological functions return to normal (Table 12.1) [1–6]. It is usually complete by six weeks. Lactation is the most obvious exception, in association with anaemia as a consequence of its haemopoietic demands.

Immediately after separation of the placenta, there is a significant increase in venous return as a result of uterine contraction and the relief of compression of the inferior vena cava. A volume of more than 500 mL (depending on

Table 12.1 Summary of physiological changes in the puerperium.

Systems	Effects
Cardiovascular	*Immediate*: autotransfusion. Elimination of placental arteriovenous shunt. Increased venous volume and venous return. Central venous pressure increases. Pulmonary blood volume increases (compounded by vasoconstrictive drugs) *Intermediate*: diuresis *Longer term*: cardiac output, heart rate changes and stroke volume return to non-pregnant levels by 2–4 weeks
Respiratory	*Immediate*: mechanical effects reduced *Intermediate*: functional residual capacity, residual volume, carbon dioxide tension and alveolar ventilation return to normal *Longer term*: haemoglobin and haematocrit return to normal at 2–4 weeks
Haematological	Effects altered by antepartum and postpartum haemorrhage
Gastrointestinal tract	*Short term*: mechanical effects reduced *Intermediate*: gastric emptying returns to normal by 24 hours
Renal	Glomerular filtration rate and creatinine return to normal at 1–3 weeks
Carbohydrate metabolism	*Immediate*: insulin requirements markedly reduced *Longer term*: Glucose response should be normal by 8 weeks postpartum
Hepatic	*Immediate*: plasma cholinesterase activity is reduced further for 2–3 days postpartum
Skeletal	*Immediate*: ligament laxity

the blood loss at delivery) may be released into the circulation at this time, a form of autotransfusion [7]. It has been postulated that this acute blood volume change is responsible for the significant increase in plasma atrial natriuretic peptide (ANP), with stretching of the atrial wall stimulating release of ANP. However, natriuresis and diuresis continue for longer than the rise in plasma ANP. In the first few days postpartum, the 24-hour creatinine clearance increases, reaching a peak on postpartum day 3, with a significant diuresis between days 3 and 4 [8]. A sustained increase in brain natriuretic peptide (BNP) occurs for three days in the postpartum period, and this may in part explain the continued postpartum diuresis. BNP is a cardiac hormone secreted mainly by the ventricles that produces natriuresis, vasodilation and inhibition of the renin–angiotensin–aldosterone system in the same manner as ANP [9].

Circulatory changes are associated with this puerperal diuresis. Cardiac output studies using Doppler and cross-sectional echocardiography at the aortic valve found that mean cardiac output in 30 parturients remained elevated for 24 hours after delivery, and then decreased over two to six days as a result of decreases in both heart rate and stroke volume [4]. The effects of postpartum haemorrhage in 10% of patients were also studied. In this group of women, who clinically had lost more than 500 mL of blood and had a haematocrit < 30%, there was a significant decrease in stroke volume and increase in heart rate such that it compensated for the reduction in stroke volume. Cardiac output was similar to the control group without blood loss. These physiological responses to haemorrhage are no different from the non-pregnant state. However, postpartum stroke volume can be affected not only by reductions in preload, such as haemorrhage, but also by a decrease in myocardial contractility [4,10], which may be secondary to a decreased end-diastolic volume. Many general anaesthetic drugs depress the myocardium, and if they are given without careful consideration, this situation may cause cardiac decompensation.

Postpartum haemorrhage (see Chapter 23) usually occurs in the first 24 hours after delivery. A mother who has not started her diuresis should therefore have an adequate blood volume to tolerate a haemorrhage of 500–1000 mL. If the normal increase in blood volume has not occurred, as in pre-eclampsia, or in patients with cardiac disease in whom a normal physiological response to haemorrhage cannot be achieved—particularly those with valve stenosis or pulmonary hypertension—haemodynamic instability and circulatory failure may develop.

One of the reasons for the swift return to normal physiological balance is the rapid elimination from the circulation of placental hormones. The steroid and protein hormones of the fetoplacental unit fall to very low levels in the first hour after delivery [11]. Uterine evacuation and involution rapidly reduce the compression on the lungs and gastrointestinal system. Mechanical effects resolve, and the lung residual volume and functional residual capacity quickly return to normal. Alveolar ventilation returns to normal by two to three weeks postpartum [12].

Investigations of the pelvic region in the normal puerperium using ultrasound [13] and computed tomography [14] found uterine artery vasoconstriction and intrauterine blood in the majority of women between one and two days after delivery. Widening of the pubic symphysis was present in half of the women. Creatine kinase and creatine kinase isoenzymes have been found in longitudinal studies to be increased on the first postpartum day [15] to levels compatible with myocardial infarction in about 40% of women [16].

12.2 Postpartum morbidity

Collection of morbidity data in the puerperium is not routine on postnatal wards, yet much of the morbidity of parturition presents in the weeks after childbirth. Postpartum morbidity is not adequately recognized by professionals [17], partly because it is not part of official statistics. Pain is experienced frequently after delivery, as are difficulties with micturition and defaecation. Pain and discomfort have a variety of causes.

- Uterine contractions. As the uterus involutes, severe cramps can be generated, which increase in severity with parity [18].
- Haemorrhoids. Constipation is a common problem, and can be exacerbated by opioid drugs given during labour or delivery. A laxative may need to be administered to prevent this. Haemorrhoids starting after delivery persisted for more than six weeks in 5–7% of women in a large postal survey [19]. A long second stage, forceps delivery and large babies increased the risk.
- *Headache.* Causes of headache can be numerous. The differential diagnosis is listed on p. 117.
- *Backache.* Bruising in the lumbar region following regional analgesia is not uncommon, but is transient and should be treated by graded exercises, analgesia and reassurance. Persistent backache must be investigated.
- *Breast engorgement.* If a breast-feeding mother is not able to feed her baby at appropriate intervals, painful breast engorgement will result. Careful timing of anaesthesia or feeding, or both, will usually overcome the difficulty. Expressing breast milk may be needed if separation of mother and baby is prolonged.

The use of regional anaesthesia, if possible, will avoid the excretion of depressant anaesthetic and analgesic drugs in breast milk, and should not interrupt the developing or existing rhythm of feeding, provided that adequate hydration is provided. If general anaesthesia must be used, it should start as soon as possible after completion of a feed. This allows the maximum postanaesthetic recovery period for the mother before she recommences feeding. Alternatively, anaesthesia could be scheduled just prior to a feed. This gives less opportunity for the build-up of a depressant drug in the breast milk. Feeding should then commence as soon as possible after surgery (see p. 443).

- *Episiotomy/Caesarean section.* An episiotomy can vary in size and can generate as much pain as a Caesarean section incision, especially when associated with forceps delivery. It may reflexly cause retention of urine [20]. Tissue swelling around the episiotomy can be relieved by posture and adequate analgesia with mild or moderate oral analgesics such as paracetamol, codeine or non-steroidal anti-inflammatory analgesics. Postoperative analgesia after Caesarean section is discussed in Section 16.14.1, pp. 307–8.

- *Musculoskeletal symptoms.* Pain in the neck and shoulders, together with tingling in the limbs, occurred in 8% of women in a large postal survey [19]. Some of these cases were associated with general anaesthesia and may have been related to the administration of suxamethonium for intubation. An adequate explanation of 'scoline pains' should be given to the mother before general anaesthesia, and the explanation may need to be repeated postoperatively when the pains are experienced. Pain may also develop after acute injury to the shoulder girdle muscles at birth due to excessive neck flexion. Physiotherapy and even orthopaedic advice may be essential in the puerperium. After epidural analgesia, meningism has to be distinguished from these cervical muscular problems. A history of abnormal posture can often be elicited. Heat and massage are useful therapies, and can prevent problems from becoming chronic. They speed recovery and optimize the mother's fitness level for looking after her baby.

Women frequently do not present postpartum symptoms of dysfunction to a doctor. Long-term postpartum stress incontinence occurs in 11% of women, as reported from a postal health questionnaire of 11 701 women [19], but only 14% of sufferers had consulted a doctor for help. Stress incontinence is thought to occur through injury to the pudendal nerves [21], and is associated with long second-stage labours, large babies and increasing maternal age. Caesarean section delivery may confer a degree of protection from this problem.

References

1 Lind T, Harris VG. Changes in oral glucose tolerance test during the puerperium. *Br J Obstet Gynaecol* 1976; **83**: 460–3.
2 Hansen JM, Ueland K. The influence of caudal analgesia on cardiovascular dynamics during normal labour and delivery. *Acta Anaesthesiol Scand* 1966; **23** (Suppl): 449–52.
3 Ueland K. Maternal cardiovascular hemodynamics, 8: intrapartum blood volume changes. *Am J Obstet Gynecol* 1976; **126**: 671–7.
4 Robson SC, Hunter S, Moore M, Dunlop W. Haemodynamic changes during the puerperium: a Doppler and M-mode echocardiograph study. *Br J Obstet Gynaecol* 1987; **94**: 1028–39.
5 Davison JM. The physiology of the renal tract in pregnancy. *Clin Obstet Gynecol* 1985; **28**: 257–65.
6 Leighton BL, Cheek TG, Gross JB *et al*. Succinylcholine pharmacodynamics in peripartum patients. *Anesthesiology* 1986; **64**: 202–5.
7 Ueland K, Ferguson JE. Cardiovascular physiology of pregnancy. In: Sciarra JJ, ed. *Gynecology and Obstetrics*, vol. 3. Philadelphia: Lippincott, 1988: 1–7.
8 Davison JM, Dunlop W. Changes in renal hemodynamics and tubular function induced by normal human pregnancy. *Semin Nephrol* 1984; **4**: 1987–2007.

9 Yoshimura T, Yoshimura M, Yasue H et al. Plasma concentration of atrial natriuretic peptide and brain natriuretic peptide during normal human pregnancy and the postpartum period. *J Endocrinol* 1994; **140**: 393–7.
10 Burg JR, Dodek A, Kloster FE, Metcalf J. Alteration of systolic time intervals during pregnancy. *Circulation* 1974; **49**: 560–4.
11 Klopper A, Buchan P, Wilson G. The plasma half-life of placental hormones. *Br J Obstet Gynaecol* 1978; **85**: 738–47.
12 Cugell DW, Frank NR, Gaensler EA. Pulmonary function in pregnancy, 1: serial observations in normal women. *Am Rev Tuberc* 1953; **65**: 568–97.
13 Tekay A, Jouppila P. A longitudinal Doppler ultrasonographic assessment of the alterations in peripheral vascular resistance of uterine arteries and ultrasonographic findings of the involuted uterus during the puerperium. *Am J Obstet Gynecol* 1993; **168**: 190–8.
14 Garagiola DM, Tarver RD, Gibson L, Rogers RE, Wass JL. Anatomic changes in the pelvis after uncomplicated vaginal delivery: a CT study on 14 women. *Am J Roentgenol* 1989; **153**: 1239–41.
15 Satin AJ, Hankins GD, Patterson WR, Scott RT. Creatine kinase and creatine kinase isoenzymes as a marker of uterine activity. *Am J Perinatol* 1992; **9**: 456–9.
16 Leiserowitz GS, Evans AT, Samuels SJ, Omand K, Kost GJ. Creatine kinase and its MB isoenzymes in the third trimester and the peripartum period. *J Reprod Med* 1992; **37**: 910–16.
17 Drife JO. Assessing the consequences of changing childbirth: better data are needed. *Br Med J* 1995; **310**: 144.
18 Murray A, Holdcroft A. Incidence and intensity of postpartum lower abdominal pain. *Br Med J* 1989; **298**: 1619.
19 MacArthur C, Lewis M, Knox EG. Health after childbirth. *Br J Obstet Gynaecol* 1991; **98**: 1193–5.
20 [Editorial.] Pain after birth. *Br Med J* 1973; **iv**: 565–6.
21 Snooks SJ, Swash M, Mathers SG, Henry MM. Effect of vaginal delivery on the pelvic floor: a five-year follow up. *Br J Surg* 1990; **77**: 1358–60.

13: Drug Abuse

13.1 General considerations

Substance abuse is occuring in an increasing number of women of reproductive age. Alcohol and cannabis (marijuana, hemp) are the substances most often abused by women of childbearing age. Most abusers deny drug use, but the recognition that one substance is being abused makes it more likely that other substances have been tried. More than one drug of abuse may be combined in one injection. Cocaine abuse has the greatest impact on obstetric morbidity, and is frequently used in combination with cannabis, alcohol, amphetamines and heroin. Stimulant drugs are often used in binges, rather than the daily dosage associated with alcohol and opioid abuse [1]. When a woman presents with a lack of prenatal care, preterm labour or abruptio placenta, drug abuse should be suspected (Table 13.1) [2,3]. Early identification of the problem is the most important step in management. The abuse of drugs during pregnancy may precipitate life-threatening problems that require

Table 13.1 Recognition of factors associated with drug abuse in the parturient.

History (abuse is usually denied)
Social
    Urban home
    Cigarette smoking
Obstetric
    Lack of prenatal care
    Preterm labour
    Intrauterine growth retardation
    Unexplained neonatal depression at birth

On examination
Behavioural abnormalities
General
    Thrombotic veins
    Scarring
    Tattoos
    Malnutrition
    Subcutaneous abscesses
Pupillary constriction
Cardiovascular (differential diagnosis is pre-eclampsia)
    Hypertension
    Tachycardia

Retrospective in baby
Drug-induced withdrawal symptoms

high-dependency or intensive care. In addition, patients should be considered to be at high risk for maternal, fetal and neonatal disorders. In late pregnancy, maternal behavioural effects can predominate. The anaesthetist should be aware that 47% of women whose urine tested positive for cocaine denied substance abuse [2].

When occurring in the first eight weeks of pregnancy, drug abuse may cause fetal dysmorphology. Drug levels can change with alterations in maternal physiology. For example, cocaine is metabolized by cholinesterases. In pregnancy, its activity is reduced, and this reduces the clearance of cocaine. Hormonal changes, alterations in plasma proteins and shifts in body water, and changes in gastrointestinal motility all alter drug pharmacodynamics and pharmacokinetics—for example, through changes in oral drug absorption from the gastrointestinal tract or alterations in the volume of distribution. Fetal exposure to drugs may not only cause teratogenic effects and intrauterine growth retardation, but can also have significant effects on the newborn and on later life.

The prevalence of drug abuse in the United States varies between inner-city areas [4], where 24% of parturients screen positive for illicit drugs, and urban and rural areas, with rates of 8% [5] and 11% [6]. In Scotland and London, opiate drugs predominate amongst intravenous drug users, and are commonly accompanied by benzodiazepines [7,8]. Less often, cannabis, amphetamines, cocaine (5% in the Scottish group), and barbiturates are self-administered, in descending order of frequency. A more recent survey carried out by a laboratory service for drug screening in Scotland [9] in a population of suspected drug users identified cannabinoids and benzodiazepines in 68% and 69%, respectively, opiates in 45%, methadone in 52% and small amounts of amphetamines (8%) and cocaine (0.1%). The small amount of cocaine detected may have been the result of the laboratory method used. A report from Australia [10] indicates that the majority of drug-abusing patients use opioids and not cocaine. The pattern of drug abuse changes from country to country and within a country over time.

Speciality clinics have developed in some large obstetric centres to manage the medical, obstetric and paediatric problems that arise. The clinics aim to reduce the maternal and perinatal morbidity and mortality by encouraging regular antenatal visits and maintaining a social worker to help with housing, legal and financial problems and drug rehabilitation, especially methadone replacement in narcotics users [11,12]. Late presentation for antenatal care may occur, because amenorrhoea is a common occurrence with narcotic abuse, symptoms of pregnancy may be interpreted as withdrawal symptoms, and psychiatric disorders and mistrust may hinder self-referral. Cocaine-induced cardiovascular disorders may mimic pregnancy-induced hypertension in the actively intoxicated patient. Fortunately, the drug has a relatively short half-life, and symptoms decrease within one to two hours after use. During this time, or on repeated use, the risks of anaesthesia are greatly

Table 13.2 Urine analysis for drugs and metabolites.

	Time up to which the drug can be detected
Alcohol	8–16 h
Cannabis	1–4 weeks
Cocaine	1–3 days
Opioids	2–4 days
Benzodiazepines	2–3 weeks
Amphetamines	variable (1–11 days)
Phencyclidine	7 days
Lysergic acid diethylamine	2–3 days

increased. Drug abuse must be included in the differential diagnosis of a parturient who presents for anaesthesia with an uncertain diagnosis, or when unexpected hypertension or dysrhythmias complicate anaesthesia.

13.1.1 Detection of drug abuse

If the diagnosis is suspected, a urinary drug screen should be obtained. Urine toxicology will often detect only recent drug use (Table 13.2) [13]. It is unlikely to detect the occasional drug user or the experienced abuser who refrains from the drug for a few days prior to antenatal visits. Cannabinoids are the exception, since metabolites of Δ^9-tetrahydrocannabinol can be detected in the urine for up to a month after use. Detectable metabolites from cocaine abuse disappear from the urine within two or three days.

Most of the relevant toxicological methods (e.g. gas chromatography, mass spectroscopy) are not rapid. There is a useful, fast method for cocaine metabolites (OnTrak Abuscreen, Roche Diagnostic Systems) [14].

13.1.2 Complications of drug abuse

Medical complications of drug abuse are as described in Table 13.3 [10], and are often the result of the route of entry of the drug, and the socio-economic effects of drug addiction. Almost half of the women who abuse drugs have at least one significant complication. Although many drug abusers come from lower socio-economic groups, cocaine abuse occurs among all social groups. The general peripartum care of drug abusers is summarized in Table 13.4.

Investigation of drug abusing parturients should include a full blood count for anaemia and infection, a blood profile screen for abnormal liver function and renal dysfunction, urine sample for routine tests, drug screen and culture, cervical swab, hepatitis B and HIV screen. Any specific symptoms should be investigated further.

Table 13.3 Common medical problems accompanying drug abuse.

Dietary
Anaemia
Malnutrition

Infections
Vascular (septicaemia, endocarditis, thrombophlebitis/emboli)
Hepatitis
Sexually transmitted disease
HIV
Pneumonia
Urinary tract

Behavioural

Psychiatric

Table 13.4 Considerations for general peripartum care in a high-dependency or intensive-care unit.

Routine monitoring: Sao_2, electrocardiogram
Maintain i.v. access
Intra-arterial pressure if haemodynamic instability
Central venous pressure if fluid deficit, cardiac failure
Consider drug interactions
Assess for known complications: drug screen, hepatitis B, HIV, renal and hepatic failure
Fetal distress: administer 100% oxygen to the mother, consider using a vasodilator, have fetal resuscitation available

13.2 Alcohol

Alcohol is probably the most abused substance worldwide. In the United States, between 8% and 11% of childbearing women are drinkers who consume enough alcohol to have complications, or alcoholics with dependence problems [15].

Alcohol is a known teratogen. Fetal abnormalities are dose-dependent, and are seen frequently when the consumption is greater than 90 mL of absolute alcohol per day (equivalent to six glasses of wine). This leads to the fetal alcohol syndrome, which includes a characteristic facies, growth retardation, microcephaly and mental retardation.

Maternal complications include cardiac dysrhythmias, sudden death, cardiomyopathy, pulmonary aspiration of stomach contents, gastritis, hepatitis, cirrhosis (with associated hypoalbuminaemia affecting drug pharmacokinetics), malnutrition and pancreatitis.

13.2.1 Anaesthetic problems

The acutely intoxicated patient presents anaesthetic difficulties (Table 13.5). Regional techniques may have advantages if the patient is conscious and cooperative, but peripheral neuropathies may be present. These should be elicited prior to anaesthesia. When levels of consciousness vary, the risk of pulmonary aspiration will be increased and general anaesthesia with a cuffed endotracheal tube is indicated. However, in addition to airway problems, gastric emptying is delayed by alcohol, and gastric volume is increased because alcohol is a powerful stimulant of gastric acid secretion. Blood volume deficits should be assessed prior to analgesia, especially if vomiting accompanies intoxication. Inability of the patient to co-operate during induction of anaesthesia will add to the anaesthetic difficulty. Metabolic drug interactions occur in acute intoxication, by inhibiting hepatic metabolism. These can increase the

Table 13.5 Anaesthetic problems in acute and chronic alcoholism.

Acute
Withdrawal (mother and baby)
Stage 1: tremor, anxiety, hypertension
Stage 2: autonomic hyperactivity
Stage 3: seizures and coma

Treatment:
    Phenobarbital and clonidine
    Chlomethiazole
    (Benzodiazepines are possible teratogens)
    (Phenothiazines do not prevent delirium tremens)

Overdose/ingestion:
Airway management: gastric contents present, potentiation of central nervous system
    depression by barbiturates (as induction agents)
Beware: maternal reactive hypoglycaemia

Chronic
Neuropathy: relative contraindication for regional anaesthesia
Myopathy: prolonged neuromuscular blockade (general or regional)
Cardiomyopathy: avoid cardiac depressant anaesthetics
Hepatic dysfunction
    Decreased albumin*
    Coagulation defects†
    Portal hypertension/ascites/oesophageal varices/liver failure‡
Convulsions: avoid ketamine, enflurane

* Consider pharmacokinetic drug effects.
† May require vitamin K, platelets, fresh frozen plasma.
‡ Consider increased volume of distribution of drugs, sodium load, bleeding with oral and nasal tubes, avoidance of halothane, effect of liver failure on drug metabolism (both general and local anaesthetics).

concentration of drugs (e.g. lidocaine), or other substances (e.g. cocaine) in the plasma [16]. Acute withdrawal in both the mother and baby may only present postoperatively.

Chronic abuse induces hepatic enzymes, and so decreases the drug availability of agents that are metabolized by the liver. It may also enhance the formation of toxic metabolites in multiple drug abuse; for example, cocaethylene is formed from cocaine [17]. Anaesthetic agents with any hepatotoxic effects, or which depend on liver metabolism, should be avoided if possible.

13.3 Opioids [18]

The narcotic abuser can use most routes of drug administration, but prefers to achieve peak effects rapidly, as with the intravenous injection of heroin or inhalation of fentanyl. Narcotic cross-tolerance is usual, so higher doses of narcotics are needed to achieve the desired therapeutic effect. All opioids rapidly cross the placenta, and recurrent episodes of maternal drug withdrawal may lead to increased uterine muscle tone and, as a consequence, a reduction in placental blood flow. This can lead to intrauterine growth retardation, premature labour and fetal death *in utero*.

Recognition of withdrawal symptoms or overdosage is important (Table 13.6). Rapid drug withdrawal in the first trimester can cause spontaneous abortion, so it should be avoided. Opioids are indicated in pregnancy and labour (even when regional analgesia is used) to prevent the symptoms of drug withdrawal. Methadone replacement should be considered in opioid-addicted women in the second trimester. Antenatally, there are advantages to the use of methadone. There is a constant blood level at a known dosage, drug purity is maintained, and fetal morbidity from intermittent periods of withdrawal is minimized. However, at delivery, neonatal drug withdrawal effects are severe [19].

In the case of a parturient with a history of narcotic abuse who has stopped taking opioid drugs, the therapeutic use of opioids should be avoided as far as possible. This can be achieved by regional analgesia and the use of non-opioid analgesics.

13.3.1 Labour

The early stages of labour may have been misinterpreted by the mother as withdrawal symptoms, so she may present late and may have taken additional illicit narcotics to cover her symptoms. However, the onset of labour may interrupt the supply of drugs, and withdrawal symptoms may complicate the subsequent progress of parturition. Withdrawal symptoms begin approximately 12 hours after the last dose of narcotic, and peak at 48–72 hours. Methadone is an inadequate treatment for labour pain, but if a mother is receiving methadone as a regular opioid replacement or is withdrawing,

Table 13.6 Narcotic abuse.

Overdose
Coma
Miosis
Respiratory depression

Naloxone is contraindicated for both mother and fetus. It may precipitate:
(a) withdrawal symptoms
(b) fetal distress
(c) fetal death *in utero*

Withdrawal signs and symptoms
Stomach cramps, tachycardia, mydriasis, tachypnoea, yawning, sweating, lacrimation, dehydration, rhinorrhoea, restlessness, diarrhoea, piloerection, nausea and vomiting

Treatment: methadone
Either convert a woman's usual 24-h dose of opioid to equivalent methadone dose
Or 15–20 mg orally and observe for withdrawal symptoms and adjust the daily dose accordingly.

Neonatal abstinence syndrome
Central nervous system irritation: (convulsions, high-pitched cry, hypertonia)
Gastrointestinal dysfunction: (vomiting, diarrhoea)
Respiratory distress
Vague autonomic symptoms: (yawning, sneezing)

---

methadone therapy should be given. Fentanyl given intravenously or epidurally can supplement methadone maintenance in labour as a short-acting opioid. Pethidine can be administered as an analgesic for labour pain, but mixed agonist–antagonist drugs must be avoided, as they may precipitate acute withdrawal. Recognition of complications (Table 13.3) is important so that drugs detoxified in the liver can be given cautiously. Complications such as coagulopathy or infection should be sought before choosing a regional anaesthetic. Regional anaesthesia is indicated in women who are consuming high doses of opioids prior to labour. They often show reduced pain tolerance and have delayed gastric emptying.

Postoperative analgesia for women receiving methadone maintenance therapy can be provided by a regional nerve block and non-steroidal anti-inflammatory analgesics given if there are no contraindications (e.g. peptic ulcer). When additional opioids are required, continuous infusions rather than intermittent doses of opioids are preferred for postoperative pain relief, as they provide a more constant blood concentration.

13.4 Cocaine

When prepared as the hydrochloride salt for local anaesthetic use, cocaine decomposes on heating, but the plant alkaloid (cocaine base extracted from

Erythroxylon coca leaves) does not. It can be smoked (as 'crack'), producing a rapid onset and short duration of effect [20]. It is absorbed slowly from the mucous membranes, with a half-life of 0.5–1.5 hours, and can be detected in the plasma for up to six hours. Multiple drug abuse with alcohol and cocaine can lead to the formation of a potent and more lethal cocaine metabolite, cocaethylene [21]. Other metabolites may be toxic, e.g. benzoylecgonine [22].

Its local anaesthetic and addictive stimulant properties have been known for over 100 years. When used as a local anaesthetic, cocaine blocks the sodium channel in the nerve membrane. Systemically, it blocks norepinephrine and dopamine re-uptake by nerve synapses in the central and sympathetic nervous systems. Excess of these neurotransmitters in the limbic system produces euphoria, restlessness and excitement; activation of the sympathetic nervous system results in vasoconstriction, tachycardia, hypotension and hypertension, dysrhythmias, mydriasis and hyperglycaemia. Higher doses may cause tremors and convulsions. Myocardial irritability and heart failure are also associated with high levels of cocaine. Cocaine and its metabolites may cause vasoconstriction of coronary or umbilical vessels directly and independent of epithelial factors [17]. Acute myocardial infarction, subarachnoid haemorrhage, aortic rupture, stroke (from cerebral vasoconstriction), and bowel ischaemia can result. The most common renal complication is myoglobinuric renal failure secondary to rhabdomyolysis, but renal infarction can also occur. With chronic use, presynaptic neurotransmitters are depleted, and depression and poor maternal health behaviour result. Response to indirect sympathomimetics, such as ephedrine, will be attenuated.

Cocaine is metabolized rapidly by liver and plasma cholinesterases to water-soluble substances that are excreted in the urine. Plasma cholinesterase activity is reduced during pregnancy, and this may contribute to the altered pharmacokinetics of cocaine and its greater toxicity during gestation. Pregnancy enhances the cardiovascular effects of cocaine in pregnant ewes. Systemic vascular resistance, heart rate and mean arterial blood pressure were higher after intravenous cocaine than in non-pregnant control animals [23]. Obstetric complications caused by cocaine abuse include both direct and indirect effects of vasoconstriction [24] (Table 13.7). There is an increased incidence of spontaneous abortion. Cocaine has not been associated with an increased risk of birth defects, but it crosses the placenta rapidly, and fetal cerebrovascular accidents can occur [25].

13.4.1 Choice of anaesthetic technique (Table 13.8)

There may be no choice of technique except general anaesthesia for the scenario of hypotension and hypovolaemia complicating placental abruption induced by cocaine. Management of haemodynamic instability is more difficult under general anaesthesia than regional. Severe hypertension and dysrhythmias triggered by intubation are commonly encountered problems.

Table 13.7 Obstetric effects of cocaine intoxication.

Mother
Placental abruption
Increased uterine contractility (premature labour)

Fetus
Reduced placental blood flow (vasoconstriction)
    Prematurity
    Intrauterine growth retardation
Direct effects
    Tachycardia
    Hypotension

Table 13.8 Anaesthetic problems in acute cocaine intoxication.

	Management
Vasoconstriction	Direct arterial pressure
Fluid deficit	Central venous line/pressure
Hypertension	Labetalol (use before intubation)
Local anaesthetic toxicity	Reduce dose: spinal (*care*! the blood pressure is labile, so there is an increased risk of hypotension)
Catecholamine alterations, acute and chronic	
Dysrhythmias	Labetalol
	Electrocardiogram monitoring
	Avoid epinephrine, halothane, ketamine
Myocardial ischaemia	I.v. nitroglycerine
Hypotension	Indirectly acting vasopressors, e.g. ephedrine, may be ineffective
Coagulation problems	Platelets (and clotting screen)
Convulsions/excitation	Control airway; benzodiazepines

Hypertension is best treated before induction of anaesthesia. Intraoperative drug interactions commonly occur. Propranolol is contraindicated, because its beta blockade may leave alpha stimulation unopposed and worsen the hypertension. Labetalol, with both alpha and beta effects, is effective in treating the hypertension and potential dysrhythmias of acute intoxication [26]. Halothane should be avoided, because it can sensitize the myocardium to dysrhythmias. Lidocaine is not recommended, because cocaine lowers the seizure threshold. If intense alpha stimulation continues the hypertensive crisis, sodium nitroprusside can be used cautiously to reduce the blood pressure to safer levels.

    There are no pharmacological treatments to reverse the effects of cocaine. Regional anaesthesia should be considered for non-emergency surgery, providing the mother is co-operative and cardiovascular effects have worn off. In the presence of intense vasoconstriction associated with acute intoxication, the woman's volume status is unknown, and the response to vasodilation will be unpredictable. As cocaine intoxication subsides, hypotension may follow if the woman is not rehydrated, and a sympathetic blockade can make this hypotension difficult to manage. Sympathomimetic and vasoconstrictive drugs, which act as substrates for neuronal amine uptake, should be avoided. It is theoretically possible that indirectly acting vasoconstrictors such as ephedrine will be less effective. Dysrhythmias will be more frequent in the presence of exogenous or endogenous epinephrine, so adequate pain relief and a calm, relaxed atmosphere should accompany either regional nerve block or general anaesthesia and be maintained postpartum. It may not be so easy to protect the newborn from these influences, and irritability and distress is common in neonates delivered by mothers who misuse cocaine.

13.5 Cannabis

Although many women of childbearing age have used cannabis before becoming pregnant, its use during pregnancy tends to decline [27]. Cannabis is usually smoked in combination with tobacco, so symptoms of bronchitis can be a complication. Anaesthetic agents that could precipitate bronchoconstriction should be avoided. There are no clear effects of cannabis on anaesthetic or obstetric outcome, but intrauterine growth retardation has been reported [28].

13.6 Benzodiazepines

Benzodiazepines stimulate opioid receptors and depress central autonomic outflow by potentiating GABAergic activity. They therefore enhance narcotics or relieve ethanol withdrawal. Maternal acute intoxication produces drowsiness, ataxia and hostility. Mortality from benzodiazepine use is rare, because the effects of other abused substances predominate [29].

The high rate of teratogenicity reported after heavy maternal benzodiazepine abuse [30] may not be due to benzodiazepine exposure alone, as the benzodiazepines are used with alcohol and other substances. Acute neonatal effects from maternal ingestion are prolonged because desmethyldiazepam, the active metabolite of diazepam, has a neonatal half-life of four days.

13.7 Amphetamines

These drugs are commonly used for their mood-elevating and stimulating properties. Cocaine and amphetamines are neuropharmacologically similar [3]. Amphetamines release catecholamines from adrenergic nerve terminals (α- and β-agonist) and inhibit their reuptake. Multiple drug use is common, either for synergistic mood-altering effects, or for controlling withdrawal symptoms in addiction. The agitation of amphetamine withdrawal is often reduced by self-medication with benzodiazepines.

The stimulant properties of amphetamines can mimic eclampsia [31]. Presenting symptoms are convulsions and hypertension. Drug interactions with sympathomimetic agents used during anaesthesia must be considered.

Chronic use of amphetamines causes an impaired sympathetic response, and cardiac failure and arrest have been reported. It may be difficult to know whether acute or chronic ingestion prevails, so invasive cardiovascular monitoring may be indicated if a positive history or drug screen of amphetamine ingestion is obtained.

13.8 Solvent abuse

Inhalation of toluene-based solvents (in spray paint and glue) is practised by young adults [32], and sniffing such vapours is associated with acute renal abnormalities, causing reversible renal tubular acidosis. Severe deficiencies of bicarbonate, potassium, phosphate and magnesium lead to cardiac dysrhythmias and muscle weakness. Early recognition and correction of electrolyte abnormalities is required in the solvent-abusing obstetric patient. Beta-sympathomimetics for premature labour and intravenous fluid therapy can potentially exacerbate the electrolyte abnormalities. Chronic sniffing of solvents is associated with a significantly increased incidence of premature labour, intrauterine growth retardation and perinatal death. Chronic use can result in irreversible neurotoxic damage with cerebellar degeneration and cortical atrophy.

The choice of anaesthetic techniques depends on renal and hepatic function. Renal tubular acidosis at the time of delivery is associated with significant neonatal acidosis.

General anaesthesia may be necessary in the comatose patient to protect the airway and facilitate oxygenation.

13.9 Hallucinogens

13.9.1 Phencyclidine

This compound binds to low-affinity σ-opioid receptor sites. It is usually smoked together with tobacco or cannabis. It has autonomic side effects and causes seizures. Severe psychotic reactions occur, and can complicate emergence from anaesthesia. Hallucinating patients require general anaesthesia, but a hypertensive response to intubation may complicate the induction of anaesthesia. Vasopressors must be used with caution.

13.9.2 Lysergic acid diethylamine (LSD)

LSD is a potent hallucinogen. It reduces central 5-hydroxytryptamine turnover, and produces congenital abnormalities. Anaesthetic agents can be potentiated, and psychoses recur postoperatively. During acute intoxication, anticholinergic agents should be avoided and body cooling may be required to counteract hyperthermia.

References

1. Gawin FH, Ellinwood EH. Cocaine and other stimulants: actions, abuse and treatment. *N Engl J Med* 1988; **318**: 1173–82.
2. McCalla S, Minkoff HL, Feldman J, Glass L, Valencia G. Predictors of cocaine use in pregnancy. *Obstet Gynecol* 1992; **79**: 641–4.
3. Spence MR, Williams R, DiGregorio GJ, Kirby-McDonnell A, Polansky M. The relationship between recent cocaine use and pregnancy outcome. *Obstet Gynecol* 1991; **78**: 326–9.
4. Matera C, Warren WB, Moomjy M, Fink DJ, Fox HE. Prevalence of use of cocaine and other substances in an obstetric population. *Am J Obstet Gynecol* 1990; **163**: 797–801.
5. Buchi KF, Varner MW, Chase RA. The prevalence of drug abuse among pregnant women in Utah. *Obstet Gynecol* 1993; **81**: 239–42.
6. Sloan LB, Gay JW, Snyder SW, Bales WR. Substance abuse in pregnancy in a rural population. *Obstet Gynecol* 1992; **79**: 245–8.
7. Skidmore CA, Roberson JR, Robertson AA, Elton RA. After the epidemic: follow up study of HIV seroprevalence and changing patterns of drug use. *Br Med J* 1990; **300**: 219–23.
8. Strang J, Griffiths P, Abbey J, Gossop M. Survey of use of injected benzodiazepines among drug users in Britain. *Br Med J* 1994; **308**: 1082.
9. Simpson D, Greenwood J, Jarvie DR, Moore FML. Experience of a laboratory service for drug screening in urine. *Scott Med J* 1993; **38**: 20–6.
10. O'Connor M. Drugs of abuse in pregnancy: an overview. *Med J Aust* 1987; **147**: 180–3.
11. Kliman L. Drug dependence and pregnancy: antenatal and intrapartum problems. *Anaesth Intensive Care* 1990; **18**: 358–60.
12. Caunnaughton JF, Reeser D, Schut J, Finnegan L. Perinatal addiction: outcome and management. *Am J Obstet Gynecol* 1977; **129**: 679–86.
13. Evans AT, Gillogley K. Drug use in pregnancy: obstetric perspectives. *Clin Perinatol* 1991; **18**: 23–32.
14. Birnbach DJ, Stein DJ, Grunebaum A, Danzer BI, Thys DM. Cocaine screening of parturients without prenatal care: an evaluation of a rapid screening assay. *Anesth Analg* 1997; **84**: 76–9.
15. Pietrantoni M, Knuppel RA. Alcohol use in pregnancy. *Clin Perinatol* 1991; **18**: 93–111.
16. Farre M, de la Torre R, Llorente M *et al.* Alcohol and cocaine interactions in humans. *J Pharmacol Exp Ther* 1993; **266**: 1364–73.
17. Isner JM, Chokshi SK. Cocaine and vasospasm. *N Engl J Med* 1989; **321**: 1604–6.
18. Hoegerman G, Schnoll S. Narcotic use in pregnancy. *Clin Perinatol* 1991; **18**: 51–76.
19. Zelson C, Lee SJ, Casalino M. Neonatal narcotic addiction: comparative effects of maternal intake of heroin and methadone. *N Engl J Med* 1973; **289**: 1216–20.
20. Cherukuri R, Minkott H, Feldman J, Parekh A, Glass L. A cohort study of alkaloidal cocaine ('crack') in pregnancy. *Obstet Gynecol* 1988; **72**: 147–51.
21. Katz JL, Terry P, Witkin JM. Comparative behavioural pharmacology and toxicology of cocaine and its ethanol-derived metabolite, cocaine ethyl-ester (cocaethylene). *Life Sci* 1992; **50**: 1351–61.
22. Madden JA, Powers RH. Effect of cocaine and cocaine metabolites on cerebral arteries *in vitro*. *Life Sci* 1990; **47**: 1109–14.

23 Wood JR, Scott KJ, Plessinger MA. Pregnancy enhances cocaine actions on the heart and within the peripheral circulation. *Am J Obstet Gynecol* 1994; **170**: 1027–35.
24 Handler A, Kitsin N, David F, Ferre G. Cocaine use during pregnancy: perinatal outcomes. *Am J Epidemiol* 1991; **133**: 818–25.
25 Chasnoff IJ, Bussey ME, Savich R, Stack CM. Perinatal cerebral infarction and maternal cocaine use. *J Pediatr* 1986; **108**: 456–9.
26 Cheng D. Perioperative care of the cocaine-abusing patient. *Can J Anaesth* 1994; **41**: 883–7.
27 Day NL, Richardson GA. Prenatal marijuana use: epidemiology, methodology issues and infant outcome. *Clin Perinatol* 1991; **18**: 77–91.
28 Zucherman B, Frank DA, Hingson R *et al*. Effects of maternal marijuana and cocaine use on fetal growth. *N Engl J Med* 1989; **320**: 762–8.
29 Woods JH, Katz JL, Winger G. Benzodiazepines: use, abuse, and consequences. *Pharmacol Rev* 1992; **44**: 151–347.
30 Bergman U, Rosa FW, Baum C, Wiholm B-E, Faich GA. Effects of exposure to benzodiazepine during fetal life. *Lancet* 1992; **340**: 694–6.
31 Elliot RH, Rees GB. Amphetamine ingestion presenting as eclampsia. *Can J Anesth* 1990; **37**: 130–3.
32 Wilkins-Haug L, Gabow PA. Toluene abuse during pregnancy: obstetric complications and perinatal outcomes. *Obstet Gynecol* 1991; **77**: 504–9.

Section 3
Regional Anaesthesia

14: Anatomy

Regional anaesthetic techniques are used in obstetric patients to produce a blockade of sensory nerves for the relief of pain during labour, and for operative interventions. The techniques currently in use include epidural nerve block, subarachnoid nerve block (SAB), and a combination of the two techniques referred to as a combined spinal/epidural nerve block (CSE). Epidural nerve blocks are usually performed in the United Kingdom via the lumbar region of the spinal column. The caudal epidural route was formerly popular, and may still occasionally be used when nerve blockade of the sacral spinal nerves is desired. Caudal nerve block, however, carries a greater risk of infection and has an increased failure rate compared with the lumbar route. In the labouring woman, the close proximity of the fetal head to the point of insertion also introduces the risk of fetal cranial puncture by an incorrectly directed needle.

The vertebral canal, for the purposes of regional nerve blockade, can be regarded as consisting of two spaces: the subarachnoid space and the epidural space. Knowledge of the anatomy of the vertebral column and an ability to visualize in three dimensions the spinal structures beneath the parturient's skin will help obstetric anaesthetists to perform regional anaesthesia accurately with minimal difficulty or parturient discomfort. The anatomical features described below apply principally to the lumbar region of the spine, and can be considered in two groups: first, the anatomy of the structures surrounding and forming the vertebral canal—this is the perivertebral anatomy; and secondly, the anatomy of the vertebral canal and its contents.

14.1 Perivertebral anatomy

Surface markings and bony landmarks help the anaesthetist to identify, with reasonable accuracy, the lumbar vertebral spines and the interspaces between them, as shown in Fig. 14.1. The vertebral spines in the non-obese parturient are usually easy to feel as hard protuberances running in the midline of the back. They identify the axis of the vertebral column, and are important landmarks. The straight line drawn between the most superior points of the right and left iliac crests usually passes across the third lumbar interspace, i.e. the space between the spines of L3 and L4. This landmark is commonly used to identify a suitable surface point for the insertion of an epidural or subarachnoid needle.

In the obese parturient, bony landmarks may be difficult to identify, but some landmarks will almost always be identifiable, although by slightly

C7 Vertebra prominens
T3 Spine of the scapula

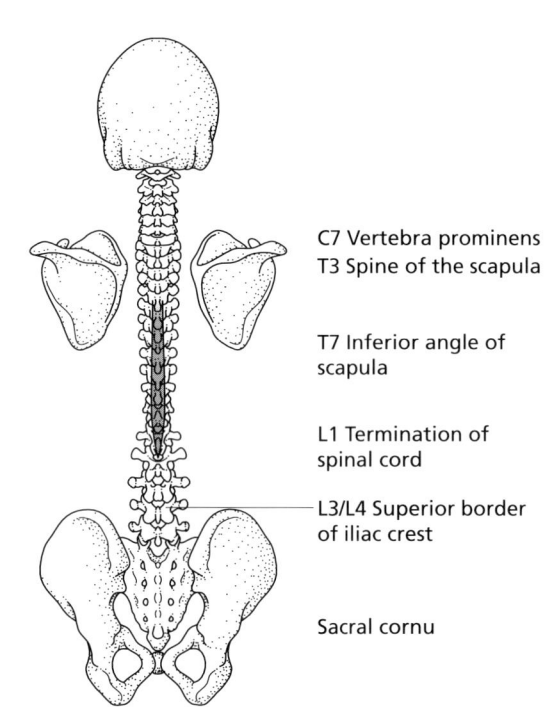

T7 Inferior angle of scapula

L1 Termination of spinal cord

L3/L4 Superior border of iliac crest

Sacral cornu

Fig. 14.1 Surface markings and bony landmarks used during regional analgesia in obese and non-obese parturients.

different techniques. With the patient in an erect sitting position, the prominent seventh cervical vertebra or the spines of thoracic vertebrae confirm the midline, which can be extrapolated downwards to the lumbar region. In the absence of visible or palpable landmarks in the lumbar region, the vertebral spines can be located carefully using a thin (e.g. 25-gauge) needle of an appropriate length. The obese patient should maintain a sitting position during the performance of epidural or subarachnoid nerve block, since it allows the midline to be more easily and accurately identified. In the lateral decubitus position, a discrepancy can develop between the apparent midline delineated by the cephalad continuation of the natal cleft and the actual midline of the bony spine. The skin, subcutaneous tissue and posterior ligaments that lie between the skin and the vertebral canal will be penetrated, or encountered, by a needle directed towards the vertebral canal in the midline. A needle inserted between the vertebral spines will therefore pass through the supraspinous ligament, the interspinous ligament, and the ligamentum flavum (Fig. 14.2). However, the ligamentum flavum is made up of two ligaments, one on either side of the midline. If an advancing needle is truly in the midline when it reaches the ligamentum flavum, it may pass between the left and right components, piercing neither. Identification of this series of tissues and ligaments is vital for the accurate insertion of an epidural needle, and for this reason blunt needles are used, because the resistance forces opposing the passage of the needle and the tactile feedback that results are greater than with sharp needles.

ANATOMY 215

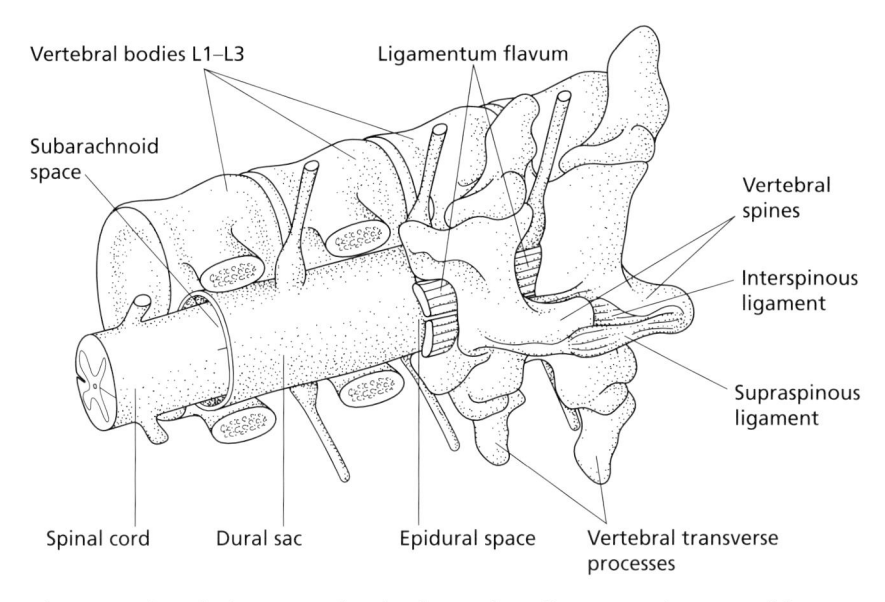

Fig. 14.2 Perivertebral anatomy, showing the vertebrae, ligaments and contents of the vertebral canal.

The distance from the skin to the epidural space varies considerably from individual to individual. Logically, smaller individuals should have a shorter skin-to-epidural space distance than larger people. One reason why this does not occur in practice is that the apparent depth of the space from the skin is also affected by the angle at which an epidural needle is introduced. A reported distribution curve of skin–space distances [1] showed that 95% of individuals had a skin-to-epidural space distance of between 3 and 6 cm. The lower limit of this range may not be expected by the anaesthetist, and inadvertent dural puncture can result.

14.2 Vertebral canal

The vertebral canal in the lumbar region is roughly triangular in cross-section, with the apex of the triangle situated dorsally in the midline. It contains the spinal cord, the origins of the ventral and dorsal spinal nerve roots, the subarachnoid space, the dural sac and the epidural space. The spinal cord enlarges in its lumbar region, because it contains the nerve supply to the lower limbs. The enlarged lumbar cord occupies the lower thoracic spinal canal, beginning at the ninth thoracic vertebra and enlarging to a maximum at the twelfth thoracic vertebra. Thereafter, the cord tapers gradually to the conus medullaris. The size of the epidural space thus varies from one vertebral level to another, and indeed within one level. The distance between the ligamentum flavum and the dura in the midline at the second lumbar interspace is said to be approximately 5–6 mm in adult males [2]. However, in the pregnant woman,

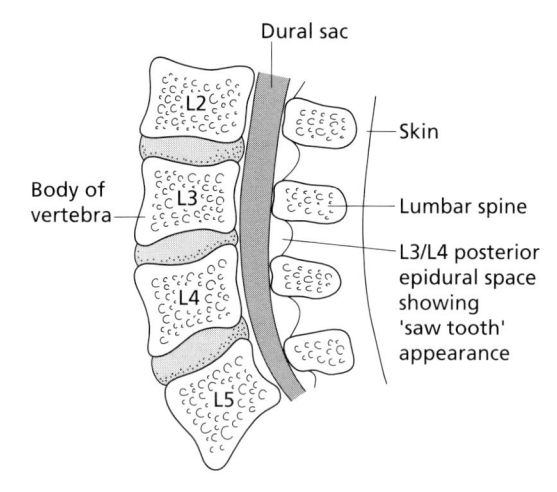

Fig. 14.3 Diagrammatic representation of the posterior epidural space on a midline sagittal section.

clinical experience teaches us that the anteroposterior size of the space may be as little as 1–2 mm or as much as 10 mm. Magnetic resonance imaging in midline sagittal sections also shows that the posterior epidural space is sawtoothed in shape (Fig. 14.3) [3]. The depth of the epidural space at any one level obviously varies depending on the angle of approach. The pattern of narrowing is quite abrupt at the cranial end of each vertebral level, where the lamina may approach the dura closely. The introduction of an epidural needle at this point must therefore increase the possibility of inadvertent dural puncture. An epidural catheter may also meet an obstruction at this point of narrowing, as the inferior surface of the lamina blocks its cephalad passage in the epidural space.

The epidural space is not an empty cavity. It contains blood vessels, lymphatics, nerves, fat and connective tissue septa (Fig. 14.4). These contents form barriers to the spread of local anaesthetic agents in the epidural space, and separate the drug from the neural tissues. They are probably the cause of patchy or uneven blocks and missed segments. The nature and distribution of the contents were clearly identified in cadavers [4], and have been confirmed during epiduroscopy [5,6] and using computed tomography (CT) (Fig. 14.4) [7].

The vertebral canal is lined by periosteum, which covers bony vertebral surfaces and ligaments joining adjacent vertebrae. The epidural space lies between this lining of the vertebral canal and the dural sac, and extends into the paravertebral space (Fig. 14.5). The dural sac contains the spinal cord and cerebrospinal fluid (CSF) and is made up of two layers of connective tissue, the dura and the arachnoid mater. The former is the tougher and more superficial of the two layers, between which lies the subdural space. The subdural space is a potential space comprising a thin fluid layer between the two dural membranes that allows movement and communication between them. It is limited above by the attachments of the dura and arachnoid membranes to the foramen magnum, and has no obvious communication with the subarachnoid

ANATOMY 217

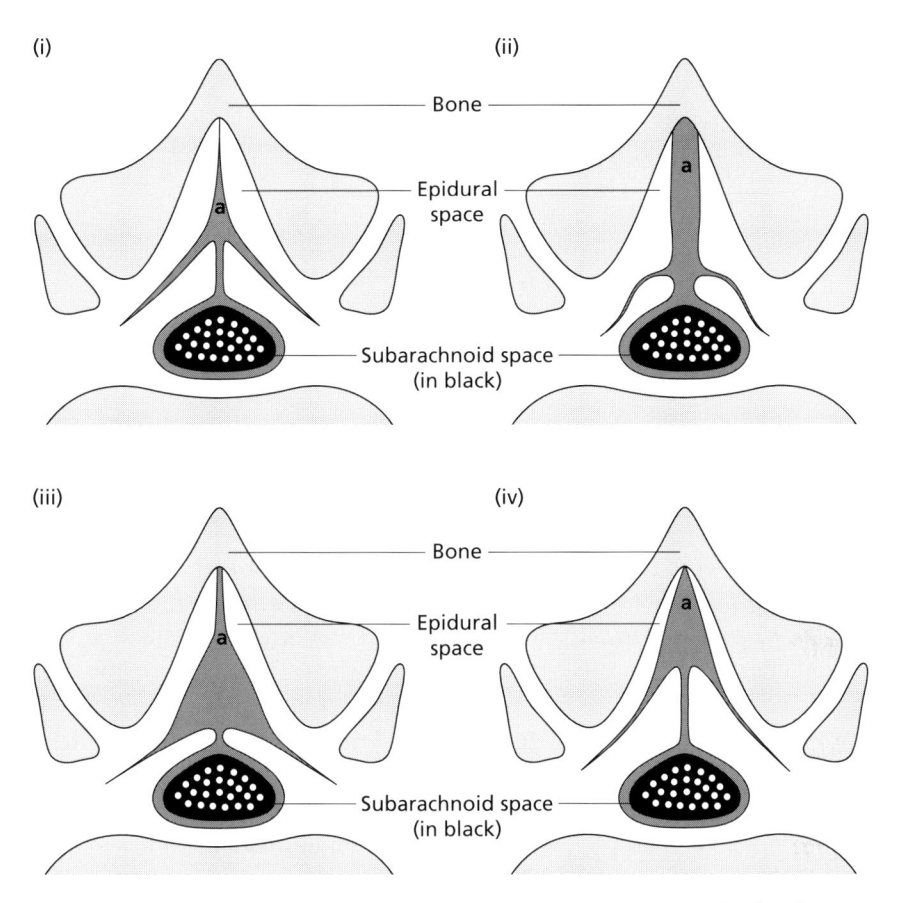

Fig. 14.4 The four patterns of epidural septa in transverse section [7]; 'a' is the dorsal midline septum.

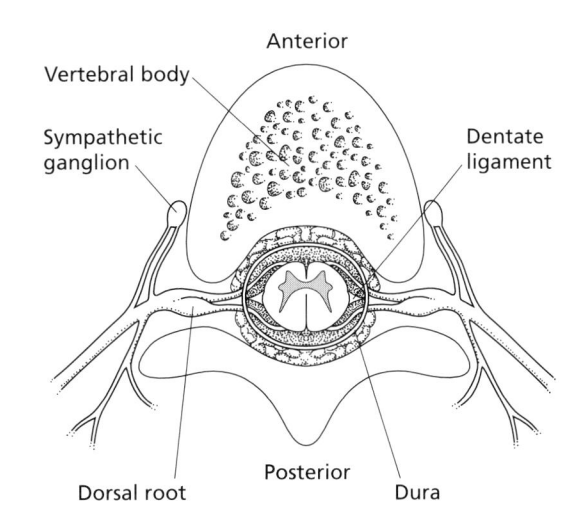

Fig. 14.5 Cross-section of the spinal column, showing the anatomical relationships of the epidural space.

space. However, microscopy of the arachnoid membrane shows that it contains many fluid-filled lacunae, which probably do allow communication between the fluid in the subdural space and the CSF. Local anaesthetic solutions and epidural catheters can occasionally accidentally pass into the subdural space. The small capacity of this potential space allows a relatively small volume of local anaesthetic solution to spread widely and affect many spinal nerves. The resulting anaesthesia is extensive, but of slow onset. Radiological evidence of the distribution of subdural spread of injected solutions is rare. The case described by Boyes and Norman [8] shows the spread of solution into the high thoracic and low cervical regions of the space, with dye extending mainly in the cephalad direction along the dorsal aspect of the space from the point of injection.

The subarachnoid space lies within the dural sac, and is filled with CSF. It surrounds the spinal cord and communicates above with the intracranial subarachnoid space surrounding the brain. Drugs injected into the CSF can therefore diffuse directly to the higher centres contained within the brain, especially if the drug concerned is water-soluble. In addition to CSF, the subarachnoid space also contains connective tissue septa and blood vessels that supply and drain the spinal cord. Spinal nerve roots pass through the subarachnoid space, and at this point in their course they have yet to acquire their dural coverings, which are derived from the dural sac itself. The exposed nerve roots are therefore more easily penetrated by local anaesthetic solutions. This accessibility of neural tissue is one reason for the rapid onset and density of block when subarachnoid, as compared with epidural, anaesthesia is used.

14.2.1 Connective tissue in the vertebral canal

The presence of connective-tissue coverings and septa in the subarachnoid and epidural spaces has clinical significance for regional anaesthetic techniques. The single largest connective-tissue structure lying in the vertebral canal is the dural sac itself. In addition to the sac, extensive septa and connective-tissue bands lie within the epidural and subarachnoid spaces. The combination of connective tissue together with fat and blood vessels gives protection to the spinal cord. Apart from a mechanical supportive and cushioning role, it has a dynamic pathophysiological effect, providing protection against infection, thermal regulation, nutrition and waste disposal for the tissues of the spinal cord.

The spinal meninges and septa link and anchor the dural sac within the vertebral canal. The fibrous trabeculations in the epidural space also contain nerves radiating from a plexus in the anterior longitudinal ligament to the dura mater. The spaces between the trabeculations contain fat and the internal vertebral venous plexus. This combination of tissues and structures provides a flexible cushion for the dural sac. The sac itself, together with the CSF and the contents of the vertebral venous plexus, provides a pliable hydraulic buffer for the spinal cord. The dural sac was for many years thought to be a simple sheet of connective tissue with most of its fibres running in the longitudinal axis of the sac. Although a general latticing effect can be seen [9], the majority of the thicker fibres do run longitudinally rather than transversely. This longitudinal disposition of fibres in the dural sac had long been thought to be the reason for the correlation of the incidence of postdural puncture headache (PDPH) and Quincke spinal needle bevel orientation [10]. In spite of the more recent recognition of the variability of fibre direction in the dural sac, it is still clear that puncture of the dura by a Quincke tipped needle with its bevel in the same axis as the fibres perforated (compared with an axis at right angles) does create a narrower hole that retracts more quickly. There is therefore both anatomical and clinical evidence for the fact that dural puncture with spinal needle bevels in the long axis of the spine produces less PDPH than puncture by needles with their bevels at 90° to the long axis of the spine. It is also logical that the oval dural holes demonstrated by Dittman and colleagues [9] are more likely to be kept open by patient movement, especially flexion of the spine, if the long axis of the hole is at 90° to the long axis of the patient.

The epidural septa and trabeculations shown in cadaveric specimens by early anatomists have been re-examined by *in vivo* radiological and CT scanning techniques. The recurring patterns of fibrous bands within the epidural space were clearly described by Savolaine and colleagues [7] (Fig. 14.4). They all have a dorsal midline septum, the plica mediana dorsalis, connected anteriorly to the dural sac and posteriorly to the lining of the vertebral canal. The fatty content of this septum varies markedly, so that in some individuals the septum is quite bulky (ii, iii, iv in Fig. 14.4), whereas in others it is quite thin (i in Fig. 14.4). The size and position of lateral projections of the septa are also variable. The bulky type of septum with long lateral projections is more likely to deflect or even be penetrated by an epidural catheter. Either eventuality is likely to lead to incomplete or failed epidural blockade. The four patterns occurred in (i) 5%, (ii) 45%, (iii) 33% and (iv) 17% of cadavers, respectively. Using the commonest patterns shown by Savolaine, Fig. 14.6 shows how an epidural catheter or local anaesthetic solution injected into the epidural space may be trapped or deviated to one side of the space, or even deflected from the space into paravertebral tissues. Given the lack of anatomical constancy of the septation within the epidural space, it is prudent to ask any parturient requesting an epidural whether she has had an epidural sited before and whether the subsequent nerve block was inadequate. A previous patchy or unilateral block may indicate the presence of bulky epidural septa and the option of CSE rather than a purely epidural technique must be considered.

A similar complexity of fibrous bands and septa exists in the subarachnoid space. Detailed observations of subarachnoid septa have been reported by Nauta and colleagues [11]. Their work confirmed the presence of a fenestrated posterior midline dorsal septum, probably related to the midline dorsal vein

220 CHAPTER 14

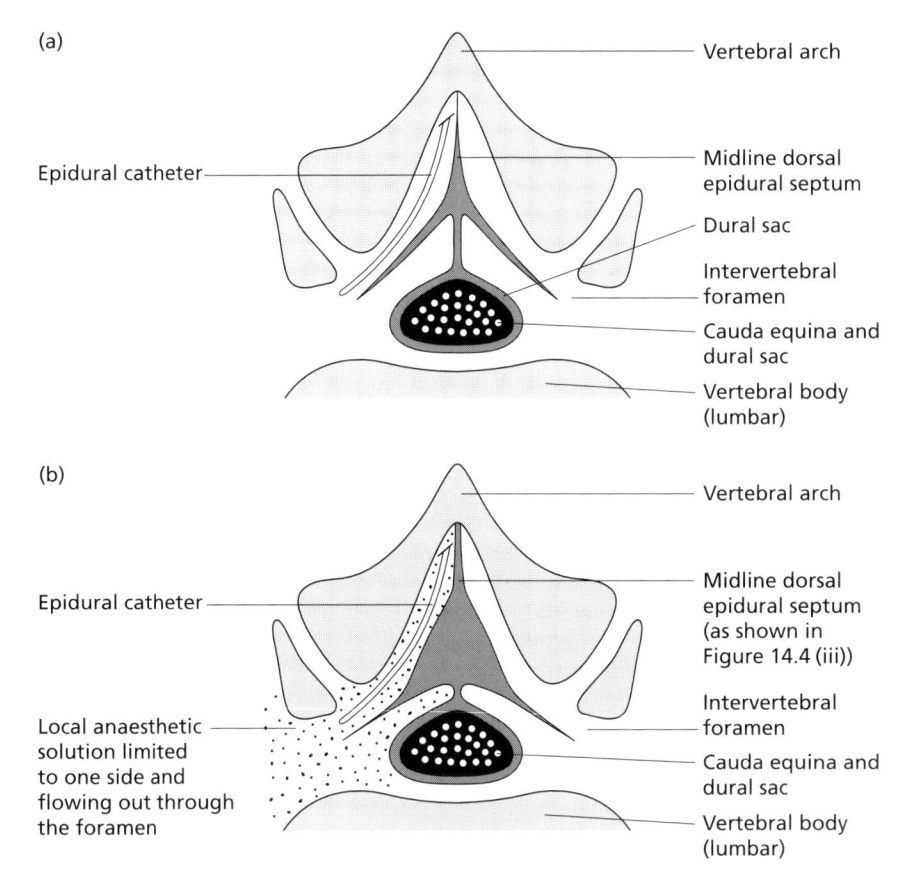

(a) [diagram with labels: Vertebral arch, Midline dorsal epidural septum, Dural sac, Intervertebral foramen, Cauda equina and dural sac, Vertebral body (lumbar), Epidural catheter]

(b) [diagram with labels: Vertebral arch, Midline dorsal epidural septum (as shown in Figure 14.4 (iii)), Intervertebral foramen, Cauda equina and dural sac, Vertebral body (lumbar), Epidural catheter, Local anaesthetic solution limited to one side and flowing out through the foramen]

Fig. 14.6 Two patterns of membranes in the posterior epidural space, showing possible lateral deflection of (a) the epidural catheter and (b) the local anaesthetic solution (hatched area).

and connecting the arachnoid and pia mater (Fig. 14.7). The septum they identified followed a variable course, and was sometimes incomplete. In addition to the dorsal midline structure, a dorsolateral septum and some transverse septa were also described. Unlike those in the epidural space, the subarachnoid septa do not impede the spread of local anaesthetic solutions, because the septa themselves are fenestrated and incomplete, and the subarachnoid space is filled with a liquid medium through which diffusion of local anaesthetic molecules may occur freely. Incomplete or inadequate blocks are therefore much less common with subarachnoid, as opposed to epidural, techniques.

The subarachnoid dorsolateral septum (Fig. 14.8) is carried laterally as an extra layer of connective tissue covering the dorsal sensory nerve roots of spinal nerves as they emerge from the subarachnoid and pass through the epidural space. The variability of the subarachnoid septal pattern makes it

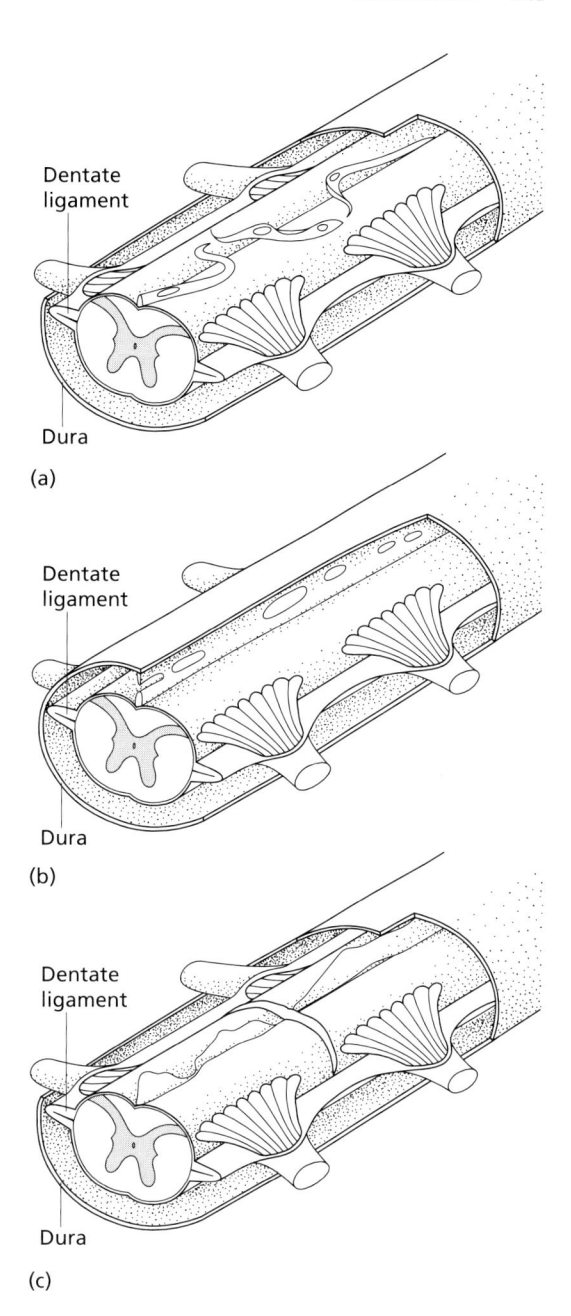

Fig. 14.7 Patterns of subarachnoid septa, showing dorsal and lateral variations.

difficult to know which sensory nerve roots will carry the additional layer of connective tissue. The additional nerve covering, when it is present, may be yet another reason why some nerve roots are more difficult to block with epidural local anaesthetic solutions, whereas they are vulnerable to subarachnoid injections of local anaesthetic solution.

222   CHAPTER 14

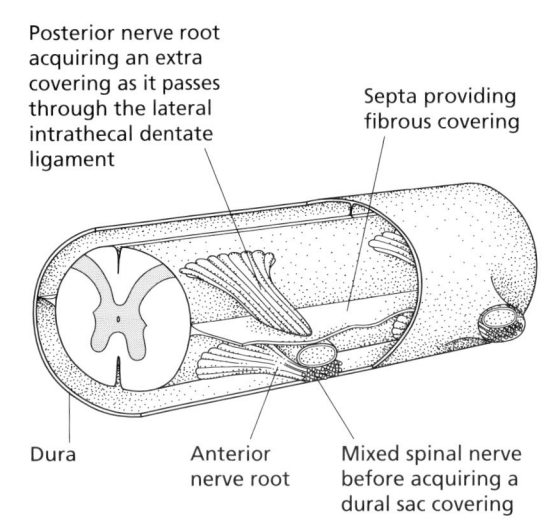

Fig. 14.8 The acquisition of additional fibrous coverings by the sensory component of a mixed spinal nerve.

14.2.2 Arterial blood supply to the spinal cord

The blood supply to the spinal cord is derived from three main sources:
1 the *pia mater* blood vessels;
2 the single anterior spinal artery;
3 the two posterior spinal arteries.

Pial blood vessels provide an important blood supply to the developing spinal cord. In adult life, however, they supply only the surface and superficial structures of the cord. The anterior spinal artery runs in the anterior median fissure for the length of the spinal cord. It originates as a branch of the vertebral artery, but as it descends it receives additional blood supply from the ascending cervical, posterior intercostal and lumbar arteries. Branches from these sources pass backwards through intervertebral foramina to the anterior spinal artery, which supplies approximately the anterior two-thirds of the spinal cord, including the anterior horn and its neighbouring grey matter (Fig. 14.9). The posterior spinal arteries, two in number, descend along the posterior surface of the spinal cord adjacent to the dorsal nerve roots. They derive their blood supply from the same arterial sources as the anterior spinal artery. They then supply the posterior third of the spinal cord, including dorsal horns and adjacent sensory pathways.

The blood supply to the spinal cord is therefore quite vulnerable to damage in the abdominal cavity, and can be markedly affected by pressure changes within the vertebral canal. A reduction in blood pressure—for instance, following a major obstetric haemorrhage or extensive regional anaesthetic block—can critically reduce blood flow to the anterior section of the spinal cord. This will mainly affect motor functions. The lumbar spinal cord seems particularly susceptible to ischaemia, because it derives its arterial supply from only one intercostal artery. This, the artery of Adamkiewicz, can arise from

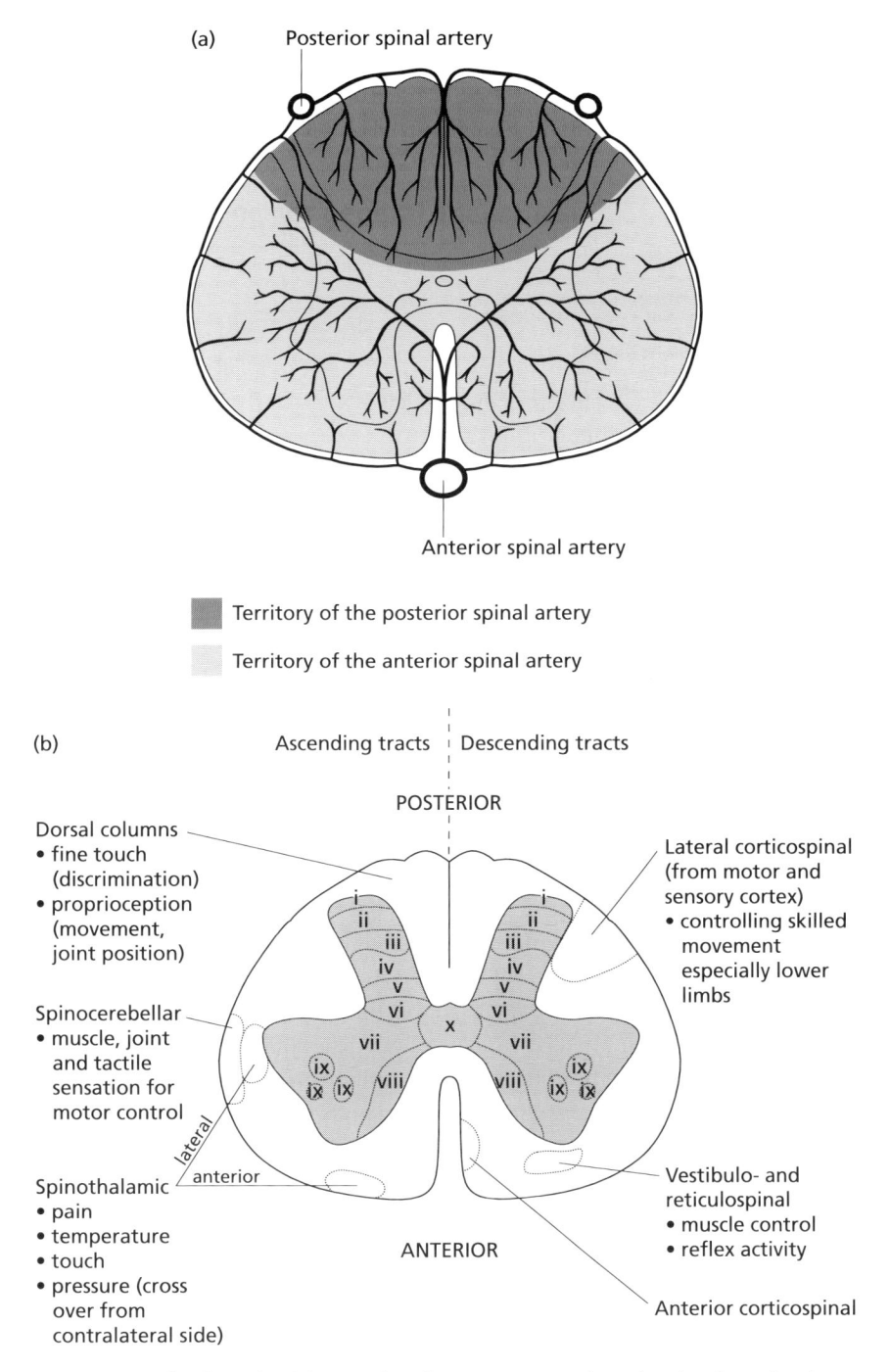

Fig. 14.9 (a) Blood supply of the spinal cord in transverse section, showing the regional distribution of supply from anterior and posterior spinal arteries. (b) The functional anatomy of the spinal cord. Rexed's laminae are numbered i–x. Their function can be grouped as follows: dorsal horn: i–iii, substantia gelatinosa (nociception); vii, Clarke's column (spinocerebellar tract, preganglionic sympathetic and parasympathetic fibres for autonomic and visceral function and postural from muscles). Ventral horn: ix, motor neurones (innervate skeletal muscle).

any intercostal artery between T8 and L3. The single vessel provides the blood supply for the majority of the lumbar and sacral segments of the spinal cord via the anterior and posterior spinal artery branches. Blood flow through this one source, together with the enlarged tissue bulk which it supplies, makes the balance of supply and demand for oxygen in this part of the spinal cord quite critical.

14.2.3 Venous drainage

The epidural space contains a dense valveless venous plexus known as the system of Batson. Its connections with the inferior vena cava and the azygous and hemiazygous veins allow it to act as a bypass for the venous blood draining from the lower half of the body. The plexus comprises two main anterior longitudinal venous channels and a series of posterior internal veins that drain via the intervertebral foramina to the paravertebral venous channels. During pregnancy, the venous plexus dilates, so that it effectively reduces the capacity of the epidural space by up to 30%. Further venous distension occurs during inferior vena caval obstruction and uterine contraction. The dilated veins increase the risk of inadvertent venous puncture by a needle or epidural catheter. Fortunately, distension of the epidural venous plexus does not lead on to venous engorgement within the spinal cord: valves have been identified in radicular veins passing from the cord through the dura mater to the epidural space [12], which are considered to provide some protection to the spinal cord.

14.3 Applied anatomy

14.3.1 Immunology

Immunologically, the pia and arachnoid membranes forming the meninges are involved in the induction of an inflammatory response, and the dura mater plays a major role in lymphatic drainage and clearance of inflammatory products from within the dural sac. Reabsorption of inflammatory cells from the CSF seems to take place at meningeal pockets found close to dorsal nerve roots. The meninges are rich in blood vessels, which drain via many anastomoses to the epidural venous plexus. Absorption of CSF and cellular debris occurs via fluid lacunae in the arachnoid mater, dural capillaries [13] and arachnoid villi that protrude into dural or epidural vessels. Many blood-borne cells, such as mast cells, T lymphocytes and monocytes are found in the dura and arachnoid mater. These immunologically active cells serve as scavengers, and cells lining the meninges have degrading enzymes and antigens on their surfaces. The dura and arachnoid mater therefore provide important protection against infection of the central nervous system [14], which is bypassed by perforation of the dura. Subarachnoid block must therefore only be carried out under the strictest aseptic conditions. It must be emphasized that great care must be taken to achieve asepsis, and a no-touch technique should be used during the performance of subarachnoid anaesthesia, not only to prevent bacterial penetration but also to avoid a chemical inflammatory response. Even when bacterial infection cannot be detected, the immunological reactivity of the arachnoid mater may respond to foreign substances acting as antibodies. This so-called 'aseptic meningitis' is the likely mechanism of the meningism seen occasionally after subarachnoid anaesthesia.

14.3.2 Thermal regulation

The rich meningeal blood supply and free drainage via the epidural venous plexus, together with the insulating properties of fat deposits in the epidural space, guarantee temperature homeostasis for the central nervous system under normal circumstances. In addition, this excellent blood supply guarantees good nutrition and removal of waste substances from the CSF. The arterial blood supply to the spinal cord itself is more tenuous than its venous drainage.

14.3.3 Configuration of the spinal column in pregnancy

An exaggeration of the lumbar lordosis during pregnancy is one of the compensatory mechanisms of the skeletal system to maintain the woman's centre of gravity when erect. It has been postulated that this change enhances cephalad spread of subarachnoid local anaesthetic solutions when a parturient is placed in a supine position. Magnetic resonance studies in late pregnancy [15] showed that in the tilted supine position, the highest point of the lumbar lordosis was located more caudally in the lower lumbar region in the pregnant women studied (36–37 weeks) than in non-pregnant individuals. This change may be due to pressure from the uterus, combined with joint and ligament laxity. Some changes in spinal curvature are also age-related, with the lowest part of the thoracic curve in the supine position lying at T8–9 in teenagers and slightly higher in young adults [16]. Visual comparison of the illustrations in these two studies shows similar flattening or straightening of the thoracic curvature in both adolescents and pregnant subjects. Individuals in both of these groups are known to have a higher cephalad spread of the effects of hyperbaric local anaesthetic agents during subarachnoid anaesthesia. A combination of a lower apex of lumbar lordosis and a flatter thoracic curve in the pregnant patient are likely to contribute to this higher spread.

References

1 Bromage PR. *Epidural Analgesia* Philadelphia: Saunders, 1978: 197.
2 Bromage PR. *Epidural Analgesia* Philadelphia: Saunders, 1978: 14.

3 Westbrook JL, Renouden SA, Carrie LES. Study of the anatomy of the extradural region using magnetic resonance imaging. *Br J Anaesth* 1993; **71**: 495–8.
4 Key EAH, Retzius MG. *Studien in der Anatomie des Nervensystems und des Bindegewebes.* Stockholm: Samson and Wallin, 1875.
5 Blomberg RG, Olsen SS. The lumbar epidural space in patients examined with epiduroscopy. *Anesth Analg* 1989; **69**: 157–60.
6 Möllmann M, Holst D, Lübbesmeyer H, Lawin P. Continuous spinal anesthesia: mechanical and technical problems of catheter placement. *Reg Anesth* 1993; **18**: 469–72.
7 Savolaine ER, Pandya JB, Greenblatt SH, Connover SR. Anatomy of the human lumbar epidural space; new insights using CT-epidurography. *Anesthesiology* 1988; **68**: 217–20.
8 Boyes JE, Norman PF. Accident subdural analgesia. *Br J Anaesth* 1975; **47**: 1111.
9 Dittman M, Schaeffer HG, Ulrich J, Bond-Taylor W. Anatomical re-evaluation of lumbar dura mater with regard to post-dural puncture headache. *Anaesthesia* 1988; **43**: 635–7.
10 Mihic DM. Post-spinal headache and relationship of needle bevel to longitudinal dural fibres. *Reg Anesth* 1985; **10**: 76.
11 Nauta HJW, Dolan E, Yasagill MG. Microsurgical anatomy of spinal subarachnoid space. *Surg Neurol* 1983; **19**: 431–7.
12 Clemens HJ, Von Quast H. Untersuchungen über die Gefässe des menschlichen Rückenmarkes. *Acta Anat* 1960; **42**: 277–306.
13 Zinker W. The dura mater from the view point of modern anatomy. In: Van Zundert A, ed. *Highlights in Regional Anaesthesia and Pain Therapy*, vol. 4. Barcelona: Permanyer, 1995: 107.
14 Lassman H. The meninges and immunology: a barrier to infection. In: Van Zundert A, ed. *Highlights in Regional Anaesthesia and Pain Therapy*, vol. 4. Barcelona: Permanyer, 1995: 110.
15 Hirobayashi Y, Shimizu R, Fukuda H, Saitoh K, Furuse M. Anatomical configuration of the spinal column in the supine position, 2: comparison of pregnant and non-pregnant women. *Br J Anaesth* 1995; **75**: 6–8.
16 Hirabayashi Y, Shimizu R, Saitoh K *et al.* Anatomical configuration of the spinal column in the supine position, 3: comparison of adolescent and adult volunteers. *Br J Anaesth* 1996; **76**: 508–10.

15: Regional Anaesthetic Techniques

A regional nerve blockade is used to produce pain relief or complete anaesthesia within a limited segmental distribution in a parturient. The nerve block can be controlled by varying the type of drug or drugs used, the dosage of drug, the patient's position and the route of administration. Epidural analgesia is used principally for pain relief during labour, or postoperatively if the technique has been part of the intraoperative anaesthetic management. A pre-existing epidural block can be modified so as to increase the density and extent of the anaesthetic effect. 'Topping up' an epidural in this way is frequently used when labour pain relief needs to be enhanced to allow operative delivery. Subarachnoid techniques are used for operative intervention because a profound anaesthetic effect is achieved very rapidly with a low incidence of failure. The speed of onset of subarachnoid analgesia makes the technique suitable for pain relief in labour when a rapidity of effect is sought. This has led to the development of a combined spinal–epidural (CSE) method that attempts to provide the benefits of both techniques and minimize their limitations.

In the United Kingdom, epidural analgesia and anaesthesia have been used increasingly in the last 25 years, and more recently subarachnoid anaesthesia has become more popular. It is estimated that some 20% of all parturients now receive epidural analgesia for pain relief in labour. The use of subarachnoid anaesthesia is increasing, principally for Caesarean section anaesthesia, but also as part of a CSE technique in labour. The decrease in the use of general anaesthesia has been welcomed with enthusiasm by many parturients, who prefer to remain awake with a regional anaesthetic technique. Obstetric anaesthetists are now able to offer anaesthesia that avoids the profound systemic maternal and fetal effects of opioid and general anaesthetic agents. Mothers suffer less from the stress responses arising from pain and operative intervention, and are able to cope with their baby and 'mother' it immediately after delivery, often returning home after a short hospital stay.

The technical developments in regional anaesthesia usage have not been matched by an increased availability of new drugs or by changes in the licences of existing drugs for their use by either epidural or subarachnoid routes. Drug usage outside the limits of licences is a phenomenon that is based on individual professional responsibility. However, given these circumstances, an obstetric anaesthetist must be absolutely certain that each particular form of drug usage is supported by a responsible body of the profession, and that clear benefits can be shown to be conferred on the woman receiving the treatment.

In keeping with professional standards, the first approach to any parturient should be a medical assessment, identification of any risks or contraindications to anaesthesia and an explanation of the procedure that is planned. Before initiating regional anaesthesia, the obstetric anaesthetist should check that appropriate facilities are available, that staffing levels are satisfactory, and that training of all staff in the unit meets or exceeds nationally defined minimum standards. The continuing availability of all of these factors for the duration of the procedure must also be guaranteed.

15.1 Indications for epidural analgesia in labour

Epidural analgesia is the most effective form of pain relief. It will prevent or minimize the effects of pain on the cardiovascular and endocrine systems, placental perfusion, acid–base balance and end-organ blood flow, such as renal blood flow. The indications for use of this form of pain relief are any need of complete pain relief and any situation in which there is a need to prevent labour pain responses that may adversely affect existing conditions in the parturient. Indications therefore include:

1 Maternal stress:
   (a) maternal request because of anticipated distress;
   (b) maternal distress.
2 Systemic disease: e.g. hypertensive disorders of pregnancy, some types of cardiac disease; pulmonary disease.
3 Disorders of labour:
   (a) abnormalities of labour, such as incoordinate uterine action; failure to progress, requiring augmentation of labour; inappropriate pushing when the cervix has not fully dilated; premature labour;
   (b) a high pre-existing risk of instrumental or operative intervention.

15.2 Contraindications to epidural analgesia

Specific contraindications should be excluded once a general medical assessment has been carried out and been found to be satisfactory.
   Absolute contraindications are:
- patient refusal (see consent);
- blood coagulopathies;
- infection at the intended site of puncture;
- generalized septicaemia;
- allergy to local anaesthetic agents/opioids;
- a lack of adequate facilities or staff.

15.2.1 Consent

Proceeding with any form of treatment without the patient's consent will expose the doctor to an accusation of assault, unless:

1   the patient is unable to give consent and is suffering from a life-threatening condition which the treatment is likely to improve;
2   the patient is not mentally competent to understand either the health problem or treatment;
3   the patient is a minor under the protection of a court order addressing the problem of the moment.

However, women refuse regional analgesia for a variety of reasons, and time should be spent explaining the other choices for pain relief. A woman should be able to change her mind after discussion of the balance of risks and benefits. A full note should be made of any such discussions and agreements lest amnesia for the events should occur later.

15.2.2 Coagulopathies

The presence of coagulation abnormalities increases the risk of epidural haematoma and its serious neurological sequelae. It is commonly agreed that the increased risk of epidural haematoma outweighs any benefits that may accrue from the use of regional techniques in these circumstances. Some special conditions may change the balance of risk/benefit—for instance, expected or proven difficulty of intubation when Caesarean section is needed. Each such case must be judged on its individual merits and the risks and benefits must be explained to the patient. If the woman is adamant that she must have regional anaesthesia, or if general anaesthesia is contraindicated, the signs and symptoms of a space-occupying lesion from an epidural haematoma must be sought at hourly intervals for at least six hours after the nerve blockade has ended and the epidural catheter removed.

15.2.3 Infection (local or general)

The presence of local infection at or near to the site of puncture exposes the patient to a high risk of epidural abscess formation and its sequelae. An abscess may take days to develop, unlike a haematoma, and the parturient may have already been discharged from anaesthesia follow-up care. Detection of the late-onset neurological signs then depends on the midwifery staff or the woman herself, and delay may occur because they are not trained to recognize such signs.

The presence of general septicaemia as a contraindication is based on the hypothesis that the bacteraemia present may predispose the parturient to bacterial accumulation at the site of epidural or subarachnoid puncture, particularly if there is a collection of blood. Evidence of the presence of such a degree of generalized septicaemia will include pyrexia and a raised white blood cell count and C-reactive protein level. In the absence of these signs, it is unlikely that significant septicaemia exists.

15.2.4 Staffing

Lack of suitable facilities or staff is sometimes difficult to assess. The facilities and staffing needed for anaesthesia services in general are reviewed elsewhere (see Chapter 1). Guidelines and minimum standards have been published by the Obstetric Anaesthetists Association and the Association of Anaesthetists and are recommended [1,2,3]. It must be remembered that initiating and maintaining regional anaesthesia or analgesia is a process that can have serious side effects. The responsibility for the regional technique will remain with the obstetric anaesthetist. He or she must therefore be satisfied that the local facilities and staff are adequate to deal with the known complications.

In addition to absolute contraindications, a number of relative contraindications to regional techniques exist in parturients. These include:

1 acute central nervous system disorders. In the presence of an undiagnosed central or peripheral nerve lesion, it is unwise to attempt epidural or subarachnoid analgesia, because the patient may deteriorate during or following the regional nerve block;

2 hypovolaemia. Maternal haemorrhage, hypotension, or low circulating blood volume are all relative contraindications, because the 'size' of the cardiovascular abnormality and the extent of the regional nerve block may summate and cause significant hypotension. However, if suitable prophylactic measures are taken, regional techniques can be used in these circumstances, e.g. a blood loss of 500–1000 mL of blood and low-dose epidural analgesia are not incompatible, provided that there are no maternal factors apart from a blood loss that has been replaced;

3 cardiac lesions that severely limit cardiac output. It is the tightly stenotic cardiac valve defect that is the main risk factor with regional nerve blockade.

15.3 Preparation for epidural or subarachnoid block

Checklist before epidural analgesia in labour.
- Consent.
- Trained midwife.
- Resuscitation equipment.
- Intravenous access.
- Monitoring of the fetus.
- Stage of labour.
- Bladder empty.
- Maternal pulse and blood pressure.
- History of allergies (including pruritus).
- Previous administration of opioids.
- Vasopressor (ephedrine) and anticholinergic drugs freshly prepared in labelled syringes.

The patient's consent for the procedure should be obtained. Ideally, the consent should be written, but in many obstetric situations written consent is not always feasible and verbal consent is all that can be obtained. In the latter circumstance, the anaesthetist should record the fact, the information, and if possible obtain a witnessed signature to the verbal consent. For any consent to be valid, the parturient must have been told of the potential risks, limitations and complications of the procedure, as well as the potential benefits.

The anaesthetist should be accompanied by a suitably trained member of staff. Whether the assistant is an operating department assistant/practitioner, nurse or midwife is less important than the assistant's training and experience. Resuscitation equipment for oxygen administration and ventilation of the lungs, together with relevant drugs such as vasopressors, must be immediately available. Equipment for general anaesthesia must also be to hand in the area in which the regional nerve block is to be done.

Intravenous access must be secured and confirmed by the free and rapid flow of crystalloid solution into a vein. Control of the volume and type of fluid given to help prevent or reduce hypotension is important. Large volumes of crystalloid or colloid are usually unnecessary, and can overload the circulation in susceptible parturients such as those with cardiac problems or those who have received β-sympathomimetic agents as tocolytics. Water intoxication can complicate the administration of fluids, particularly when 5% dextrose is used either as a prophylactic preload or as a diluent for oxytocin, which has antidiuretic properties. In the absence of any contraindications to a fluid load, the first 500 mL of crystalloid should be administered while surface markings and the lumbar anatomy are carefully identified. Whether a midline or paramedian approach is contemplated, clear identification of the lumbar spines and interspaces should be made whenever possible. At the same time, the anaesthetist should identify any local cutaneous infection or other lesions that might influence the decision to perform an epidural or the site at which it is carried out.

15.3.1 Patient position

The mother can be positioned either in the lateral decubitus position or in the sitting position. The choice may depend on the mother's preference, the anaesthetist's experience, or a perceived benefit in the particular patient. The lateral position, for instance, will provide more support for a woman in severe pain who has already received systemic analgesia. In addition, it can avoid an increase in hydrostatic pressure in the dural sac. The sitting position, on the other hand, is preferable in the obese parturient in whom accurate identification of the midline is required. Careful consideration should be given to the parturient's position before starting a regional technique, because it is difficult to move from one position to another half-way through the procedure. Such a move may desterilize the site of puncture, and can easily reduce the parturient's confidence in her anaesthetist. The advantages of the two positions are summarized in Table 15.1.

Table 15.1 Maternal position for regional nerve block.

Sitting
Provides good flexion
Makes the midline easier to identify
Increases hydrostatic pressure within the dural sac
   Aids identification of the subarachnoid space
   Speeds CSF flashback in very small-calibre needles
   Assists in dural perforation by tensing the dural sac
Is contraindicated in:
   Prolapsed cord
   Distressed or sedated mother
   Low or abnormal presenting part

Lateral decubitus
Reduces hydrostatic pressure in the dural sac
Allows the mother to use Entonox analgesia during contractions
Is useful in many emergency situations where the mother is in great distress

CSF, cerebrospinal fluid.

The most popular interspaces used for regional nerve blocks are those between the second and third or third and fourth lumbar vertebrae. These spaces are often chosen because the spinal cord in the adult terminates at the lower border of the first or at the upper border of the second lumbar vertebra. Entry into the epidural space below the L1–L2 interspace should therefore preclude direct trauma to the spinal cord. However, it must be remembered that the lower end of the cord may be found to be as low as the upper border of the third lumbar vertebra. In addition, the spinal cord's position varies with movements of the vertebral column, rising to a higher level when the patient is in the flexed position. It is for this reason, as well as the increased gap posteriorly between adjacent laminae and spines, that having the patient in a flexed position when carrying out an epidural is so important. In the lateral position, flexion is best achieved by allowing the upper leg to abduct and rest on pillows, rather than simply raising the knee towards the chin. The latter movement, if unaccompanied by abduction, will be impeded by the mass of the gravid uterus. It may be easier to achieve spinal flexion if the parturient is in the sitting position. Even then, however, abducting the thighs to allow the gravid uterus to rest between them helps to achieve good flexion. If the sitting position is uncomfortable, a pillow can be placed across the thighs to improve comfort and support the uterus. In each individual parturient, a balance must be achieved between patient comfort and technical requirements, which include maintaining fetal monitoring as well as expeditious placement of the epidural.

15.3.2 Asepsis

Maintaining asepsis throughout regional nerve blockade is vital, because infection in the epidural or subarachnoid space is such a serious complication.

The anaesthetist must undertake a surgical scrub and wear a 'theatre' cap, sterile gown and gloves for the procedure. It is recommended that face masks should be worn to prevent droplet spread. Face masks should be kept dry to be fully effective, and should only be placed over the mouth and nose immediately before undertaking the procedure. Similarly, surgical sterility of the skin of the parturient must be guaranteed by maximizing the bactericidal effect of any skin preparation. The area to be covered by skin preparation should extend from a line joining the lower angle of both scapulae to the natal cleft and laterally on each side to a line projected cephalad from the posterior superior iliac spines. Alcoholic solutions of 0.5% chlorhexidine or povidone-iodine are probably equally effective skin preparations. Both should be left in contact with the skin for three to four minutes before proceeding, and it is prudent to wipe any excess solution from the skin prior to inserting the epidural or spinal needle, in order to prevent alcohol or iodine from being carried into the vertebral space. Iodine solutions are coloured, making it easier to see the limits of skin application, but they carry a small risk of sensitivity. The patient must be questioned to exclude known iodine allergy or sensitivity before use. Once the skin is prepared, a sterile towel can be draped over the woman's back so as to leave the lumbar area exposed. Confirmation of the level of the interspace selected can be obtained by palpating the iliac crests through the drapes; a line joining the crests usually passes through the third lumbar interspace (i.e. L3–L4).

15.3.3 Epidural technique

Epidural puncture is usually performed using a 16- or 18-gauge Tuohy needle. Prior to insertion, a skin weal of local anaesthetic should be raised at the intended point of puncture. If the midline approach is to be used, a small volume (0.5 mL) of local anaesthetic solution can be deposited between the skin and the posterior surface of the supraspinous ligament. This small volume should not obscure the bony landmarks, because it can be easily dispersed by gentle fingertip massage. Further injections of local anaesthetic solution (1–2 mL) immediately lateral to the interspinous ligament will produce a block of the nerves supplying that ligament. One method is to make a small incision or hole through the skin weal before inserting the Tuohy needle, in order to prevent small pieces of skin from being cored out and carried into the epidural space, with a subsequent risk of dermoid cyst formation. Whether a hole is made or not, the close-fitting stylet that is supplied with the Tuohy needle must be kept fully inserted during the early stages, since this also reduces the risk of 'coring' pieces of skin or ligament into the tip of the Tuohy needle.

The epidural (or subarachnoid) space can be approached using midline or paramedian techniques. The lateral approach is rarely used in parturients, because the epidural venous plexuses lie to either side of the midline and may be traumatized by a needle approaching laterally. The anatomical structures that will be encountered during a midline insertion have been described

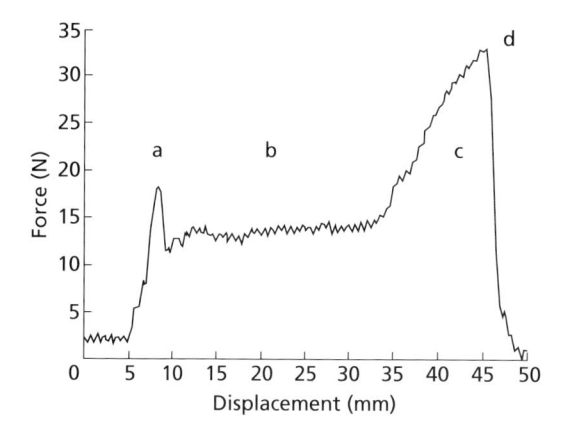

Fig. 15.1 Resistance forces encountered during insertion of a 16-gauge Tuohy needle in the midline. (a) Skin and supraspinous ligament. (b) Passage through interspinous ligament. (c) Passage through the ligamentum flavum. (d) Entering into the epidural space.

above. Each tissue encountered by the tip of the advancing needle has a characteristic resistance, which can be sensed by the anaesthetist. This tactile feedback helps identify the position and track of the needle. The forces involved in advancing an epidural needle through the tissues have been measured in cadavers [4]. A typical trace showing these forces is shown in Fig. 15.1. The forces experienced depend on two main factors: first, the resistance of tissue to penetration by the needle tip, and secondly, a drag factor caused by tissue friction on the shaft of the needle. The first varies with needle sharpness and tissue density, and the second varies with the length of the needle shaft embedded in tissue and the needle's diameter and surface polish, as well as tissue density. The forces shown in Fig. 15.1 represent puncture of the skin, entry into the supraspinous ligament, passage through the interspinous ligament, entry and passage through the ligamentum flavum, and finally entry into the epidural space. Two peaks are shown on the trace, the first representing puncture of the supraspinous ligament and the second representing needle entry into and passage through the ligamentum flavum. The increase in resistance with passage through the ligamentum flavum is commonly used as a warning sign that the epidural space is about to be entered. However, it is worth reiterating the fact that the ligamentum flavum is made up of two parts, one on either side of the midline. If the advancing needle is truly in the midline, the increase in resistance described may not be encountered. Needle entry into the epidural space may therefore occur unexpectedly, and a dural puncture may result. It is unusual for the needle point to be so accurately placed that it does not penetrate the ligamentum flavum, however. Recognition of the commonly described pattern of change allows the anaesthetist to determine whether the needle is moving in the correct path. It is particularly important to avoid deviation from the midline during insertion of an epidural using this approach. A variation in angle of approach by as little as 10° can bring about a failure to find the epidural space. Narang and Linter [5] demonstrated that the greater depth from skin to epidural space in an obese parturient leads to an exaggeration of the spatial error produced by each

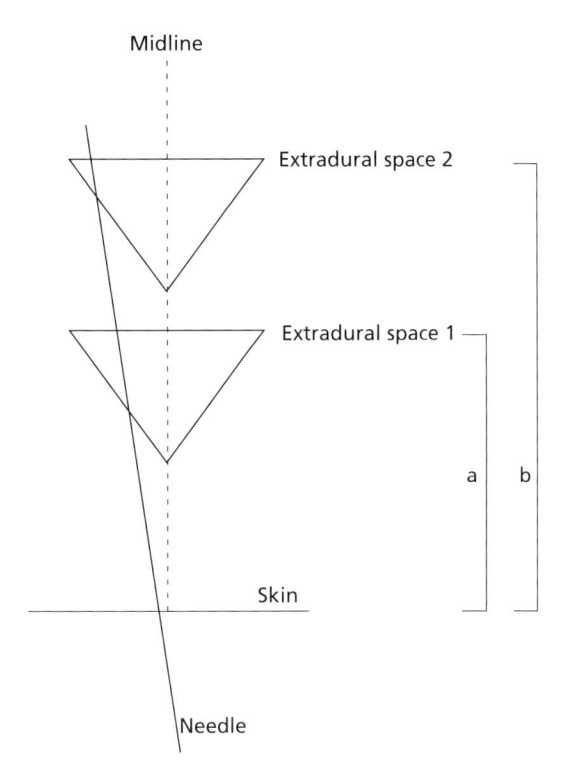

Fig. 15.2 Effects of deviation of the needle path from the midline in (a) non-obese and (b) obese patients.

degree of deviation from an exact midline approach (Fig. 15.2). Errors in the angle of approach to the epidural space are caused by a number of factors. The failure to insert the epidural needle perpendicular with the skin in the transverse plane is perhaps the commonest. However, if a woman moves or is malpositioned, the change in position can also disturb the angle of approach. Movement is more common during insertion of epidurals for the relief of labour pain than in elective procedures, so an obstetric anaesthetist must be vigilant and constantly aware of the angle formed between the epidural needle and the midline structures when a parturient is restless.

Verbal contact must be maintained between the anaesthetist and the woman throughout the procedure. The woman should be kept informed of progress and, most importantly, told what she may expect to feel from moment to moment. She should also be encouraged to report any unusual or painful sensations, particularly when the Tuohy needle is approaching or entering the epidural space or, subsequently, during insertion of the epidural catheter. Any reports of pain, feelings of electric shock, tingling, or pins and needles should alert the anaesthetist to the possibility of direct neural contact. If this warning sign is ignored, nerve trauma may occur. Complaints of local pain around the site of the procedure during needle insertion may simply indicate that the Tuohy needle is not in the midline, having either emerged from the interspinous ligament or passed lateral to it, touching the sensitive periosteum.

Identification of the epidural space

There is commonly a useful, identifiable change of resistance to advancement of the Tuohy needle when it passes from the interspinous ligament into the ligamentum flavum. However, as explained above, the ligamenta flava do not meet in the midline, so that the Tuohy needle that is truly in the midline will pass almost directly from the interspinous ligament into the epidural space without encountering the increased resistance. Entry into the space can therefore occur without the anaesthetist feeling either an increase in resistance or a click as the space is entered. A more reliable method of identifying the point of entry is therefore essential in order to minimize the risk of inadvertent dural puncture. A number of methods have been described. Some of them, such as the hanging drop technique, rely on the presence of negative pressure in the epidural space. However, negative pressure may not be present in the labouring parturient due to engorgement of the epidural veins and increases in intrathoracic pressure, especially during contractions. Obstetric anaesthetists therefore usually identify the epidural space by a loss of resistance to the injection of air or normal saline. The underlying principle of this method is as follows. A syringe or loss of resistance device containing 3–5 mL of air or 0.9% normal saline is connected to the hub of the Tuohy needle once the tip of the latter has passed into the interspinous ligament and the stylet has been withdrawn. Partial or complete resistance is felt to the injection of either air or saline through the Tuohy needle, and continues for as long as the tip of the Tuohy needle remains within the ligaments. When the tip of the needle enters the epidural space, however, resistance to injection of the contents of the syringe is abruptly lost. The end point is said to be easier to detect when saline is used, and the incidence of inadequate pain relief or missed segments following the first dose of local anaesthetic is lower with loss-of-resistance saline injection [6]. It has been suggested that local anaesthetic solutions themselves might be used to detect loss of resistance. The argument seems to be that injection of a test dose or the full dose of a single-shot epidural can be expedited. This practice cannot be recommended. If rapid analgesia or anaesthesia is required, subarachnoid anaesthesia should be employed instead of epidural.

There are therefore only two substances that can be recommended for use in loss of resistance techniques—air and saline. The advantage gained from the use of air is simply that any clear fluid seen issuing from the hub of the Tuohy needle or refluxing along the epidural catheter after entry into the epidural space can only be cerebrospinal fluid (CSF). Inadvertent dural puncture is therefore more easily and reliably detected when air is used. When saline is used to identify the epidural space, clear or blood-tinged fluid may flow from the hub of the Tuohy needle or reflux along the epidural catheter. If the fluid is in fact saline, the flow is usually slight and limited to a few drops, provided the anaesthetist has injected only a small volume of saline into the space.

It is in any case unnecessary to inject more than one or two millilitres of fluid when identifying the epidural space. Many novice anaesthetists feel the need to inject larger volumes—5–10 mL are not uncommon. This practice stems from a lack of confidence or a lack of control of the plunger of the loss-of-resistance syringe. Two methods of applying pressure on the plunger are common. Some obstetric anaesthetists use a 'stop/go' type of approach. In this technique, the anaesthetist advances the Tuohy needle a millimetre at a time and tests for resistance to injection between episodes of advancement. Others prefer to maintain a constant pressure on the plunger of the syringe whilst advancing the Tuohy needle through the ligamentous structures. Much of the advancing pressure pushing the needle onwards is therefore lost on entering the epidural space, especially when saline is used as the fluid in the syringe. It is not always possible to apply pressure constantly. When patients have particularly tough ligaments, it is sometimes necessary intermittently to steady and advance the needle with both hands. Whichever technique is used, good control should be maintained over the action of the plunger and thereby over the volume of fluid injected into the epidural space. When saline is used, identification of the epidural space is said to be easier, and a lower dural tap rate is achieved among less experienced anaesthetists.

Once the epidural space has been entered, its depth from the skin must be noted. One-centimetre marks on the Tuohy needle allow a simple estimate of the length of needle protruding from the skin. This length can then be subtracted from the total length of the needle to give the depth of the space from the skin. An epidural catheter can now be passed into the epidural space.

If the tip of the Tuohy needle comes to rest in the subarachnoid space, the flow of CSF will usually be quite free and continuous. If the anaesthetist is uncertain as to the nature of the fluid emerging, a number of tests are available to differentiate between CSF and normal saline.

- Temperature test. If a few drops of the fluid are dripped onto the anaesthetist's exposed wrist, the temperature of the fluid can be assessed. If the fluid is cold, it is saline; if it is warm, it is CSF. This test is subjective, and involves a small risk to the sterility of the technique.
- Glucose test. If a few drops of the fluid are dropped onto a glucose test paper, the presence or absence of glucose can be assessed. The concentrations of glucose in CSF are similar to those of plasma, but slightly lower, so a positive result will be produced. Saline contains no glucose and will produce a negative result. However, if a small quantity of blood is present in the saline, a false-positive result will be observed.
- Thiopental precipitation test. If a few drops of CSF are added to a solution of thiopental, a precipitate will form. Saline will have no visible effect. This test is perhaps less immediately practical than the previous two.

If an inadvertent dural puncture has occurred, replace the stylet before withdrawing the needle [7], inform the woman, and follow a management plan (Fig. 15.3).

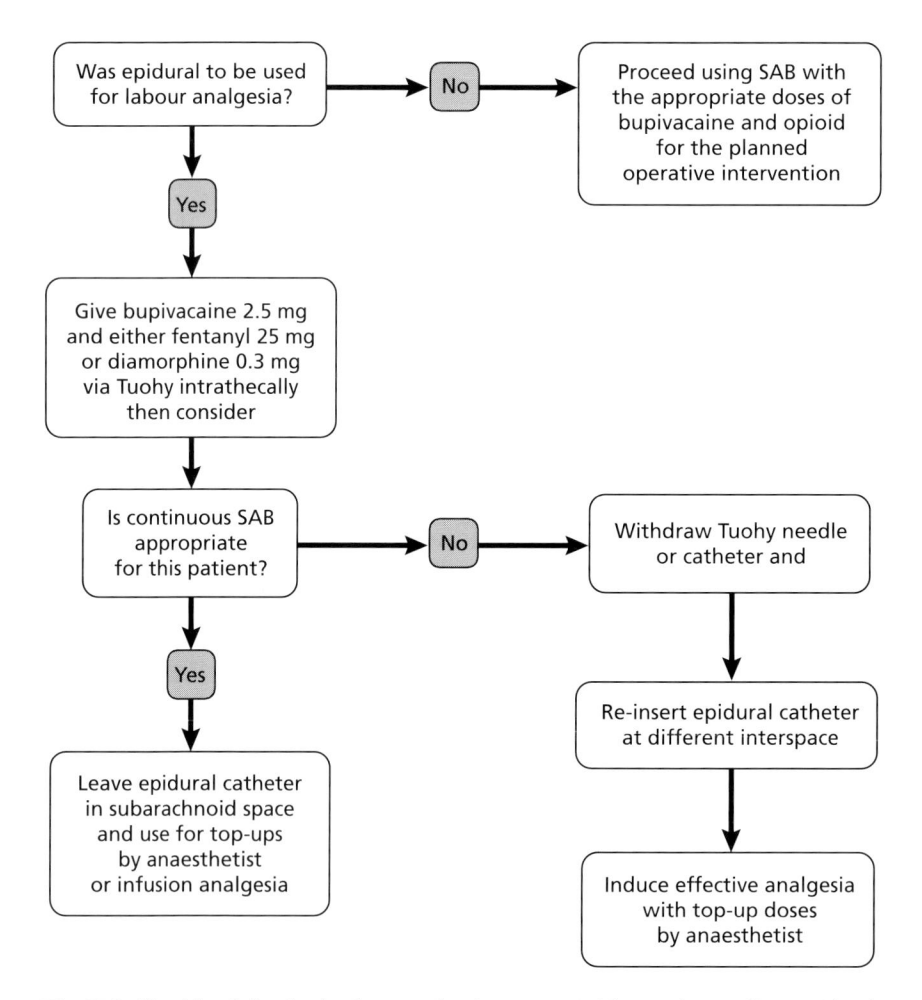

Fig. 15.3 Algorithm following inadvertent dural puncture (with a Tuohy needle or epidural catheter). SAB: subarachnoid block.

Needle bevel orientation

The orientation of the bevel of any needle introduced into the spinal canal is of importance, particularly if dural puncture is either planned or likely. The importance increases with the size of needle being used. Studies using 22-gauge and 25-gauge Quincke spinal needles [8] or 17-gauge and 18-gauge Tuohy epidural needles [9] both found a reduced incidence of postdural puncture headache associated with orientation of the needle bevel parallel to the long axis of the dural sac. However, entry into the epidural space by a Tuohy needle tip with its bevel in the long axis of the spine must inevitably be followed by rotation of the needle so as to allow epidural catheter insertion in the cephalad or caudal direction. To date, there is no good evidence comparing the net risk–benefit balance between a transverse and a longitudinal entry.

Paramedian approach

When a paramedian approach to the epidural space is chosen, certain differences in technique are required. The skin puncture site in a paramedian approach lies close to the lateral edge of the spinous process (within 1 cm of it). The advantage of the paramedian approach is that the Tuohy needle is passed down to the bony landmark of the selected vertebral lamina. Identification of the bony lamina with the tip of the Tuohy needle gives the anaesthetist an alternative landmark from which to approach the epidural space. It also estimates the approximate depth of the epidural space from the skin puncture site. Infiltration with 2–5 mL of 1% lidocaine along the planned axis of insertion and on the sensitive periosteum of the bony lamina to be used is essential if pain is to be prevented during insertion. Once the bony landmark of the vertebral arch has been identified, the tip of the needle can be 'walked' cephalad and medially towards the midline, with the bone of the lamina being tapped until the junction of the superior border of the lamina and the ligamentum flavum is discovered by the disappearance of the bony resistance. At this point, a syringe or loss-of-resistance device is connected to the hub of the Tuohy needle, as in the midline approach. The epidural space is identified by loss of resistance to injection. When the paramedian approach is used, the Tuohy needle tends to enter the epidural space with a steeper cephalad angulation. The steeper angle is said to reduce the rate of CSF leakage if inadvertent dural puncture occurs. Theoretically, a reduction of CSF loss should reduce the incidence of postdural puncture headache [10]. It also assists in directing the epidural catheter towards the midline and in a cephalad direction. The paramedian technique is useful in the obese parturient in whom anatomical landmarks are difficult to establish. The novice epiduralist would be well advised to develop some skill with the approach once confidence using the midline approach has been gained.

The epidural catheter

The parturient must be warned before the catheter is passed that she may feel some tingling or shooting sensations in her back, hip, buttock or leg. She must be asked to report these sensations at once whilst trying not to move. Any occurrence of the symptoms should alert the obstetric anaesthetist to the possibility of causing neural tissue damage. A fresh insertion may be required if symptoms persist or if there is an increase in the pressure needed for catheter insertion. Provided no warning symptoms occur, the catheter may be passed so that approximately 3 cm of its length come to lie in the epidural space. Some anaesthetists prefer to introduce greater lengths of catheter to begin with, because some of the catheter may be withdrawn inadvertently when the Tuohy needle is removed, and again when the woman straightens up from flexion. Great care should be taken to support the catheter in position during withdrawal of the Tuohy needle. Once again, the physical technique used to effect this manoeuvre varies from one anaesthetist to another. The general principle is that one hand steadies the catheter and exerts gentle pressure on it towards the hub of the Tuohy needle as the needle is withdrawn from the patient's back. In most cases, using this technique the catheter will not be withdrawn with the Tuohy needle. Once the tip of the Tuohy emerges from the skin, the epidural catheter can be gripped at this point by a finger and thumb and the Tuohy needle can be slid gently along and off the catheter.

Once any length of catheter has been passed, it should not be withdrawn through the Tuohy needle, even though improvements to the needle have reduced the possibility of shearing the catheter tip. Any adjustment of the length of the catheter to be left in the epidural space should be carried out only after the Tuohy needle has been removed. Whatever the method of insertion and adjustment used, the general principle controlling the length ultimately remaining in the space is 'not too much but not too little'.

A longer length will increase the chances of the catheter tip lying laterally in the epidural space, or even passing through a vertebral foramen to lie outside the epidural space [11]. Nerve root entrapment with epidural catheters has also been reported with greater lengths of catheter [12]. Some 20 years ago, Doughty recommended that only 2 cm of catheter should be left in the epidural space [13]. This is the very minimum length that can be left when using a side-hole catheter. In this—the commonest type of catheter in UK practice—the most proximal hole lies about 1.5 cm from the tip of the catheter. Doughty's recommendation therefore leaves a margin for error of only 0.5 cm. The risk of displacement of catheters is greater when shorter lengths are left in the space [14], whereas with greater lengths there is a higher risk of kinking, knotting and tracking outside the epidural space [15–17]. The potential for movement and misplacement has led to the recommendation that up to 4 cm of catheter should be left in the epidural space.

Dural puncture with an epidural catheter probably occurs with similar frequency to dural puncture with a Tuohy needle, and has been reported in 0.7% of obstetric epidural catheter placements [18]. In order to test for this eventuality before fixation of the bacterial filter, the catheter end should be held below the level of the puncture site for about 30 seconds. If the catheter tip has perforated the dura, CSF will reflux along the catheter and drip from the end. If CSF is detected, the anaesthetist must decide whether to continue with the procedure as a continuous subarachnoid technique (Fig. 15.3) or to withdraw the catheter and attempt entry into the epidural space at a different level. In any case, the woman should be informed of the change of technique.

During their insertion into the epidural space, catheters puncture epidural veins more frequently than they puncture the dura. The incidence of this complication may be as high as 9% in obstetric patients [19], a similar incidence to that of puncture of an epidural vein with the epidural needle [20,21].

The incidence of this complication may be reduced by using a non-rigid catheter. Such catheters may incorporate silicone, but this adds to their cost.

If venous catheterization occurs, blood may be seen refluxing along the catheter. The epidural should then be re-sited in an adjacent space. Flushing and withdrawing the catheter a few millimetres in the hope that it will be drawn out of the vein is very dangerous, especially when using side-hole catheters. The side holes may be freed from the vein while the tip of the catheter remains in the lumen during the first injection of local anaesthetic. Sufficient length of catheter can subsequently re-enter the vessel to bring one or more orifices into the lumen. Intravenous administration of the next top-up dose can then occur and will be followed by hypotension, convulsions and unconsciousness [22].

Once a catheter has been seen to be free of CSF and blood, it must be attached to a bacterial filter which should be filled with local anaesthetic solution before attachment. Gentle aspiration of the assembled parts serves as a further test for subarachnoid or intravenous placement. The catheter should then be fixed firmly to the skin of the patient's back. The use of transparent dressings over the puncture site and the catheter itself is advisable, to allow inspection for signs of movement or blood. With the catheter secured, the parturient can now be placed in a comfortable posture, avoiding the supine position, and the epidural nerve block can be started. There is a principle that every dose is a test dose, but where large doses are planned, a test dose is still the initiating dose. If this test dose has no effect within five minutes, the completion of the full dose of local anaesthetic, with or without additional agents, can be given.

Test doses

Test doses in the context of obstetric analgesia and anaesthesia are controversial, because their reliability during labour is questionable and because the doses of local anaesthetic currently used for pain relief in labour can be smaller than a test dose itself. A test dose of 15 mg bupivacaine (as the 0.5% solution) may negate the advantages of using low-dose epidural top-ups or infusions of bupivacaine, or CSE techniques. A test dose is given in order to detect either intravascular or subarachnoid placement of an epidural catheter. An ideal test dose, when positive, should produce an effect that is harmless, easily detectable and brief. It should produce the effect in all cases of subarachnoid or intravenous placement and in no cases of epidural placement. The detection of inadvertent subarachnoid placement of an epidural catheter is probably more important if intermittent bolus injections rather than infusions are to be used, especially because boluses may be sufficiently large to produce sudden significant cardiovascular and central nervous system effects. A dose of local anaesthetic that is usually of the same magnitude as the dose used to produce subarachnoid anaesthesia for Caesarean section—e.g. bupivacaine 12.5–15.0 mg

(2.5–3.0 mL of 0.5%)—has been advocated. If such a dose is injected into the subarachnoid space, it will produce spinal anaesthesia from T4 to S5. If it is injected into a vein, it will produce systemic manifestations of local anaesthetic agents, such as circumoral tingling and a light-headed feeling.

The sensory and motor changes that accompany subarachnoid block can be appreciated by the parturient within five minutes. She will tell her anaesthetist, if asked, that one or both lower limbs feel warm, numb, tingling or heavy. Sensory changes precede motor effects, and sensory rather than motor effects should be sought initially following a test dose. The confirmatory motor effects will follow quite rapidly, but by that time the positive sensory test result should have alerted the anaesthetist to the subarachnoid position of the epidural catheter.

The addition of epinephrine 15 µg to the test dose in young, healthy surgical patients improves the effectiveness and specificity of the test for the detection of intravascular placement, as epinephrine produces an increase in heart rate of approximately 20 beats/min [23,24]. The relevance of this test to women in labour is doubtful, because of variable changes in heart rate during labour itself. Van Zundert et al. [25] observed that administration of epinephrine 12.5 µg intravenously to labouring parturients rapidly increased maternal heart rate and blood pressure and briefly slowed uterine contractions. However, the epidural administration of epinephrine 15 µg increased maternal heart rate by more than 25 beats/minute in five out of 10 labouring women studied by Chestnut et al. [26]. The use of epinephrine in clinical practice is not widespread [27], particularly because false-positive results may be obtained from epinephrine-containing test doses, in labouring women, and the drug may have a deleterious effect on the progress of labour and on fetal condition. The unreliability and possible harmful effects of epinephrine have led many consultant obstetric anaesthetists in the United Kingdom to exclude it from their test doses. Fractionation of the initiating dose of local anaesthetic minimizes systemic changes resulting from inadvertent intravascular injection, and maintenance of the epidural with an infusion will prevent any subsequent peaks of blood concentration that may be associated with bolus injections. However, test doses are still used in obstetric patients, particularly when large doses of local anaesthetic drugs are administered for anaesthesia. Care must always be taken to observe and record the effects of the top-up doses in labour used currently, because they have in effect become a 'test dose'.

15.4 Epidural analgesia in labour

Ideally, pain relief with epidural techniques should be produced with the minimum disturbance to the progress of labour or to sympathetic functions, other sensory functions (e.g. proprioception) and motor functions of the central nervous system. This objective can only be achieved by careful and considered selection of a therapeutic regimen. Above all, a flexible approach by the anaes-

Table 15.2 Pharmacokinetic properties of opioid drugs.

Opioid	Lipid partition coefficient 20°C	pK_a	% free base at pH 7.35	% unbound in plasma	$t\frac{1}{2}\beta$ (min)	Onset latency (min)
Morphine	1.4	7.9	22	70	177	30–60
Pethidine	39	8.5	7	30	222	12–30
Diamorphine	280	7.6	34	60	177	n.a.
Fentanyl	813	8.4	8	16	185	6–9
Sufentanil	1778	8.0	18	8	98	2–8

thetist is essential, judging each parturient as an individual with specific needs and expectations. The analgesia to be provided depends on the stage of labour, the segmental distribution of the pain experienced, the severity of the pain and any previous analgesia, such as systemic opioids. The regimens that are used for obstetric analgesia are for the most part not suitable for postoperative pain relief, with the possible exception of pain relief after Caesarean section or related gynaecological surgery. In the absence of a deliberate test dose, the first bolus of local anaesthetic solution to be given through the epidural catheter is always a test dose. It should therefore comprise no more than 15 mg of bupivacaine, or its equivalent if another drug with local anaesthetic properties is to be used. In fact, a test dose alone may have enough analgesic effect to initiate an epidural nerve block to relieve pain in early labour. Greater analgesia is reliably produced by larger doses of local anaesthetic agent, either alone or mixed with an opioid or other adjuvant, but more sensory and motor effects will accompany higher doses. The changing spinal segments that may need to be blocked in order to produce adequate analgesia during labour are discussed in Chapter 18. Once satisfactory pain relief has been achieved, it must be maintained either by repeated injections (top-ups), or by continuous infusion, alone or with top-ups. Many regimens of different concentrations of bupivacaine with and without one or other opioid have evolved over the years. Bupivacaine dilutions as low as 0.03% have been studied, although most units use 0.06–0.1% solutions. A number of opioids have been used as adjuvants in the more dilute mixtures (Table 15.2). The choice of opioid is influenced not only by efficacy but also by national availability or licence. For instance, diamorphine is available in the United Kingdom, whereas sufentanil is not. Other adjuvants such as α_2-agonists are not used routinely. The newer local anaesthetic ropivacaine may prove to have advantages over bupivacaine because of its motor-sparing properties, its lower systemic toxicity and perhaps adequate quality of analgesia without opioids. Clinical comparisons are awaited.

15.4.1 History of epidural regimens

When epidural analgesia was being introduced into obstetric practice in the

Table 15.3 The Bromage Score for motor nerve blockade.

Score	Clinical assessment
1 No block	Full power in flexion of knees and feet
2 Partial block	Full flexion of feet possible. Only just able to flex knees
3 Almost complete block	Unable to flex knees. Some flexion of feet
4 Complete	Unable to move legs or feet

United Kingdom in the 1960s and 1970s, bupivacaine 0.5% and 0.25% was given as top-up injections in volumes of 5–10 mL. Anaesthetists realized that motor blockade was an inevitable accompaniment to these regimens, and sought to reduce this effect. In the 1980s and 1990s, more dilute solutions of bupivacaine, usually combined with an opioid, have been advocated. The intention has always been to limit motor effects and restrict the spread of sensory block only to those segments transmitting pain.

Doughty developed this concept by using doses as small as 4 mL of bupivacaine 0.5% [13]. The intention was to limit the spread of local anaesthetic drug to those spinal segments conducting nociceptive information. This was called 'segmental analgesia'. The motor effects from such small volumes were often slight for the first few top-ups. However, as labour progressed, a degree of motor block was produced in most parturients. Its assessment led to the development of the Bromage scoring system (Table 15.3) [28]. Gradually, the volume and concentration of bupivacaine used was changed, and the method of administration was extended to include continuous infusions by electronic volumetric pumps designed specifically for high-risk infusions, which were capable of delivering small volumes accurately. Concentrations of bupivacaine from 0.125% to 0.0625% were studied [29], but the total dosage of local anaesthetic was maintained by infusing volumes of dilute solution sometimes as large as 25 mL per hour of 0.08% bupivacaine [30]. The intention was to create a 'liquid sleeve' of local anaesthetic drug in the epidural space, so that a wide segmental spread of epidural effect could be maintained. Considerable motor blockade accompanied such regimens but, at the time, relatively little importance was accorded to this side effect.

A significant development was the first report of pain relief for parturition in the rat using spinal morphine in 1979 [31]. This was followed by trials of opioids for pain relief in labour. It was soon apparent that opioids alone did not provide good pain relief in labour, but that the synergism of action that allowed analgesia to be maintained with lower doses of local anaesthetic agents when mixed with opioid drugs was the best option. Encouraging reports of fentanyl and bupivacaine mixtures being used for analgesia in labour began to appear in the early 1980s [32]. Many papers comparing regimens of bupivacaine and various opioids then appeared from workers on both sides of the Atlantic [33–39].

Table 15.4 The concentrations of bupivacaine and opioids in general use for epidural analgesia in labour with simplified bupivacaine dilution ratios in saline.

Local anaesthetic	Opioids
Bupivacaine 0.0625% (15 mL 0.25% in 60 mL*) 0.08% (10 mL 0.5% in 60 mL*) 0.1% (10 mL 0.5% in 50 mL*) 0.125% (15 mL 0.5% in 60 mL*)	Diamorphine 25–50 µg/mL (1.5–3 mg in 60 mL) Fentanyl 1–2 µg/mL (2 mL 50 µg/mL in 50 mL = 2 µg/mL)

* signifies total volume

Table 15.5 The times (min) to peak plasma and CSF concentrations and CSF $t_{1/2\beta}$ of opioids given by the epidural route and the CSF $t_{1/2\beta}$ for the same drugs given after a subarachnoid dose.

	After an epidural dose			After subarachnoid dose
	Peak plasma concentration	Peak CSF concentration	CSF $t_{1/2\beta}$	CSF $t_{1/2\beta}$
Morphine	5	90	369	90
Pethidine	10–15	15–30	900	68
Sufentanil (dogs)	6	6	110	–
Diamorphine	–	–	–	7

CSF, cerebrospinal fluid.

15.4.2 Systematic approach

The range of alternative regimens has become so great that a systematic approach is needed when deciding what is the most appropriate therapy for any individual parturient. The options are as follows.

1 *Technique:*
  - Epidural.
  - Combined spinal–epidural (CSE).
  - Intermittent doses (top-ups).
  - Continuous infusion, with or without intermittent doses.
  - Patient-controlled epidural analgesia (PCEA): continuous/intermittent.
2 *Local anaesthetic agents:*
  - Drug, e.g. bupivacaine, ropivacaine.
  - Dilution (Table 15.4).
3 *Pharmacological adjuvants:*
  - Opioids, e.g. fentanyl, diamorphine, sufentanil (Tables 15.2, 15.4, 15.5).
  - Other non-opioid adjuvants have been reported, but are not in widespread use for obstetric analgesia. They include α_2-agonists such as clonidine and dexmedetomidine, which potentially enhance the effects of

opioids, reduce opioid requirements and hence respiratory depressant side effects. Low doses are required to avoid hypotension and fetal heart abnormalities.

The type of nerve block planned will influence the choice of drugs to be administered and the administration technique to be used. For example, the presence of incompetent cardiac valve disease will encourage the use of infusion techniques, lower local anaesthetic dosage (both in volume and concentration) with opioid adjuvants, because this combination avoids the cardiovascular variability that accompanies intermittent techniques and high doses of local anaesthetic drugs. The choice of regimen will also be greatly influenced by staffing numbers and experience, equipment and drug availability, and patient co-operation, request and expectations. Minimum standards have been defined for staffing levels and availability of monitoring and resuscita-tion equipment needs in units offering epidural pain relief [1,2,3] (and see Chapter 1). Specific equipment for different epidural techniques must also be available, e.g. infusion pumps suitable for the administration of high-risk drugs. Parturients requesting 'mobile' epidurals will need low dose regimens and/or CSE techniques. Limited patient co-operation or understanding will discourage the use of techniques such as PCEA. CSE might be the method of choice if pain is very severe and a rapid onset and low risk of inadequate block needs to be achieved.

15.4.3 Equipment

In order to achieve a high quality of care with minimum risk, properly designed and sterilized disposable equipment is necessary. This equipment should be available, assembled and ready for use before beginning to site an epidural nerve block. The anaesthetist must wear suitable clothing to enable a sterile technique to be performed. A theatre cap, mask, sterile gown and sterile gloves should be worn. A dressing pack containing at least a sterile towel for draping the parturient's back, sterile gauze swabs, gallipot and forceps for skin disinfection can be provided separately or as part of a disposable epidural set. The contents of epidural sets vary a little, but typically include a sterile disposable epidural needle (usually a Tuohy needle with Huber tip), loss-of-resistance syringe or device, an epidural catheter and a bacterial and particulate filter, plus an assortment of syringes, needles and swabs.

Preferred syringe sizes are a matter for individual anaesthetists, and for most purposes are not critical. However, when a subarachnoid block is being carried out, accurate measurement of local anaesthetic volumes and opioid doses is important. Equally, the loss of an unknown volume of solution halfway through a subarachnoid injection because of needle–syringe disconnection is disconcerting, and may lead to low block height. A 3-mL Luer-Lok syringe can avoid these problems. It measures the relevant volumes more accurately than a 5-mL syringe, and the Luer–Lok makes a secure fastening to the hub of the subarachnoid needle, so that accidental leakage of local anaesthetic solution is prevented. It also avoids disconnection of the syringe from the needle when aspiration of CSF is undertaken during subarachnoid injection.

Needles

Epidural needles. Identification of the lumbar epidural space is most readily achieved by recognizing the ligaments traversed. This is best assessed using a large blunt needle. Space for passing a catheter through the needle is also required, so a size of preferably 16–18 gauge is required. The most commonly used is undoubtedly the Tuohy needle—which ironically was introduced in the first instance for continuous subarachnoid anaesthesia [40], and was only subsequently adapted for continuous lumbar epidural blockade [41]. The original needles used for epidural puncture were straight with end openings. Curving the tip effectively creates a lateral hole. This Huber tip is associated with a lower dural puncture rate, and guides the epidural catheter as it emerges from the needle shaft. Tuohy needles have the common function of imparting a change of direction to the epidural catheter as it emerges into the epidural space. The shape of the Huber tip, and in particular the angle of the orifice at the end of the needle, varies slightly from manufacturer to manufacturer. These small differences do not appear to affect the performance, quality or complications of epidural analgesia. Most Tuohy needles in current use incorporate Lee's or Doughty's modifications [42,43] with respect to 1-cm markings at intervals along the shaft of the needle, beginning 3 cm from the proximal edge of the bevel. They help to estimate the depth of the epidural space from the skin.

Spinal needles. When subarachnoid injections are to be made, either as the sole regional technique or as part of a CSE nerve block, a suitable spinal needle must be chosen. Quincke established lumbar puncture as a simple clinical procedure in 1891. His spinal needle had a characteristic short bevelled tip, each side of which was sharp—making the needle, essentially, a cutting implement. To minimize damage to the dura, he introduced the needle with its bevel in the long axis of the dural sac. The Quincke needle was the most widely used spinal needle until the late 1980s. However, in parturients, the incidence of postdural puncture headache following its use was very high. Smaller-gauge needles were introduced to reduce the incidence of this problem. Improving needle technology allowed needle gauges as fine as 29–30 gauge to be made, although 27 gauge was, and probably still is, the smallest calibre in common use. Needles smaller than 27 gauge are much more difficult to use, because they deform easily and deviate from the path of insertion. CSF 'flashback' flow through them is slow, which delays confirmation of subarachnoid position. They have a higher 'failed technique' rate unless the anaesthetist is experienced in their use.

A new design of atraumatic needle with a point tip was described by Hart

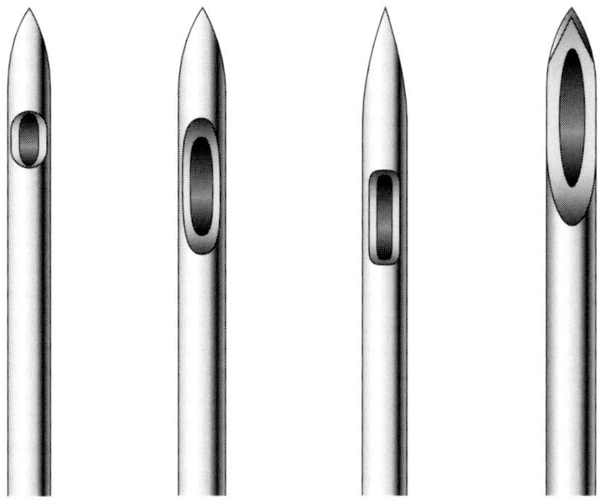

Fig. 15.4 A selection of needles for spinal anaesthesia. (a) Gertie Marx; (b) Sprotte; (c) Whitacre; (d) Quincke.

and Whitacre [44]. This needle had a sharp conical or pencil point. A similar tip was described by Sprotte, the only difference being that the shoulders of the tip are curved, making it into a bullet shape rather than a cone. Both needle types have solid tips, lateral side holes and no cutting edges. Dural fibres are therefore split away from one another in the same way that fabric fibres are split during sewing, instead of being severed as they are with Quincke tips. The resulting hole closes and heals faster. Variations on these two types of needle tip have been developed, and are shown in Fig. 15.4. The main differences between the types are the precise shape of the shoulders of the tip and the position and size of the lateral hole. The hole is larger in the Sprotte needle, and this confers an advantage in the speed of reflux of CSF for the identification of subarachnoid placement during subarachnoid block. However, the larger hole reduces the strength of the needle tip and increases the risk of loss of local anaesthetic solution into the epidural space if the hole lies partially in the subarachnoid and partially in the epidural spaces. This may account for a failed subarachnoid block. It is probably better to use a needle with a relatively small hole placed as close as possible to the tip, which is why the Gertie Marx needle was developed. The only disadvantage of such a needle, particularly in the labouring woman, is the relative slowness of reflux of CSF into the hub.

Epidural catheters. Epidural catheters can be divided into two categories: closed-end catheters with three lateral holes, or open-end catheters with a single end hole. The closed-end type of catheter was developed in order to improve the spread of local anaesthetic solution and reduce the incidence of unilateral blocks and missed segments. The open-end design has the theoretical advantage of improved detection of intravenous or subarachnoid placement. A comparison of the two types [45] confirmed that open-end catheters are associated with a higher incidence of unsatisfactory blocks, particularly unilateral blocks and difficult or painful placements. The closed-end catheters were associated with more frequent intravenous siting. All manufacturers attempt to design catheters that are soft at the tip but rigid enough for easy insertion. Catheters also have a tensile strength allowing withdrawal without breakage. The softness of the tip is important, because the catheter may touch a nerve root during insertion.

The main properties and qualities of a good epidural catheter are that it must be sufficiently stiff to facilitate introduction, but sufficiently flexible not to damage tissue, especially nervous tissues and the dura. The tip should be smoothly machined in both the end-hole and side-hole types. It should be constructed of inert, non-irritating material with good tensile strength, so that it is not easily broken during withdrawal. Centimetre markings should be clearly identifiable for at least the first 10 cm at the distal end of the catheter. Further markings at 15 cm or 20 cm, or both, should also be present. It is usual for the markings at 10 cm and 15 cm to consist of double and treble rings, respectively. These markings serve two functions: initially to inform the anaesthetist how much catheter has been passed through the Tuohy needle, and subsequently to calculate how much catheter lies within the epidural space. In addition, the markings provide an easy method of checking whether the catheter has moved in or out after it has been fastened to the patient's skin (provided the original position has been recorded). Many manufacturers include some method of rendering the catheter radiopaque. Whether this is essential is open to question, because the ability to identify catheter fragments by radiographic investigation may encourage surgical attempts to remove them. A compromise must be reached by the manufacturer such that the external diameter of the catheter matches the internal diameter of the Tuohy needle closely, with the wall of the catheter being thick enough to prevent kinking while leaving a sufficient lumen to allow easy injection of local anaesthetic solutions. Non-kinking catheters are available that incorporate a rigid spring structure.

15.4.4 Local anaesthetic agents

Recently, our understanding of the relative efficacy of local anaesthetic solutions has been improved by the introduction of the concept of minimum local analgesic concentration (MLAC) [46]. The minimum local analgesic concentration is defined as the median effective concentration (EC_{50}) for the production of epidural pain relief in the first stage of labour. The concentration vs. response estimates are derived from the up/down sequences of sequential allocations of concentrations of the drug under investigation. A recently reported meta-analysis of these investigations in a number of European centres using volumes of 20 mL [47] has provided some indication of the minimum effective concentrations of plain bupivacaine alone in obstetric patients. The results from the four centres showed MLAC values ranging from 0.065% to 0.141% bupivacaine, with a weighted overall MLAC of 0.093% and a 95% effective concentration of 0.119%. The effective concentration varied with cervical dilatation, with higher concentrations being required later in labour to produce an equivalent degree of pain relief. The reported results relate to the use of bupivacaine alone and not to the use of mixtures of bupivacaine and opioids. They do, however, confirm the appropriateness of bupivacaine concentrations of 0.06–0.1% being used for the relief of pain in labour.

Until recently, bupivacaine was, in effect, the only feasible local anaesthetic agent available for the maintenance of pain relief during the protracted periods of labour. Lidocaine has been used, but tachyphylaxis limits its clinical duration of action. Recently, ropivacaine has become available in the United Kingdom for this purpose. Ropivacaine is a long-acting amide local anaesthetic that is structurally closely related to bupivacaine. It is a single *S*-enantiomer rather than a racemic mixture. The two drugs are similar not only structurally, but also in their clinical effects. At any given concentration, the analgesic effects are not significantly different. However, ropivacaine has less central nervous system and cardiovascular toxicity than bupivacaine [48,49]. The pharmacodynamic and pharmacokinetic similarity of the two drugs has also been clearly identified [50,51]. Many of the comparative studies of these two agents have indicated that motor block is less with ropivacaine than with bupivacaine when the drugs are used in equal concentration [52,53]. Whether the differences are clinically significant when the drugs are used for pain relief in labour seems in doubt [54,55]. It is equally doubtful whether any differences in motor blockade identified by the Bromage scale actually produce any difference in the mode of delivery. The results of studies of combinations of ropivacaine with opioids are awaited with interest, particularly with regard to whether or not they show benefits from the addition of opioids. This may make ropivacaine an alternative local anaesthetic in situations in which opioids should be avoided, e.g. recent systemic opioid administration.

15.4.5 Epidural/subarachnoid opioids

Administration of an opioid drug into the epidural or subarachnoid space is so far unlicensed in the United Kingdom. However, the technique is logical if evidence exists that the drug will have increased efficacy and reduced side effects when given by this route rather than systemically. In other words, improved pain relief will be achieved without any concomitant increase in respiratory depression, nausea or other unwanted side effects. The central depressant complications of opioid administration, which may be life-threatening, result from actions of the drug within the brain, which may follow either raised CSF or plasma concentrations. Some opioid agents are highly lipophilic, so that uptake of the drug from cerebrospinal fluid into the spinal cord will be very rapid (Table 15.2, Fig. 15.5). These lipophilic agents are less likely to be

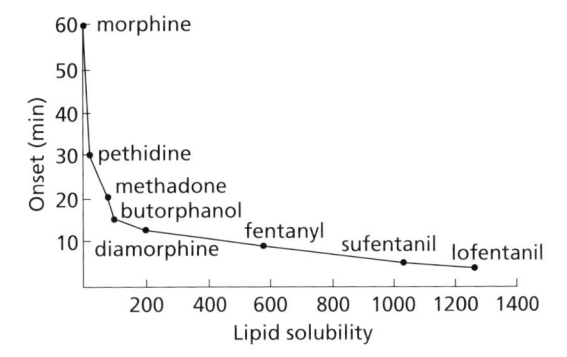

Fig. 15.5 A graph of the onset time of intrathecal opioids in relation to their lipid solubility.

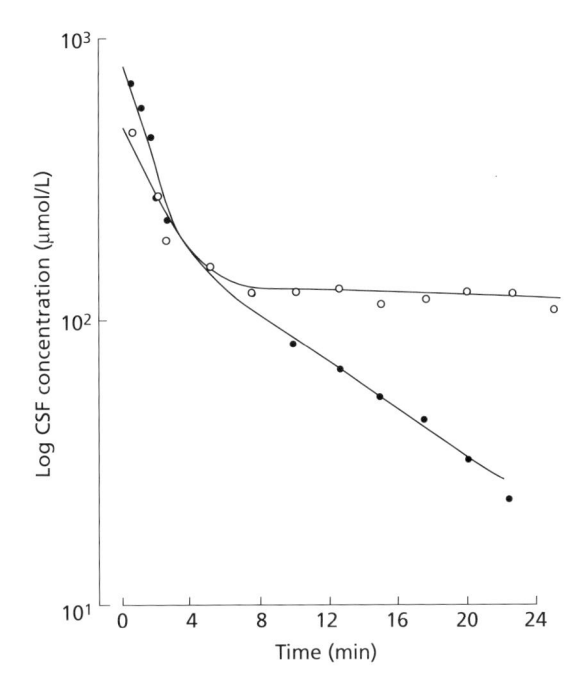

Fig. 15.6 Cerebrospinal fluid concentrations over 24 minutes of (o) morphine and (•) diamorphine following subarachnoid injection of morphine sulphate 2.5 mg and diamorphine 2 mg.

associated with prolonged high concentrations in CSF than are agents that are more hydrophilic. The CSF concentrations resulting from a subarachnoid injection of morphine compared with diamorphine show these differences clearly (Fig. 15.6) [56]. The wide disparity in the rate of decline of CSF concentrations of the two drugs was considered to be the result of different rates of uptake into the spinal cord. The rapid decline of diamorphine concentration suggests that any residual diamorphine is unlikely to be sufficient to spread rostrally and cause late-onset respiratory depression. In contrast, the sustained CSF concentration of morphine means that any rostral movement of CSF could easily result in significant opioid concentrations occurring in the brainstem and medulla. Diamorphine's lipophilicity and mode of action may mean that it has a unique advantage. It is certainly a very effective opioid adjuvant in labour analgesia, and gives prolonged pain relief after Caesarean section when administered by subarachnoid injection [57].

Fentanyl is also a lipophilic opioid. It is probably the opioid most widely used internationally for epidural pain relief in labour, particularly because of the limited availability of diamorphine. Like diamorphine, it can be combined with dilutions of bupivacaine that range from 0.0625% to 0.125%. In practice, the rates of administration of the two opioids reported have varied, but their individual concentrations have been similar. Diamorphine is used at a concentration of 50 µg/mL, whereas fentanyl is commonly diluted to a concentration of 1 or 2 µg/mL. Used in this dilution, fentanyl can provide good analgesia for the first few hours of labour, although its effects seem to fade with time—unlike diamorphine analgesia, which is well maintained over many hours [37–39]. This decrease in analgesic effects with fentanyl may be the result of tachyphylaxis, but studies have so far not confirmed this.

Epidural alfentanil has been compared with fentanyl [58]. Analgesia was found to be acceptable, but alfentanil is well absorbed from the epidural space into the bloodstream and then crosses the placenta freely because of its low pK_a and lipid solubility compared to fentanyl. It is therefore unsuitable for prolonged administration, because of the likelihood of fetal side effects [59].

Sufentanil is a more recently introduced opioid adjuvant for epidural analgesia. It has been widely used in the United States and mainland Europe, but it is not presently available in the United Kingdom. It is a highly potent fentanyl analogue, and the addition of sufentanil 10–13 µg/mL to bupivacaine 0.125% solution with epinephrine 1 : 800 000 significantly improved the quality and duration of analgesia and reduced instrumental delivery rates in one report [60]. Sufentanil should, hypothetically, be the ideal epidural opioid because of its very high lipid solubility and affinity for the µ-opioid receptor. However, when given via this route, sufentanil appears to be only two to three times more potent than fentanyl, whereas systemically, it is 5–10 times more potent. The inadvertent intravenous injection of an epidural bolus dose of sufentanil (30 µg) would cause significant maternal and fetal respiratory depression. The drug has also been associated with maternal dizziness and lowered one-minute Apgar scores [59]. It is also associated with significantly more maternal nausea and hypotension than other opioids. At present, it seems to offer no advantage over fentanyl.

Some of the relevant characteristics, properties and pharmacokinetics of spinal opioids are shown in Fig. 15.6 and Tables 15.2 and 15.5. In theory, opioids alone administered into the epidural or subarachnoid space should provide prolonged pain relief and avoid the hypotension and impaired motor block that results from local anaesthetic nerve blockade. In clinical practice, spinal opioids alone have yielded disappointing results, although subarachnoid administration produces better results than epidural injection. The doses required are associated with troublesome side effects; less lipid-soluble opioids have a delayed onset of action, and opioids alone do not produce the type of pain relief that might have been expected. Their real advantage is only realized when they are combined with local anaesthetic agents. Such combinations, often as an infusion into the epidural space, are now commonplace. Low concentrations of both local anaesthetic and opioid dosage allow parturients to retain more motor power than with less concentrated solutions, and the low opioid dosage reduces the incidence of opioid-related side effects. The most useful concentrations of local anaesthetic and opioid infusions for pain relief in labour are summarized in Table 15.4.

15.4.6 Epidural infusions

Continuous infusion of local anaesthetic drugs into the epidural space was described in 1963 [61] but the method was not widely used in obstetric practice until the introduction of reliable 'high-risk drug' infusion pumps some 15 years later. Infusion analgesia is probably the most widely used method of providing epidural pain relief at present, because infusions have obvious advantages over intermittent top-ups. The continuous infusions avoid peaks and troughs of pain relief. They reduce the need for top-up injections, which have the associated risks of hypotension, total spinal block and intravenous systemic local anaesthetic toxicity. Infusions can therefore reduce the demands on both medical and midwifery staff time. However, infusions must not be left to run unattended. The method demands frequent assessments of the level of neural blockade. The extent of cephalad and caudad spread of effects, as well as the completeness of neural block between the two limits, must be checked regularly, e.g. hourly. The extent of caudad spread is often ignored, but it is an important factor in the maintenance of pain relief in late first-stage and second-stage labour, when pain is mediated via the sacral nerves and the sacral spinal segments. An infusion may miss these nerve roots unless steps are taken to overcome the problem. For example, the parturient can be encouraged to adopt a sitting position while the epidural infusion continues. In spite of reports indicating that gravity does not govern the spread of epidural injections, clinical experience would indicate that the sitting position during epidural infusion can help the caudad spread of pain relief during the later stages of labour.

Midwives are able to chart the progress of epidural infusions if properly trained to do so. They can use either ethyl chloride spray or ice to detect the loss of cold sensation discrimination as an assessment of the block. A dermatome diagram can be included as part of the epidural chart, so that the assessing midwife has a reference source to which she can refer should she be in any doubt as to the levels involved (see Chapter 18, p. 345). In addition to the midwife's assessment of blockade, the attending anaesthetist should, together with the parturient, review the progress of the infusion and labour at regular intervals of one to two hours. Regular reviews can confirm the presence and extent of problems, such as inadequate sacral nerve blockade, and allow timely modifications of the infusion rate or patient position, or both.

Even when mixed with an opioid, the more dilute solutions of bupivacaine, such as 0.031%, 0.0625% or 0.08%, may require supplementation from time to time with top-up doses of more concentrated local anaesthetic solution. The need for supplementation will increase with time, particularly if fentanyl rather than diamorphine is used [39]. Typical advantages and disadvantages identified by workers using the range of infusions shown in Table 15.4 are as follows.

1 Epidural infusion of bupivacaine 0.125% alone provides poor analgesia when compared to 0.125% with an opioid. When using the plain solution, more top-up supplements are requested and given.

2 Epidural infusion of bupivacaine 0.062% and 0.031%, both with fentanyl 2 µg/mL, produces poorer-quality pain relief than bupivacaine 0.125% with fentanyl 2 µg/mL.

3 The number of top-ups requested by parturients receiving bupivacaine 0.062% with fentanyl 2 µg/mL was the same as in those receiving bupivacaine 0.125% with fentanyl 2 µg/mL. This may seem to contradict item 2 above. The difference between the two is that the 'amount' of pain relief as judged by the various scoring systems, e.g. visual analogue scores (VAS), does not equate with the 'amount' of pain relief desired by parturients. The latter is better judged by their request for top-ups (or use of patient-controlled analgesia). In a proportion of labouring women, the total dosage of bupivacaine can be reduced without obvious subjective detriment to the parturient.

4 Epidural infusions of bupivacaine 0.125%, 0.062% and 0.031% with diamorphine 25 µg/mL produce similar degrees of pain relief. However, those parturients receiving the two more dilute solutions only obtain equal relief by receiving more top-up supplements.

5 Epidural infusions of bupivacaine 0.125%, 0.062% and 0.031% all produced similar degrees of motor block when mixed with fentanyl 2 µg/mL.

6 Less motor block was detected in patients receiving bupivacaine 0.062% and 0.031% with diamorphine 25 µg/mL than in those receiving bupivacaine 0.125% with diamorphine 25 µg/mL.

In most of the studies used to derive this information, top-ups of 5–10 mL bupivacaine 0.25% were used as escape medication. There seemed to be no correlation in any of the studies between the presence of motor block and the incidence of top-ups with these concentrations of bupivacaine. Overall, motor block was greater with fentanyl-containing than with diamorphine-containing solutions, and this difference may perhaps be due to enhancement of neural blockade by the reported local anaesthetic effects of fentanyl [62]. The decrease in motor blockade observed in many studies using infusion analgesia does not significantly change spontaneous vaginal delivery rates. Motor effects are usually measured using the Bromage scale, and it is possible that this scale is actually measuring an inappropriate motor effect in the context of vaginal delivery. The Bromage test assesses lower limb strength. Vaginal delivery demands abdominal and pelvic muscle function, and the legs have little input. A measure of rectus abdominis muscle activity would perhaps be more useful. An epidural solution is still awaited that will be associated with high spontaneous vaginal delivery rates while still maintaining good pain relief. Interestingly, parturients who received 0.062% bupivacaine solutions in two of the studies already quoted [34,37] had the relatively high spontaneous vaginal delivery rates of 59% and 58%. These groups also had higher pain visual analogue scale (VAS) scores without an increase in top-up request rates. It would seem that in some circumstances, parturients are content with less effective pain relief provided that motor and other sensory functions are retained. It may well be that the feeling of being 'in control', together with some awareness of contractions, is the desired situation for many parturients. This can only be achieved if analgesia regimens are tailored to suit individual requirements by adjusting dosages, concentrations, etc. There is still, however, a proportion of parturients who wish to have complete pain relief and who will need higher doses of local anaesthetic to achieve their desired level of comfort. Such women have to be clearly identified by an anaesthetist, and their choices should be recorded in each patient's notes.

15.4.7 Testing the block

Testing the upper and the lower limits of a regional anaesthetic block, whether from epidural or subarachnoid injections, must be carried out as a routine on every occasion these forms of anaesthesia are used. Thorough testing is obviously vital prior to surgery under regional anaesthesia. The tests should also be performed when epidural pain relief is used, because they will define the extent of epidural effect initially and, when repeated, any changes in its spread. For instance, once good pain relief has been attained, ascending or descending sensory loss should alert an obstetric anaesthetist to review drug dosages and infusion flow rates.

A number of sensory modalities can be tested, and the tests themselves can be performed in a number of ways. The modalities that are commonly tested include cold temperature discrimination, light touch and pinprick. A loss of cold temperature discrimination, tested using either an ethyl chloride spray or ice, indicates a block of the sympathetic nervous system at the level tested. Loss of light touch and pinprick sensation indicates a block of sensory nerve supply. For any given regional anaesthetic block, tests of these three modalities will give different results. Brull and Greene [63] reported the differences detected in the cephalad spread of epidural effect when tested with light touch, pinprick and cold temperature discrimination. Their results showed that a block would be judged to have risen highest when tested by cold discrimination. The block height would be one to two dermatomes lower if tested by pinprick, and two to three dermatomes lower if tested by light touch (Fig. 15.7). They termed these differences 'zones of differential block'. These zones exist for the whole duration of both an epidural and a subarachnoid block.

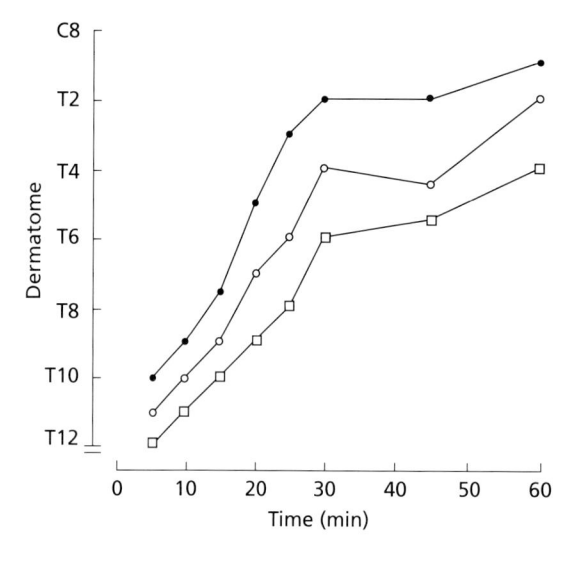

Fig. 15.7 The development of denervation for cold (●), pinprick (o) and light touch (□) during epidural anaesthesia. (With permission from [63].)

The modalities test different afferent neuronal functions, so it is not surprising that such zones exist. An important clinical consequence is that loss of appreciation of light touch at T4 will equate with a sympathetic block (loss of cold discrimination) to T1. The cardiovascular consequences of a T1 sympathetic block will obviously be greater than those from a T4 sympathetic block. Brull and Greene carried out their tests by comparing the skin of unblocked dermatomes with blocked skin testing from unaffected to affected patches of skin. Testing from above downwards is a very convenient way of performing the test for loss of cold sensation. It gives the patient a clear indication of what they should be feeling, and most parturients are easily able to inform the anaesthetist when the cold stimulus feels less cold. Testing from below (anaesthetized dermatomes) to unaffected areas of skin does in fact give a block height that is ostensibly one or two dermatomes lower.

Testing is probably most critical before operative interventions begin. Both cephalic and caudal limits of any regional anaesthetic must be detected and recorded. Completeness of block between the limits must also be confirmed. It is also necessary to test more than one modality when a Caesarean section is to be performed. A painful stimulus should be applied to the skin at the site of intended surgical incision in order to ensure that surface anaesthesia is adequate and complete at this level. Measures of the extent of a nerve block will inform the anaesthetist whether adequate anaesthesia has been achieved for the individual patient and the surgical intervention. Inadequacy in the density, completeness or spread of epidural or subarachnoid blocks should alert the obstetric anaesthetist to the possibility of patient discomfort or frank pain during future procedures. A failure to recognize the deficiencies of a block and take appropriate steps will inevitably lead to the unexpected need for further intervention by the anaesthetist. If emergency general anaesthesia proves necessary during a Caesarean section, it may be hazardous for the patient and fetus (if present *in utero*), and difficult and stressful for the staff involved. The safety benefits of the regional anaesthetic will be lost and, at best, the mother may have memories of the birth.

15.4.8 Top-up injections

In the early 1970s, epidural analgesia pain relief was provided almost entirely using intermittent epidural injections of local anaesthetic agents or top-ups. The first injections through an epidural catheter were, and still are, given by a doctor. Second and subsequent injections were, and still are, usually given by midwives acting under regulations originally formulated by the then Central Midwives' Board. In a few centres, all top-up injections continued to be given by obstetric anaesthetists. The reasons for this practice were that each top-up was considered to carry with it the risk of systemic toxicity or total spinal anaesthesia. The presence of an anaesthetist at the top-up would make resuscitation immediately available, and this advantage was considered to outweigh the logistical difficulties in providing sufficient obstetric anaesthetic staff. Although such risks still exist, midwifery skills have developed, resuscitation training has improved, and the use of fractionated injections has reduced the danger. Top-up injections can be of any concentration from bupivacaine 0.5% to 0.0625%. Most need contain no more mass of bupivacaine, whatever the concentration, than would a test dose. Bupivacaine 15 mg, i.e. 3 mL of bupivacaine 0.5% or 6 mL of 0.25% or 12 mL of 0.125%, is considered suitable as a maximum test dose. Top-ups can therefore be divided into fractions, each containing no more than 15 mg of the drug. This principle is important, because a single dose of local anaesthetic drug given in the presence of a functioning epidural block is unreliable as a test dose for the detection of subarachnoid placement of the epidural catheter. If top-ups consist of very dilute solutions, they may have to be given frequently—half-hourly intervals are not uncommon in order to maintain a reasonable quality of pain relief. In such circumstances, increasing the concentration of bupivacaine may extend the duration of effect, whereas an increase in opioid concentration in a mixture is not usually helpful. The peaks and troughs of pain relief that are encountered with top-up methods, together with the repeated risk of hypotension, toxicity and total spinal anaesthesia, have encouraged the development of infusion analgesia. Obviously, top-up injections are still needed from time to time even when infusions are used, but many studies show that well-chosen infusion regimens reduce the demand for top-up supplementation to one or two top-ups in a labour lasting many hours. The improvements in risk management, pain relief and efficiency make both continuous and patient-controlled epidural infusions a popular form of epidural pain relief in labour.

Table 15.6 Care during regional analgesia in labour (based on guidelines from St Michael's Hospital, Bristol).

- The woman must not lie supine, because of the risk of hypotension from vena cava compression
- If the BP falls below 90 mmHg systolic, or the pulse rate below 50 b.p.m.:
  1. Place patient in lateral position—usually left
  2. Give oxygen to breathe at 10 L/min
  3. Raise foot of bed
  4. Increase the intravenous drip rate to the maximum possible
  5. Switch the epidural infusion off
  6. Call the anaesthetist

  NB, if the woman is in the lateral position and the BP cuff is on the uppermost arm, the BP reading may be 10–15 mmHg lower than in other positions—if the woman is asymptomatic and the FHR trace is unchanged, try repositioning the cuff on the dependent arm before following the above steps:
- Measure and chart the respiratory rate if an opioid is used. If respiratory rate is less than 10, call the anaesthetist
- If forceps delivery is required and perineal analgesia is inadequate, contact the anaesthetist
- At the end, remove the catheter from the back with a steady pull and inspect it. Confirm that the catheter is intact with your dated signature. Apply a small dressing to the puncture site. If in doubt, contact the anaesthetist

Care of patients having top-ups
- Each top-up should commence with the administration of a test dose, followed after 5 min (if there is no untoward event) by the main dose. Following the test dose, measurement of BP and pulse must be at 5-min intervals up to 20 min, at 30 min, and thereafter every 30 min

Care of patients with epidural infusions
- The infusion delivers a weak solution of bupivacaine and diamorphine mixture constantly. This usually provides good pain relief throughout labour, but may become inadequate if:
  1. The pain of contractions increases—a top-up may be needed
  2. The block wears off on one side—the woman may have to lie on her side with the painful side down
- Measure and chart the BP half-hourly
- Check and chart the height of the block every hour. If the patient has pain at any time, first check the block level. Use cold ethyl chloride spray to test height of block on each side of the chest and abdomen, four inches from the midline, using the nipple level (T4), xiphoid process (T7), umbilicus (T10) and groin (L1) as surface landmarks (see dermatome chart). Test the sensation of cold ethyl chloride spray on the patient's arms first, to give the patient a point of reference, then apply spray to each side of the abdomen. If the spray is felt as a sensation, but not as cold as felt on the arm, then that segment is regarded as blocked
- Take the following actions:

The block is at T4 or above	Stop infusion and call anaesthetist immediately
The block has not changed and the patient has no pain	No action required
The block has gone down the body, e.g. T4–T10 but the patient has no pain	No action required
The block has gone down the body, is below T10 and/or the patient has pain	Give a top-up dose if prescribed or call anaesthetist
The block has gone further up the body, or differs significantly on the two sides	Inform anaesthetist

BP, blood pressure; FHR, fetal heart rate.

15.4.9 Maintaining epidural analgesia in labour

Once pain relief in labour has been established with epidural analgesia and any initial hypotension has been treated, management often passes to the midwife caring for the woman, although the ultimate responsibility remains with the anaesthetist. Safety during epidural analgesia dictates that the midwife should have received appropriate training and have been found to be competent in the subject. The midwife should not nurse another patient at the same time. The midwife will be expected to maintain verbal contact with the woman and to measure the maternal pulse and blood pressure at appropriate regular intervals, which should be defined by local guidelines (Table 15.6). These guidelines should reflect professional practice for both anaesthetists and midwives. The fetal heart rate and uterine contractions should be monitored, and the mother should be encouraged to empty her bladder regularly, preferably by moving to the toilet if an absence of motor block allows this.

If a continuous infusion is being used, the infusion device must be checked for volume infused on an hourly basis, and the extent of the sensory and sympathetic block must be recorded. The midwife should notify an anaesthetist if the block extends above the umbilicus, or if it does not provide adequate pain relief. If top-ups are being administered by the midwife, these must be recorded as prescribed on the prescription sheet, in addition to the nursing and/or epidural form. Again, if pain relief is inadequate, an anaesthetist must be called and the stage of labour assessed in relation to the extent and quality of the nerve block.

When an anaesthetist is called to a woman whose pain has returned after an initial satisfactory block, the following checks should be made.

1 Assess the progress of labour (cervical dilatation, presenting part, delay in labour). If these are abnormal, obstetric advice should be sought. The back pain associated with an occipitoposterior position can be continuous and difficult to treat. Larger or more concentrated doses of local anaesthetic may be needed.
2 Define the position of the pain by talking to the mother, and test the sensory dermatomes blocked by the epidural. If the pain is outside the sensory segmental distribution of the epidural, a top-up is indicated, and the mother's position may require adjustment. If it is within the sensory segmental distribution, the quality of the nerve block may require adjustment. Pain felt within the limits of an otherwise apparently satisfactory block should be discussed with the obstetrician to exclude serious labour complications, e.g. ruptured uterus.
3 Palpate the bladder. A full bladder will increase painful sensations.
4 Check the maternal pulse and blood pressure. A top-up should not be given if the mother has cardiovascular instability. Obstetric and anaesthetic complications should be considered, e.g. placental abruption or uterine rupture.
5 Check the fetal heart rate and observe the fetal heart rate tracing. If there is

fetal distress, a top-up may have to be given slowly in order to avoid any hypotension.

If the mother's pain is severe, she should be encouraged to use Entonox for alternative pain relief while these assessments are completed and before the epidural top-up has its effect.

If a top-up is unable to achieve analgesia, the position of the epidural catheter must be checked. A transparent dressing over the site of insertion will allow the anaesthetist to assess the number of centimetres of catheter still inside, and gentle palpation around the catheter entry may detect subcuticular excursion of the catheter. If the catheter has migrated out of the epidural space, it should be replaced. Occasionally, the catheter migrates within the epidural space towards the paravertebral space, producing a unilateral nerve block (Fig. 14.6, p. 220). Under such conditions, the catheter may be withdrawn by 1–2 cm (dependent on how much was left in the space initially) under aseptic conditions. A fresh transparent occlusive dressing should then be applied. A further top-up dose can be given, usually with good effect.

In prolonged labour, the administration of local anaesthetic and opioid drugs into the epidural space may have cumulative effects in the fetus through placental transfer. The doses of bupivacaine used are not associated with significant fetal or maternal effects. The total dose of opioid used should be considered. In a study of 40 nulliparous women after CSE in the first stage of labour, maternal and umbilical blood samples for fentanyl concentrations did not reach a value compatible with respiratory depression, and no clinical effects were detected using the Apgar score or Neurologic and Adaptive Capacity Score (NACS) [64]. The mean total dose of fentanyl administered epidurally was 105 ± 61 μg, and only four women received more than 200 μg. For those women who have received prolonged analgesia, neonatal depression should be assessed regularly postpartum, and if necessary opioid antagonists should be given.

15.5 Epidural anaesthesia for Caesarean section

Epidural anaesthesia was recommended for Caesarean section as an alternative to general anaesthesia in the late 1970s. The recommendation was made because of the risks of failed intubation and aspiration of gastric contents, clearly identified in the *Confidential Enquiries into Maternal Deaths* reports of the 1960s and 1970s. Epidurals have been largely superseded by subarachnoid anaesthesia whenever possible, as the latter produces a better block more reliably and more quickly, and pencil-point needles have reduced the incidence of postdural puncture headache. However, there are still some circumstances in which an epidural is the preferred method of anaesthesia for Caesarean section. There are two main circumstances:
- when an effective epidural is already in place;
- when a regional nerve block needs to be established slowly.

15.5.1 Extension of an existing epidural

The existing nerve block will usually have been given for pain relief in labour. The density of such blocks is inadequate for operative abdominal delivery. The existing distribution of effect will, however, give the obstetric anaesthetist some indication of what can be achieved with the particular parturient and epidural by administering more concentrated injections of local anaesthetic solution. A word of caution is appropriate at this point. If the existing epidural has been patchy or only intermittently effective, it is probably better to abandon it and use subarachnoid or even general anaesthesia. Attempting to fill in missed segments and to compensate for low or inadequate blocks will inevitably lead to a stormy intraoperative course and a dissatisfied patient postoperatively. Pain during Caesarean section under regional anaesthesia is one of the more common causes of litigation against obstetric anaesthetists. However, if the epidural has provided good analgesia throughout labour, without deficiencies such as missed segments or unilateral blocks, it is reasonable to attempt to modify it for a Caesarean section. The density of block and its distribution will both need to be increased. A block that is complete bilaterally from T4 to S4/S5 should be established before surgical intervention begins. Testing the block must be thorough, in particular, the site of the surgical incision should be tested for loss of sensation to a painful needle prick or a hard pinch with a pair of forceps, as well as loss of cold sensation, which will only provide evidence of sympathetic nerve blockade. Testing for sacral block is important, because if the sacral segments remain unaffected by the epidural local anaesthetic solution, the patient will experience severe discomfort and autonomic effects when viscera or peritoneum innervated by these segments are manipulated. The most obvious example is stretching of the bladder and its associated peritoneum, both of which are almost inevitably affected by traction during Caesarean section. If there is any doubt as to the adequacy of effect, the patient must be told and should be offered either subarachnoid block or general anaesthesia, whichever is most appropriate for that individual parturient and her circumstances.

When extension of an existing epidural is being considered, a number of factors must be assessed:
- the urgency and cause of the Caesarean section, e.g. haemorrhage;
- the existing spread of block;
- the density and completeness of block (e.g. all segments blocked bilaterally);
- the dose of local anaesthetic already administered, to avoid toxicity.

If Caesarean section is very urgently required, e.g. in the case of a prolapsed cord accompanied by fetal heart rate decelerations, extension of an epidural may not be feasible. At least 15 minutes must be available if the anaesthetist is to have a reasonable chance of achieving a sufficient block for operation. The only exception to this rule of thumb is the local anaesthetic agent chloroprocaine. This ester-based local anaesthetic will achieve satisfactory

Table 15.7 The physicochemical properties of local anaesthetic drugs.

	Partition coefficients	Protein binding	pK_a
Lidocaine	2.9	70%	7.9
Ropivacaine	6.1	92%	8.1
Bupivacaine	27.5	96%	8.1

epidural blockade within 5–10 minutes of its being administered. However, it is not available in the United Kingdom, where the choice of drugs lies between: bupivacaine 0.5% plain; bupivacaine 0.5% plain plus lidocaine 2% (in equal volumes); lidocaine 2% with epinephrine 1 : 200 000; ropivacaine 0.75%; and levobupivacaine.

These local anaesthetic solutions can be mixed with an opioid such as fentanyl 50–100 µg or diamorphine 2.5–3.0 mg. The speed of onset can be increased by raising the pH of the local anaesthetic solution and thereby increasing the proportion of non-ionized drug present. The theory behind this practice is that most local anaesthetics are weak bases with a pK_a varying from 7.7 to 8.9 (Table 15.7). When supplied in plain solutions, they are slightly acidic in order to improve the stability of the local anaesthetic. To be effective, the drug must cross the perineural sheath and nerve membrane, and it can only do so when it is in its non-ionized form. Lidocaine 2% is usually supplied at a pH of 6.4, bupivacaine 0.5% at a pH of 6. Less than 5% of the drug is present in the non-ionized form at these pH values. Raising the pH of lidocaine to 7 increases the proportion of non-ionized drug to 11% [65], and theoretically should markedly increase the speed of onset of action of this drug. Results that conflict with this hypothesis have, however, been reported [66,67] and it would appear that there is little advantage in alkalinizing lidocaine solutions.

Bupivacaine has a pK_a value of 8, which is greater than that of lidocaine, so the increase in the proportion of non-ionized drug when the solution is alkalinized should be even larger than that for lidocaine. However, studies on bupivacaine have shown similar disparities. One report on epidural blockade for Caesarean section [68] showed an improvement of onset time from a mean of 6.4 minutes to 3.2 minutes. A number of other studies on both Caesarean section [69] and lower limb surgery patients [70] have failed to confirm this benefit. Care must be taken with preparing an alkalinized bupivacaine solution. If the pH rises above 7, precipitation may occur. Some difficulty may therefore be encountered in assessing the dose of sodium bicarbonate to be added to bupivacaine 0.5%. Sodium bicarbonate 8.4% can only be added in very small quantities. Approximately 0.1 mL can be added to 20 mL bupivacaine without causing precipitation. The improvement in onset time for the resulting solution is only some three minutes when a loss of cold sensation at L1 is used as the end point. Clinically, this difference is of little importance when compared with the eventual quality of the blockade. Thus, there is no indication that adding sodium bicarbonate to either bupivacaine or lidocaine local anaesthetic solution will dependably improve the quality of block obtained.

The results obtained by mixing bupivacaine and lidocaine have also been varied. A comparison has been reported between four local anaesthetic solutions [71]: lidocaine 2% with epinephrine 1 : 200 000; bupivacaine 0.5% with epinephrine 1 : 200 000; bupivacaine 0.5% plain; and a mixture of equal volumes of bupivacaine 0.5% with lidocaine 2%. Lidocaine 2% with epinephrine produced a significantly less effective block than the other solutions. Bupivacaine 0.5% with epinephrine produced the most consistent block, and was judged to be very good or excellent by all mothers receiving it. There was no difference between the four solutions in the time to readiness for surgery. Given this uncertainty, the choice would be to use a single agent rather than a mixture. Since the duration of action of lidocaine is shorter than bupivacaine, the benefits obtained from lidocaine are far from clear. Thus, if an existing epidural is to be extended for Caesarean section, at least 10–15 minutes must be available to achieve an adequate block. Bupivacaine is a safe and well-tried drug which, when mixed with an opioid (and possibly epinephrine 1 : 200 000), will usually produce sufficient nerve blockade to allow Caesarean section to be undertaken. The newer single-enantiomer local anaesthetics, *S*-bupivacaine (levobupivacaine) and ropivacaine, may have advantages for the extension of existing epidural blocks because of their wider therapeutic index and relative safety from cardiotoxicity [72]. The isomer *R*-bupivacaine stays in the sodium channel for a prolonged period compared with the *S* isomer, and hence is more cardiotoxic. In addition, levobupivacaine has a higher protein binding than its isomer, and this would also tend to reduce cardiotoxicity [73].

The slower onset time of epidural nerve block compared to subarachnoid nerve block can be advantageous. The rapid onset time and greater density of block from the latter lead to a greater speed and incidence of hypotension. Epidural blockade, either alone or combined with a low subarachnoid block to T12, gives the advantage of greater cardiovascular stability in patients with cardiac problems or untreated hypovolaemia. Varying the technique of injection into the epidural space can change both the onset time and the incidence of hypotension. Laishley and Morgan found that slow injection of a single bolus ensured a rapid onset of block but was associated with hypotension in 27% of parturients receiving it [74]. On the other hand, fractionating the dose of local anaesthetic is associated with a slower onset and a lower incidence of hypotension [75]. Prevention of hypotension by intravenous preload or volume expansion prior to epidural blockade was first suggested in 1968 [76], but its value has been questioned [77]. Moderate preloading with up to 10 mL/kg is, however, a simple and usually safe technique which, when combined with the judicious use of ephedrine to treat hypotension when it occurs, can lead to cardiovascular stability during extension of epidural blocks—just as it can when an epidural is used for Caesarean section when no pre-existing block exists.

If the woman begins to complain of pain during surgery, the nature of the pain should be determined. Is it pain, fear, tugging or pulling? The woman must be reassured that it will be treated, and if necessary the surgery must be stopped. The following alternatives should be offered: epidural top-up (e.g. 2% lidocaine, with or without opioid), intravenous boluses of fentanyl, a mixture of nitrous oxide and oxygen from the anaesthetic machine, local anaesthetic infiltration by the surgeon (lidocaine using non-toxic doses), or conversion to general anaesthesia.

15.5.2 Slow establishment of an epidural nerve block

This is the other indication for epidural analgesia as distinct from subarachnoid block. Sympathetic nerve blockade will occur in both, but the spread of onset using the epidural route is slower and so therapeutic measures and maternal cardiovascular compensation can occur without acute blood pressure changes. The technique is to inject volumes of 5 mL 0.5% bupivacaine intermittently over 30 minutes up to 25 mL. Normal precautions must be taken to manage hypotension, because rare complications such as intrathecal or intravascular injection can still occur.

15.6 Subarachnoid anaesthesia

The terms 'spinal anaesthesia', 'intrathecal anaesthesia', 'subarachnoid anaesthesia' and 'subarachnoid block' (SAB) are frequently used synonymously. A combination of epidural and subarachnoid anaesthesia, whether using the needle-through-needle method or two separate punctures, is called CSE (combined spinal–epidural). The distinction between SAB and CSE is of some importance, because SAB is most frequently used as a single-shot technique for Caesarean section. CSE combines a single-shot subarachnoid injection with an epidural catheter that can be used for labour or Caesarean section, and allows incremental top-up injections or infusions to be made into the epidural space to increase the spread of the subarachnoid block or its duration.

15.6.1 History

In the United Kingdom, SAB has had a chequered history, particularly in the context of obstetric anaesthesia. The first successful clinical SAB was performed in 1898 by August Bier. The method was subsequently developed and popularized by Théodore Tuffier in France. SAB was pioneered in the United Kingdom by Arthur E. Barker of University College Hospital, London, who introduced hyperbaric local anaesthetic solutions. Using these solutions, he reported on the use of the anatomical curves of the vertebral column as a means of influencing the distribution and spread of the local anaesthetic effects [78]. The method fell into disrepute in the United Kingdom due to litigation, notably the Woolley and Rowe case and related articles that appeared shortly thereafter [79]. Additional problems complicated the use of the method in pregnant patients, in some cases due to a lack of understanding of the pathophysiological changes of pregnancy, particularly the supine hypotensive syndrome. Other problems were due to equipment limitations. The large-calibre needles with Quincke points gave rise to a very high incidence of postdural puncture headache in parturients. The true value of the technique in obstetric anaesthesia has only become firmly established in the last decade.

15.6.2 Advantages and disadvantages

SAB can be performed rapidly, has a short onset time, and produces a dense block of motor and sensory nerves with a finite duration. The expected duration of surgery must be estimated with some accuracy, since extension of the block is not possible with the single-shot technique. The characteristically dense block and low risk of missed segments or unilateral block have always made SAB an effective method of anaesthesia. However, the significant risk of hypotension and high incidence of postdural puncture headache in obstetric patients limited its widespread use. The magnitude of hypotension in pregnant women is the result of the combination of vena caval occlusion and rapid sympathetic blockade accompanying the onset of subarachnoid anaesthesia. Vasodilation occurs quickly, causing a fall in systemic vascular resistance. Venous return decreases—markedly, if caval occlusion is present—and this decrease may trigger the Bezold–Jarisch reflex, which can cause slowing of heart rate and more pronounced hypotension because of a decrease in cardiac output. Intravenous preload, vasopressors and lateral tilt positioning have mainly overcome the problem of hypotension. Use of small-diameter, conically tipped needles has largely resolved the longer-term effects of postdural puncture headache. Even with these needles, the obstetric anaesthetist must proceed with caution.

The dangers of neural damage with the needle are still present. Verbal contact must be maintained with the woman, and particular enquiries must be made during insertion about shooting pains, discomfort, tingling or electric shock-like sensations. If the patient complains of any of these symptoms, or if CSF is not detected at the hub of the needle, the introducer and needle should be withdrawn and the patient reappraised. The position of the woman should be checked and flexion of the spine confirmed. The same or an adjacent space can be used, but the site of introduction and angulation of the needle must be reassessed. The anatomy is essentially the same as for epidural insertion, the main difference in technique being the click or pop felt as the spinal needle pierces the dura. When that has been felt, the stylet can be withdrawn and the needle hub inspected for CSF.

Once CSF has appeared, a dose of local anaesthetic can be injected slowly into the subarachnoid space. During the injection, care must be taken to control and steady the spinal needle and ensure that it does not move. Maintenance of subarachnoid positioning should be confirmed by aspirating CSF into the syringe containing local anaesthetic solution on three occasions: first, before injection begins; secondly, half-way through the injection; and thirdly, after the injection of local anaesthetic solution is complete. Use of a Luer–Lok syringe is recommended to make these checks easier and to guard against any leakage of local anaesthetic solution during injection.

15.6.3 Doses and volumes

The anaesthetic agent most commonly used for Caesarean section anaesthesia in the United Kingdom is hyperbaric bupivacaine 0.5% in a volume of 2.5–3.0 mL. Opioid agents can be mixed with this solution in order to improve the quality of intraoperative anaesthesia and postoperative analgesia. Diamorphine 0.3 mg or fentanyl 10–25 μg can be added without disturbing the hyperbaricity of the solution. Diamorphine 0.1–0.2 mg confers little postoperative benefit, but 0.3 mg makes postoperative systemic opioid administration unnecessary in a significant number of women [80]. Other authors [81] have reported similar dose-related benefits, although they have not found the significantly better pain relief with 0.3 mg or more compared with smaller doses. Doses larger than 0.3 mg are unnecessary and should be avoided.

Isobaric bupivacaine is less frequently used in obstetric patients than the hyperbaric formulation. When it was first used for Caesarean section, the isobaric solution produced a much less predictable height of block than the hyperbaric solution, but Russell and Holmqvist subsequently showed that there is little difference between the two solutions [82]. Historically, given the degree of reluctance to use SAB, it is not surprising that doses as small as 1.5 mL of bupivacaine 0.5% were initially used. It slowly became apparent that doses as large as 3 mL of the hyperbaric solution could be used to produce a subarachnoid block with an upper limit of T2 to T4, provided that patients were carefully positioned during initiation of the block to prevent cephalad spread.

It is essential that in the supine/tilt position, the long axis of the patient's vertebral column is arranged so that the bolus of hyperbaric solution will flow from the point of injection to the mid-thoracic part of the subarachnoid space. To ensure that spread reaches this point and does not extend further cephalad, the upper thoracic vertebrae must be elevated towards the neck. A number of anatomical factors must be understood if this position is to be achieved. If the parturient lies in the lateral position with knees drawn up, on a horizontal surface the long axis of the spine will run in a 5° head-down tilt because of the width of the female pelvis (Fig. 15.8). Great care must therefore be taken to ensure that the head, neck and shoulders are supported to bring the upper

Fig. 15.8 A diagram to show the 'head-down' tilt which results if a parturient is placed in a lateral position on a flat horizontal surface.

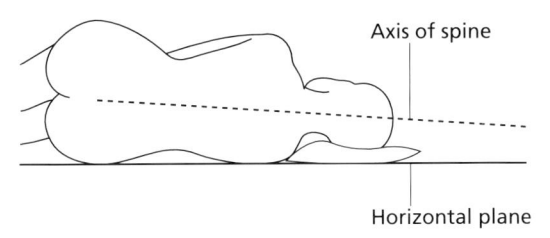

Fig. 15.9 Limitation of cephalad spread of hyperbaric solution, (a) in the lateral position and (b) in a wedged/tilted supine position, both with suitable support beneath head, neck and shoulders to produce curvature of the thoracic spine and dural sac.

thoracic and cervical vertebrae above the level of the mid-thoracic part of the vertebral column (Fig. 15.9). If this curvature is not achieved, the hyperbaric bupivacaine injected will flow too far in a cephalad direction, and this flow—combined with diffusion of bupivacaine through the CSF—can result in very high or even total spinal block. The anaesthetist is then faced with a difficult decision on whether and when to intervene with general anaesthesia, endotracheal intubation and ventilatory support. If the intervention proves necessary at a time when the parturient's blood pressure is unstable, the combination of anaesthetic manoeuvres and cardiovascular effects will produce such profound changes that the patient's life can be placed in jeopardy.

Provided that a patient is placed in an appropriate position, the volume of bupivacaine to be used is less critical. Doses of 12.5–15.0 mg of hyperbaric bupivacaine (2.5–3.0 mL of bupivacaine 0.5%) rarely produce motor block above T4, and they are also unlikely to be associated with blocks that are inadequate either in completeness, spread or duration. High blocks do occur, often unrelated to the patient's size or height. Fortunately, they are usually limited to a high sensory blockade. The parturient (and anaesthetist) may be alarmed at the onset of numbness in hands and arms, but bupivacaine has the distinction of having a useful differential between sensory and motor block of several spinal segments, and it is most unusual to see motor effects spreading to cervical segments.

The use of smaller volumes will not necessarily be associated with less spread, but merely shorter duration of anaesthesia. In order to achieve a lower block for operative vaginal delivery, the sitting position must be adopted and will need to be maintained for about 10 minutes if the majority of the dose of local anaesthetic solution is to settle into the sacral curvature and limit the effect on the thoracic segments of the cord. Moving to a wedged supine position earlier will not prevent sacral block, but will encourage thoracic spread and hypotension.

The woman's systolic and diastolic blood pressure and heart rate must be recorded before the subarachnoid injection is made and then at one-minute intervals during the onset of anaesthesia and until delivery of the fetus. During the early stages of the technique, while the height of local anaesthetic block is increasing, the patient should be closely observed for any signs of facial pallor or sweating, which often precede the onset of hypotension by a short interval. Verbal contact should be maintained throughout this period, and the patient should be encouraged to report any feelings of discomfort, nausea or faintness. Ephedrine injections must be immediately available for intravenous administration to treat hypotension. The dose can be most easily titrated if the drug has already been diluted, to a concentration of 3 mg/mL in a 10-mL syringe. A decrease in blood pressure occurs so frequently during SAB with a block height above T10 that many anaesthetists administer prophylactic i.v. ephedrine as soon as the subarachnoid injection of local anaesthetic is completed. If ephedrine is given as an additive in intravenous crystalloid solution, it is impossible to gauge the dose given. Bolus injection of ephedrine into a fast-flowing infusion of intravenous crystalloid solution is therefore preferred. The ephedrine and intravenous fluid can then be administered independently. In the United Kingdom, ephedrine is invariably the sympathomimetic agent of choice for obstetric patients prior to delivery, unless contraindicated. There have been reports of tachyphylaxis to its repeated use, so alternative vasopressors should be available. Alternative agonists such as methoxamine or phenylephrine can be used after delivery of the fetus, and should be used preferentially if tachycardia needs to be avoided—for example, in cases of ischaemic heart disease.

15.6.4 Block height

The extent of spread of local anaesthetic effect that is sought will vary depending on the procedure to be undertaken. For instance, to achieve good-quality analgesia for Caesarean section, a block that is complete bilaterally from T4 to

S5 is needed. If this spread is not achieved and surgery is undertaken, some degree of patient discomfort or pain should be anticipated. As a general rule, the amount of discomfort will vary inversely with the height of the block, and a woman with a block limited to T8 will suffer substantial pain or discomfort, particularly once the abdominal cavity is open and viscera are stimulated. A block that does not spread downwards to include the sacral segments is likely to be associated with discomfort whenever sacrally innervated viscera are handled. The bladder is one such organ, and pain fibres pass from it in the pelvic splanchnic nerves to ganglia on the posterior roots of the sacral nerves. Although some innervation of the bladder passes via the sympathetic and superior hypogastric plexus and spinal segments between T11 and L2, absence of local anaesthetic block of the sacral segments will expose the patient to a considerable risk of pain when the obstetrician places a retractor over the bladder, as is inevitable early in a Caesarean section. If deficiencies in local anaesthetic spread are suspected, the patient should be told of their extent and the likely consequences of proceeding with surgery. It is better in most circumstances to have a mutually agreed plan between patient and anaesthetist that anticipates problems, rather than adopting a 'hope-for-the-best' attitude and shirking the responsibility of telling the woman and her attendant of the possible inadequacy of the block.

Other forms of obstetric operative intervention may require rather less extensive block. Any procedures involving only the vagina or perineum, or both, can be easily and successfully carried out when a regional anaesthetic block is secured from S1 to S5. However, if any manipulation of the cervix or body of the uterus is to be undertaken, a regional block extending to and including T10 (as assessed by pinprick) will be necessary. It must be emphasized that the spread of nerve block when using subarachnoid techniques depends more on the patient's position at the beginning and during the early stages of the procedure than it does on the volume and milligram dose of local anaesthetic employed.

15.7 Combined spinal–epidural technique

15.7.1 Labour

The combined spinal–epidural (CSE) method was introduced as a technique for labour analgesia that provided a faster onset of analgesia and decreased motor block, and hence a better sense of maternal control (Table 15.8). It heralded the concept of 'mobile' epidural analgesia, and its development coincided with the epidural use of low doses of local anaesthetic agents combined with opioids.

Comparisons of CSE and epidural analgesia [83,84] have found no difference in maternal satisfaction between the two techniques, nor in the rate of Caesarean section. In a proportion of women with both techniques there is a

Table 15.8 Advantages and disadvantages of combined spinal–epidural for labour analgesia.

Advantages
Rapid onset
Safety: less fetal drug transfer
Less motor block

Disadvantages
Technical failures
Intrathecal transfer (theoretical)
Epidural catheter migration (theoretical)
Reports of meningitis after combined spinal–epidural

continual increase in motor block throughout labour, and this may influence the number of women achieving spontaneous or instrumental vaginal delivery. Unfortunately, studies of motor block with low-dose techniques have as yet not differentiated the confounding variables of multiple top-ups or longer-term continuous infusions.

CSE for labour is slowly gaining acceptance in the United Kingdom, but reservations still exist because of the additional technical requirements of the spinal component and its associated complications—in particular, the reports of meningitis after CSE [85]. As with any anaesthetic, CSE risks should be discussed antenatally so that a woman is aware of the difference between a 'mobile' epidural and a 'mobile' CSE. The CSE technique may use either the 'needle-through-needle' technique or separate epidural and spinal needle insertions at a different space, or the same space. The needle-through-needle technique can achieve pain relief quickly, with effectively a single insertion through the spinous ligaments. It is technically more difficult to learn, and therefore has a higher failure rate until the necessary experience has been gained. Equipment developments have made the technique more accessible. They allow the position of the spinal needle within the epidural needle to be fixed in order to prevent movement between the needles—for example, during a contraction—so that access to the intrathecal space is not lost. The spinal needle has to be longer than the epidural needle by about 1.5 cm to allow at least 1 cm to extend beyond the tip of the epidural needle and pierce the dura. The range of distances which the spinal needle is inserted past the end of the epidural needle was found to vary from 2.5 to 14.5 mm, with a mean distance of 7.0 mm [86]. Paraesthesiae are felt more commonly with pencil-point needles than with Quincke needles, and more commonly with the needle-through-needle technique than with separate insertions.

The main indication for CSE in labour is the situation in which a mother has developed severe pain before requesting 'epidural' analgesia. The separate techniques of spinal and then epidural nerve block are also appropriate—for example, an SAB with bupivacaine 2.5 mg plus fentanyl 25 µg will produce good pain relief within minutes. The mother can then gain control of her situation, and the epidural can be sited in a calmer atmosphere. The CSE technique, as described previously, allows extra pain relief through the intrathecal injection prior to epidural analgesia. This may have no overall effect on patient satisfaction, but it can allow more rapid assessment of the progress of labour in an uncontrollable mother. Where a mother has had a failed epidural in a previous labour and requests epidural analgesia again, a CSE technique may be recommended as the preferred method of pain relief.

The risk of intrathecal spread of epidural injections or infusions via the dural hole is more a theoretical risk than practical, since the hole is small. However, there may be times when more than one dural puncture is made. This should be considered to be an additional risk factor for intrathecal side effects, or more extensive effects than expected after epidural injections. Appropriate action should be taken by an anaesthetist to maintain vigilance in assessing the nerve block and its segmental spread, especially when more than one needle insertion has been made to establish the SAB.

15.7.2 Caesarean section

A CSE is commonly used for Caesarean section when specific advantages are sought for the mother by the anaesthetist. It has been mentioned earlier that SAB is now a successful and common anaesthetic for Caesarean section. CSE it increases the flexibility of the regional technique, because the addition of the epidural catheter allows the anaesthetic effects of the SAB to be extended over more spinal segments, or to be prolonged if the operating time is greater than normal. CSE can also be recommended to a mother when she has experienced a previous failed regional technique, where there are surgical difficulties expected, or when problems become apparent during the siting of a spinal—for example, when a 'dry tap' is experienced.

The subarachnoid dose can be varied to suit the circumstances. When 2.5–3.0 mL of 0.5% heavy bupivacaine with diamorphine 0.3 mg or fentanyl 25 µg is given, further epidural doses are usually unnecessary, unless the duration of the nerve block is inadequate or surgery is prolonged. At the end of surgery, however, there is the option for epidural opioids for postoperative pain relief.

15.8 Complications of regional nerve block in obstetrics

15.8.1 Maternal hypotension

Ideally, maternal blood pressure should be measured regularly every 15 minutes during labour, particularly if a regional nerve block is in progress. After top-up injections, the arterial blood pressure should be measured at five-minute intervals for 20 minutes, and then at 30 minutes after top-up before resuming 15-minute recordings. During regional nerve block for surgery, especially SAB, blood pressure should be measured at one-minute intervals until it is stable. Hypotension can occur throughout Caesarean section, and in addition to blood pressure recordings, maternal complaints of nausea, vomiting or dizziness should be taken as indicators of hypotension until proved otherwise.

The definition of hypotension varies. The best relates the change to a 'control' value, and a change of 25% of 'control' systolic pressure is often used, because an absolute figure may not reflect pre-nerve block values. A satisfactory rule of thumb is to consider a blood pressure decrease of more than 20 mmHg to be significant. In all cases of hypotension, if the mother is bradycardic an anticholinergic drug is indicated, and must be given intravenously. However, maternal position is important—particularly because a decrease in left atrial filling will exacerbate bradycardia via the Bezold–Jarish reflex—so parturients must be tilted in order to avoid aortocaval compression, and if one lateral position is unsatisfactory, the other side should be tried. If hypotension occurs an intravenous infusion should be given rapidly if a fluid load (up to one litre) has not already been administered. Oxygen should be administered to the mother and the fetal heart rate should be checked. If the hypotension does not respond to these measures, a vasopressor is indicated, and intravenous ephedrine is the drug of choice. It is usually diluted to 3 or 5 mg/mL, and given as 1–2 mL increments until a satisfactory blood pressure is achieved. Failure to respond should alert an anaesthetist to other causes of hypotension that may be obstetric in origin. These include:
- aortocaval occlusion;
- sympathetic nerve block;
- haemorrhage (concealed or revealed);
- others, e.g. amniotic fluid embolus.

15.8.2 Pruritus after epidural or spinal opioids

Itching is very common after epidural or subarachnoid opioids, and the mother should be reassured about its cause and the likelihood that it will not get worse, but instead will settle with time. If it persists and is unacceptable, naloxone 50 µg intravenously can be administered every 10 minutes until it diminishes, up to a maximum dose of 400 µg. Other drugs, such as the antihistamines, may have antipruritic effects. They also have sedative side effects. Where patients are at high risk of pruritus—such as those with eczematous or psoriatic skin conditions, or when there is a history of pruritus with previous regional nerve blocks—spinal opioids should be avoided.

15.8.3 Respiratory depression

Whenever opioids are administered by any route, there is a risk of respiratory depression. A clinical guide to this complication is a decrease in the respiratory rate to less than 10 breaths per minute, but this is an insensitive measure and a late clinical manifestation of respiratory depression. Care should therefore be taken in the administration and monitoring of opioid use. In labour, respiration is often not regular, and episodes of oxygen desaturation occur. Subclinical respiratory depression after intrathecal opioids has been monitored using end-tidal carbon dioxide levels [87], and increases of up to 2 kPa (13 mmHg) were observed. In addition to epidural or subarachnoid opioids, women frequently request intramuscular pethidine before considering epidural analgesia. Epidural and subarachnoid opioids are not given if pethidine has been used within the previous four hours in some units. Unfortunately, this decision may affect the quality of regional nerve blockade. Where this is considered important, close monitoring of respiration should be instituted for the duration of opioid action. Additional risk factors will include the use of other sedative drugs, including general anaesthesia, and pathological conditions affecting the nervous and muscular systems. Cardiorespiratory disease must also be assessed when opioids are prescribed. Once the decision to use opioids is made, monitoring of respiratory depression and sedation is necessary in the post-delivery period.

15.8.4 Epidural catheter removal

Most epidural catheters are removed by the midwife attending the mother. The midwife should check that the catheter is intact, and should record this event. Where a catheter has been sited and the mother is receiving drugs with anticoagulant properties, catheter removal should be timed by the anaesthetist to avoid the risk of bleeding on withdrawal. If any difficulty is experienced on withdrawal of the catheter, the woman should be encouraged to flex her back. Knots occur occasionally, and withdrawal should then only be attempted by an anaesthetist. Most catheters are radiopaque, but retrieval of a sheared catheter is not advised.

15.8.5 Postpartum bladder disturbance

When epidural analgesia techniques in labour were first advocated in the 1960s, there were reports of bladder distension leading to postpartum bladder dysfunction. Despite the advent of low-dose epidural regimens, this complication can still occur, and subarachnoid opioids may increase the risk. Distension may also be associated with obstetric complications rather than aspects of epidural management. Whatever the cause, a full bladder can cause suprapubic discomfort and increase the pain of contractions, so maintenance of normal bladder activity should be encouraged in labour. Bladder distension must be prevented so catheterization is necessary if normal micturition fails.

15.8.6 Outcome of labour: spontaneous or operative delivery

Progress in epidural analgesia has focused on achieving spontaneous vaginal delivery of the infant together with a satisfactory sensory nerve block. Studies of delivery outcome following epidural analgesia lag behind developments in analgesia regimens by a number of years. This is inevitable. It is not only the different regimens of regional nerve block that require randomized controlled outcome studies, but also comparisons with women randomly assigned to receive no regional nerve block.

15.8.7 Nausea and vomiting

Labour itself is associated with nausea and vomiting, but opioids have the potential to delay gastric emptying and induce nausea and vomiting. This is particularly troublesome with intramuscular pethidine, but may occur with epidural or spinal opioids. Where a regional nerve block is functional, hypotension must be excluded as a cause.

15.8.8 Meningitis

Meningitis is a rare complication of regional analgesia or anaesthesia. It can present as a medical emergency with severe headache, neck stiffness and signs of sepsis. It may present with neurological deficits, and meningitis is only one of several different diagnoses [88]. Irritation and inflammation of the meninges are potential complications of spinal anaesthesia. All the barriers to infection surrounding the nerves and spinal cord are bypassed by subarachnoid injections, and disposable equipment and sterile drugs together with full aseptic precautions on the part of the operator are therefore essential to keep the incidence of meningitis very low. Symptoms of meningitis arise from bacterial infection, viral infection and chemical contamination, and can be drug-induced (non-steroidal anti-inflammatory drugs and H_2-receptor blocking drugs). The infection may also be blood-borne. Bacteria in the woman's blood can gain access to the subarachnoid space due to microscopic bleeding caused by insertion of the needle. This mechanism is a risk in obstetrics, because genital tract infection and bacteraemia occur, particularly in relation to chorioamnionitis and puerperal sepsis. The usual precaution is not to site an epidural or subarachnoid block if a woman has a fever and she has not received therapeutic blood levels of antibiotics. This type of haematogenous spread can complicate both epidural anaesthesia, with the possible formation of an epidural abscess, and subarachnoid anaesthesia, where the flow of CSF can spread infection in the intrathecal space. The other risk in regional nerve block is where an accidental dural puncture produces a headache, requiring a blood patch. It is recommended that blood cultures should be taken at the time of the blood patch, so that any bacteria can be identified and the correct antibiotic regimen can be used if infection occurs.

In the majority of cases of meningitis after regional nerve block, a causative organism cannot be identified, and the condition is probably aseptic in origin [89]. Chemicals used in sterilization procedures were identified in the 1950s as being causative factors, and these have been removed. Contamination with glove powder necessitates either washing it off before touching a needle, or using powder-free gloves. An aseptic picture can also present in drug-induced meningitis [90]. This is particularly important in obstetric anaesthesia, because non-steroidal anti-inflammatory agents can induce aseptic meningitis, and these drugs are used commonly after both labour and operative delivery. Symptoms worsen with drug administration. Meningitis can also be induced by ranitidine, another drug commonly used before regional nerve block in obstetrics.

15.8.9 Accidental dural puncture

If accidental dural puncture occurs, the parturient should be told and the fact should be entered into her notes to assist appropriate follow-up and, if necessary, treatment.

A survey of the management of accidental dural puncture revealed considerable variation between maternity units in the United Kingdom [91]. In the majority, epidural catheters were re-sited, usually in an adjacent space. In a few units, a catheter was placed intrathecally and a subarachnoid technique was selected. There was a conflict of opinion as to whether or not second-stage of labour should be assisted. The insistence on an operative delivery without evidence that it protects against postdural puncture headache is irrational. The practice is based on the hypothesis that cerebrospinal fluid (CSF) leakage will increase with pushing. However, other tissue pressures change, and the overall differential pressure at the puncture site may not increase. A prospective randomized trial has shown that the incidence of headache was not influenced by preventing bearing down or by the method of delivery [92]. The placement of an epidural catheter intrathecally at the time of puncture can reduce the incidence of postdural puncture headache—although why this should be so is unclear.

Once delivery has occurred, prophylactic action is required by the mother and the anaesthetist designed to diminish the flow of cerebrospinal fluid and allow healing to occur (Table 15.9). An epidural infusion of 1000 mL of crystalloid solution in 24 hours can produce an increase in epidural and subarachnoid pressures that are associated with relief of the headache, but its efficacy has been disputed. The epidural catheter must be removed after this manoeuvre. It cannot be used for blood patch because of the risk of infection. It is possible that epidural crystalloid washes off any accumulated inflammatory reaction around the hole.

The major complication of accidental dural puncture is headache, and this is manifest once the woman tries to mobilize. For this reason, mobilization is often delayed for 24 hours, but there is no evidence that the incidence of

Table 15.9 Prophylaxis and symptomatic treatment for postdural puncture headache.

Epidural crystalloid infusion
Avoid constipation
Oral hydration (especially if breast feeding), including caffeine-containing drinks. Instant coffee or tea provides 30–40 mg caffeine/100 mL. Caffeine induces vasoconstriction, which may relieve the reflex vasodilation induced by reduced CSF pressure
Analgesia (mild, moderate, or strong)
Bed rest if headache occurs up to 24 h only (will delay onset of headache). Caution: thromboembolism, muscle or joint disorders

CSF, cerebrospinal fluid.

headache is reduced by such delay. Pathophysiologically, the headache is secondary to traction on pain-sensitive intracranial structures through a reduction in CSF. The lumbar CSF pressure increases from about 10 cmH$_2$O in the horizontal position to over 40 cmH$_2$O on sitting. Coupled to this is a lack of change of pressure in the epidural space, so that a pressure differential favours CSF leakage. Flow of CSF from the intrathecal to epidural space will depend on this pressure difference, the size of the hole in the dura and the rate of CSF production. In time, the hole naturally decreases in size, but this can take a week or more.

The dural hole can be sealed by an epidural blood patch. If carried out 24 hours or more after puncture, this procedure has a success rate of 85–95% [93]. During the waiting period of 24–48 hours, other symptomatic therapies can be tried, and a full discussion can be undertaken with the patient concerning the risks and benefits (Table 15.10). A headache is common after delivery, and a complete neurological history and examination should be performed to exclude other pathology. In particular, signs of infection should be sought, if necessary with a white cell count. The signs and symptoms characteristic of postdural puncture headache are listed in Table 15.11. These may occur after accidental dural puncture, or following spinal anaesthesia, or after

Risks
Backache (usually transient)
Recurrence of headache after variable period
Repeat blood patch (25%)
Epidural abscess (rare)
Radicular pain

Benefits
Complete abolition of headache
Mobilization
    Faster discharge
    Fetal–maternal bonding

Table 15.10 Risks and benefits of epidural blood patch of postdural puncture headache.

Table 15.11 Characteristics of postdural puncture headache.

Severe headache
   Frontal (from traction above the tentorium on the trigeminal nerve)
   Occipital (from traction below the tentorium)
Depressive reaction: tearful, miserable, bedridden
Dizziness (traction on vagus)
Nausea (traction on vagus)
Neckache (involvement of traction on upper cranial nerves)
Double vision (traction on 6th cranial nerve)
Auditory symptoms (acuity and tinnitus) (possible pressure changes between
   intracochlear fluid and CSF)
Severity increased by
   Upright position (abdominal compression in the sitting position can reduce or abolish
     headache and has been used as a diagnostic sign)
   Coughing
   Sudden movements of the head
Decreased by lying down

epidural anaesthesia when there is no clinical indication that the dura has been punctured.

The method used for epidural blood patch can be summarized as follows.

1 Asepsis:
maternal check: no fever, or leucocytosis;
carry out in an operating theatre.
Two anaesthetists scrubbed, capped, gowned and masked. Anaesthetist 1 prepares the patient's forearm with surgical preparation and drapes; anaesthetist 2 introduces the epidural needle with full aseptic precautions. Blood cultures sent at the time of withdrawal of blood.

2 20 mL × 2 venous blood samples taken by operator (1) and given to operator (2). Blood is slowly injected epidurally at the interspace of the dural puncture or the one below, until either the woman complains of backache or other discomfort or a total of 20 mL has been introduced [94]. The second (20 mL) is used for the blood cultures.

3 Remove blood from the shaft or the epidural needle before removing it, to reduce backache.

The woman will often want to mobilize quickly afterwards, but should be encouraged to do so gradually over the next 6 hours. Failure of the blood patch to relieve the headache may be caused by improper identification of the epidural space or an error in diagnosis. Although the headache may be relieved immediately, the action does not relate to a rapid production of CSF. The dural tear can take 48 hours to heal, and on magnetic resonance imaging studies of women after blood patch, the injected blood was observed to move mainly cephalad in the epidural space and to leak into subcutaneous tissues [95]. Clot retraction occurred by seven hours, leaving a thick layer of mature clot over the thecal sac. The mechanism for the rapidity of symptomatic relief is still not clear. It is usual to allow the woman home after a blood patch within hours, but with the caution that if the headache returns she is to report promptly to the labour ward for reassessment. Subdural haematoma presenting as a headache has been described after dural puncture [96]. If a woman requires epidural analgesia in a subsequent pregnancy, she can be reassured that having had an epidural blood patch is not a contraindication.

15.8.10 Total spinal block

This occurs rapidly within the first 30 minutes after epidural local anaesthetic injection. There is transmission of the epidural dose of local anaesthetic into the CSF. The condition usually presents as an acute emergency, with altered level of consciousness, hypotension, bradycardia, reduced or absent respiration and vasodilation with a reduction in central venous pressure. If management is immediate, the woman should come to no harm. Support for the respiratory and cardiovascular system is required until the local anaesthetic concentration decreases. If the fetus is *in utero*, immediate Caesarean section should be considered.

Management of total spinal block.
1. Left lateral position if the fetus is *in situ*.
2. Ventilate with 100% oxygen with a cuffed endotracheal tube.
3. Cardiac massage if carotid pulses absent.
4. Vasopressors: ephedrine 15 mg i.v.
5. Volume replacement with colloids, if possible.
6. Atropine 0.6 mg i.v. to treat bradycardia.

If hypotension persists, diagonists should be given and central venous pressure should be monitored to confirm and manage fluid balance.

References

1. *Anaesthetic Services for Obstetrics – A Plan for the Future*. Association of Anaesthetists of Great Britain and Ireland and Obstetric Anaesthetists Association; London, 1987.
2. *Recommended Minimum Standards for Obstetric Anaesthesia Services*. Obstetric Anaesthetists Association; London, 1995.
3. *Guidelines for Obstetric Anaesthesia Services*. Association of Anaesthetists of Great Britain and Ireland and The Obstetric Anaesthetists Association; London, 1988.
4. Brett PN, Parker PJ, Harrison AJ *et al.* Simulation of resistance forces acting on surgical needles. *Proc Inst Mech Eng* 1997; **211**: 335–47.
5. Narang VPS, Linter SPK. Failure of extradural blockade in obstetrics: a new hypothesis. *Br J Anaesth* 1988; **60**: 402–4.
6. Valentine SJ, Jarvis AP, Shutt LE. Comparative study of the effects of air or saline to identify the extradural space. *Br J Anaesth* 1991; **66**: 224–7.
7. Strupp M, Brandt T. Should one reinsert the stylet during lumbar puncture? *N Engl J Med* 1997; **336**: 1190.
8. Mihic DN. Post spinal headache and relationship of needle bevel to longitudinal dural fibres. *Reg Anesth* 1985; **10**: 76–81.

9. Norris MC, Leighton BL, De Simone CA. Needle bevel direction and headache after inadvertent dural puncture. *Anesthesiology* 1989; **70**: 729–31.
10. Ready LB, Couplin S, Haschke RH, Nessle M. Spinal needle determinants of rate of transdural fluid leak. *Anesth Analg* 1989; **69**: 457–60.
11. Usubiaga JE, Reis A Jr, Usubiaga LE. Epidural misplacement of catheters and mechanisms of unilateral blockade. *Anesthesiology* 1970; **32**: 158–61.
12. Sidhu MS, Asrani RV, Bassell GM. An unusual complication of extradural catheterisation in obstetric anaesthesia. *Br J Anaesth* 1983; **55**: 473–5.
13. Doughty A. Lumbar epidural analgesia: the pursuit of perfection. *Anaesthesia* 1975; **30**: 741–51.
14. Mourisse J, Geilen MJM, Hassenbos MAWM, Heystraten FMJ. Migration of thoracic epidural catheters: three methods for evaluation of catheter position in the thoracic epidural space. *Anaesthesia* 1989; **44**: 574–7.
15. Sanchez R, Acuna J, Rocha F. An analysis of the radiological visualisation of the catheters placed in the epidural space. *Br J Anaesth* 1967; **39**: 485–9.
16. Scott DB, Wilson J. Insertion of epidural catheters. *Anaesthesia* 1983; **38**: 1108–9.
17. Kumar CM, Dennison B, Lawlor PGP. Excessive dose requirements of local anaesthetic for epidural analgesia: how far should an epidural catheter be inserted? *Anaesthesia* 1985; **40**: 1100–2.
18. Moir DD, Willocks J. Epidural analgesia in British obstetrics. *Br J Anaesth* 1968; **40**: 129–38.
19. Verniquet AJW. Vessel puncture with epidural catheters. *Anaesthesia* 1980; **35**: 660–2.
20. Crawford JS. Observations on one thousand epidural blocks given in labour. In: Doughty A, ed. *Proceedings of the Symposium on Epidural Analgesia in Obstetrics, Kingston Hospital, Kingston upon Thames, 18 March 1971*. London: Lewis, 1972: 83–8.
21. McNeil MJ, Thorburn J. Cannulation of the epidural space. *Anaesthesia* 1988; **43**: 154–5.
22. Ravindra R, Albrecht W, McKay M. Apparent intravascular migration of epidural catheter. *Anesth Analg* 1979; **58**: 252–3.
23. Moore DC, Batra MS. The components of an effective test dose prior to epidural block. *Anesthesiology* 1981; **55**: 693–6.
24. Guinard JP, Mulroy MF, Carpenter RL, Knopes KD. Test doses: optimal epinephrine content with and without acute beta-adrenergic blockade. *Anesthesiology* 1990; **73**: 386–92.
25. Van Zundert A, Vaes L, Soetens M *et al*. Every dose given in epidural analgesia for vaginal delivery can be a test dose. *Anesthesiology* 1987; **67**: 436.
26. Chestnut DH, Owen CL, Brown CK, Vandewalker GE, Weiner CP. Does labour affect the variability of maternal heart rate during induction of epidural anesthesia? *Anesthesiology* 1988; **68**: 622–5.
27. Holdcroft A. Use of adrenaline in obstetric analgesia. *Anaesthesia* 1992; **47**: 987–90.
28. Bromage PR. A comparison of the hydrochloride and carbon dioxide salts of lidocaine and prilocaine in epidural analgesia. *Acta Anaesthesiol Scand Suppl* 1965; **55**: 55–69.
29. Li DF, Rees GAD, Rosen M. Continuous extradural infusion 0.0625% or 0.125% bupivacaine for pain relief in primigravid labour. *Br J Anaesth* 1985; **57**: 264–70.
30. Tunstall ME, Ramamoorthy C. Continuous epidural infusion with 0.08% of bupivacaine. *Anaesthesia* 1984; **39**: 939–40.
31. Yaksh TL, Wilson PR, Kaiko RF, Inturrisi CE. Analgesia produced by a spinal action of morphine and its effects upon parturition in the rat. *Anesthesiology* 1979; **51**: 386–92.
32. Jungstrom E, Eastwood D, Patel H *et al*. Epidural fentanyl and bupivacaine in labour: double-blind study. *Anesthesiology* 1984; **61**: A414.
33. Cowan ES, Tan S, Albright GA, Halpern J. Epidural fentanyl/bupivacaine mixtures for obstetric anaesthesia. *Anesthesiology* 1987; **67**: 403–7.

34 Chestnut DH, Owen CL, Bates JN et al. Continuous infusion epidural analgesia during labor: a randomized, double-blind comparison of 0.0625% bupivacaine/0.0002% fentanyl vs. 0.125% bupivacaine. *Anesthesiology* 1988; **68**: 754–9.

35 McGrady EM, Brownhill DK, Davis AG. Epidural diamorphine and bupivacaine in labour. *Anaesthesia* 1989; **44**: 400–3.

36 Jones G, Paul DL, Elton RA, McLure JH. Comparison of bupivacaine and bupivacaine with fentanyl in continuous extradural analgesic during labour. *Br J Anaesth* 1989; **63**: 254–9.

37 Ennever GR, Noble HA, Kolditz D, Valentine S, Thomas TA. Epidural infusion of diamorphine with bupivacaine in labour: a comparison with fentanyl and bupivacaine. *Anaesthesia* 1991; **46**: 169–73.

38 Noble HA, Ennever GR, Thomas TA. Epidural bupivacaine dilution for labour: a comparison of the three concentrations infused with a fixed dose of fentanyl. *Anaesthesia* 1991; **46**: 549–52.

39 Lowson SM, Eggars KA, Warwick JP, Moore WJ, Thomas TA. Epidural infusions of bupivacaine and diamorphine in labour. *Anaesthesia* 1995; **50**: 420–2.

40 Tuohy EB. Continuous spinal anesthesia: a new method of utilizing a ureteral catheter. *Surg Clin North Am* 1945; **25**: 834.

41 Curbelow MM. Continuous peridural segmental anesthesia by means of a ureteral catheter. *Curr Res Anesth Analg* 1949; **28**: 13–16.

42 Lee JA. Specially marked needle to facilitate extradural block. *Anaesthesia* 1960; **15**: 186.

43 Doughty A. A precise method of cannulating the lumbar epidural space. *Anaesthesia* 1974; **29**: 63–5.

44 Hart JR, Whitacre RJ. Pencil point needle in prevention of post-spinal headache. *JAMA*, 1951; **147**: 657–8.

45 Michael S, Richmond MN, Birks RJS. A comparison between open end and closed end epidural catheters: complications and quality of sensory blockade. *Anaesthesia* 1989; **44**: 578–80.

46 Columb MO, Lyons G. Determination of the minimum local analgesic concentrations of epidural bupivacaine and lidocaine in labor. *Anesth Analg* 1995; **81**: 833–7.

47 Capogna G, Celleno D, Lyons G, Columbo MO, Fusco P. Minimum local analgesic concentration of extradural bupivacaine increases with progression of labour. *Br J Anaesth* 1998; **80**: 11–13.

48 Scott DB, Leigh A, Fagan D et al. Acute toxicity of ropivacaine compared with that of bupivacaine. *Anesth Analg* 1989; **69**: 563–9.

49 Rutten AJ, Nancarrow C, Mather LE et al. Hemodynamic and central nervous system effects of lidocaine, bupivacaine and ropivacaine in sheep. *Anesth Analg* 1989; **69**: 291–9.

50 Katz JA, Bridenbaugh PO, Knarr DC, Helton SH, Denson DD. Pharmacodynamics and pharmacokinetics of extradural ropivacaine in humans. *Anesth Analg* 1990; **70**: 16–21.

51 McCrae AF, Westerling P, McClure JH. Pharmacokinetic and clinical study of ropivacaine and bupivacaine in women receiving extradural analgesia in labour. *Br J Anaesth* 1997; **79**: 558–62.

52 Brown DL, Carpenter RL, Thompson GE. Comparison of 0.5% ropivacaine and 0.5% bupivacaine for extradural anesthesia in patients undergoing lower extremity surgery. *Anesthesiology* 1990; **72**: 633–6.

53 Brockway MS, Bannister J, McClure JH, McKeown D, Wildsmith JAW. Comparison of extradural ropivacaine and bupivacaine. *Br J Anaesth* 1991; **66**: 31–7.

54 McCrae AF, Joswiak H, McClure JH. Comparison of ropivacaine and bupivacaine in extradural analgesia for the relief of pain in labour. *Br J Anaesth* 1994; **74**: 261–5.

55 Stienstra R, Jonker TA, Boudrez P et al. Ropivacaine 0.25% versus bupivacaine 0.25% for continuous extradural analgesia in labor: a double-blind comparison. *Anesth Analg* 1995; **80**: 285–9.

56 Moore A, Bullingham R, McQuay H et al. Spinal fluid kinetics of morphine and heroin. *Clin Pharmacol Ther* 1984; **35**: 40–5.
57 Kelly MC, Carabine UA, Mirakhur RK. Intrathecal diamorphine for analgesia after Caesarean section: a dose-finding study and assessment of side effects. *Anaesthesia* 1998; **53**: 231–7.
58 Ray N, Datta S, Jolson MD et al. Low dose alfentanil v. fentanyl with bupivacaine for continuous epidural infusion for labor. *Anesthesiology* 1990: **73**.
59 Van Steenburg A, de Broux HC, Noorduin H. Extradural bupivacaine with sufentanil for vaginal delivery: a double-blind trial. *Br J Anaesth* 1987; **59**: 1518–22.
60 Vertommen J, Van der Meulen E, Vanneken H et al. The effects of the addition of sufentanil to 0.125% bupivacaine on the quality of analgesia during labor and on the incidence of instrumental deliveries. *Anesthesiology* 1991; **74**: 809–14.
61 Scott DB, Walker LR. Administration of continuous epidural analgesia. *Anaesthesia* 1963; **18**: 82–3.
62 Power I, Brown DT, Wildsmith JA. The effect of fentanyl, meperidine and diamorphine on nerve conduction *in vitro*. *Reg Anesth* 1991; 16: 204–8.
63 Brull SJ, Greene NM. Zones of differential sensory block during extradural anaesthesia. *Br J Anaesth* 1991; **66**: 651–5.
64 Fernando R, Bonello-Gill P, Urquhart J, Reynolds F, Morgan B. Neonatal welfare and placental transfer of fentanyl and bupivacaine during ambulatory combined spinal–epidural analgesia for labour. *Anaesthesia* 1997; **52**: 517–24.
65 Difazio CA, Carron H, Grossleit KR et al. Comparison of pH-adjusted lidocaine solutions for epidural anesthesia. *Anesth Analg* 1986; **65**: 760–4.
66 Gaggero G, Meyer O, Van Gessel E, Kaplan R. Alkalinisation of lidocaine 2% does not influence the quality of epidural anaesthesia for elective Caesarean section. *Can J Anaesth* 1995; **42**: 1080–4.
67 Liepert DJ, Douglas MJ, McMorland GH et al. Comparison of lidocaine CO_2, two per cent lidocaine hydrochloride and pH-adjusted lidocaine hydrochloride for Caesarean section anaesthesia. *Can J Anaesth* 1990; **37**: 333–6.
68 McMorland GH, Douglas MJ, Axelson JE et al. The effect of pH adjustment of bupivacaine on onset and duration of epidural anaesthesia for Caesarean section. *Can J Anaesth* 1988; **35**: 457–61.
69 Benhamon D, Labaille T, Bonhomme L, Perrachon N. Alkalinization of epidural 0.5% bupivacaine for Cesarean section. *Reg Anesth* 1989; **14**: 240–3.
70 Verbough C, Claes MA, Camu F. Onset of epidural blockade after plain or alkalinized 0.5% bupivacaine. *Anesth Analg* 1991; **73**: 401–4.
71 Howell P, Wrigley M, Tan P, Davies W, Morgan BM. Are two better than one? A preliminary assessment of an epidural mixture of lignocaine and bupivacaine for elective Caesarean section. In: Reynolds FM, ed. *Epidural and Spinal Blockade in Obstetrics*. London: Baillière Tindall, 1990.
72 Cox CR, Faccenda KA, Gilhooly C et al. Extradural *S*(–)-bupivacaine: comparison with racemic *RS*-bupivacaine. *Br J Anaesth* 1998; **80**: 289–93.
73 Burm AGL, Van der Meer AD, van Kleef JW et al. Pharmacokinetics of the enantiomers of bupivacaine following intravenous administration of the racemate. *Br J Clin Pharmacol* 1994; **38**: 125–9.
74 Laishley RS, Morgan B. A single dose epidural technique for Caesarean section. *Anaesthesia* 1988; **43**: 100–3.
75 Thorburn J, Moir DD. Epidural analgesia for elective Caesarean section: technique and its assessment. *Anaesthesia* 1980; **35**: 3–6.
76 Wollman SB, Marx GF. Acute hydration for prevention of the hypotension of spinal anesthesia in parturients. *Anesthesiology* 1968; **29**: 374–6.
77 Murray AM, Morgan M, Whitwam JG. Crystalloid versus colloid for circulatory preload for epidural Caesarean section. *Anaesthesia* 1989; **44**: 463–70.

78 Barker AEJ. A report on clinical experiences with spinal anaesthesia in 100 cases. *Br Med J* 1907; **i**: 665–74.
79 Atkinson RS, Rushman GB, Davies NJH. *Lee's Synopsis of Anaesthesia*, II edn. Oxford: Butterworth Heinemann International 1993: 692.
80 Skilton RW, Kinsella SM, Thomas TA. Subarachnoid diamorphine for Caesarean section: a dose-finding study. *Int J Obs Anesth* 1999 (in press).
81 Kelly MC, Carabine UA, Mirakhur RK. Intrathecal diamorphine for analgesia after Caesarean section: a dose-finding study and assessment of side effects. *Anaesthesia* 1998; **53**: 231–7.
82 Russell IF, Holmqvist EL. Subarachnoid analgesia for Caesarean section: a double-blind comparison of plain and hyperbaric 0.5% bupivacaine. *Br J Anaesth* 1987; 59: 347–53.
83 Collis RE, Davies DW, Aveling W. Randomised comparison of combined spinal–epidural and standard epidural analgesia in labour. *Lancet* 1995; **345**: 1413–16.
84 Nageotte MP, Larson D, Rumney PJ, Sidhu M, Hollenbach K. Epidural analgesia compared with combined spinal–epidural analgesia during labor in nulliparous women. *N Engl J Med* 1997; **337**: 1715–19.
85 Bonhemad B, Donnas M, Mercier FJ, Benhomon D. Bacterial meningitis following combined spinal–epidural analgesia for labour. *Anaesthesia* 1998; **53**: 290–5.
86 Hoffman VLH, Vercauteren MP, Buczkowski PW, Vanspringel GLJ. A new combined spinal–epidural apparatus: measurement of the distance to the epidural and subarachnoid spaces. *Anaesthesia* 1997; **52**: 350–5.
87 Norris M, Ryan C, Fogel ST, Holtmann B. Intrathecal sufentanil increases end-tidal CO_2 in laboring women. *Anesthesiology* 1997; **87**: A885.
88 Harding SA, Collis RE, Morgan BM. Meningitis after combined spinal–extradural anaesthesia in obstetrics. *Br J Anaesth* 1994; **73**: 545–7.
89 Burke D, Wildsmith JAW. Meningitis after spinal anaesthesia. *Br J Anaesth* 1997; **78**: 635–6.
90 Marinac JS. Drug and chemical induced meningitis: a review of the literature. *Ann Pharmacol* 1992; **26**: 813–21.
91 Sajjad T, Ryan TDR. Current management of inadvertent dural taps occurring during the siting of epidurals for pain relief in labour: a survey of maternity units in the United Kingdom. *Anaesthesia* 1995; **50**: 156–61.
92 Ravindran RS, Viegas OJ, Tasch MD *et al.* Bearing down at the time of delivery and the incidence of spinal headache in parturients. *Anesth Analg* 1981; **60**: 524–6.
93 Loeser EA, Hill GE, Bennett GM, Sederberg JH. Time vs. success rate for epidural blood patch. *Anesthesiology* 1978; **49**: 147–8.
94 Szeinfeld M, Ihmeidan IH, Moser MM *et al.* Epidural blood patch: evaluation of the volume and spread of blood injected into the epidural space. *Anesthesiology* 1986; **64**: 820–2.
95 Beards SC, Jackson A, Griffiths AG, Horsman EL. Magnetic resonance imaging of extradural blood patches: appearances from 30 minutes to 18 hours. *Br J Anaesth* 1993; **71**: 182–8.
96 Whiteley SM, Murphy PG, Kirolloir RW, Swindells SR. Headache after dural puncture. *Br Med J* 1993; **306**: 917–18.

Section 4
General Anaesthesia

16: Anaesthesia for Caesarean Section

The aims of general anaesthesia for Caesarean section are to produce unconsciousness reliably, while reducing adverse changes in the mother and fetus until delivery. Short-lasting, subtle changes in the neonate can be detected following general anaesthesia [1,2]. However, careful control of anaesthesia will result in a vigorous baby and will enable the mother to start fulfilling her maternal role comfortably in as short a time as possible after surgery.

16.1 Indications for general anaesthesia

General anaesthesia is not usually the preferred method of anaesthesia for operative intervention in the pregnant patient, as it is one of the major causes of maternal morbidity and mortality. In the United Kingdom from 1982 to 1993 [3–6] there were 35 deaths related to general anaesthesia and four related to regional anaesthesia in parturients (Fig. 2.1, p. 24). In contrast, in the United States of America, out of 129 maternal deaths for the period 1979–90, 67 (52%) were associated with general anaesthesia (in which airway problems predominated) and 33 (26%) associated with regional analgesia, death in most of the latter cases being from the effects of high spinal anaesthesia [7]. Thus, the underlying risk of mortality from general anaesthesia predominates in both British and American statistics, and specific indications should be present to justify its use (Table 16.1).

Emergency general anaesthesia has been shown to be particularly hazardous for pregnant women. It is less likely to be needed when parturients have a working epidural catheter *in situ* during their labour. Regular assessment of women on the labour ward will help to identify risk factors for emergency intervention [8]. Occasionally, patients with obvious risk factors for general anaesthesia may also have contraindications for regional anaesthesia. The presence of coagulopathy due to pre-eclampsia in a patient with a history of failed intubation is an obvious example. The risks involved should be communicated to the parturient, together with the planned method of anaesthesia. Awake fibre-optic intubation may be the only safe option, and specialist consultant obstetric units should have access to both the equipment and the expertise that will be required in these very rare patients.

General anaesthesia is usually considered to be the method of choice in parturients with cardiovascular disorders, with systemic effects that arise from a high pressure gradient across a stenotic mitral or aortic valve. Regional techniques inevitably lead to sympathetic blockade, which in such cases may induce acute decreases in blood pressure and cardiac decompensation. The

Table 16.1 Indications for general anaesthesia at Caesarean section.

Woman refused regional anaesthesia
Woman is unable to co-operate (e.g. alteration of consciousness)
Failed regional anaesthesia (epidural and/or subarachnoid)
Regional anaesthesia is contraindicated in:
    Hypovolaemia and hypotension
    Coagulopathy
    Infection: generalized septicaemia; local infection at lumbar site
    Cardiovascular disorders with high risk factors for regional anaesthesia,
       e.g. tight aortic stenosis
    Allergy to local anaesthetic agents
Inadequate time for preparation of regional anaesthesia, e.g. prolapsed cord with
   fetal heart rate decelerations
When further surgery is planned immediately after the Caesarean section, e.g. removal
   of tumour
Rare neurological disorders with the potential for exacerbation, e.g. haemangioma
High risk of postoperative intermittent positive-pressure ventilation of the lungs and
   intensive care

---

pathophysiology is described in Section 3.3, p. 46 onwards. These women should be identified early in their pregnancy, and detailed preoperative discussions must be held between the obstetric anaesthetist, the cardiologist and the obstetrician responsible for the patient. The multidisciplinary team approach should be pursued in order to arrange the lowest-risk management of all three areas of care. If it is not possible to put such a team together, the patient should be referred to a specialist unit in which the appropriate expertise and team attitudes are available. The presence of cardiac dysrhythmias, such as intermittent atrial fibrillation or paroxysmal ventricular tachycardia, may also demand the use of general anaesthesia, which will allow prompt cardioversion to be performed when needed [9].

General anaesthesia is also indicated when postoperative ventilation of the lungs in an intensive-care unit is a likely sequel to Caesarean section. Parturients presenting with severe pre-eclampsia may develop multiorgan failure and are at considerable risk of developing pulmonary oedema or acute respiratory distress syndrome. The timing and place of delivery, together with the personnel to be involved, should be planned as carefully as possible and preferably close to the intensive-care unit chosen for the parturient's care following delivery.

The presence of acute neurological deficits or lesions of unknown cause will almost always preclude the use of regional anaesthetic techniques. General anaesthesia is probably indicated for both elective and emergency delivery until a firm diagnosis has been made. Chronic neurological lesions, on the other hand, present the anaesthetist and the mother with a difficult decision. The neurological deficits should be fully assessed prior to any decision about which method of anaesthesia is preferable. The risks of both regional and general anaesthesia should be discussed with the patient.

16.2 Preparation for general anaesthesia

The conduct of general anaesthesia involves a sequence of events as listed in Table 16.2 whether or not surgery is urgent. General anaesthesia administered to the parturient once gestation has passed 18–20 weeks will require the parturient to be protected against physiological changes such as inferior vena caval occlusion and gastrointestinal effects. It will usually follow a set pattern of securing intravenous access, attaching a full range of monitoring, preoxygenation, rapid-sequence induction of anaesthesia, endotracheal intubation, intermittent positive-pressure ventilation, and reversal of muscle relaxant and anaesthesia when surgery is complete.

Certain minimum requirements or standards must be met whenever general anaesthesia is to be administered. Any unit in which general anaesthesia is administered must provide the equipment, staff and facilities outlined in Chapter 1. Obstetric units that fail to meet these criteria are offering substandard care. The only excuse for general anaesthesia being initiated in such units would be a sudden, and totally unexpected, onset of life-threatening events, e.g. the occurrence of a major antepartum haemorrhage during an antenatal consultation in a satellite outpatient clinic. Even in such circumstances, it would usually be considered prudent to transfer the patient urgently to a properly equipped hospital unless the threat to the patient's life was great.

The criteria discussed in Chapter 1 are adequate for most obstetric general anaesthetics. Many obstetric theatres are staffed by midwives who are not trained to assist the anaesthetist or to 'scrub' for non-obstetric operative surgery. Skilled anaesthetic assistance must be available throughout obstetric or non-obstetric procedures in pregnant women, and properly trained and supervised recovery room staff must care for the parturient until she has fully recovered from her anaesthesia. Induction of general anaesthesia in the pregnant patient

Table 16.2 Essential aspects of general anaesthesia.

Preoperative evaluation
Discussion of risks
Aspiration prophylaxis (see Chapter 5, Section 5.5, p. 91 onwards)
Intravenous cannulation (with 14-gauge cannula)
Patient positioning—either lateral tilt or the full lateral position should be maintained whilst transferring to theatre and throughout surgery until the fetus is delivered
Monitoring
Rapid-sequence induction
Anaesthetic record
Recovery
Postoperative pain relief

Table 16.3 The minimum monitoring set for general anaesthesia. Clinical monitoring requires the presence of a trained anaesthetist at all times.

Electrocardiograph
Non-invasive blood-pressure machine with an automatic one-minute cycle
Pulse oximeter
Capnograph
Volatile agent monitor
Fresh gas oxygen monitor
Ventilation pressures and volumes monitor(s)
Disconnection alarm
Peripheral nerve stimulator
Temperature probe

---

is a particularly difficult and stressful time. The checking and application of the relevant anaesthetic, cardiovascular and respiratory monitoring (Table 16.3) should be complete before induction. The trained anaesthetic assistant may be fully occupied applying cricoid pressure when the anaesthetist requires an additional pair of hands to assist with intubation and the institution of intermittent positive-pressure ventilation. Most obstetric units lack both the facilities and the staff necessary for anaesthetizing medically complicated patients who require invasive monitoring and complex non-obstetric surgical interventions. The complex, high-risk patient is usually at less risk if anaesthetized in a general or specialist theatre near an intensive-care unit with specialist surgical assistance available.

Preparations for the rapid induction of general anaesthesia should always be in hand on a labour suite. In particular, it should be routine practice for all consultant units to have a complete set of anaesthetic equipment and drugs available for immediate use. The drugs (see below) should be drawn up and labelled with the name of the drug, its concentration and the time of preparation. This set of drugs is best kept in a refrigerator within the obstetric theatre complex. Sufficient anaesthetic equipment should be prepared and laid out to allow an immediate start and thereafter maintenance of general anaesthesia. The anaesthetist responsible for labour-ward care for that day must ensure drug and equipment availability and carry out the necessary checks of equipment function at the start of the day. These checks should not be delegated to a non-medical deputy.

The drugs to be drawn up on a daily basis are:
- thiopental;
- suxamethonium;
- atropine;
- atracurium;
- ephedrine;
- oxytocin (this may be confused with suxamethonium in an emergency, because the syringe size used is often the same; careful labelling is essential to avoid such a hazard).

16.2.1 Preoperative evaluation

The patient's medical and obstetric history must be obtained. The respiratory and cardiovascular system should be examined, with particular reference to potential difficulty with intubation, venous access or medical complications. Investigations that should be available include a full blood count, blood grouping and a sickle-cell test if indicated. The drug and allergy history should include questions about recreational agents, smoking and alcohol ingestion. It is important to ask whether the patient or her family have had any anaesthetic problems previously. Much of this information can be obtained by asking the patient to complete a simple questionnaire, which can be part of the anaesthetic record (Table 16.4).

It should be assumed that any drug given to the mother will, to some extent, transfer through the placenta to the fetus. Anxiolytics can have significant fetal depressant effects, and no preoperative medication is therefore given except what is necessary to provide aspiration prophylaxis and to maintain therapeutic requirements for medical or obstetric complications and prophylactic antibiotics, if necessary.

16.2.2 Risk information

A mother should receive sufficient information about a procedure and have time to discuss the risks involved before giving consent, except in case of dire emergency. A consensus of 523 British obstetric anaesthetists [10] considered the main risks of general anaesthesia to be pulmonary aspiration, deep vein thrombosis and postoperative pain. About half of these anaesthetists would also discuss awareness and blood pressure changes. Most anaesthetists would not mention backache, headache, hypoxia or one-lung ventilation. The majority of a smaller sample of 75 obstetric anaesthetists in the United Kingdom [11] would describe the risks of aspiration, but other aspects of general anaesthesia—such as maternal sedation, dental trauma, risk of awareness and the effect of drugs on the fetus—would only be discussed by 30–50%. This smaller study compared United Kingdom anaesthetists with a similar group in the United States.

More information on general anaesthesia was being provided by the American obstetric anaesthetists. This may be related to patient requests for more information, a pattern that may emerge in the United Kingdom. The anaesthetist must be fully aware of the risks involved with the procedure in order to brief the mother accurately. A written summary of the discussion should be made in the patient's notes, or on the anaesthetic chart if it is routinely filed in the notes. It seems likely that some form of written patient information will eventually be needed, but regular updating of any such information would be required.

Even in an emergency, it is necessary to record at some stage the information that has been given to a patient. Advance consent implies that sufficient

Table 16.4 Preoperative assessment questionnaire.

1	Do you bring up phlegm from your chest	Yes/No
	(a) Now?	Yes/No
	(b) At regular intervals during the year?	Yes/No
2	Does your chest ever sound wheezy?	Yes/No
3	Do you get more short of breath than other people of your own age:	
	(a) When climbing hills/stairs?	Yes/No
	(b) When walking on level ground?	Yes/No
4	Have you ever had pain or discomfort in your chest	
	(a) When you exercise or hurry?	Yes/No
	(b) Does it disappear on resting?	Yes/No
5	Are you or your parents of Afro-Caribbean or East Mediterranean origin?	Yes/No
	If *yes*, have you had a sickle cell test?	Yes/No
6	Do you smoke?	Yes/No
	If *yes*, how much?	
7	Do you drink alcohol?	Yes/No
	If *yes*, how much?	
	Have you had or do you suffer from:	
8	Heart trouble	Yes/No
9	High blood pressure	Yes/No
10	Asthma/bronchitis	Yes/No
11	Heartburn/indigestion/hiatus hernia	Yes/No
12	Jaundice/liver disease	Yes/No
13	Kidney disease	Yes/No
14	Diabetes	Yes/No
15	Thyroid disorder	Yes/No
16	Bleeding tendency	Yes/No
17	Thrombosis (blood clots)	Yes/No
18	Severe anxiety/depression	Yes/No
19	Blackouts/epilepsy/convulsions	Yes/No
20	Sciatica/back trouble	Yes/No
21	Neck/jaw problems	Yes/No
22	Are you allergic to anything?	Yes/No
	If *yes*, what?	
23	Has any member of your family had a serious problem with an anaesthetic?	Yes/No
24	Have you taken any drugs or medicines within the last 3 months?	Yes/No
	If *yes*, please list:	
25	Do you have any loose, capped, crowned or false teeth?	Yes/No
26	Have you had any previous anaesthetics or operations?	Yes/No
	If *yes*, please list:	
27	Is there anything you would like to discuss with your anaesthetist?	Yes/No

information has been given to the patient to allow her to decide whether or not she is willing to receive an anaesthetic. Then, if the circumstances of labour or an emergency should require a general anaesthetic, the patient's choice will have been established and confirmation should be all that is necessary [12].

16.2.3 Provision of monitoring

The full range of minimum monitoring for the mother defined by professional bodies in the United Kingdom, the United States and Australia [13–16] must be available for all obstetric general anaesthetic procedures, as it is for anaesthesia for all forms of surgery. The minimum requirements are listed in Table 16.3. However, additional forms of monitoring, such as invasive intra-arterial and central venous pressure monitoring, should be available and should be used whenever maternal medical or obstetric complications develop that indicate it. The fetal heart rate should also be measured prior to induction of anaesthesia and commencement of surgery. In an emergency, induction may need to proceed simultaneously.

Some aspects of pregnancy, obstetrics and obstetric anaesthesia can affect measured values and ranges detected by monitors. These variations from non-pregnant values must be remembered if correct interpretation of monitoring systems is to be ensured. Changes relating to obstetrics are summarized systematically below.

Capnography

It is especially important to connect the capnograph to confirm the position of the endotracheal tube in parturients, because oesophageal placement has been a significant cause of maternal death. The adequacy of ventilation must also be confirmed, because the normal pregnant woman at term has a lower arterial carbon dioxide tension (Pa_{CO_2}) than the non-pregnant adult. This is reflected in reduced end-tidal CO_2 values of 4.3 kPa (32–33 mmHg), which should be maintained during general anaesthesia at least until the fetus is delivered.

Electrocardiogram

Although S–T segment changes have been reported at Caesarean section with general or regional anaesthesia, they have not been accompanied by evidence of significant myocardial ischaemia on echocardiography [17,18]. The changes have been associated with higher heart rates. High spinal anaesthesia may block the cardiac sympathetic innervation and prevent tachycardias, but in a study using continuous electrocardiogram monitoring in which a sensory level of T6 was achieved, there were brief but clinically insignificant S–T segment changes [19].

Pulse oximeter

Desaturation has been associated with venous air embolism during Caesarean section [20] with both epidural and general anaesthesia. The embolic phenomenon can be diagnosed by precordial ultrasound Doppler monitoring, and can be prevented by a slight head-up tilt. It occurs between uterine incision and delivery, and is less common with general anaesthesia [21] because intermittent positive-pressure ventilation increases venous and intrathoracic pressures.

Nerve stimulator

The assessment of neural blockade at the end of a general anaesthetic for Caesarean section is important, because pregnancy can change the individual's response to both depolarizing and non-depolarizing muscle relaxants. When evaluating recovery from neuromuscular blockade, a train-of-four ratio between the height of the first and fourth twitch of > 0.7 should be achieved, together with a head lift of five seconds before extubation is performed [22]. A number of maternal deaths have occurred because these simple criteria have not been applied.

Agent monitor

Awareness is probably more common during general anaesthesia for Caesarean section than other surgery, and knowledge of expired concentrations of volatile anaesthetic agent can help to prevent this terrifying possibility. Maintenance of end-tidal concentrations at approximately minimum alveolar concentration (MAC) for the chosen agent from the beginning of anaesthesia will make awareness unlikely and will reduce the chance of uterine relaxation. MAC levels for volatile anaesthetic agents are affected by pregnancy and vary during the course of Caesarean section, decreasing markedly once the post-delivery dose of opioid has been given.

16.3 Preoxygenation

One of the safety features of a rapid-sequence induction is the avoidance of positive-pressure inflation of the lungs before intubation. Pressurization of gas in the airway may move air along the oesophagus and into the stomach, especially if there is difficulty maintaining a patent airway. Gas in the stomach may force stomach contents back along the oesophagus, so that regurgitation occurs.

The goal of preoxygenation is to fill the alveoli and air passages with 100% oxygen and to achieve a high P_{AO_2}. A reservoir of oxygen is produced that will prevent hypoxaemia and make manual ventilation of the lungs unnecessary in the period of apnoea during rapid-sequence induction of general anaesthesia and tracheal intubation. The reservoir is created by breathing 100% oxygen from an anaesthetic breathing system. The face mask must be closely applied to the face to achieve an airtight seal and guarantee 100% oxygen concentration. Parturients are often unable to achieve the appropriate seal, and better preoxygenation can be secured if the anaesthetist holds the face mask.

Nitrogen is gradually replaced by oxygen (nitrogen washout) in the air passages. The time taken for complete nitrogen washout is considerable, but sufficient washout in the non-pregnant state is achieved with three minutes' tidal breathing of 100% oxygen to allow several minutes of apnoea to occur without signs of peripheral oxygen desaturation. However, the rate of nitrogen washout and the duration of apnoea without hypoxaemia are both affected by changes during pregnancy. The nitrogen washout rate is faster, because the functional residual capacity is reduced, improving ventilation and mixing of gases. More importantly, the size of the oxygen reservoir is reduced, and together with the increased oxygen consumption of pregnancy this leads to more rapid apnoeic desaturation [23]. The net effect in the parturient is therefore that three minutes' tidal breathing will only give about 60 seconds of apnoea without hypoxaemia. If there is a grave obstetric emergency, four vital capacity breaths may achieve high Pa_{O_2} levels and be adequate [24] in such difficult situations.

16.4 Rapid-sequence induction

Induction of anaesthesia is performed, after preoxygenation, in such a way as to guard against regurgitation and aspiration of gastric contents. Intravenous injection of the anaesthetic agent is followed, just before consciousness is lost, by the application of cricoid pressure and by the intravenous injection of the rapidly acting depolarizing muscle relaxant suxamethonium. Endotracheal intubation should then be performed. It is important to wait until muscle relaxation has occurred before attempting intubation. Pre-empting the relaxant's action will lead to difficulty or failure of intubation, with all the attendant risks. Waiting for good relaxation can be a very stressful period, especially for inexperienced anaesthetists. No attempt should be made to ventilate the patient via the face mask during this time, and the 30–45-second wait is best used in ensuring that the head and neck are still in the optimum position with the neck flexed on the thorax and the head extended on the neck.

Intubation is often made easier by the routine use of a lubricated guide wire inside a tracheal tube or bougie, either through a tracheal tube or alone (in which case the tracheal tube can be threaded onto it once the bougie has entered the trachea). The use of a bougie alone may enable a clicking sensation to be felt on tracheal placement. Whether a gum elastic bougie, a Portex guide wire (incorporating a protective plastic coat), or some other device is chosen is a matter of personal preference. Whichever is used, it should be readily available, the anaesthetist should be familiar with it, and the anaesthetic assistant should place it into the anaesthetist's hand so that the latter need not lose concentration on the laryngoscopy.

Once the endotracheal tube has been passed and its cuff inflated, the intra-tracheal position of the tube must be confirmed. Detection of end-tidal carbon dioxide in the expired gases of six consecutive breaths is the most reliable method of confirming the endotracheal tube's position. Auscultation should be performed to exclude or detect unilateral placement in a bronchus. When success is confirmed and the cuff on the endotracheal tube is inflated sufficiently to exclude leaks and seal the airway, then—and only then—may the cricoid pressure be released.

16.5 Cricoid pressure

16.5.1 Technique

The cricoid cartilage is the only cartilage in the upper airway to form a complete ring. Cricoid pressure is a backward pressure on this cartilage, with the head extended on the neck. The pressure occludes the oesophagus by pinching it between the ring of the cricoid in front and vertebral bodies behind, and thus prevents regurgitation [25]. It is a manoeuvre that is performed only at the induction of anaesthesia. However, regurgitation can also occur on recovery from anaesthesia, when the ability of cricoid pressure to prevent aspiration is limited. Its usefulness has been called into question [26], as the technique is not always performed to a standard that ensures effective pressure [27], and incorrect timing has occurred [28]. These are issues concerning the quality of practice and training rather than the method itself, which has been shown to prevent regurgitation. It is not usually an anaesthetist who administers cricoid pressure during general anaesthesia for Caesarean section, so the correct technical standard has to be taught and practised both by anaesthetists and by their assistants. The difficulties are summarized in Table 16.5.

In the fully conscious patient, control over regurgitation of material refluxed into the oesophagus is achieved by closing the upper oesophageal sphincter, which is formed from the cricopharyngeus muscle and is under voluntary control (i.e. striated muscle). The normal resting pressure of the upper oesophageal sphincter (UOS) is about 40 mmHg. It can decrease to a mean of 8 mmHg during sleep (Fig. 16.1) [29–38]. After thiopental administration, just before loss of consciousness the UOS pressure decreases to less than 10 mmHg, at a time when protective laryngeal cough reflexes have been

Table 16.5 Difficulties experienced in using cricoid pressure.

General
Difficult to monitor
May be applied inaccurately
Can contribute to difficult intubation
Can contribute to oesophageal rupture

Two-handed
Requires two assistants, one dedicated to cricoid pressure

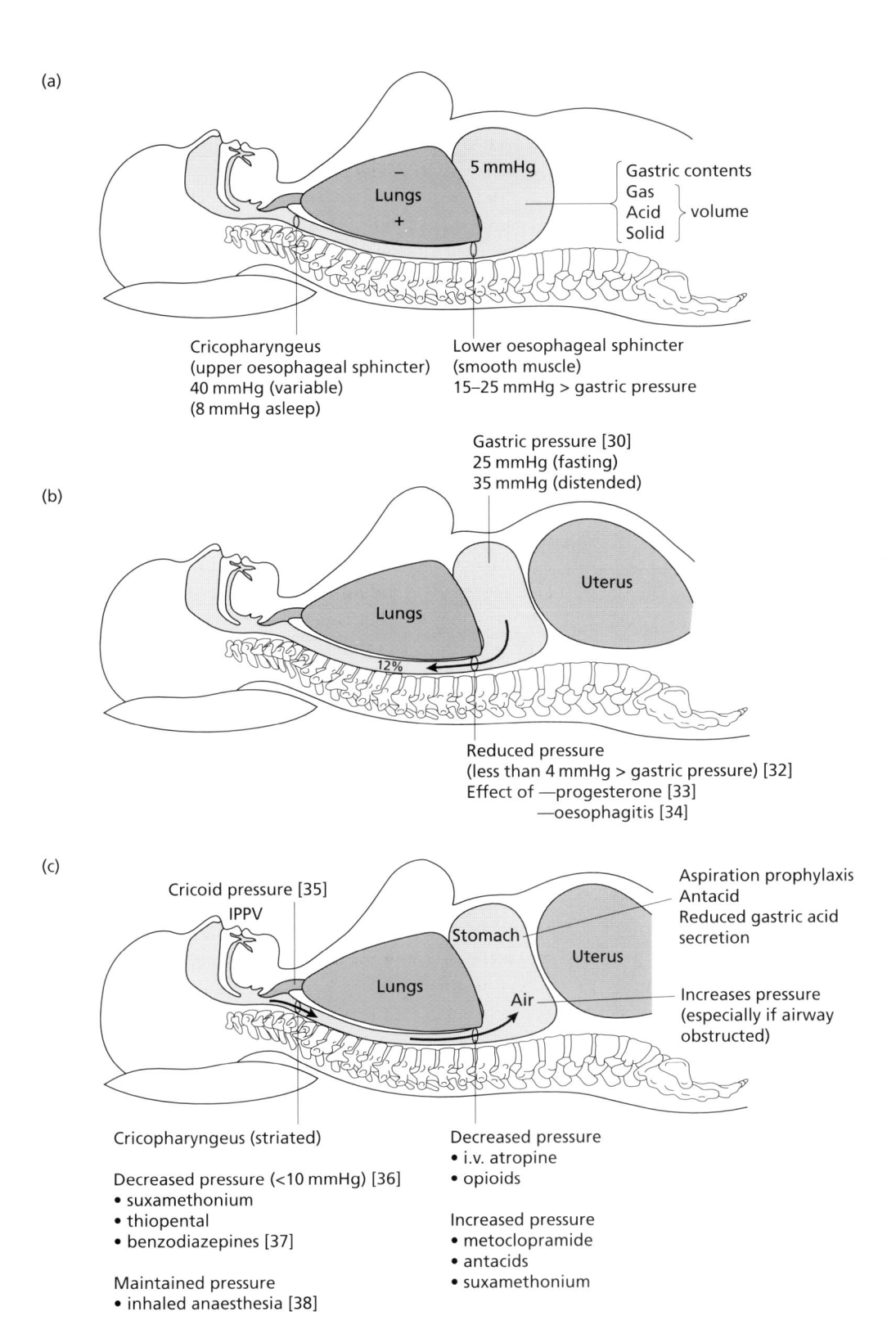

Fig. 16.1 Factors affecting regurgitation. (a) Normal conditions. (b) Passive movement of gastric secretions (regurgitation) at term occurs in 12% of awake women [2]. (c) Effect of anaesthetics on the mechanisms of regurgitation. IPPV, intermittent positive pressure ventilation.

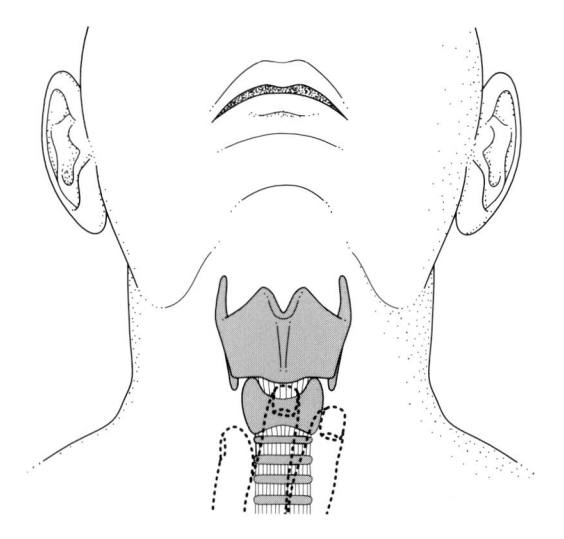

Fig. 16.2 The correct placement of the hands and fingers during cricoid pressure.

abolished. Regurgitation will occur when the UOS pressure decreases below the pressure of the oesophageal contents. A cricoid 'pressure' of 20 N (9.81 N = 1 kg = 2.2 lb) has been shown to prevent the regurgitation of oesophageal contents with a pressure of 25 mmHg in cadavers. When the oesophageal pressure was increased to 40 mmHg, a cricoid pressure of 30 N prevented passage of the material into the pharynx [39]. The correct amount of force to be applied for effective cricoid pressure is said to be 30 N (3 kg, or 6.6 lb). The digital sensation of applying this force can be mimicked by pressing on weighing scales to produce a reading of 3 kg. Cricoid pressure should be applied just before consciousness is lost, and should be maintained until tracheal placement of the endotracheal tube is confirmed and the cuff has been inflated. This is an important concept to stress when training supporting staff.

Staff must also be taught to identify the cricoid cartilage accurately. It is common for some part of the thyroid cartilage to be mistaken for the cricoid. Pressure will then be applied at too high a point in the neck, making intubation very difficult or impossible. The easiest and best way of identifying the cricoid cartilage is as follows:

1 position the patient with neck flexed on the thorax and head extended on the neck;
2 palpate the sternal notch;
3 keeping the palpating finger in the midline, move it cephalad until the first hard tracheal bump is felt. This is the cricoid cartilage;
4 confirmation of the cartilage can be achieved by moving the finger a few millimetres cephalad, where the cricothyroid gap/membrane can be felt as a small depression between the lower cricoid and higher thyroid cartilages.

The other aspect of cricoid pressure is the correct positioning of the hands and fingers. The original manoeuvre was described with one hand, as shown in Fig. 16.2. The use of two hands has been recommended [40] to prevent the head flexing on the neck during cricoid pressure. One hand is positioned comfortably behind the neck to maintain neck flexion and head extension. Three digits of the other hand are required, usually the thumb and first and second fingers—two to maintain the trachea in the midline and one finger to exert the force (Fig. 16.2). If an adequate neck support is provided, one-handed cricoid pressure should not distort the anatomical position required to achieve intubation.

Cricoid pressure should only be released when the airway is sealed by expanding the tracheal tube cuff and checking that a leak does not occur, or else when active vomiting occurs. In the latter circumstance, the vomitus will be under high pressure and can cause oesophageal rupture [41].

16.5.2 Complications (see Table 16.5, p. 294)

It was originally recommended that a cricoid pressure (force) of 40 N should be applied while the patient was awake [25]. However, a conscious patient does not tolerate more than 20 N without discomfort and nausea, so it has been suggested [42] that this lower pressure should be used until loss of consciousness occurs, when pressure can be increased. If vomiting occurs whilst cricoid pressure is being applied, oesophageal rupture may result. A study in cadavers has shown that when the oesophagus is occluded by a force of 40 N, a rise in pressure in the lumen of the oesophagus can cause oesophageal rupture [39]. Cricoid pressure has been shown to produce mechanical distortion of the airway during laryngoscopy and distortion of a laryngeal mask airway [43]. The distortion of tissues may take the form of actual indentation of the tracheal lumen or lateral displacement of the larynx. It may make intubation impossible and manual ventilation difficult after failed intubation. The positioning of a laryngeal mask airway during a failed intubation drill may be hindered by correctly applied cricoid pressure (see p. 317). On occasions, therefore, it may be necessary to release cricoid pressure momentarily in order to complete intubation or establish an airway. This is a difficult decision to make, but increasing severe hypoxia and absence of an airway when other measures have failed is an indication for a trial release of cricoid pressure.

16.6 Intravenous induction agents

16.6.1 Thiopental

Thiopental is the standard anaesthetic induction agent [44]. It is a thiobarbiturate that is about 75% bound to albumin and highly lipophilic. The maternal concentration decreases rapidly by redistribution in body tissues. The drug passes to the fetus within 30 seconds. Peak umbilical venous levels occur in 2–3 minutes, but fetal tissue concentrations gradually rise as redistribution occurs. Peak fetal tissue levels are much lower than maternal ones. A maternal dose of 4 mg/kg (term weight) or 5 mg/kg (pre-pregnant weight) has no significant effect on the clinical status of the neonate at birth.

16.6.2 Ketamine

Ketamine is a phencyclidine derivative that has potent analgesic effects without respiratory depression. It is less than 50% protein-bound, and crosses the placenta rapidly. At a dose of 2 mg/kg it has been associated with neonatal depression [45], but placental perfusion was well maintained in the study. It has been used for its vasopressor effects in the presence of hypovolaemia. The side effect of hallucinations means that there are few indications for its use in the developed world, where many alternatives are available. In the developing countries, it is an invaluable drug.

16.6.3 Etomidate

Etomidate administration produces a high incidence of pain on injection and involuntary muscle movement, especially in unpremedicated patients such as women undergoing Caesarean section. It can also depress cortisol production in the neonate [46]. As a consequence, it is not used routinely as an induction agent for Caesarean section, but it is useful when thiopental is contraindicated.

16.6.4 Methohexital

Methohexital is an oxybarbiturate with a shorter elimination half-life than thiopental. When doses of 1.0 and 1.4 mg/kg were compared, the higher dose was associated with clinical neonatal depression [47]. The lower dose may be associated with maternal awareness. Methohexital has excitatory side effects and causes pain on injection. It has no particular advantages over thiopental.

16.6.5 Propofol

In the fit, non-pregnant adult, propofol, in doses of 2–3 mg/kg, is a reliable induction agent that is associated with rapid recovery and a low incidence of postoperative nausea and vomiting. It has been used both to induce and to maintain general anaesthesia for Caesarean section [48–50]. An induction dose of 2 mg/kg has been shown to obtund the nor-epinephrine response to endotracheal intubation [51]. However, propofol as an induction agent has been associated with a risk of maternal awareness with low doses and neonatal depression if larger doses are used [52]. The umbilical venous : maternal venous blood ratios lie between 0.62 and 0.86 [50], and the value may increase if induction and delivery time is prolonged. Propofol is therefore unsuitable for induction or maintenance of general anaesthesia for Caesarean section except in special circumstances in which other intravenous agents are contraindicated, for instance in porphyria [53].

16.7 Intubation

Cuffed endotracheal intubation is required at Caesarean section for two reasons: first, to allow intermittent positive-pressure ventilation, and secondly to prevent pharyngeal contents from soiling the trachea. Before starting a general anaesthetic for Caesarean section, it is necessary to have a range of sizes of endotracheal tubes, including cuffed tubes down to 6.0 mm and a smaller uncuffed tube of adequate length. Variability in tracheal and laryngeal diameter may result from oedema or external pressure, and unexpectedly small-diameter endotracheal tubes may be needed. Clinical evidence of tracheal placement is confirmed by the following signs:

- visible passage of the endotracheal tube through the vocal cords;
- bilateral visible chest movement;
- audible breath sounds on manual inflation in the right and left upper zones and axilla;
- absence of gas entry into the stomach;
- capnographic confirmation (six breaths) of appropriate end-tidal carbon dioxide concentration. (NB, expired air forced into the stomach can present an inaccurate picture of tracheal placement for one or two breaths if the tube is in the oesophagus.)

It is necessary to have a trained anaesthetic assistant available (i.e. not applying cricoid pressure) when an anaesthetist is intubating a woman at Caesarean section, so that the necessary equipment for a difficult intubation can be made available without delay.

The position of the head and neck at intubation is important to produce the best conditions for the first attempt. The ideal position, 'sniffing the morning air', originally described by Magill [54] is achieved by placing a pillow beneath the neck and occiput to achieve the required flexion of the neck on the thorax together with extension of the head on the neck.

16.7.1 Cardiovascular responses to laryngoscopy and intubation

Tachycardia and arterial hypertension can be induced by laryngoscopy and tracheal intubation at Caesarean section. The average increase in systolic pressure has been observed to be 56 mmHg in hypertensive parturients [55]. These effects are dangerous and must be prevented. Adequate antihypertensive therapy should start before induction of anaesthesia if it is to be effective. Fetal effects of any drug administered must be considered. If opioids are used, transient neonatal respiratory depression should be expected, and facilities for neonatal ventilation and reversal with naloxone of the opioid depression should be available. There are a number of drugs which have been observed to block the hypertensive response, but which are not recommended for this use by their manufacturers.

Methods of reducing the hypertensive response to intubation

Short-acting opioid drugs can reduce both the hypertensive and heart rate responses to intubation, particularly in combination with other drugs that rapidly cross the placenta. In hypertensive parturients, the use of fentanyl 2.5 µg/kg or alfentanil 10 µg/kg after 5 mg droperidol attenuated the response in most women [56], and in a comparative study of alfentanil 10 µg/kg, magnesium sulphate 40 mg/kg, and lidocaine 1.5 mg/kg given separately on induction of anaesthesia, up to a quarter of women developed an increase in systolic arterial blood pressure and alfentanil resulted in significant fetal depression [57]. Lidocaine was the least effective agent, but it requires a longer time for its action than was allowed in this study.

Beta-adrenergic receptor blocking drugs are not used as first-line prophylaxis. Doses of labetalol (20 µg/kg followed by 10 mg intravenous increments) have been used to reduce the hypertensive response to intubation [58] with no adverse fetal effects, but β-adrenergic receptor blocking drugs generally have limited use, because they can obtund the heart rate response and still have little effect on the pressor response, which is mediated by adrenergic receptor mechanisms. In contrast, calcium-channel blockers such as nifedipine [59] may attenuate the pressor response but not heart rate responses. Glyceryl trinitrate, a direct vasodilator, has also been used to prevent the hypertensive response [60].

Combinations of drugs have been tried in non-pregnant patients, mainly involving the addition of an opioid to an antihypertensive agent so that the dose of each can be reduced. In obstetric anaesthesia, it would therefore be advisable to start antihypertensive therapy in women with hypertensive disorders preoperatively in good time in order to allow adequate dosage and effect to be established prior to anaesthesia.

16.8 Oxygenation

Adequate ventilation of the lungs with appropriate concentrations of oxygen is required to ensure tissue oxygenation. Compliance is lower in pregnant patients than in normal individuals, and a ventilator that can generate adequate inspiratory pressures is therefore required. Measurement of the volume and content of inspired and expired gases is an essential part of the basic monitoring to be used during Caesarean section.

An increase in F_{IO_2} from 33% to 50% has been advocated for women having an operative delivery in order to improve fetal and maternal conditions. Comparisons between these two inspired concentrations [61,62] have detected no significant differences in the clinical outcome for the fetus. The reduction in nitrous oxide concentration in preference for more oxygen, coupled with a minimal amount of other anaesthetic agents in order not to depress the baby, has caused an unacceptably high incidence of maternal awareness [62]. It is possible that the fetus can become acidotic as a result of uterine artery vasoconstriction following 100% oxygen if accompanied by sympathetically mediated effects of an inadequate depth of anaesthesia. An increase in maternal inspired oxygen tension from 50% to 100% can, however, improve the umbilical vein Po_2 and reduce the time to sustained respiration [63,64], so it has been suggested that in an emergency a higher inspired oxygen concentration should be administered to the mother, together with adequate concentrations of a volatile inhalational agent in order to prevent awareness and reduce the need for neonatal resuscitation [65,66].

16.9 Induction–delivery interval

An induction–delivery interval of less than three minutes is not advised, because the fetal blood concentrations of the intravenous induction agent are high at this time. In the same period, maternal concentrations are declining and the inhalational agents have not achieved an effective brain concentration. Maternal awareness of skin incision and memory of a painful event is more likely to occur at this time [67].

A prolonged time between uterine incision and neonatal delivery can occur because of an abnormal presentation, uterine hypertonus and other difficulties. During this time, uterine manipulations may occur that can cause restriction of uterine blood flow. A uterine incision to delivery time of less than 90 seconds compared with 90 seconds or more during general anaesthesia was associated with a better Apgar score [68]. Nitrous oxide is transferred to the fetus continuously [69], so that if the induction-to-delivery time is prolonged for more than 15 minutes, fetal depression may occur. This situation can arise when a woman has had previous surgery and access to the uterus requires division of adhesions. Similarly, transfer of a volatile agent also occurs, and a 'sleepy' baby may result (see below).

16.10 Inhalational agents

Inhalational anaesthetic agents are given to parturients following intravenous induction. The objective is to prevent maternal awareness during surgery without harming mother or fetus. Combining nitrous oxide with volatile inhalational agents can prevent maternal awareness prior to delivery of the fetus if used appropriately together with an agent monitor and a breathing system that allows rapid variation of the concentration of anaesthetic agents. In particular, a closed system should not be used, because of the time delay in

Table 16.6 Properties of inhalational agents [72].

	MAC* (in 100% O$_2$)	MAC* (70% N$_2$O in O$_2$)	Boiling point °C	Saturated vapour pressure at 20°C	Blood–gas partition coefficient	Oil–gas partition coefficient	% metabolized
Halothane	0.75	0.3	50.2	240	2.4	220	15–20
Isoflurane	1.15	0.6	48.5	236	1.4	98	0.2
Enflurane	2.0	0.6	56.5	172	1.0	97	2.4
Desflurane	6.0	3.0	22.8	664	0.45	28	0.02
Sevoflurane	2.0	0.8	58.5	170	0.65	47	3.0
Nitrous oxide	104	–	–	–	0.47	–	0.004

* Non-pregnant. MAC, minimum alveolar concentration.

achieving the desired concentration of agents in the system, while washout of any remaining anaesthetic gases or air in the system prior to anaesthesia may be slow. A breathing system which allows an immediate response to changes in the fresh gas mixture and will achieve the desired end-tidal CO$_2$ reliably is preferred. The fetus is usually exposed to volatile agents for a short time before delivery, so any long-term cardiovascular depressant effects that might theoretically enhance acidosis in an already compromised fetus can be ignored [70]. The choice of volatile agent does not affect fetal outcome [71].

The physical characteristics of the inhalational agents are described in Table 16.6 [72]. The MAC of a volatile agent describes the concentration of vapour in a steady state required to achieve a lack of response to a surgical stimulus in 50% of patients. It is reduced by nitrous oxide and pregnancy [73]. A reduction in MAC has been observed as early as 8–12 weeks' gestation [74]. Various mechanisms have been proposed for this decrease, including the sedative effects of progesterone and the production of endogenous opioids. A woman in labour may also have received exogenous opioids or regional analgesia, and the anaesthetist should take this into account when considering anaesthetic requirements.

Among the volatile agents, isoflurane has theoretical advantages over halothane. It has a lower blood–gas partition coefficient, so that its uptake by the mother and elimination from the fetus are more rapid; it should therefore provide better protection against maternal awareness, and should reduce neonatal depression. Uptake of halothane 0.5% has been compared with isoflurane 0.8% in supplementing anaesthesia with nitrous oxide 50% and oxygen 50% at elective Caesarean section [75]. The arterial partial pressure as a fraction of the inspired gas was significantly greater for isoflurane than halothane at five minutes after induction but not at 10 minutes. Fetal uptake of the two agents was similar, so the partial pressure of isoflurane was higher in the fetus at delivery. The fetal effects of general anaesthetic agents may manifest as a lower Apgar score at one minute because the neonate is 'sleepy' or sedated, but they are readily reversed by the neonate's own spontaneous respiratory function, which removes the volatile agent.

The volatile inhalational agents halothane, enflurane and isoflurane decrease uterine muscle tone when blood levels are > 0.5 MAC [76], but the oxytocic response is not lost until blood levels are > 0.9 MAC. This reversible uterine relaxation is only useful if there is uterine spasm obstructing delivery. If uterine tone is reduced, haemorrhage can occur from the placental site after delivery.

Nitrous oxide, when used as a 70 : 30 mixture with oxygen and no volatile agent in pregnant ewes, induced light anaesthesia that was not deep enough to prevent uterine artery vasoconstriction due to the release of catecholamines [77]. Measured uterine blood flow decreased by 18–30% from control values. The addition of volatile agents may prevent this. The addition of nitrous oxide to an inhaled oxygen/volatile agent gas mixture in the first few minutes of anaesthesia for Caesarean section is valuable. It will produce a 'second gas effect' because the rapidity of uptake of nitrous oxide enhances the uptake of the volatile agent. The use of nitrous oxide is advisable also, because it is a good analgesic and produces minimal uterine depression. The presence of N_2O will contribute to the total MAC of the inspired gases and allow the use of a lower concentration of volatile agents.

An additional high concentration of inspired volatile agent during the first few minutes of anaesthesia will produce effective blood levels more quickly than a constant moderate concentration. This 'over-pressure' principle can readily be used in a paralysed patient with no respiratory reflex disturbance from an irritant concentration. Isoflurane has been administered for five minutes in a 2% concentration, then reducing to 1.5% for five minutes and 0.8% subsequently. Effective maternal arterial blood levels of isoflurane were achieved more rapidly with this regimen than when a constant inspired concentration of isoflurane of 1% was used [78]. Fetal effects of this technique have yet to be measured.

The choice of volatile agent may depend on the woman's medical condition. Enflurane should not be used in parturients who have epilepsy, because of the risk of worsening the disease. It should also be avoided in any mother with pre-eclampsia or chronic pre-existing hypertensive disorders, where there is a potential for renal function to deteriorate due to the problem of enflurane impairment of renal function.

16.11 Muscle relaxants

16.11.1 General principles

Muscle relaxants are used in general anaesthesia for obstetrics for two reasons: first, to expedite and facilitate endotracheal intubation; and secondly, to improve surgical access while maintaining relatively light levels of general anaesthesia. The first objective can only be achieved by the use of a rapidly acting drug that produces complete muscle relaxation and good conditions for intubation. The drug must also have a short duration of action, so that spontaneous respiration is re-established quickly in the event of a failure to intubate. The only drug that currently meets these criteria is suxamethonium (usually as the chloride salt).

The second objective of improving surgical access is less important because, once the baby is delivered by Caesarean section, the parturient's stretched anterior abdominal wall offers little resistance to surgical intrusion. Delivery is often completed before muscle tone returns after suxamethonium administration, and subsequently muscle relaxation dosage should be given sparingly. Almost any relaxant will produce the desired effect, but recommendations for the choice of muscle relaxant and dosage for this situation are as follows.

1   The drug need only have a moderate duration of action, because the duration of surgery is usually limited to 30–45 minutes. Long-acting relaxants should not be used because of the risk of residual effects during extubation and recovery. A number of maternal deaths have occurred because of residual muscle relaxant effects, particularly following pancuronium usage. The problems included respiratory insufficiency, inability to maintain an airway, inability to intubate following loss of the airway and subsequent aspiration of gastric contents.

2   The drug should have a clear end point, either from spontaneous degradation or following reversal of its effects. Similarly, it should have a low risk or no risk of residual effects re-emerging during recovery.

3   It should have a low risk of cumulative effects if additional doses prove necessary.

4   It should have minimal side effects, especially in terms of anaphylactic reactions and cardiovascular consequences.

5   When considering the dose to be used, the previous drug regimen of the individual patient should be considered. Suxamethonium given for intubation can potentiate subsequent doses of both depolarizing and non-depolarizing relaxants.

6   The relaxant and its metabolites should either not cross the placenta, or should cross it in insignificant quantities that do not affect the neonate.

16.11.2 Choice of neuromuscular blocking drugs

Depolarizing neuromuscular blocking drugs

Suxamethonium is still the only fast-acting muscle relaxant with a short recovery time that is suitable for rapid-sequence anaesthetic induction. In the case of failed intubation, which is more common in late pregnancy than in non-pregnant individuals, quick recovery of spontaneous respiration and muscle tone within five minutes allows the mother to regain her airway and spontaneous ventilation, and reduces the risk of hypoxia. The pharmacokinetics of suxamethonium can therefore be life-saving at times.

The effects of an initial dose of suxamethonium should be seen to be wearing off before any other (non-depolarizing) relaxant is given. If the duration of suxamethonium is prolonged the second relaxant may not be needed, and if the prolonged action is present the anaesthetist should give early consideration to a likely diagnosis. The complication of an additional drug will make diagnosis and treatment decisions more difficult. Variation in the duration of the block and prolonged paralysis can occur following suxamethonium for a number of reasons.

- Abnormal genotype (suxamethonium apnoea).
- Interaction with other drugs:
  metoclopramide [79];
  ester local anaesthetics.
- Low plasma cholinesterase levels (which may be exacerbated by pregnancy).

The rate of metabolism of the drug cannot be easily increased if prolonged paralysis occurs, and in this circumstance the patient should be transferred to an intensive-care unit for sedation and lung ventilation until the effects of suxamethonium wear off. Theoretically, the administration of fresh blood or fresh frozen plasma can reverse the action of suxamethonium, as they are both sources of plasma cholinesterase. Fresh blood is no longer available from blood banks, and the possibility (albeit low) of transmitted viral infection in fresh frozen plasma tilts the risk–benefit balance in favour of intermittent positive-pressure ventilation for a few hours until the suxamethonium effects wear off. During this period, very light levels of anaesthesia or sedation should be used to prevent awareness. Peripheral neuromuscular monitoring can then be performed regularly to assess the reversal of the neuromuscular block.

The use of suxamethonium can cause postoperative morbidity, with up to one in five women experiencing muscle pains [80], which are usually felt in the neck, shoulders or back. These pains can be quite disabling for a few days, so patients should be told of this possibility before they receive a general anaesthetic. Contraindications to suxamethonium include hyperkalaemia, e.g. renal failure, a history of sensitivity to the drug and a family history of malignant hyperpyrexia. The method of intubation if general anaesthesia is required is then open to debate, and an awake intubation should be considered.

Non-depolarizing neuromuscular blocking drugs

Atracurium and vecuronium are the two main non-depolarizing neuromuscular blocking agents in use. Their duration of action is 25–40 minutes, suitable for Caesarean section. Atracurium has a particular advantage in its end point, since it is rapidly metabolized, leaving little or no risk of residual paralysis. Longer-acting agents such as pancuronium are no longer used, particularly since residual effects of the drug in the postoperative period have been identified as a cause of maternal death.

The non-depolarizing muscle relaxant should only be administered after the neuromuscular blocking effects of suxamethonium have worn off, as determined by a nerve stimulator, and the dose used can be less than normal, e.g. 20 mg atracurium for a 70-kg pregnant woman prior to delivery of her baby. If the effect using a nerve stimulator is inadequate, a further small incremental dose can be given. All non-depolarizing muscle relaxants must be adequately reversed before recovery from anaesthesia, and a peripheral stimulator with a train-of-four stimulation should be used to confirm reversal before awakening and extubation. In clinical situations in which residual paralysis may be expected, such as in renal failure or myasthenia gravis, atracurium and its isomer cisatracurium, which lacks most of atracurium's side effects, are indicated.

Non-depolarizing muscle relaxants can cross the placenta from the mother to the fetus. The ratio of drug concentration in the umbilical vein compared with maternal venous blood is between 0.1 and 0.2 for atracurium [81], vecuronium and pancuronium [82]. The atracurium metabolite, laudanosine, is found in the fetus but also in low concentration [83]. Pancuronium is mainly protein-bound, so the increase in total plasma protein in pregnancy will produce a larger blood reservoir and possibly delay reversal. It is therefore not a suitable agent in obstetrics. Vecuronium and atracurium are 30% and 37% protein-bound, respectively.

Other neuromuscular blocking drugs such as rocuronium and mivacurium are available, but are not recommended in obstetrics. For example, rocuronium 0.6 mg/kg has been used together with thiopental for rapid-sequence induction [84], but its use as the sole muscle relaxant for Caesarean section should be avoided, because intubating conditions were not satisfactory in 10% of patients and neuromuscular recovery is slower than from suxamethonium, so that inevitably a situation of failed intubation will be accompanied by no return of maternal spontaneous ventilation—a potential disaster. Mivacurium is eliminated almost exclusively by plasma cholinesterase, so its duration of action is affected by the activity of this enzyme. There are now several reports of prolonged block following its use, and there are no indications for its use in obstetrics [85,86].

16.12 Perioperative analgesics—opioids

After delivery of the neonate, sedative and analgesic drugs can be administered to the mother without concern about placental transfer. Since the woman has usually received no opioids prior to delivery, it is essential to start their administration. Boluses of alfentanil or fentanyl can be given intravenously. Opioids are given not only as part of the anaesthetic technique, but also to maintain analgesia in the early recovery period. Morphine can be titrated intravenously (e.g. 1–2 mg increments) so that on waking, the mother is pain-free. Further increments are usually necessary immediately on recovery. An assessment of the maternal response to intravenous morphine during and after surgery will assist in the establishment of satisfactory patient-controlled analgesia postoperatively.

If there are no contraindications to non-steroidal anti-inflammatory drugs and consent to rectal administration has been given, they should also be administered before the patient wakens in order to allow early mobilization with minimal discomfort and reduce morphine demand. It is not unusual for the dose of postoperative morphine used to be larger than expected; this is partly because the mother will have received no preoperative opioid medication, and there is also a difference in the pharmacokinetics, mainly as a result of hormonal effects (similar to the effects that occur during the use of oral contraceptives).

16.13 Blood transfusion and Caesarean section

Obstetric haemorrhage is rarely predictable, so all obstetric patients should be grouped and blood should be saved for cross-matching. If risk factors are identified, cross-matching is indicated, especially if the patient has a placenta praevia or a coagulopathy. Planned surgical access should also be taken into consideration. Vertical incision or classical Caesarean section is more likely to cause greater blood loss. The amount of blood required may vary, and two to six units may be ordered, depending on the risks or estimated preoperative anaemia. Additional venous access should also be secured in parturients who are at risk. Early placement of intravenous cannulae while peripheral veins are visible and available will make the replacement of major blood loss faster. A blood-warming infusion set is required for these rapid infusions.

Risk factors for haemorrhage have been identified. A 12-year review of 1668 women who underwent Caesarean section [87] found that 2.5% of patients received perioperative blood transfusions. The main risk factors were placenta praevia, abruptio placenta and coagulopathies. A similar number of women at Caesarean section were studied retrospectively [88], 7.9% of whom suffered either an estimated blood loss of more than 1.5 L, a blood transfusion to maintain haemodynamic stability, or a decrease in postoperative haematocrit of > 10%. The risk factors associated with this blood loss were pre-eclampsia, disorders of active labour, previous postpartum haemorrhage and obesity of over 114 kg.

16.14 Postoperative care

16.14.1 Pain relief

Postoperative pain relief after general anaesthesia for Caesarean section requires varying amounts of analgesia. Some women complain of difficulty in mobilizing because of pain, whereas others only demand oral analgesics. Mothers who plan to breast-feed often express concerns about drug effects on the baby. In the initial postoperative period, they should be advised that neonatal effects will be slight, and that good pain relief will allow them to mobilize more quickly and reduce the risk of deep venous thrombosis—a major cause of maternal death. The choice of drugs for acute postoperative pain after operative delivery depends on the severity of the pain complained of, as well as other factors such as patient preference, time after surgery and the availability of the oral route of administration. Morphine is the opioid of choice for severe somatic pain, and is best made available as intravenous patient-controlled analgesia [89]. The transfer of the opioids morphine and pethidine into breast milk has been studied in patients receiving patient-controlled analgesia with one or other of these opioids. Neonates in the morphine group had significantly higher neurobehavioural scores [90], so pethidine is unsuitable in nursing mothers. When opioids are administered in the postpartum period gastric emptying will be delayed, and patient-controlled analgesia is associated with nausea and vomiting in over half of the parturients receiving it [91]. This side effect may be important if the woman requires further surgery postpartum, because of the renewed risk of acid aspiration.

The most effective drugs for oral medication have been determined in systematic reviews, and ibuprofen was claimed to be the best, closely followed by a combination of paracetamol 600 mg and codeine 60 mg [92]. The choice between these agents will depend on the relative risks of adverse effects. Non-steroidal anti-inflammatory analgesics (NSAIDs), such as diclofenac, prevent the release of peripheral mediators of pain and inflammation and reduce the requirements for opioids. They do not require parenteral access and are not associated with unwanted opioid side effects such as nausea, constipation and respiratory depression. When a mother is to return home soon after surgery, NSAIDs are often the analgesic of choice. Contraindications to non-steroidal anti-inflammatory drugs can, however, severely limit their use in high-risk parturients, particularly those women with renal disorders, pre-eclampsia, haemorrhage or a history of asthma. Diclofenac is commonly used, 100 mg either given rectally or orally, preferably in a modified-release preparation to prolong its effect. Potential risks of non-steroidal drugs, such as increased bleeding and transfer to the neonate through breast milk, are not troublesome in clinical practice [93].

16.14.2 Anti-emetic drugs

The potential danger of aspirating vomit means that preventing this risk is part of the anaesthetic technique. Postoperative nausea and vomiting are particularly undesirable in parturients, as they delay ambulation and interfere with the mother's care of her baby. Vomiting is not only unpleasant, but delays resumption of oral intake. The increased use of non-steroidal anti-inflammatory

Table 16.7 Receptor site affinities and half-life of some antiemetic drugs.

Drug groups	Dopamine (D$_2$)	Muscarinic (cholinergic)	Histamine	Serotonin (5-HT$_3$)	T$_{1/2}$ hours
Antihistamine, e.g. prochlorperazine	+++	+	++	0	7
Butyrophenones, e.g. droperidol	++++	0	+	+	2
Anticholinergic, e.g. hyoscine	+	++++	+	0	2–4
Benzamides, e.g. metoclopramide	+++	0	+	++	4
Serotonin antagonists, e.g. ondansetron	0	0	0	++++	3

0, no affinity; +, 10-fold increases in drug potency at neurotransmitter receptor site.

analgesic drugs has helped to reduce the incidence of postoperative nausea and vomiting by reducing the amount of opioid drugs that may be required for analgesia.

There are at least four receptor types involved in the emetic response, and four sites of action of anti-emetic drugs (Table 16.7). No single agent that is available can antagonize all four receptor sites. There seems to be great individual patient variation in emetic reflexes and the response to anti-emetic drugs. Some patients respond better to one or other anti-emetic, and may know which drug is best for them. If one drug is found to be inadequate for a patient, sequential or combination therapy should be considered, provided that central nervous system depression or extrapyramidal effects are not enhanced. For example, if the initial anti-emetic acted mainly on cholinergic receptors, then one that blocked histamine receptors may be used, followed by a serotonin (5-hydroxytryptamine (5-HT)) antagonist. No particular order of use has been studied or found to be more effective than another, but it seems logical to use a sequential method based on pharmacological activity. The most common anti-emetic given before a Caesarean section is metoclopramide, which has mixed actions. It is both a gastrointestinal prokinetic and an antidopaminergic drug. Occasionally, extrapyramidal side effects can limit its use. Postoperatively, phenothiazines have antihistamine properties that may be useful, e.g. prochlorperazine, and these should be administered intramuscularly. If these two drug types have failed, there is little point in giving another drug with the same action. Either a 5-HT$_3$ antagonist may be used, such as ondansetron, which is effective but expensive, or hyoscine, an anticholinergic antagonist. Once a mother has received the four drug types, the main emetic pathways should be blocked, and in the majority of cases the problem will have been controlled.

16.15 Complications of general anaesthesia

16.15.1 Difficult intubation

A difficult intubation is still the major cause of morbidity and mortality in general anaesthesia for Caesarean section.

Predictors of difficult intubation

The assessment of a patient's airway is summarized in Table 16.8. Soft-tissue assessments as described by Mallampati [94] and subsequently modified [95] as shown in Fig. 16.3, have a high incidence of false-positive results and predict about 50% of difficulties. The same limitations apply to Wilson's score [96], which uses five risk factors: weight, head and neck movement, mouth opening, receding mandible and buck teeth. The thyromental distance, measured as the distance from the thyroid notch to the mental prominence with the neck fully extended, is a rule of thumb to assess head extension, laryngeal position and the depth of the mandible. A measurement of 7 cm or more suggests there will be no difficulties with viewing the larynx. The combined use of the Mallampati test and the thyromental distance improves the sensitivity of detecting a difficult intubation [97]. Mouth opening is also another important observation, and can be tested using a patient's fingers such that three fingers between the incisors is adequate but any less could herald difficulty in mouth opening due to soft-tissue or bone and joint diseases. The Mallampati score

Table 16.8 Patient assessment for difficult intubation.

History	Previous difficult intubation (check anaesthetic records if available)
	Rheumatoid arthritis
	Facial trauma/operations
	Problems with the voice, tracheostomy, thyroidectomy
	Assess risk of vomiting, e.g. full stomach
Examination (anatomy)	Soft tissues: mouth, tongue (Mallampati)
	Pharynx
	Bones:
	Mandible: size, shape
	Neck: thyromental distance
	Teeth: protusion, absence
	Joints: mouth opening, bite
Function	Neck movements: flexion, extension
	Jaw movements (temporomandibular joint)
General examination	Body mass index (weight and height)

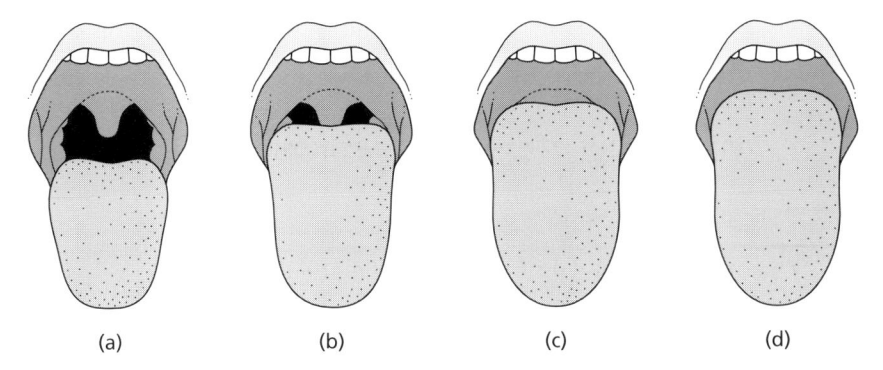

Fig. 16.3 The preoperative modified Mallampati score, measured with the patient upright, the tongue protruding and no phonation. (a) A class 1 airway with full view of all soft-tissue structures. (b) A class 2 airway, with loss of part of the uvula but some posterior pharynx visible. (c) A class 3 airway, with loss of the posterior pharynx to vision, while the soft palate is still seen. (d) A class 4 airway, with only the hard palate visible. This is sometimes difficult to distinguish from (c).

has been observed to change during labour [98], and airway assessment immediately prior to anaesthesia is therefore important.

A prospective relative risk analysis by Rocke *et al.* [99] in 1606 women presenting for elective or emergency Caesarean section found that difficult intubation could be predicted if a number of subjective abnormalities (Table 16.9) were present in one patient. Obesity was a factor that had the same risk as a short neck, and since the two conditions were usually both present, obesity itself was not analysed. Morbid obesity in another study of women above 136.4 kg [100] was associated with a 35% incidence of difficult intubations, and may be a factor to include in any clinical assessment by obstetric anaesthetists. The limitations of all the practically useful scoring systems so far reported are typified by the sensitivity and specificity of the modified (Samsoon and Young [95]) Mallampati score, sensitivity being the ability of the score to identify a problem and specificity being the accuracy of identification, i.e. if the score identifies all patients with a problem and none of those who do not have a problem, it is 100% sensitive and 100% specific. The modified Mallampati scoring system used by Rocke *et al.* [99] failed to detect difficult or failed intubations in 13 women, one in 100 intubations with graded scores of 1 or 2. Among those with a score of 3 or 4, 21% proved to be easy intubations. Other factors such as pre-eclampsia and its associated oedema, as well as head and jaw mobility, have to be considered. The finding that there is an increased probability of difficult intubation in parturients with a greater number and severity of risk factors, as shown in Table 16.9, makes a full airway assessment necessary. It is therefore important to decide at what level of probability the choice of an alternative anaesthetic technique is made. This may depend on the anaesthetist's experience and the availability of equipment. All trainee anaesthetists should seek assistance in intubation if a higher than normal risk is suspected.

Table 16.9 Predictors of difficult intubation [99]. Class 3 and 4 refer to the modified Mallampati score [95].

	Probability of difficult intubation (%)
Class 4	3
Class 4 and short neck	> 10
Class 4 and receding mandible	> 20
Class 3 and short neck and receding mandible	> 50
Class 4 and receding mandible and prominent incisors	> 70
Class 4 and receding mandible, short neck and prominent incisors	> 90

The reported risk of difficult intubation in obstetric patients of all types is at least one in 300 [95,101,102] and increasing. It is more common than that reported in the general population (one in 2000) [95], and skills and procedures for managing difficult and failed intubation are therefore more likely to be needed in parturients. The teaching and regular practice of these skills is an important facet of obstetric anaesthesia. Every unit should have protocols to meet these demands, and a simple algorithm should be learned for both difficult and failed intubation [102]. A wide range of equipment to be used for both events must be immediately available whenever and wherever anaesthetics are to be given in the obstetric unit. Usage of such equipment will be dictated by the experience and skills of individual anaesthetists, but a full range of intubation equipment must be available so that individual anaesthetists can use their skills in the most effective manner.

Equipment for difficult intubation

All items needed for a difficult intubation should be kept together. They should be immediately accessible when anaesthesia is to be given (even if regional analgesia is used, because of the small risk of excessively high or total spinal block and because the regional block may need to be converted to general anaesthetic if it is not fully effective).
1 *Laryngoscope.* 'Hook-on' pattern handles and blades allow total interchangeability, which can be helpful when difficulty is experienced. This pattern also allows the blade to be inserted separately and then clipped to the handle, a manoeuvre that overcomes obstacles such as large breasts, or hands applying cricoid pressure.
Handles:
    Normal length
    Short
    Polio
Blades:

Macintosh adult.
Macintosh long.
Macintosh polio.
Straight adult.

Miller or Robertshaw are preferred patterns for the straight adult and straight long types, because of their slim vertical profile, which allows access when mouth opening is restricted.

Straight long.
Special pattern McCoy.

2 *Introducers.* Introducers must always be lubricated before use. If they are guide wires, they must be coated to allow atraumatic insertion, and they should fit inside and shape the endotracheal tube. Gum elastic bougies can guide a tube into the trachea, and are either positioned inside the tube or usually used with the short *coudé* tip protruding. They can be used alone and positioned first before railroading the endotracheal tube over it into the trachea. The latter method is extremely valuable in difficult intubation.

Flexible gum elastic bougies.
'Bendable' plastic-coated wire introducers.

3 *Airways*:

Guedel (all sizes).

Nasopharyngeal (4.0–6.0 mm). Plain (uncuffed) Portex endotracheal tubes cut to 10–12 cm length and with a Portex connector inserted are effective nasopharyngeal airways. However, they are rather too hard in texture and may cause bleeding in the nose. Using a smaller size will minimize this possibility, as will warming and softening of the tube (e.g. under the hot-water tap).

Laryngeal mask airways (sizes 2–4).

4 *Endotracheal tubes* of varying sizes (those below 6 mm having no cuff) and cut to adult length (approximately 23 cm or slightly longer for the adult woman). Tubes must be marked in centimetre lengths, because if they are too long they will track into the right main bronchus, and if they are too short they can dislodge.

5 *Magill forceps*, to grip an endotracheal tube or to remove foreign objects.

6 *Disposable cricothyrotomy set.* Both Quick Trach and Transtracheal Catheter single-thrust devices with built-in 21-mm connectors are available. The latter resembles a curved intravenous cannula, and is therefore particularly easy to use.

7 *Bronchoscope*, to remove solid particles with suction.

Fibre-optic intubation equipment may not be available solely for obstetric use. However, all obstetric anaesthetists should have immediate access to it if required, and should be experienced in its use.

16.15.2 Failed intubation

Every obstetric unit in which general (or regional) anaesthetics are given must

314   CHAPTER 16

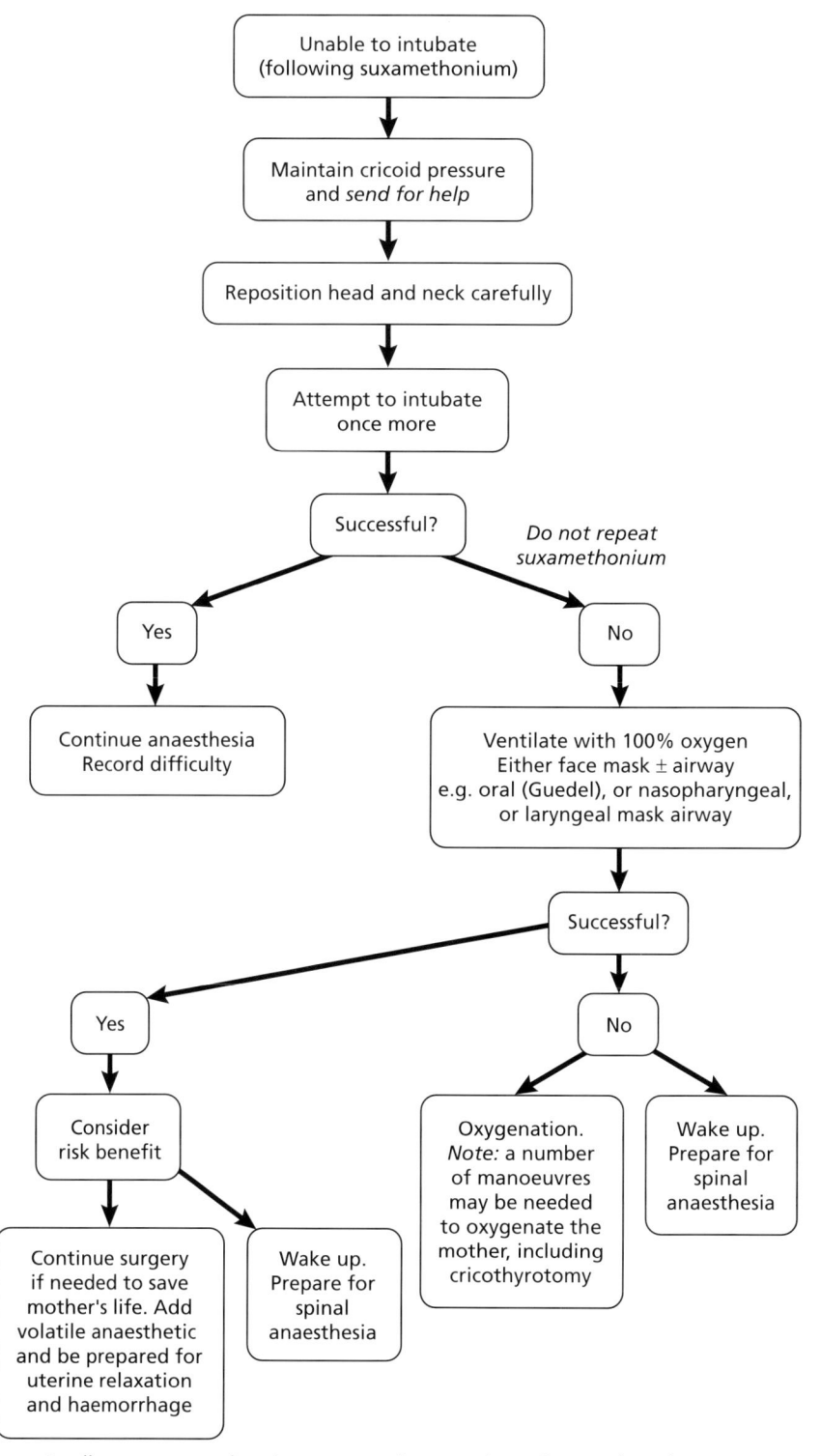

```
┌─────────────────────────────┐
│     Unable to intubate      │
│  (following suxamethonium)  │
└──────────────┬──────────────┘
               ▼
┌─────────────────────────────┐
│  Maintain cricoid pressure  │
│     and send for help       │
└──────────────┬──────────────┘
               ▼
┌─────────────────────────────┐
│ Reposition head and neck carefully │
└──────────────┬──────────────┘
               ▼
┌─────────────────────────────┐
│     Attempt to intubate     │
│         once more           │
└──────────────┬──────────────┘
               ▼
         ╱ Successful? ╲              Do not repeat
        ╱               ╲             suxamethonium
      Yes                No
       │                 │
       ▼                 ▼
┌──────────────┐   ┌─────────────────────────────┐
│  Continue    │   │ Ventilate with 100% oxygen  │
│  anaesthesia │   │ Either face mask ± airway   │
│  Record      │   │ e.g. oral (Guedel), or      │
│  difficulty  │   │ nasopharyngeal, or          │
└──────────────┘   │ laryngeal mask airway       │
                   └──────────────┬──────────────┘
                                  ▼
                            ╱ Successful? ╲
                           ╱               ╲
                         Yes                No
                          │               ╱ ╲
                          ▼              ▼   ▼
                   ┌──────────┐   ┌──────────┐  ┌──────────┐
                   │ Consider │   │Oxygenation│ │ Wake up. │
                   │  risk    │   │Note: a   │  │Prepare   │
                   │ benefit  │   │number of │  │for spinal│
                   └────┬─────┘   │manoeuvres│  │anaesthesia│
                        │         │may be    │  └──────────┘
                   ┌────┴────┐    │needed to │
                   ▼         ▼    │oxygenate │
           ┌──────────┐ ┌────────┐│the mother│
           │Continue  │ │Wake up.││including │
           │surgery if│ │Prepare ││cricothy- │
           │needed to │ │for     ││rotomy    │
           │save      │ │spinal  │└──────────┘
           │mother's  │ │anaes-  │
           │life. Add │ │thesia  │
           │volatile  │ └────────┘
           │anaes-    │
           │thetic and│
           │be        │
           │prepared  │
           │for uterine│
           │relaxation│
           │and       │
           │haemorrhage│
           └──────────┘
```

In all cases, ensure that the woman subsequently carries an 'alert' document

Fig. 16.4 Failed intubation drill.

have a failed intubation protocol. The protocol should be simple and easily understood (Fig. 16.4). Staff should be familiar with it and should practise implementing it regularly. When endotracheal intubation has failed, the woman should be woken up and an alternative anaesthetic method used if at all possible. In certain circumstances, it is possible to proceed with surgery using general anaesthesia being maintained with face mask or laryngeal mask airway and inhalational anaesthetic agents. In this difficult and dangerous situation, the anaesthetist and surgeon must agree that the imperative is to continue in spite of the serious risk to the mother's life from aspiration into or obstruction of the unsecured maternal airway. Few risks outweigh the latter; those that do may include maternal haemorrhage and an imminent threat to life. Fetal survival may also fall into this category. Whether the latter priority outweighs maternal risk is a matter for individual conscience and circumstance. It should be remembered when making this decision that losing a mother who has an existing family to care for can be a greater tragedy than losing a baby.

If the decision to proceed is made, this form of general anaesthesia demands (in the 1990s) unusual skills and judgement. The depth of anaesthesia must be carefully and continuously assessed. Anaesthesia that is too light will be accompanied by active laryngeal reflexes, coughing, straining and a degree of obstruction. These reactions produce marked negative intrathoracic pressure, which in turn causes reflux and regurgitation of gastric contents. Maintenance of a clear airway is equally important. Obstruction of the airway when the depth of anaesthesia is adequate also tends to create negative intrathoracic pressures, reflux and regurgitation. Anaesthesia that is too deep should also be avoided. Increasing depth of anaesthesia is synonymous with high blood and tissue levels of inhaled volatile anaesthetic agents, unless other agents have been used to maintain anaesthesia, such as ketamine. High concentrations of volatile agents cause uterine relaxation, and excessive blood loss will occur. A careful combination of hypnotics, opioids, dissociative drugs and inhalational anaesthetics is essential in order to minimize the risks.

Management of difficult and failed intubation

Management plans (Fig. 16.4 and Table 16.10) should be available for failed intubation and when difficulty is encountered in both intubation and extubation [103]. Consideration should be given not only to intubation but also to ventilation of the lungs during periods of apnoea. If difficulty is encountered during endotracheal intubation the responses outlined below should be followed.

When the first attempt at intubation has failed, and before the second intubation, check and secure the following.

1   Correct head position: 'sniffing the morning air' (neck flexed on the thorax and extension of the head at the atlanto-occipital joint).
2   Reconsider the laryngoscope blade, choosing a more suitable one if necessary.

Table 16.10 Management plans for intubation and extubation.

Intubation	Extubation
Choices	
Awake or anaesthetized	Awake or anaesthetized
Muscle relaxation or not	Position: lateral preferable
Non-surgical or surgical tracheal approach	
Guidelines	*Plan for*
Failed intubation drill	Reintubation

3 If cricoid pressure has distorted the laryngeal anatomy, readjust the direction and amount of pressure.

4 Endotracheal tube and bougie curvature at end (lubricated). Use a smaller tube, e.g. 7 mm, to ensure that the difficulty is not due to a small laryngeal opening or laryngeal oedema.

5 Assess the laryngoscopic appearance, grading the view as below on the Cormack–Lehane (C & L) scale [104]. Take action as follows:

C & L grade 1. *Whole laryngeal aditus visible*. Intubate using a gum elastic bougie in the endotracheal tube.

C & L grade 2. *Posterior extremity of glottis visible*. Use pressure vertically on the larynx to bring the arytenoid cartilages into view, use a bougie or guide.

C & L grade 3. *No glottis, only epiglottis visible*. Check the position of cricoid pressure. Pass the endotracheal tube or gum elastic bougie, followed by the endotracheal tube blindly behind the epiglottis.

C & L grade 4. *No glottis or epiglottis visible*. The laryngeal opening may have been moved by cricoid pressure; recheck the grade by altering the direction and force of cricoid pressure. Use a bougie alone and pass behind the tongue with the *coudé* tip directed anteriorly, blindly, when clicks should be felt.

Send for senior help before a second intubation attempt, and warn the obstetrician of the possibility of a failed intubation. Only turn the woman in the lateral position if she is actively vomiting or if an airway cannot be established in the tilted supine position. The full lateral position will relieve some airway obstruction and any residual aortocaval compression, and is the position most likely to achieve good cardiac output and placental perfusion. The main disadvantages of the lateral position are the difficulties of good intermittent positive-pressure ventilation and cricoid pressure maintenance. Both can be overcome if this is practised beforehand and if sufficient pairs of hands are made available to squeeze breathing bags and pass equipment to the anaesthetist. If cricothyrotomy is to be undertaken, the patient must be placed in the supine position.

If the second intubation fails, follow the guidelines for failed intubation (Fig. 16.4).

Emergency techniques to establish an airway: the laryngeal mask airway (LMA). The LMA should be considered in a failed intubation when adequate ventilation with a face mask cannot be maintained. Cricoid pressure can still be applied, and LMA insertion should probably be tried while a single-handed cricoid pressure technique is used. If this fails, the cricoid pressure should be released and LMA insertion attempted again [105]. If this fails, ventilation with a face mask without cricoid pressure should be tried before any other manoeuvres. If the anaesthetic is wearing off, the woman should be allowed to wake up and another LMA insertion should not be attempted.

When correctly positioned, the tip of the LMA lies behind and slightly above the cricoid cartilage. When cricoid pressure is applied, double-handed pressure appears to make LMA insertions more difficult than the single-handed manoeuvre [106]. In a study of cases in which an LMA was used, cricoid pressure could usually be maintained without obstructing the airway [105]. The cricoid pressure had to be reduced to achieve airway patency before insertion in one case, and then it was re-applied. Cadaveric studies have confirmed that cricoid pressure helps to prevent regurgitation with an LMA *in situ* [107]. The laryngeal mask does not protect the lungs from regurgitated gastric contents, but if it has to be used in an emergency and there is a risk of regurgitation, the risk of aspiration is probably low [105]. The upper oesophageal sphincter usually remains competent [38].

If the LMA establishes the airway, the mother should be kept in the tilted supine position and cricoid pressure should be continued. Spontaneous respiration hopefully will have started, and inhalational anaesthesia can be continued or the patient can be woken up. Controlled ventilation through the LMA may cause gaseous gastric dilation [108], especially in the presence of increased ventilation pressures. If general anaesthesia is to be continued via the LMA, spontaneous respiration is preferable and is satisfactory for Caesarean section. Blind intubation via the LMA is more difficult with cricoid pressure applied [109], and glottic distortion occurs with double-handed cricoid pressure [43]. Using the LMA to intubate the mother may be technically difficult [110], but it has been used with good effect after delivery of the fetus [111]. An obstetric patient with a full stomach and difficult airway may be better managed by continuing with the LMA [112] and spontaneous respiration if ventilation and anaesthesia are progressing satisfactorily. The LMA is removed after surgery, with the patient in the left lateral position when she is responding and awake and able to protect her own airway.

Emergency techniques to establish an airway: cricothyrotomy. Percutaneous cricothyrotomy or mini-tracheostomy is a useful technique when indicated electively, but in the emergency situation it is significantly more difficult, and a number of complications can occur. The Seldinger technique allows the insertion of a catheter that is larger in diameter than the needle used to place a guide wire. Dilation of the access route can then occur along the track of the guide wire prior to placing the tracheal tube. Faster access requires an all-in-one insertion and dilation, and there are disposable specialist kits (Quick Trach and Transtracheal Catheter) with which all members of the anaesthetic staff should have received training if they are available for use. Training on cadavers is probably better than the plastic manikin alternative. The single-thrust insertion devices are very quick to establish access to the airway, and can be life-saving when all less invasive methods have failed.

Emergency techniques to establish an airway: surgical intervention. Surgical intervention to secure the airway requires expertise in the technique, the availability of equipment and good access to the trachea by positioning the patient with the neck fully extended, shoulders lifted and the table tilted head-up. The thyroid gland lies near to the tracheal site of tracheostomy, and haemorrhage leading to death has complicated this procedure [3]. The time factor for this technique to be put into practice is also important. It is not, therefore, usually attempted as first-line management of failed intubation.

Transtracheal intermittent jet ventilation may be used with most cricothyrotomy devices, but there is always a risk of barotrauma [113]. A patent upper airway is essential to allow adequate expiration and to reduce the risk of barotrauma. Occlusion of the airway can lead to an increase in intrathoracic pressure and hypoventilation with hypercarbia and hypoxia, and the increased intrathoracic pressure can impede venous return [114].

16.15.3 Awake fibre-optic intubation

Fibre-optic intubation needs to be learned and practised if it is to be used successfully in a difficult situation. It is not the easy answer to a failed intubation, because blood and secretions in the pharynx can cover the tip of the fibre-optic scope and obstruct vision. It is doubtful whether it has any place in the response to unexpected failure to intubate the trachea. However, it is useful when difficulty is anticipated and awake intubation is planned. In these circumstances, some variations are advisable from the techniques used in non-pregnant patients. It is preferable to administer atropine or hyoscine as an antisialagogue prior to the procedure. Three early stages in the procedure are:
1 topical anaesthesia of the upper airways;
2 vasoconstriction of the nasal cavity (if the nasal route is chosen), especially important in the parturient;
3 anaesthesia of the larynx.

A number of topical local anaesthetics can be used either as lozenges to be sucked or as solutions and gels to be sprayed or gargled. Lidocaine and prilocaine are available for topical anaesthesia of oral, pharyngeal and nasal mucous membranes. These upper airway passages should be treated as the first step of the procedure. The doses used should be kept within toxic limits, a very important factor if either lidocaine 4% or a metred spray of 10 mg/spray are used. In the non-pregnant patient, cocaine is often used to produce both vasoconstriction and topical anaesthesia of the nasal cavity. However, the drug may cause vasospasm of the uterine vessels after systemic absorption from the nose, and its use in the pregnant patient is not necessary.

If the oral route is used, the tongue is anaesthetized with a local anaesthetic spray or gargle. The oral pharyngeal mucosa is therefore prepared using a spray-as-you-go technique with lidocaine or prilocaine. The split oral airway that is used to guide and protect the fibre-optic scope should not be inserted until satisfactory anaesthesia of tongue, pharynx and larynx has been achieved. Local anaesthesia of the larynx is achieved either with a bilateral laryngeal nerve block or by the faster method of injecting 4% lidocaine, 2 mL into the lumen of the larynx via the cricothyroid membrane. Coughing is stimulated, and spreads the local anaesthetic over the laryngeal mucosa and vocal cords. Supplementation of laryngeal local anaesthesia can be achieved by injecting a further 2 mL of lidocaine or prilocaine via the endoscope when the cords are closely visualized.

16.15.4 Awareness

The incidences of recall of awareness and dreaming are 0.9% and 6.0%, respectively when inspired fresh gas mixtures containing < 1 MAC of inhalational anaesthetics are used for Caesarean section [115]. This can be reduced by the use of higher doses of thiopental (5 mg/kg) for induction, followed by maintenance with 1% isoflurane using an initial over-pressure of the volatile agent to achieve rapid increases of alveolar and blood concentrations. The MAC of a volatile agent decreases with pregnancy and with the addition of nitrous oxide. However, the recall of awareness can be terrifying [116] and the importance of adequate depth of anaesthesia for Caesarean section is undoubted.

There is no reliable method by which to detect awareness. If muscle relaxants are given, the possibility of purposeful movements is lost. Tunstall pioneered and developed the isolated forearm technique to investigate wakefulness during muscle relaxation. In a study of 32 women for elective Caesarean section [117] there were significant within-patient variations up to 10 minutes after induction of anaesthesia, with both positive and negative responses in the same mother. The majority of women responded to a command by squeezing the anaesthetist's hand during anaesthesia, but no mother had recall or dreaming. A more recent study of 30 patients in the induction-to-delivery interval did not elicit explicit recall [118], yet up to 97% of women responded positively using the isolated forearm technique. The induction dose in this study was 3 mg/kg thiopental, smaller than the recommended dose and known to be associated with higher risk of awareness.

It is not easy to explain the apparent paradox of awareness detected by a purposeful response to questions which is later not recalled. However, there is a difference between information processing in the brain (i.e. perception of stimuli and their processing) and consciousness. Anaesthetics gate sensory information flow at the level of the thalamus, but other afferent pathways are left relatively untouched, such as the spinothalamic and auditory pathways [119]. The P300 auditory evoked response is associated with changes in incoming information. However, a lack of P300 response cannot be used as a sign of lack of awareness [120]. Lower oesophageal contractility has not proved to be a reproducible indicator either [121], and none of the methods described is used routinely except postoperative recall, which is diagnostic rather than preventative. It is hoped that a measure of the depth of anaesthesia may be developed in the future. Until then, it is essential to use an adequate dose of intravenous induction agent followed by monitored use of a suitable concentration of inhalational agent to maintain end-tidal concentrations of volatile agent at the MAC level, together with nitrous oxide. Postoperatively, a visit from the anaesthetist should elicit any remembered events or dreams. It is simple to ask a woman what she last remembers before going to sleep and what she remembers on waking up. A direct question on awareness is not usually necessary, but a question on dreaming may open an avenue for discussion or the acknowledgement that people often hear things before they waken fully. Any suggestion that awareness has occurred should be treated seriously, and a cause should be sought. The equipment used must be checked for leaks and gas calibration, the episode should be documented, and a full explanation should be given to the mother. She should also be followed up in puerperium until the anaesthetist is confident that long-term psychological help is not needed.

References

1 Abboud TK, Nagappalla S, Murakawa K et al. Comparison of the effects of general and regional anaesthesia for Caesarean section on neonatal neurologic and adaptive capacity scores. *Anaesthesia Analg* 1985; **64**: 996–1000.
2 Hodgkinson R, Bhatt M, Kim SS, Grewal G, Marx GF. Neonatal neurobehavioral tests following Cesarean section under general and spinal anesthesia. *Am J Obstet Gynecol* 1978; **132**: 670–4.
3 Department of Health. *Report on Confidential Enquiries into Maternal Deaths in England and Wales, 1982–1984.* London: HMSO, 1989.
4 Department of Health. *Report on Confidential Enquiries into Maternal Deaths in the United Kingdom, 1985–1987.* London: HMSO, 1991.
5 Department of Health. *Report on Confidential Enquiries into Maternal Deaths in the United Kingdom, 1988–1990.* London: HMSO, 1994.
6 Hibberd BM, Department of Health. *Report on Confidential Enquiries into Maternal Deaths in the United Kingdom, 1991–1993.* London: HMSO, 1996.
7 Hawkins JL, Koonin LM, Palmer SK, Gibbs CP. Anesthesia-related deaths during obstetric delivery in the United States 1979–90. *Anesthesiology* 1997; **86**: 277–84.
8 Morgan BM, Magni V, Goroszenuik T. Anaesthesia for emergency Caesarean section. *Br J Obstet Gynaecol* 1990; **97**: 420–4.

9 Field LM, Barton FL. The management of anaesthesia for Caesarean section in a patient with paroxysmal ventricular tachycardia. *Anaesthesia* 1993; **48**: 593–5.

10 Lanigan C, Reynolds F. Risk information supplied by obstetric anaesthetists in Britain and Ireland to mothers awaiting elective Caesarean section. *Int J Obstet Anaesth* 1995; **4**: 7–13.

11 Bush DJ. A comparison of informed consent for obstetric anaesthesia in the USA and the UK. *Int J Obstet Anaesth* 1995; **4**: 1–6.

12 Knapp RM. Legal view of informed consent for anesthesia during labor. *Anesthesiology* 1990; **72**: 211.

13 Eichhorn JH, Cooper JB, Cullen DJ et al. Standards for patient monitoring during anesthesia at Harvard Medical School. *JAMA* 1986; **256**: 1017–20.

14 Beemer GH, Cass NM. Monitoring the neuromuscular junction. *Anaesth Intensive Care* 1988; **16**: 62–6.

15 Association of Anaesthetists of Great Britain and Ireland. *Recommendations for Standards of Monitoring During Anaesthesia and Recovery.* London: AAGBI, 1988.

16 Winter A, Spencer AA. An international consensus on monitoring? *Br J Anaesth* 1990; **64**: 263–6.

17 Mathew JP, Fleisher LA, Rinehouse JA et al. S–T segment depression during labor and delivery. *Anesthesiology* 1992; **77**: 635–41.

18 McLintic AJ, Pringle SD, Lilley S, Houston AB, Thorburn J. Electrocardiographic changes during Cesarean section under regional anesthesia. *Anesth Analg* 1992; **74**: 51–6.

19 Trotter TN, Langton JA, Barker P, Rowbotham DJ. Perioperative continuous monitoring of S–T segment changes in patients undergoing elective Caesarean section. *Br J Anaesth* 1992; **69**: 352–5.

20 Fong J, Gadalla F, Druzin M. Venous emboli occurring during Caesarean section: the effect of patient position. *Can J Anaesth* 1991; **38**: 191–5.

21 Matthews NC, Greer G. Embolism during Caesarean section. *Anaesthesia* 1990; **45**: 964–5.

22 Eriksson LI. Ventilation and neuromuscular blocking drugs. *Acta Anaesthesiol Scand* 1994; **38** (Suppl 102): 11–15.

23 Archer GW, Marx GE. Arterial oxygenation during apnoea in parturient women. *Br J Anaesth* 1974; **46**: 35–60.

24 Norris MC, Kirkland MR, Torjman MC, Goldberg ME. Denitrogenation in pregnancy. *Can J Anaesth* 1989; **36**: 523–5.

25 Sellick BA. Cricoid pressure to control regurgitation of stomach contents during induction of anaesthesia. *Lancet* 1961; **ii**: 404–6.

26 Benhamou D. Cricoid pressure is unnecessary in obstetric general anaesthesia. *Int J Obstet Anaesth* 1995; **4**: 30–3.

27 Howells TH, Chamney AR, Wraight WJ, Simons RS. The application of cricoid pressure: an assessment and a survey of its practice. *Br J Anaesth* 1983; **38**: 457–60.

28 Warner MA, Warner ME, Webster JG. Clinical significance of pulmonary aspiration during the perioperative period. *Anesthesiology* 1993; **78**: 56–62.

29 Kahrilas PJ, Dodds WJ, Dent J et al. Effect of sleep, spontaneous gastroesophageal reflux and a meal on upper esophageal sphincter pressure in normal human volunteers. *Gastroenterology* 1987; **92**: 466–71.

30 Smith G, Dalling R, Williams TIR. Gastro-oesophageal pressure gradient changes produced by induction of anaesthesia and suxamethonium. *Br J Anaesth* 1978; **50**: 1137–43.

31 Vanner RG, Goodman NW. Gastro-oesophageal reflux in pregnancy, at term and after delivery. *Anaesthesia* 1989; **44**: 808–11.

32 Dent J, Dodds WJ, Hogan WJ, Toouli J. Factors that influence induction of gastroesophageal reflux in normal human subjects. *Dig Dis Sci* 1988; **33**: 270–5.

33 Van Thiel DH, Gavaler JS, Stremple J. Lower esophageal sphincter pressure in women using sequential oral contraceptives. *Gastroenterology* 1976; **71**: 232–5.

34 Dent J, Holloway RH, Toouli J, Dodds WJ. Mechanisms of lower oesophageal sphincter incompetence in patients with symptomatic gastro-oesophageal reflux. *Gut* 1988; **29**: 1020–8.

35 Vanner RG, O'Dwyer JP, Pryle BJ, Reynolds F. Upper oesophageal sphincter pressure and the effect of cricoid pressure. *Anaesthesia* 1992; **47**: 95–100.

36 Vanner RG, Pryle BJ, O'Dwyer JP, Reynolds F. Upper oesophageal sphincter pressure and the intravenous induction of anaesthesia. *Anaesthesia* 1992; **47**: 371–5.

37 Groves ND, Rees JL, Rosen M. Effects of benzodiazepines on laryngeal reflexes. *Anaesthesia* 1987; **42**: 808–14.

38 Vanner RG, Pryle BJ, O'Dwyer JP, Reynolds F. Upper oesophageal sphincter pressure during inhalational anaesthesia. *Anaesthesia* 1992; **47**: 950–4.

39 Vanner RG, Pryle BJ. Regurgitation and oesophageal rupture during cricoid pressure: a cadaver study. *Anaesthesia* 1992; **47**: 732–5.

40 Crowley DS, Giesecke AH. Bimanual cricoid pressure. *Anaesthesia* 1990; **45**: 588–9.

41 Ralph SJ, Wareham CA. Rupture of the oesophagus during cricoid pressure. *Anaesthesia* 1991; **46**: 40–1.

42 Vanner RG. Tolerance of cricoid pressure by conscious volunteers. *Int J Obstet Anaesth* 1992; **1**: 195–8.

43 Brimacombe JR, Berry AM. Cricoid pressure. *Can J Anaesth* 1997; **44**: 414–25.

44 Holdcroft A, Morgan M. Intravenous induction agents for Caesarean section. *Anaesthesia* 1989; **44**: 719–20.

45 Meer FM, Downing JW, Coleman AJ. An intravenous method of anaesthesia for Caesarean section, 2: ketamine. *Br J Anaesth* 1973; **45**: 191–6.

46 Reddy BK, Pizer B, Bull PT. Neonatal serum cortisol suppression by etomidate compared with thiopentone for elective Caesarean section. *Eur J Anaesthesiol* 1988; **5**: 175–6.

47 Holdcroft A, Robinson MJ, Gordon H, Whitman JG. Comparison of the effect of two induction doses of methohexitone on infants delivered by elecure Caesarean section. *Br Med J* 1974; **2**: 472–5.

48 Moore J, Bill KM, Flynn RJ, McKeating KT, Howard PJ. A comparison between propofol and thiopentone as induction agents for obstetric anaesthesia. *Anaesthesia* 1989; **44**: 753–7.

49 Yau G, Gin T, Ewart MC *et al.* Propofol for induction and maintenance of anaesthesia at Caesarean section. *Anaesthesia* 1991; **46**: 20–3.

50 Gin T, Yau G, Jong W *et al.* Disposition of propofol at Caesarean section and in the postpartum period. *Br J Anaesth* 1991; **67**: 49–53.

51 Gin T, O'Meara ME, Kan AF *et al.* Plasma catecholamines and neonatal condition after induction of anaesthesia with propofol or thiopentone at Caesarean section. *Br J Anaesth* 1993; **70**: 311–16.

52 Celleno D, Capogna G, Tomassetti M *et al.* Neurobehavioural effects of propofol on the neonate following elective Caesarean section. *Br J Anaesth* 1989; **62**: 649–54.

53 Kantor G, Rolbin SH. Acute intermittent porphyria and Caesarean delivery. *Can J Anaesth* 1992; **39**: 282–5.

54 Magill IW. Technique in endotracheal anaesthesia. *Br Med J* 1930; **ii**: 817–19.

55 Connell H, Dalgleish JH, Downing JW. General anaesthesia in mothers with severe pre-eclampsia/eclampsia. *Br J Anaesth* 1987; **59**: 1375–80.

56 Rout CC, Rocke DA. Effects of alfentanil and fentanyl on induction of anaesthesia in patients with severe pregnancy-induced hypertension. *Br J Anaesth* 1990; **65**: 468–74.

57 Allen RW, James MF, Uys PC. Attenuation of the pressor response to tracheal intubation in hypertensive proteinuric pregnant patients by lignocaine, alfentanil and magnesium sulphate. *Br J Anaesth* 1991; **66**: 216–23.

58 Ramanathan J, Sibai BM, Mabie WC, Chauhan D, Ruiz AG. The use of labetalol for attenuation of the hypertensive response to endotracheal intubation in pre-eclampsia. *Am J Obstet Gynecol* 1988; **159**: 650–4.

59 Kumar N, Batra YK, Bala I, Gopalan S. Nifedipine attenuates the hypertensive response to tracheal intubation in pregnancy-induced hypertension. *Can J Anaesth* 1993; **40**: 329–33.

60 Hood DD, Dewan DM, Jones FM, Floyd HM, Bogard TD. The use of nitroglycerin in preventing the hypertensive response to tracheal intubation in severe pre eclampsia. *Anesthesiology* 1985; **63**: 329–32.

61 Lawes EG, Newman B, Campbell MJ et al. Maternal inspired oxygen concentration and neonatal status for Caesarean section under general anaesthesia: comparison of effects of 33% or 50% oxygen in nitrous oxide. *Br J Anaesth* 1988; **61**: 250–4.

62 Wilson T, Turner DJ. Awareness during Caesarean section under general anaesthesia. *Br Med J* 1969; **i**: 280–3.

63 Marx GF, Mateo CV. Effects of different oxygen concentrations during general anaesthesia for elective Caesarean section. *Can Anaesth Soc J* 1971; **18**: 587–93.

64 Bogod DG, Rosen M, Rees GAD. Maximum F_{IO_2} during Caesarean section. *Br J Anaesth* 1988; **61**: 255–62.

65 Piggott SE, Bogod DG, Rosen M, Rees GA, Harmer M. Isoflurane with either 100% oxygen or 50% nitrous oxide in oxygen for Caesarean section. *Br J Anaesth* 1990; **65**: 325–9.

66 Thorp JA, Trobough T, Evans R, Hedruck J, Yeast JD. The effect of maternal oxygen administration during the second stage of labor on umbilical cord blood gas values: a randomized controlled prospective trial. *Am J Obstet Gynecol* 1995; **172**: 456–74.

67 Magno R, Selstram U, Karlsson K. Anaesthesia for Caesarean section, 2: effects of the induction–delivery interval on the respiratory adaptation of the newborn in the elective Caesarean section. *Acta Anaesthesiol Scand* 1975; **19**: 250–9.

68 Crawford JS, James FM, Davies P, Crawley M. A further study of general anaesthesia for Caesarean section. *Br J Anaesth* 1976; **48**: 661–7.

69 Marx GF, Joshi CW, Orkin LR. Placental transmission of nitrous oxide. *Anesthesiology* 1970; **32**: 429–32.

70 Mokriski BK, Malinow AM. Neonatal acid–base status following general anesthesia for emergency abdominal delivery with halothane or isoflurane. *J Clin Anesth* 1992; **4**: 97–100.

71 Warren TM, Datta S, Ostheimer GW et al. Comparison of the maternal and neonatal effects of halothane, enflurane and isoflurane for Caesarean delivery. *Anaesth Analg* 1983; **62**: 516–20.

72 Eger EI II. New inhaled anesthetics. *Anesthesiology* 1994; **80**: 806–22.

73 Palahniuk RJ, Shnider SM, Eger EI II. Pregnancy decreases the requirements for inhaled anesthetic agents. *Anesthesiology* 1974; **41**: 82–3.

74 Gin T, Chan MT. Decreased minimum alveolar concentration of isoflurane in pregnant humans. *Anesthesiology* 1994; **81**: 829–32.

75 Dwyer R, Fee JPH, Moore J. Uptake of halothane and isoflurane by mother and baby during Caesarean section. *Br J Anaesth* 1995; **74**: 379–83.

76 Marx GF, Kim YI, Lin CC, Halevy S, Schulman H. Postpartum uterine pressures under halothane or enflurane anesthesia. *Obstet Gynecol* 1978; **51**: 695–8.

77 Palahniuk RJ, Cumming M. Foetal deterioration following thiopentone–nitrous oxide anaesthesia in the pregnant ewe. *Can Anaesth Soc J* 1977; **24**: 361–70.

78 McCrirrick A, Evans GH, Thomas TA. Overpressure isoflurane at Caesarean section: a study of arterial isoflurane concentrations. *Br J Anaesth* 1994; **72**: 122–4.

79 Turner DR, Kao J, Bivona C. Neuromuscular block by suxamethonium following treatment with histamine type 2 antagonists and metoclopramide. *Br J Anaesth* 1989; **63**: 348–50.

80 Thind CS, Bryson THL. Single dose suxamethonium and muscle pains in pregnancy. *Br J Anaesth* 1983; **55**: 743–5.

81 Frank M, Flynn PJ, Hughes R. Atracurium in obstetric anaesthesia. *Br J Anaesth* 1983; **55**: 1135–48.

82 Dailey PA, Fisher DM, Shnider SM et al. Pharmacokinetics, placental transfer, and neonatal effects of vecuronium and pancuronium administered during Cesarean section. *Anesthesiology* 1984; **60**: 569–74.

83 Shearer ES, Fahy LT, O'Sullivan EP, Hunter JM. Transplacental distribution of atracurium, laudanosine and monoquaternary alcohol during elective Caesarean section. *Br J Anaesth* 1991; **66**: 551–6.

84 Abouleish E, Abboud T, LeChavalier T et al. Rocuronium (Org 94–26) for Caesarean section. *Br J Anaesth* 1994; **73**: 336–41.

85 Sockalingham I, Green DW. Mivacurium-induced prolonged neuromuscular block. *Br J Anaesth* 1995; **74**: 234–6.

86 Fox MH, Hunt PCW. Prolonged neuromuscular block associated with mivacurium. *Br J Anaesth* 1995; **74**: 237–8.

87 Imberti R, Preseglio I, Trotta V, Filisetti P, Mapelli A. Blood transfusion during Caesarean section: a 12-year retrospective analysis. *Acta Anaesthesiol Belg* 1990; **41**: 139–44.

88 Naef RW, Chauhan SP, Chevalier SP et al. Prediction of hemorrhage at Cesarean delivery. *Obstet Gynecol* 1994; **83**: 923–6.

89 Howell PR, Gambling DR, Pavy T, McMorland G, Douglas MJ. Patient-controlled analgesia following Caesarean section under general anaesthesia: a comparison of fentanyl with morphine. *Can J Anaesth* 1995; **42**: 41–5.

90 Wittels B, Scott DT, Sinatra RS. Endogenous opioids in human breast milk and acute neonatal neurobehavior: a preliminary study. *Anesthesiology* 1990; **72**: 864–9.

91 Russell D, Duncan LA, Frame WT et al. Patient-controlled analgesia with morphine and droperidol following Caesarean section under spinal anaesthesia. *Acta Anaesthesiol Scand* 1996; **40**: 600–5.

92 McQuay HJ, Justins D, Moore RA. Treating acute pain in hospital. *Br Med J* 1997; **314**: 1531–5.

93 Spigs TO. Anaesthetic agents and excretion in breast milk. *Acta Anaesthesiol Scand* 1994; **38**: 94–103.

94 Mallampati SR. Clinical signs to predict difficult tracheal intubation. *Can Anaesth Soc J* 1983; **30**: 316–17.

95 Samsoon GLT, Young JRB. Difficult tracheal intubation: a retrospective study. *Anaesthesia* 1987; **42**: 487–90.

96 Wilson ME, Spiegelhalter D, Robertson JA, Lesser P. Predicting difficult intubation. *Br J Anaesth* 1988; **61**: 211–16.

97 Frerk CM. Predicting difficult intubation. *Anaesthesia* 1991; **46**: 1005–8.

98 Farcon EL, Kim MH, Marx GF. Changing Mallampati score during labour. *Can J Anaesth* 1994; **41**: 50–1.

99 Rocke DA, Murray WB, Rout CC, Gouws E. Relative risk analysis of factors associated with difficult intubation in obstetric anesthesia. *Anesthesiology* 1992; **77**: 67–73.

100 Hood DD, Dewan DM. Anesthetic and obstetric outcome in morbidly obese parturients. *Anesthesiology* 1993; **79**: 1210–18.

101 Lyons G. Failed intubation. *Anaesthesia* 1985; **40**: 759–62.

102 Hawthorne L, Wilson R, Lyons G, Dresner M. Failed intubation revisited: 17-year experience in a teaching maternity unit. *Br J Anaesth* 1996; **76**: 680–4.

103 American Society of Anesthesiologists Task Force on Management of the Difficult Airway. Practical guidelines for management of the difficult airway. *Anesthesiology* 1993; **78**: 597–602.

104 Cormack RS, Lehane J. Difficult intubation in obstetrics. *Anaesthesia* 1987; **39**: 1105–11.

105 Brimacombe J, Berry A. The laryngeal mask airway for obstetric and neonatal resuscitation. *Int J Obstet Anesth* 1994; **3**: 211–18.

106 Brimacombe J, Berry A, White A. Single versus double handed cricoid pressure for LMA insertion. *Anaesthesia* 1994; **72**: 732–3.

107 Strang TI. Does the laryngeal mask airway compromise cricoid pressure? *Anaesthesia* 1992; **47**: 829–31.

108 Devitt JH, Wenstone R, Noel AG, O'Donnell MP. The laryngeal mask airway and positive-pressure ventilation. *Anesthesiology* 1994; **80**: 550–5.

109 Heath ML, Allagain J. Intubation through the laryngeal mask: a technique for unexpected difficult intubation. *Anaesthesia* 1991; **46**: 545–8.

110 Asai T. Use of the laryngeal mask for tracheal intubation in patients at increased risk of aspiration of gastric contents. *Anesthesiology* 1992; **77**: 1029–30.

111 Hasham FM, Andrews PJD, Juneja MM, Ackerman WE III. The laryngeal mask airway facilitates intubation at Caesarean section: a case report of a difficult intubation. *Int J Obstet Anaesth* 1993; **2**: 181–2.

112 Maltby JR, Neil SG. Laryngeal mask airway and difficult intubation. *Anesthesiology* 1993; **78**: 994–5.

113 Baer GA. Prevention of barotrauma during intratracheal jet ventilation. *Anaesthesia* 1993; **48**: 544–5.

114 Schumacher P, Stotz G, Schneider M, Urwyler A. Laryngospasm during transtracheal high frequency jet ventilation. *Anaesthesia* 1992; **47**: 855–6.

115 Lyons G, McDonald R. Awareness during Caesarean section. *Anaesthesia* 1991; **46**: 62–4.

116 [Editorial.] On being aware. *Br J Anaesth* 1979; **51**: 711–12.

117 Tunstall ME. The reduction of amnesic wakefulness during Caesarean section. *Anaesthesia* 1979; **34**: 316–19.

118 King H, Ashley S, Brathwaite D, Decayette J, Wooten DJ. Adequacy of general anaesthesia for Caesarean section. *Anaesth Analg* 1993; **77**: 84–8.

119 Angel A, Lebeau F. A comparison of the effects of propofol with other anaesthetic agents on the centripetal transmission of sensory information. *Gen Pharmacol* 1992; **23**: 945–64.

120 Plourde G, Joffe D, Villemure C, Trahan M. The P3a wave of the auditory event related potential reveals registration of pitch change during sufentanil anesthesia for cardiac surgery. *Anesthesiology* 1993; **78**: 498–509.

121 Bogod DG, Orton JK, Yau HM, Oh TE. Detecting awareness during general anaesthetic Caesarean section: an evaluation of two methods. *Anaesthesia* 1990; **45**: 279–84.

17: Anaesthesia for Antepartum and Postpartum Surgery

17.1 Pregnancy

Anaesthesia is administered during pregnancy for a small variety of surgical interventions. The surgery may be necessary for the emergency treatment of conditions not connected with pregnancy—appendicitis being the commonest of these—or for correction of problems that threaten the pregnancy itself. The reported incidence of surgery during pregnancy varies from 0.36% [1] to 2.2% [2,3]. Other studies show incidences of 1.6% [4], where, in a series of 9000 deliveries, 147 operations had been undertaken antenatally, 87 of them under some type of regional anaesthesia.

Planned or elective surgery is almost never undertaken during pregnancy, because anaesthesia and surgery are associated with an increased risk of spontaneous abortion [2]. Whether the increased risk is due to the stress of surgery, the systemic effects of anaesthesia, or the presenting condition is still uncertain. Whatever the mechanism, anaesthesia and surgery are best avoided during pregnancy, but if they are unavoidable the second trimester is probably the most stable time. In addition to the risk of abortion, a hypothetical risk has been postulated of fetal dysplasia or teratogenesis following maternal exposure to some inhalational anaesthetic agents during the first trimester. The hypothesis was based mainly on the evidence that nitrous oxide is teratogenic in the rat. The first report [5] showed in the rat that administration of 70% nitrous oxide throughout the period of organogenesis resulted in increased rates of abnormality. It seems likely that the dysplasia in the rat was due to nitrous oxide interference with folate metabolism, because pretreatment with folic acid prevented some of the effects [6]. Inactivation of the vitamin B_{12} fraction of the enzyme methionine synthetase by nitrous oxide and concomitant falls in plasma methionine have also been recorded [7].

However, similar changes have not been detected in humans undergoing minor or intermediate surgery [8], and the evidence for the safety of nitrous oxide during human pregnancy is quite strong [9–12]. If a risk exists at all, it is slight. Should any doubt exist as to the wisdom of administering nitrous oxide during human organogenesis in the first eight weeks of pregnancy, the drug can be easily avoided. A mixture of oxygen, air and isoflurane produces good anaesthesia safely, and isoflurane has not so far been implicated in any fetal dysplasia. In fact, its pharmacodynamics and kinetics make it an excellent maintenance anaesthetic agent for general anaesthesia in the pregnant patient.

Local anaesthetic techniques avoid the systemic effects of general anaesthetic agents and the risks of intubation problems and aspiration of gastric contents, and they also reduce the secretion of stress-related hormones such as adrenocorticotropic hormone. The inference clearly is that this form of anaesthesia may be associated with less hormonal stress for the duration of the local anaesthetic.

When choosing the timing and method of anaesthesia for the pregnant patient, some basic principles should be remembered.
- Avoid anaesthesia and surgery during organogenesis in the first eight weeks of pregnancy, if at all possible.
- Avoid general anaesthesia, if possible.
- Avoid drugs that can cause uterine artery vasoconstriction, e.g. epinephrine.
- Consider altered physiology, with changes in circulating blood volume and drug-related effects such as changes in volume of distribution.
- Maintain normal (for each patient) cardiovascular and respiratory system functions. After 20 weeks, use a lateral wedged position.

In addition, consider whether or not the pregnancy is viable and how close delivery may be. In cases in which the pregnancy is no longer viable, the choice of anaesthesia is entirely based on the mother's needs and safety. Extreme examples of this type of situation include ectopic pregnancy. In such cases, the priorities of anaesthesia are no different from those in any other major emergency. Treating the effects of major blood loss and ensuring a clear airway and ventilation are paramount. The use of general anaesthesia is advised, because it allows full access to any part of the patient for both therapeutic and invasive monitoring. Central venous pressure, arterial pressure and possibly pulmonary artery pressures will frequently be measured in such situations. Manipulation of the cardiovascular functions of the patient can be freely undertaken without any concern for the effect that such changes might have had if the patient were conscious.

The commonest operation carried out on pregnant patients is undoubtedly termination of pregnancy. The legal gestational maturity limit at present in the United Kingdom for the termination of pregnancy is 24 weeks. Most operations are performed electively before 20 weeks. Evacuation of retained products of conception following one or other type of miscarriage places similar demands on the anaesthetist, and as far as the choice of anaesthesia is concerned, can be considered together with termination. The patient is usually starved and the evacuation is completed as a semi-elective procedure. These apparently simple procedures and anaesthetics are complicated by the question of whether the pregnancy has advanced to a maturity at which gastrointestinal function is altered. The answer to this question determines whether or not anaesthesia should include a rapid-sequence induction and endotracheal intubation.

Studies in pregnant patients with a mean gestational maturity of 15 weeks showed that their residual gastric contents volume following a period of starvation was identical with that of non-pregnant control patients [13]. Lower oesophageal barrier pressure in early pregnancy has also been shown to remain unchanged [14]. However, Bainbridge and co-workers [15] recorded a decrease in lower oesophageal pressure also during early pregnancy. Vanner [16] investigated oesophageal pH changes in 100 patients undergoing termination of pregnancy. The gestational maturity varied from six to 22 weeks, and the incidence of oesophageal reflux was the same for patients in both first and second trimester. Two patients in his series also showed low pharyngeal pH readings, but had no clinical evidence of regurgitation or aspiration of gastric contents. In the United Kingdom, all maternal deaths are reported in the triennial *Reports on Confidential Enquiries into Maternal Deaths.* Only one death has resulted from pulmonary aspiration in over one million (estimated) early pregnancy procedures. It would therefore seem to be a very low-risk anaesthetic procedure, for which a combination of rapid-sequence induction and endotracheal intubation should be reserved for pregnancy gestations in excess of 20 weeks.

If evidence of oesophageal reflux and regurgitation are present at any stage of pregnancy, prophylactic control of gastric secretions (see Chapter 5, Section 5.5, p. 91) should be given, and endotracheal intubation is likely to be needed.

In most patients requiring termination or evacuation of products of conception, general anaesthesia with an opioid/propofol induction followed by maintenance with oxygen, air and isoflurane via a laryngeal mask airway will provide smooth general anaesthesia with rapid recovery for day-case surgery.

Total intravenous anaesthesia can be used just as effectively, but the propofol infusion rate needed for these young, fit, apprehensive women is often higher than many regimens recommend. An intravenous infusion of propofol in combination with alfentanil can be used, and the inclusion of alfentanil reduces the dose of propofol needed. When women are at risk of nausea and vomiting—for example, with a previous obstetric or anaesthetic history—the use of alfentanil may be avoided. However, a dose of 1.5 µg/kg fentanyl 2–3 minute pre-induction will make induction and maintenance smoother, and has few emetic sequelae, especially if an anti-emetic combination is also given. One such combination consists of:
- metoclopramide 10 mg oral premedication;
- hyoscine 200 µg i.v., 2–3 min pre-induction;
- fentanyl 1.25 µg/kg i.v., 2–3 min pre-induction;
- propofol 1.5–2.0 mg/kg i.v. bolus;
- propofol 10 mg/kg/h i.v. infusion reducing after 5 min to 8 mg/kg/h.

Hyoscine is used for its sedative, anti-emetic, antisialagogue and mild cardiovascular anticholinergic effects. The prophylactic anti-emetic drug metoclopramide 10 mg is given orally as premedication one hour before surgery, and helps to increase gastric emptying and improve lower oesophageal sphincter tone. A brief period of apnoea may follow induction, so oxygen 100% should be given for the two to three minutes between the fentanyl and the propofol injection. During anaesthesia, it is occasionally necessary to reduce the propofol infusion rate below 8 mg/kg/h.

17.2 Postpartum surgery

Gastric function usually returns to normal by 24 hours after delivery (see pp. 88–9), unless opioids have been administered by whatever route. Prophylaxis for acid aspiration will need to be given if acid aspiration is still a risk factor.

Blood loss or ongoing losses require assessment, and haemoglobin concentration may not be a true reflection of blood volume loss. If general anaesthesia is required a difficult intubation may continue to be a risk, because fluid retention can persist until a diuresis starts. High concentrations of volatile anaesthetic agents are to be avoided due to their uterine relaxation effects. Drug dosages may start to change from their altered potency in pregnancy, and transfer of drugs to breast milk and their effects on the fetus should be considered (see Appendix 2, p. 443).

17.3 Fetal surgery

Fetal surgery has a great potential for development. Laparoscopic surgery with a restricted approach to the amniotic cavity has reduced the trauma of opening the uterus and exteriorizing the fetus. Technical aspects have been refined, and innovative methods are being used to modify fetal abnormalities. During surgery, the anaesthetist must prevent fetal movements and provide adequate analgesia. The requirements for pain relief both for the mother and the fetus extend into the postoperative period [17]. Postoperatively, the development of uterine contractions is a potential hazard, but tocolytic drugs can be administered.

17.4 Ectopic pregnancy

Most ectopic pregnancies occur in the Fallopian tube. There has been a downward trend in maternal deaths from ectopic pregnancy, and the death rate per 1000 estimated ectopic pregnancies is 0.3% [18]. All of the cases were associated with substandard care, particularly a delay in diagnosis. The management of the collapsed bleeding woman must be fast, and teamwork is essential. An experienced gynaecologist, anaesthetist and haematologist must all be involved, and the availability of intensive-care facilities is required. In some cases, resuscitation and surgery will need to be carried out simultaneously. Surgery is the curative treatment, and it is urgently needed in the collapsed patient.

The presentation of ectopic pregnancy can be considered as two distinct scenarios, depending on whether or not the tube is ruptured (Table 17.1).

Table 17.1 Presentation of ectopic pregnancy.

Unruptured
Severe pain of sudden onset
Vague tenderness

Ruptured
Shock, rigid abdomen
Too tender to palpate

There are asymptomatic women who have earlier gestations, and surgical or medical management may be chosen. The most common surgical procedure is a laparoscopy with conservative, fertility-preserving procedures. The anaesthetic management of such patients even early in gestation requires the use of a cuffed endotracheal tube in order to protect the airway inflation of, and allow surgical access to, the abdomen. These patients are not emergency cases, and adequate time can therefore be allowed for preparation and emptying gastric contents. Where there are major contraindications to anaesthesia, medical management with local injection of methotrexate is the therapy of choice.

17.4.1 Ruptured ectopic pregnancy

Where the ruptured ectopic pregnancy has haemorrhaged, with the blood loss being concealed, resuscitation with fluid and blood restoration through large-bore cannulae prior to anaesthesia is essential. Cardiovascular monitoring of pulse rate, oxygen saturation and blood pressure (invasive, if there is blood loss of more than 1.5 L) is necessary before induction of anaesthesia if possible. If the woman continues to bleed despite adequate resuscitation, she will have an unstable haemodynamic state. If the patient is collapsed with very low blood pressure, the initial steps to correct the circulating blood volume must be taken as they would be with any major obstetric haemorrhage (see Section 23.1, p. 419). Two large-bore intravenous cannulae with fast-flowing infusions and emergency blood supplies are essential. It is not necessary to return systemic blood pressure to 'normal' before inducing anaesthesia. A systolic baseline blood pressure of 80–90 mmHg will suffice. Induction of general anaesthetic is best carried out using cardio-stable drugs, and in such circumstances ketamine 2 mg/kg intravenously is an invaluable agent, providing complete anaesthesia for approximately 20 minutes, with good maintenance of blood pressure. Rapid surgical intervention is vital once the initial resuscitation has been started.

Complications can arise from laparoscopy with carbon dioxide insufflation in this situation. End-tidal carbon dioxide will increase, and may mask the underlying reduction in pulmonary blood flow. An increase in intra-abdominal pressure may further reduce a diminished venous return to the heart. Continuous monitoring of cardiac and respiratory functions are vital at the time of insufflation, so that the gas flow can be stopped if necessary and open laparotomy undertaken.

Postoperatively, pain after laparoscopy is not as severe as after laparotomy, but nausea and vomiting can be troublesome complications.

References

1 Smith BE. Fetal prognosis after anesthesia during gestation. *Anesth Analg* 1963; **42**: 521–6.
2 Brodsky JB, Cohen EN, Brown BW, Wu ML, Whitcher C. Surgery during pregnancy and fetal outcome. *Am J Obstet Gynecol* 1980; **138**: 1165–7.
3 Konieczko KM, Chapple JC, Nunn JF. Fetotoxic potential of general anaesthesia in relation to pregnancy. *Br J Anaesth* 1987; **59**: 449–54.
4 Schnider SM, Webster GM. Maternal and fetal hazards of surgery during pregnancy. *Am J Obstet Gynecol* 1965; **92**: 891–900.
5 Fink BR, Shepard TH, Blandau RJ. Teratogenic activity of nitrous oxide. *Nature* 1967; **214**: 146–8.
6 Keeling PA, Rocke DA, Nunn JF *et al.* Folinic acid protection against nitrous oxide teratogenicity in the rat. *Br J Anaesth* 1986; **58**: 528–34.
7 Koblin DD, Watson JE, Deady JE, Stokstad EL, Eger EI II. Inactivation of methionine synthetase by nitrous oxide in mice. *Anesthesiology* 1981; **54**: 318–24.
8 Nunn JF, Sharer NM, Bottiglieri T, Rossiter J. Effect of short term administration of nitrous oxide on plasma concentrations of methionine, tryptophan, phenylalanine and *S*-adenosyl methionine in man. *Br J Anaesth* 1986; **58**: 1–10.
9 Aldridge LM, Tunstall ME. Nitrous oxide and the fetus: a review and results of a retrospective study of 175 cases of anaesthesia for insertion of Shirodkar suture. *Br J Anaesth* 1986; **58**: 1348–56.
10 Crawford JS, Lewis M. Nitrous oxide in early human pregnancy. *Anaesthesia* 1986; **41**: 900–5.
11 Duncan PG, Pope WD, Cohen MM, Greer N. Fetal risk of anesthesia and surgery during pregnancy. *Anesthesiology* 1986; **64**: 790–4.
12 Park GR, Fulton IC, Shelly MP. Normal pregnancy following nitrous oxide exposure in the first trimester. *Br J Anaesth* 1986; **58**: 576–7.
13 Wyner J, Cohen SE. Gastric volume in early pregnancy. *Anesthesiology* 1982; **57**: 209–12.
14 Brock-Utne JG, Dow TG, Dimopoulos GE *et al.* Gastric and lower oesophageal sphincter (LOS) pressures in early pregnancy. *Br J Anaesth* 1981; **53**: 381–4.
15 Bainbridge ET, Nichols SD, Newton JR, Temple JG. Gastro-oesophageal reflux in pregnancy. *Scand J Gastroenterol* 1984; **19**: 85–9.
16 Vanner RG. Gastro-oesophageal reflux during general anaesthesia for termination of pregnancy. *Int J Obstet Anaesth* 1992; **1**: 123–8.
17 Lloyd-Thomas AR, Fitzgerald M. Reflex responses do not necessarily signify pain. *Br Med J* 1996; **313**: 797–8.
18 Hibberd BM, Department of Health. *Report on Confidential Enquiries into Maternal Deaths in the United Kingdom, 1991–1993.* London: HMSO, 1996.

Section 5
Labour

18: Labour

18.1 General considerations

18.1.1 Mobility

Some women in labour are concerned about their ability to move and adopt different positions for rest, relaxation and delivery. At home, women have access to many different supporting structures such as chairs and pillows, and are free to move and change position at will. In hospital, a range of chairs and pillows should be available, but the parturient may be restricted by attachments such as monitoring equipment or by her obstetric state if complications have arisen, or by anaesthetic requirements to establish a regional nerve block. The one position at home or in hospital that she should be actively discouraged from adopting is the supine position, in order to prevent aortocaval occlusion. Changes of posture should also be encouraged in order to determine the best position to relieve muscle tension and pressure on superficial nerves, such as the lateral popliteal nerve. There are many positions that have been advocated both for labour and delivery. They can broadly be divided into recumbent or upright positions. The full lateral decubitus position may be necessary—either left-sided or right-sided—if the woman becomes hypotensive, or if fetal distress occurs.

Without epidural analgesia, a woman can ambulate, provided that there is no increased risk of cord prolapse or haemorrhage. In the first stage of labour, women may wish to be active and walk around. However, the need to move and ambulate in labour has been reassessed with the advent of ambulatory epidural analgesia in labour. Movement helps bladder emptying and prevents venous stasis with the potential risk of thromboembolism. Safe ambulation requires haemodynamic stability, visual orientation, intact vestibular function and proprioception. Drugs or pathology that affect these symptoms can prevent ambulation.

The upright positions for labour and delivery are the sitting, standing, forward-leaning kneeling position and squatting. For women with known lumbar intervertebral disc abnormalities, a posture that avoids spinal flexion can be achieved using the kneeling on all fours position.

At the time of delivery, a vertical position may be considered more natural, and gravity can perhaps speed events. Thus, standing, squatting, hanging from a bar and sitting in a special bed or chair are positions for which there are enthusiasts. Some of these methods are inexpensive, but birth chairs may be elaborate and costly.

Squatting has been used for delivery over the ages in many countries. Lower limb motor power is required, so regional analgesia that protects motor activity is of value in this context. A prospective randomized controlled trial of the supported squatting posture and the conventional semi-recumbent position in 427 well-matched women found significantly fewer forceps deliveries (9% compared with 16%), significantly shorter second stages and fewer perineal tears but more labial tears in the squatting group [1]. Women with epidural analgesia were excluded from the trial. A birth chair does not offer any advantages over the recumbent position, and has been associated with vulval oedema and postpartum haemorrhage [2,3]. Such bleeding is probably perineal rather than uterine. Transfer to a bed is essential if operative delivery or other emergencies such as haemorrhage intervene. An anaesthetist attending the mother should be aware of and sympathetic to maternal wishes, but more particularly needs to be able to advise the mother on any risks or incompatibilities between the planned anaesthesia and the desire for a parturient posture.

18.1.2 Monitoring during labour

The partogram

A partogram is a graphical record of the progress of labour, and it is used to help to identify labours that are progressing normally and those which are not and may require intervention [4].

The visual presentation of clinical information is a useful mechanism for generating communication and review of an individual's labour management. The central feature of the partogram is the graphical plot of cervical dilatation with time (Fig. 18.1). Distinction is made between the latent phase of labour—up to 3 cm dilatation of the cervix—and the active phase that follows, in which at least 1 cm of cervical dilatation should be achieved per hour. Once 3 cm of dilatation has been charted, an alert line can be drawn with a 45° slope to represent expected normal progress. A second line four hours to the right of this and parallel with it is the active line up to which conservative management is recommended. The progress of labour is assessed by abdominal palpation of contraction strength and frequency, rate of oxytocin infusion, descent of head both abdominally and vaginally, and cervical dilatation.

In addition, the chart records maternal and fetal observations at least every 15 minutes.
- *Maternal condition:* heart rate, blood pressure, temperature, fluid balance (oral, intravenous, fluid output) and urinalysis (ketones, protein, glucose).
- *Fetal condition:* heart rate, presence or absence of meconium, degree of moulding and caput function.

The partogram is a monitoring tool requiring management guidelines. It is preferably combined with other forms of monitoring, e.g. a cardiotocogram, to provide a full assessment of an individual labour. In this way, it is possible to anticipate problems so that advanced planning can reduce the need for emergency interventions.

Invasive haemodynamic monitoring during labour

An electrocardiogram (ECG) with dysrhythmia and ischaemia monitoring and direct monitoring of systemic arterial blood pressure and/or central venous pressure may be required if uncomplicated labour is progressing in a woman with known cardiovascular disease, e.g. valvular incompetence or tachydysrhythmias, where alterations in cardiac performance require assessment. Complications associated with the placement of intra-arterial catheters are relatively uncommon in peripheral, non-end arteries. Placement of a central venous catheter in the internal jugular vein is associated with morbidity and a potential for major complications, particularly with staff unfamiliar with the use of these catheters. As with most interventions, the anticipated benefits should outweigh the risks, and the process with the least risk should be chosen. For example, a peripheral ante-cubital vein can be used, or when there is a danger of endocarditis the procedure should only be undertaken with specially impregnated catheters under full aseptic conditions in theatre. Assessment of clotting abnormalities may be required before central venous catheter insertion, particularly during labour associated with pre-eclampsia. Additional problems with the siting of central venous catheters in pregnant women include active muscle tone altering the depth of insertion; the use of an additional painful procedure in an awake patient; and a head-down tilt in addition to a lateral pelvic tilt, with cardiorespiratory compromise.

18.1.3 Active management of labour

The active management of labour involves continuous professional support and repeated assessment of the stage of labour. The partogram indicates that it is the intention of an obstetrician to limit the duration of labour. If progress in labour requires augmentation, the amniotic membranes may be ruptured and an oxytocin infusion commenced once clear amniotic fluid drains. Active management regimens seem to be associated with low operative delivery rates. It is unclear which component of the regimen is responsible for this result, and it may be the combination of elements that is important.

Uterine stimulants

Oxytocin. Oxytocin acts on specific receptors in the uterine muscle to activate the inositol phospholipid pathway and increase ionized calcium in human myometrial cells, so that contraction of the myometrium is enhanced.

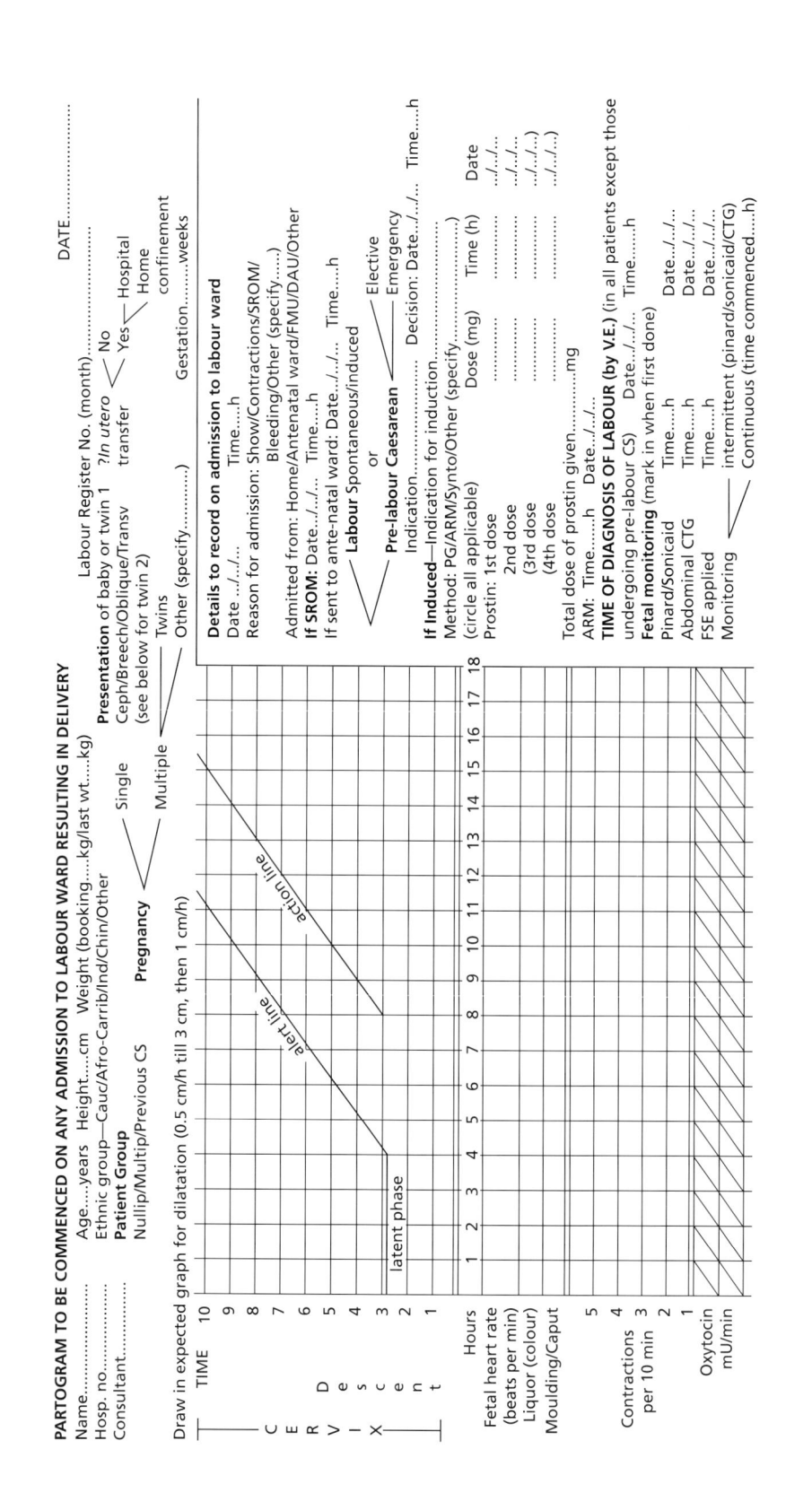

PARTOGRAM TO BE COMMENCED ON ANY ADMISSION TO LABOUR WARD RESULTING IN DELIVERY

Name.................... DATE............
Hosp. no................ Labour Register No. (month)....................
Consultant.............. Age.....years Height.....cm Weight (booking.....kg/last wt.....kg)
Ethnic group—Cauc/Afro-Carrib/Ind/Chin/Other
Presentation of baby or twin 1 ?In utero — No
Patient Group Ceph/Breech/Oblique/Transv transfer — Yes — Hospital
Nullip/Multip/Previous CS **Pregnancy** — Single (see below for twin 2) — Home
— Multiple Twins confinement
Other (specify............) Gestation......weeks

Draw in expected graph for dilatation (0.5 cm/h till 3 cm, then 1 cm/h)

Details to record on admission to labour ward
Date.../.../... Time.....h
Reason for admission: Show/Contractions/SROM/Bleeding/Other (specify.....)
Admitted from: Home/Antenatal ward/FMU/DAU/Other
If SROM: Date.../.../... Time.....h
If sent to ante-natal ward: Date.../.../... Time.....h
 — Labour Spontaneous/induced
 or
 — Pre-labour Caesarean — Elective
  Indication............ Decision: Date.../.../... — Emergency Time.....h

If Induced—Indication for induction............
Method: PG/ARM/Synto/Other (specify............)
(circle all applicable) Dose (mg) Time (h) Date
Prostin: 1st dose ..../.../...
        2nd dose ..../.../...
        3rd dose ..../.../...
        4th dose ..../.../...
Total dose of prostin given..........mg
ARM: Time.....h Date.../.../...

TIME OF DIAGNOSIS OF LABOUR (by V.E.) (in all patients except those undergoing pre-labour CS) Date.../.../... Time.....h

Fetal monitoring (mark in when first done)
Pinard/Sonicaid Time.....h Date.../.../...
Abdominal CTG Time.....h Date.../.../...
FSE applied Time.....h Date.../.../...
Monitoring — intermittent (pinard/sonicaid/CTG)
           — Continuous (time commenced.....h)

TIME
Cervix 10
       9
       8
       7
       6
       5
       4
       3
       2
       1

latent phase / alert line / action line

Hours 1 2 3 4 5 6 7 8 9 10 11 12 13 14 15 16 17 18
Fetal heart rate (beats per min)
Liquor (colour)
Moulding/Caput
Contractions per 10 min: 5 4 3 2 1
Oxytocin mU/min

Analgesia
Drugs and i.v.
fluids (inc.
epidural)

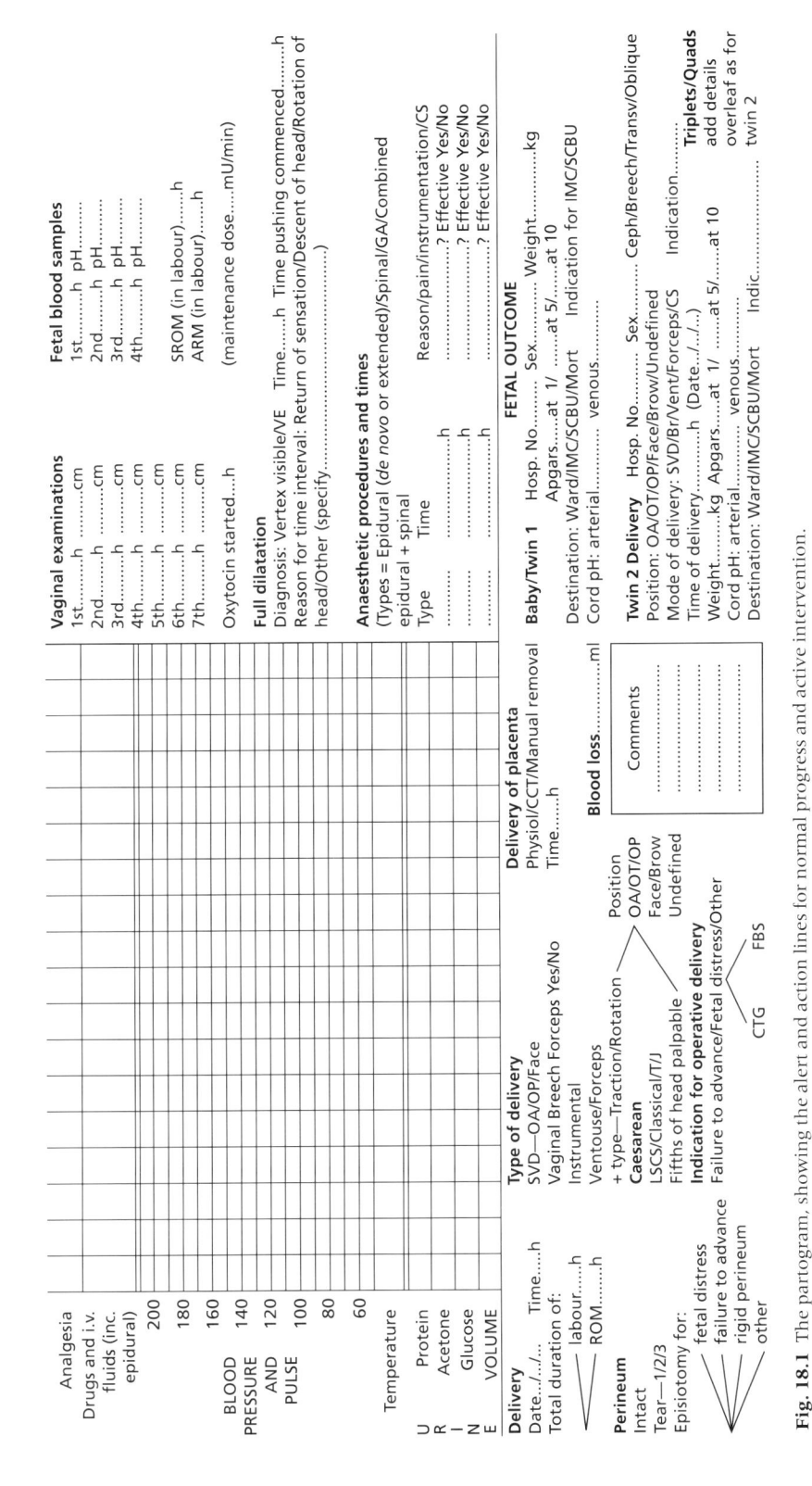

200
180
160
BLOOD 140
PRESSURE 120
AND 100
PULSE 80
60

Temperature

U Protein
R Acetone
I Glucose
N
E VOLUME

Delivery
Date..../..../.... Time.....h
Total duration of:
⎧ labour......h
⎩ ROM......h

Perineum
Intact
Tear—1/2/3
Episiotomy for:
⎧ fetal distress
⎪ failure to advance
⎨ rigid perineum
⎩ other

Type of delivery
SVD—OA/OP/Face
Vaginal Breech Forceps Yes/No
Instrumental
Ventouse/Forceps
+ type—Traction/Rotation ⎫ Position
Caesarean   ⎬ OA/OT/OP
LSCS/Classical/T/J   ⎪ Face/Brow
Fifths of head palpable   ⎭ Undefined
Indication for operative delivery
Failure to advance/Fetal distress/Other

        CTG   FBS

Delivery of placenta
Physiol/CCT/Manual removal
Time......h

Blood loss..............ml

Comments

Vaginal examinations
1st.......h ....cm
2nd.......h ....cm
3rd.......h ....cm
4th.......h ....cm
5th.......h ....cm
6th.......h ....cm
7th.......h ....cm

Oxytocin started....h   (maintenance dose.....mU/min)

Full dilatation
Diagnosis: Vertex visible/VE   Time.....h Time pushing commenced.......h
Reason for time interval: Return of sensation/Descent of head/Rotation of head/Other (specify..)

Anaesthetic procedures and times
(Types = Epidural (*de novo* or extended)/Spinal/GA/Combined epidural + spinal
Type   Time   Reason/pain/instrumentation/CS
....h ....? Effective Yes/No
....h ....? Effective Yes/No
....h ....? Effective Yes/No

Fetal blood samples
1st.......h pH........
2nd.......h pH........
3rd.......h pH........
4th.......h pH........

SROM (in labour).......h
ARM (in labour).......h

FETAL OUTCOME
Baby/Twin 1   Hosp. No............ Sex.......... Weight...........kg
               Apgars.....at 1/ ......at 5/......at 10
Destination: Ward/IMC/SCBU/Mort   Indication for IMC/SCBU
Cord pH: arterial........... venous...........

Twin 2 Delivery Hosp. No............ Sex.......... Ceph/Breech/Transv/Oblique
Position: OA/OT/OP/Face/Brow/Undefined
Mode of delivery: SVD/Br/Vent/Forceps/CS
Time of delivery..........h (Date..../..../....)
Weight.......kg Apgars.....at 1/ ......at 5/......at 10   Indication..........
Cord pH: arterial........... venous...........
Destination: Ward/IMC/SCBU/Mort   Indic..........

Triplets/Quads
add details
overleaf as for
twin 2

Fig. 18.1 The partogram, showing the alert and action lines for normal progress and active intervention.

Oxytocin is a potent vasodilator, decreasing peripheral resistance and mean arterial pressure. This reflexly induces a mild tachycardia. The hypotension occurs rapidly after a bolus intravenous injection, and can be profound if the woman has cardiac disease or is hypovolaemic. During labour, this effect is not usually observed because the oxytocin is given slowly by a controlled infusion. An obstetric anaesthetist may reduce the rate of this infusion during placement of an epidural catheter or if fetal distress is manifest. When oxytocin is required as a bolus after delivery, a dose of 5 IU will often suffice, can be given slowly and repeated if necessary.

Prostaglandins. Prostaglandins are usually given parenterally for treatment of postpartum haemorrhage, induction of labour or midtrimester abortion, rather than to augment labour. They are contraindicated in asthma, and can induce hypertension and tachycardia.

Active management of the third stage of labour

The third stage of labour is the time from delivery of the fetus to delivery of the placenta, which is usually up to 30 minutes. Active management of the third stage of labour is a routine method that significantly reduces postpartum haemorrhage [5]. It requires the administration of an oxytocic agent, umbilical cord clamping and controlled cord traction when there are signs of separation and descent of the placenta. Prophylactic administration of an oxytocic agent reduces the risk of haemorrhage by 40% [5,6]. The two most widely used agents are oxytocin and Syntometrine (a mixture of 0.5 mg ergometrine and 5 IU oxytocin). Ergometrine is contraindicated in hypertensive disorders and cardiac disease. It is also associated with an increased incidence of nausea and vomiting.

At Caesarean section, the normal practice is to defer giving an oxytocic agent until the cord has been clamped.

Complications can occur in the third stage of labour. The most acute is an acute inversion of the uterus. Nitroglycerine (glyceryl trinitrate) 100 µg i.v. is the recommended treatment to relax the uterus and allow the inversion to be replaced within the uterus. The woman will be shocked, but not in relation to amount of blood loss. Hypotension should therefore be expected and treated until the inversion is 'reverted' when cardiovascular stability will return. Trauma to the genital tract can follow vaginal delivery, but rarely requires general anaesthesia for suturing. Usually, local anaesthesia is sufficient, or an epidural top-up. However, if blood loss is persisting, a more invasive examination is required and the anaesthetist will need to assess the patient haemodynamically prior to anaesthesia (i.e. blood pressure, heart rate, fluid balance, haemoglobin, urine output). Occasionally, if a tear has extended into the broad ligament, a laparotomy is required.

When the placenta or part of it is retained, bleeding continues from the placenta site. An intravenous infusion must be established and blood sent for grouping and saving. If there is severe blood loss, cross-matching must be requested. If there is vasoconstriction compensating for hypovolaemia, severe hypotension may follow spinal anaesthesia or an epidural top-up. Adequate preoperative assessment is necessary. If the woman is haemodynamically stable she has the choice of a general or regional block. Occasionally, an epidural sited for labour may not provide adequate anaesthesia and spinal anaesthesia should be used. If the cervix is constricted during general anaesthesia, an increase in the concentration of the inhalation agent may suffice to relax it, with the woman's blood pressure always being monitored. If regional anaesthesia is being used, intravenous or sublingual glyceryl trinitrate may be used, again with cardiovascular monitoring. Where bleeding persists, a haemoglobin concentration and a coagulation screen should be measured, and if necessary the haemorrhage protocol should be activated.

18.1.4 Fluid balance in labour

Fluid may be required in labour for a number of reasons. There is discomfort for a woman in having a dry mouth during mouth breathing through painful contractions. This problem is exaggerated when Entonox is used for long periods, because it is a dry gaseous mixture. Increased evaporative loss also occurs from the lungs with hyperventilation and from the skin during sweating from exertion. Water is most easily administered orally, but in high-risk pregnancies, oral fluid is restricted in order to prevent gastric acid aspiration risk. There has to be a documented reason for choosing the intravenous route for fluid administration, because of the discomfort of its siting and the potential hazards of its use. The choice and volume of intravenous solutions has changed over the past years, as their limitations in labour have become apparent. A pregnant or labouring woman has less capacity to cope with a water load than a non-pregnant individual. Her total body water has increased by up to 7–10 L, of which 2 L can be mobilized and are not accounted for by the products of conception or maternal blood and tissue [7]. Hormonal control of pregnancy generates steroid hormones, and in labour endogenous or exogenous oxytocin can both retain sodium and inhibit water excretion. Water retention predominates, and may be part of the adaptive processes for labour, so that a short period of water restriction can be tolerated. Infusion of solutions without sodium can induce hyponatraemia because of water retention, and oxytocin effects on the kidney and the hazards of such solutions are related to the amount of fluid infused.

Ketonuria in labour used to be treated with dextrose infusions, but it is of no clinical significance because ketones occur in labour in 40% of healthy women [8] and are associated with the increase in metabolic rate in pregnancy and changes in fat utilization. Solutions containing glucose can generate fetal hyperglycaemia, the consequence of which is neonatal hypoglycaemia. Again, these harmful effects are related to the volume of solution and concentration of glucose infused [9].

18.1.5 Diet in labour

The work of labour is considerable, and the labouring mother will find the process of labour tiring. However, tiredness is produced by two factors: the actual work done and the cumulative effect of regularly recurring crescendo pain. The latter is often overlooked, but the lack of tiredness in mothers who have enjoyed excellent or complete pain relief without central nervous system depressant drugs is marked.

The availability of fat and carbohydrate stores in the adult human is sufficient to sustain the most vigorous work for many hours. Hunger pains experienced by those undertaking the work are due to a combination of central nervous system and gastrointestinal functions. Hunger centres are located in the lateral hypothalamic area. Stimulation of these centres causes intense feeding activity in animals. Inhibition of the sensation of hunger generated in the lateral hypothalamic area can be achieved by stimulating satiety centres in the ventromedial nucleus of the hypothalamus. The hypothalamus and the pituitary are involved in the process of labour, so it is hardly surprising that many parturients in labour experience no particular desire to eat, and may suffer nausea. The gastrointestinal system contributes to the sensation of hunger. Intense contractions of the stomach, which presumably are similar to the phase three contractions of the fasting interdigestive motility complex (see Chapter 5), usually do not become troublesome until 12–24 hours after the last ingestion of food. These contractions often last 2–3 minutes and are at their most intense in young, healthy persons with a high gastrointestinal tone. Their intensity is enhanced by the presence of low blood sugar levels. We have already noted that the pregnant patient, and especially the patient in labour, has a low gastrointestinal tone. This is an additional factor that probably contributes to the lack of appetite during labour. A number of other factors operate in order to increase or decrease hunger and appetite, but the labouring parturient often has a low desire for food and maintains an adequate blood glucose concentration.

Diet in labour should be small in quantity and contain no particulate material. The contents of the diet should not stimulate gastric secretions or delay gastric emptying. Fluid in small quantities seems to have a minimal effect on both gastric secretion and gastric emptying. Clear fluids can and should be continued in modest quantities. At any stage during labour, foods rich in secretagogues, such as proteins, are particularly to be avoided. Similarly, the ingestion of hyperosmolar materials, whether solid or fluid, such as very sugary drinks, is not advised.

18.2 Analgesia for labour

Pain relief in labour should be safe for the mother and fetus and should have a

Table 18.1 Methods of analgesia in labour.

Non-pharmacological
Antenatal preparation/psychoprophylaxis
Relaxation
Lamaze method
Transcutaneous nerve stimulation
Acupuncture
Hypnosis
Massage
Warm water (birthing pool)

Pharmacological
Inhalation
   Nitrous oxide
   Volatile anaesthetics
Epidural lumbar/caudal
   Local anaesthetics
   Opioids
   Other adjuvants
   Boluses, infusions, patient-controlled
Spinal
   Opioids
   Local anaesthetics
   Other adjuvants
Combined spinal–epidural
   Local anaesthetics
   Opioids
   Other adjuvants
Systemic
   Intravenous
   Intramuscular
   Subcutaneous
   Infusion
   Patient-controlled
Paracervical block
   Local anaesthetics

minimal effect on the process of labour. Effective analgesia is beneficial for the mother and baby. Many routes of analgesia are available, which vary in their ease of administration. These are summarized in Table 18.1. The ones most commonly used are the inhalational, epidural, spinal and systemic. It is often a combination of routes and drugs that provides adequate analgesia throughout the process of labour, because events are not static and changes in drugs and techniques have to be available at all stages. There is a continuous impetus to provide relief of labour pain without any side effects. Unfortunately, this goal is difficult to achieve in practice and often a compromise has to be reached. To achieve this, patient education for pain relief in labour should begin antenatally.

18.2.1 Pain and its mechanisms

An open, frank and sympathetic attitude freely expressed by members of staff will gain a woman's confidence and make her better able to cope with the stresses of labour. She should be well informed by an anaesthetist during antenatal classes about what she may expect during her labour and about the benefits and complications of pain relief in labour with regional techniques. She may then formulate a birth plan. A good understanding of the underlying anatomy, mechanisms and pathways of labour pain will help when advising a woman in labour what types of pain relief may be appropriate for her.

Physiological changes in nociception during pregnancy in humans [10] and rats [11] indicate that an increase in the nociceptive threshold occurs in late pregnancy. A spinal cord mechanism has been suggested to explain a decrease in the nociceptive threshold following the intrathecal administration of an opioid antagonist [12], which is mediated by a spinal κ-opioid mechanism. The evidence for this is the measurement of increased levels of dynorphin, an endogenous κ-agonist at parturition in rats [13] and specific κ-antagonist reversal of antinociceptive activity in late pregnancy [14]. Hormonal modification by oestrogens and progesterone also increases spinal cord dynorphin in the lumbar region [15], and oxytocin is known to be inhibited by endogenous opioids at parturition [16]. Both hormonal and neuronal factors may therefore be involved in the activation of endogenous pregnancy-induced analgesia. However, the potential benefit of these pain-inhibiting substances during labour may be negated by their effects on inhibiting oxytocin release.

Mechanisms of labour pain

The uterus is made up of bundles of smooth-muscle cells, each separated from its neighbour by thin sheets of connective tissue. The bundles appear to be arranged in several layers, and the proportions of muscle cells to connective tissue varies markedly from the body of the uterus to the cervix. The main muscle mass is found in the body of the uterus. The cervix, on the other hand, is made up principally of collagenous tissue, with an estimated muscle mass of 10% [17–19].

Labour is the active process of delivering a fetus. It is a process that the uterus has been preparing for over the months of pregnancy, and uterine muscle activity increases in frequency and duration during gestation. Spasmodic uterine pain usually indicates that labour has begun, and for many women it will be the most intense pain they will ever feel [20]. When the intensity of labour pain was compared with other pains using the McGill Pain Questionnaire, the average scores indicated an extremely high pain severity. The scores were higher in primiparous women than in multiparous women, especially if there had been no antenatal preparation. The pain of labour is an

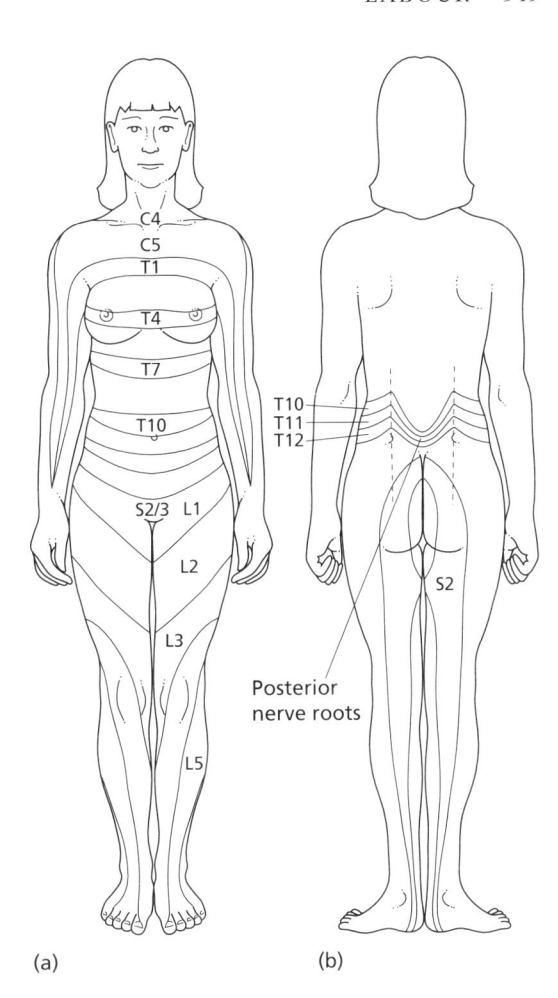

Fig. 18.2 The dermatomal distribution of spinal segments. (a) Anterior view. (b) Posterior nerve roots supply skin between lines drawn through posterior iliac spines. These dermatomes lie one to two segments more caudally when compared to those derived from the anterior nerve roots.

intermittent, crescendo pain. The intervals between painful episodes become shorter as labour progresses, and the pain increases not only in frequency but also in duration and severity. The idea that this pain may arise because of muscle ischaemia during contractions is not supported by research, which has shown that arterial blood flow into the uterus and placenta continues during contractions [21].

The pains from a woman's reproductive system can be divided into two components—somatic and visceral. Somatic sensations are those evoked by stimulation of structures such as skin and underlying tissues—that is, touch, temperature and pain—and the superficial nerves involved in this pain are described by dermatomes (Fig. 18.2). The visceral component originates from the internal organs, and the only sensation that is felt is pain. The unanaesthetized cervix can be incised without discomfort to a conscious woman having a Caesarean section under abdominal field block [22], but if it is dilated she feels pain similar in nature and distribution to that of labour. This type of study would not be repeatable today.

346   CHAPTER 18

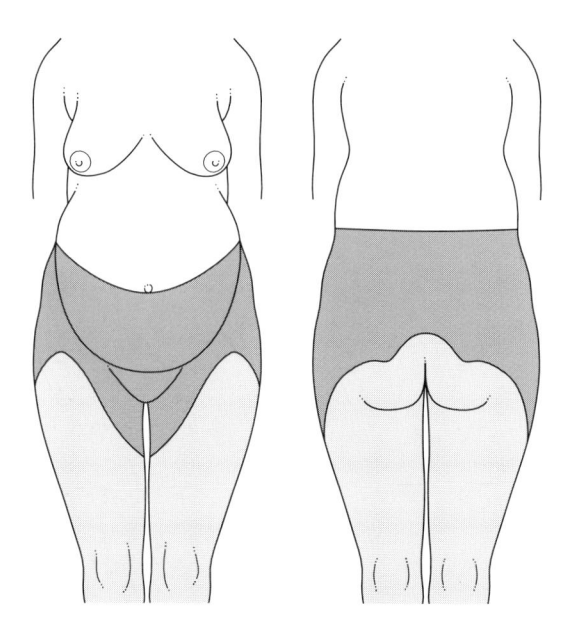

■ Area of major discomfort and pain

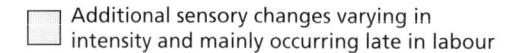

□ Additional sensory changes varying in intensity and mainly occurring late in labour

Fig. 18.3 The 'pants and stocking' distribution of pain during labour.

During the first stage of labour, most parturients experience pain from visceral stimulation. In quality, it is described as a dull ache, and it is usually poorly localized to the lower abdomen, which is the classical viscerotome region [23] (Fig. 18.3). In addition, more widespread deep somatic muscle pains have been described in association with reproductive tract structures [24], which have a similar aching and poorly localized quality. A minority of women experience pain in other areas of skin innervated from lumbar or sacral spinal segments, such as the lower limbs, especially in the thighs (L1, L2 and L3). Pain originating from visceral distension is often accompanied by autonomic effects, e.g. the nausea and vomiting that are manifest in labour.

Labour pains during the first stage of childbirth are due to dilatation of the cervix and the lower uterine segment, as well as the associated uterine contractions [25]. Nociceptive pathways from the cervix travel with sympathetic nerve pathways to T11 (not to sacral segments), with some involvement of T10 and T12 (Fig. 18.4). This can be tested by any anaesthetist who wishes to achieve cervical anaesthesia for dilation and curettage with a low subarachnoid anaesthetic that blocks only the sacral spinal segments. Extension of the block to include T11 will be necessary before continuing dilation of the cervix. The skin overlying the sacroiliac area is also innervated from T10, T11 and T12. Much back pain is therefore referred, in the same manner as anterior abdominal pain. Sacroiliac joint pain may, of course, contribute to the patient's

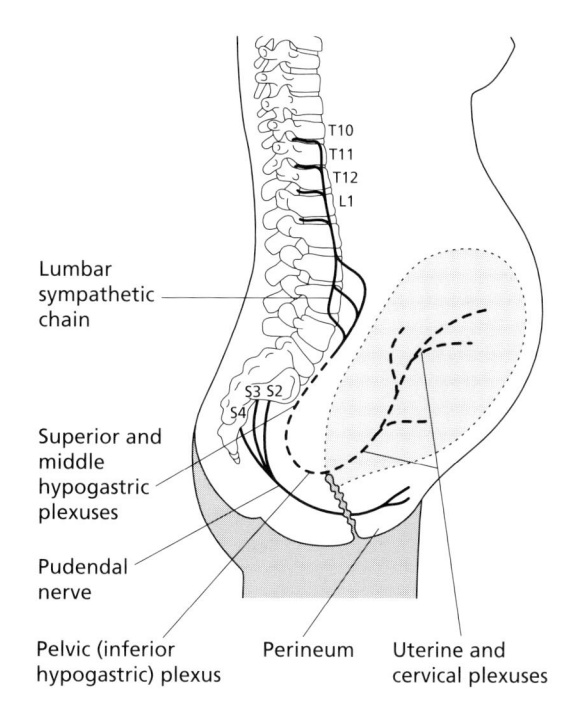

Fig. 18.4 The sensory pathways involved in parturition.

Table 18.2 A summary of labour pain in the first and second stages.

First stage	
Origin	Cervix (visceral)
Quality	Dull and aching
Site	Poorly localized to the lower abdomen
	Backache or lumbosacral discomfort
Pathways	Autonomic via T11
Second stage	
Origin	Mixed visceral (uterus) and somatic (perineal and pelvic structures, including joints)
Quality	Dull and sharp
Pathways	Autonomic: parasympathetic and sympathetic plexuses
	Lumbar and sacral spinal segments
Site	Somatic component localized to the perineum
	Referred pain felt in any corresponding spinal segment from T11 to S5

discomfort, but the principal component arises from cervical dilatation. As the presenting part descends, compression of other viscera, such as the bladder and the rectum, can add to the pain, and it changes (Table 18.2). Once the cervix is fully dilated, the amount of painful stimuli originating in this structure decreases, but uterine contractions continue and pressure effects in the pelvis and perineum become significant.

In the second stage of labour, the pain originating from somatic structures in the perineum is added to or modifies the pain of early labour. Pain of somatic origin is usually well localized, and follows a pathway through either the lumbar or sacral spinal segments. The identification of these segments is of importance when selecting pain relief. Pain from visceral origin responds to opioids, whether given systemically or as part of a regional anaesthetic technique. Pain from other structures may be more effectively blocked with local anaesthetics. This effect can be observed with mixed opioid and local anaesthetic solutions given for postoperative epidural analgesia. If the local anaesthetic is omitted, the dull aching pain is still obtunded, but pain arising during movement or coughing is often troublesome.

18.2.2 Central pathways

The appreciation of pain in labour is not a simple matter of nociceptive information transmitted through A delta fibre and C fibre activity that enters the dorsal horn. Synapses and fibres cross to relay in the thalamus and cortex. Modulation of this activity occurs both centrally and peripherally. Fear and anxiety alter pain perception, whereas psychological and cognitive preparations for labour aim to enhance transmission in the descending inhibitory pathways from the brain to the spinal cord. Transcutaneous electrical nerve stimulation (TENS), opioids and adrenergic agonists also inhibit nociception by spinal mechanisms. More peripherally in the uterus, local release of bradykinin, 5-hydroxytryptamine and prostaglandins can amplify peripheral nerve activity. Non-steroidal anti-inflammatory analgesics are therefore useful post-partum analgesics. At present, they are the only group of drugs which can prevent these tissue changes, although more specific antagonists may become available in the future.

In the spinal cord, convergence of information from somatic and visceral structures occurs at a spinal segment. This may be one mechanism for the referral of pain sensation from viscera to body wall dermatomes. It may manifest as muscle or skin sensitivity [26]. The laminae activated by visceral nociceptive fibres also receive an input from a number of other segments in the spinal cord, so that the sensation produced is diffuse. Cervical pain is therefore described as a dull ache, usually centrally placed in the part of the body wall innervated by T11. Anteriorly, this lies just below the umbilicus. Posteriorly, the T11 dermatome innervates skin over the lumbo–sacral junction. This distribution is lower than that shown on most dermatome diagrams, because it is not commonly appreciated that the segmental nerve supply to the back is by way of the medial and lateral cutaneous branches of the dorsal rami of the spinal nerves. These dorsal rami supply sensory nerves to the skin of the back between the right and left dorsolateral lines. These lines run from their origins on the back of the head down laterally to the skin over the acromion. They continue downwards to the skin over, or just posterior to, the greater trochanter of the femur. From there, they pass medially to the coccyx. Each dorsal ramus supplying the trunk has a medial and lateral cutaneous branch, and both of these branches travel caudally and overlap before innervating the skin. They may run caudally for as much as the breadth of four ribs before becoming superficial, and the lateral branch of T12 reaches the skin only a little above the iliac crest [27].

Nociceptive visceral pathways from the dorsal horn can relay on anterior horn cells to complete segmental autonomic reflex arcs. This is the mechanism that generates the skeletal muscle spasm associated with visceral distension. They also pass cephalad by many interconnecting pathways such as the spinothalamic tracts, the spinoreticular tract, the solitary nucleus and the dorsal column. The spinothalamic tracts have few synapses and large fibres, and therefore conduct impulses rapidly. The spinoreticular pathway is multisynaptic, and therefore carries information more slowly. It is a vital link in supraspinal reflexes and emotional responses to pain, and by stimulating areas of the brain in the periaqueductal grey region [28] it may be at least partially responsible for the analgesia produced by descending control system activity [29].

Midbrain structures which are sensitive to opioids such as the periaqueductal grey matter, project to the dorsal horn of the spinal cord with adrenergic or serotonergic neurones. Pain modulation can occur in the spinal cord by enkephalinergic interneurones directly inhibiting nociceptive transmission. Enkephalins and endorphins are endogenous opioid peptides. Opioid-mediated analgesia can be activated by stimulation, stress and suggestion, and may contribute to the variety of perceived labour pains. Pregnancy itself induces opioid-mediated analgesia [30].

Visceral nociceptive afferents have also been described in the dorsal column nuclei [31]. The dorsal columns transmit touch and proprioception, and dorsal column nuclei respond to gentle tactile stimulation. This conceptualization of the relationship between touch and visceral pain perceptions has implications for obstetric anaesthetists. The aim of pain relief in the first stage of labour is to obtund visceral pain. Regional nerve block may be effective if part of the dorsal column pathway is anaesthetized. This may remove proprioceptive function, and the woman thus relies on her visual and vestibular sensation for mobility.

18.2.3 Pathophysiological responses to pain

Factors listed in Table 18.3 enhance endogenous mechanisms that provide pain relief in labour. The parturient's personality and cultural background will influence her response to pain, if not her perception of it. It is, of course, a great advantage to be able to control pain. However, careful observation of the woman is necessary even in these circumstances, because the underlying adverse effects of untreated pain appear in spite of outward stoicism. Labour

Confidence
Familiar surroundings
Distraction
Warmth
Preparation, information and support
Relaxation

Table 18.3 Factors in labour that can enhance pain relief.

Table 18.4 Pathophysiological responses to uterine contractions.

System	Response to contraction	Comments
Respiration	Hyperventilation during contraction (20–40 L/min)	Increased work of breathing increases oxygen consumption Reduces $Paco_2$ from 4.3 kPa (32 mmH$_2$O), the normal value in pregnancy (by doubling the ventilation the $Paco_2$ is halved) Hypoventilation follows with a reduction in $Paco_2$
Cardiovascular	Catecholamines reduce uterine blood flow by 35–70%	Compounds the effects of hyperventilation on the oxygen supply to the fetus
Metabolic	Increased metabolic rate and oxygen consumption	Maternal acidosis accumulates, especially in the second stage of labour Metabolic acidosis is transferred to the fetus
Gastrointestinal	Delay in gastric emptying	Increased risk of acid aspiration
Urinary	Delay in bladder emptying	Obstructed labour Retention of urine (increases pain in the same spinal cord segments as the uterus)

pain is associated with physiological changes that are the result of the peripheral and central stress and energy requirements of contractions, as shown in Table 18.4. Hyperventilation occurs with hypocapnia, leading to tetany or apnoea. Catecholamines are released, which increase cardiac output and induce vasoconstriction, leading to acidosis and fetal distress and inhibiting gastric emptying. These deleterious effects can be attenuated by analgesics.

18.2.4 Choice of pain relief in labour

The methods available are summarized in Table 18.1. In 1990, the National

Birthday Trust surveyed pain relief in 4516 women nation-wide over a period of a week [32]. The report found that homeopathy, acupuncture and hypnosis are used by less than 0.5% of women. Transcutaneous electrical nerve stimulation is used more frequently, by up to 6% of women, and TENS machines are available in many units. They are battery-operated, and deliver a stimulus that can be controlled for intensity, frequency and duration, through large surface electrodes which are usually placed bilaterally in the lumbar and sacral regions. Some types of product offer a 'burst' control, whereby the frequency can be changed with a contraction. This can limit the development of tolerance to the stimulation. The survey noted disappointment with the effectiveness of TENS by the women using it. TENS did not reduce the need for other forms of analgesia [33], but it may assist women early in labour, particularly with backache, because they were prepared to wait for longer periods before asking for systemic or regional pain relief. This effect may be beneficial in reducing the total dose of any analgesic agent used.

A birthing pool can be used to assist in pain management during both labour and delivery. It provides a warm environment in which to relax. Almost half of the women who enter the pool leave it before delivery, and the majority seek alternative analgesia [34]. If epidural analgesia is required, an assessment of maternal temperature and fetal heart rate should be made and normal values obtained before commencing an epidural nerve block, which involves a blockade of sympathetic effects and interference with temperature regulation.

Pethidine may be given by a midwife without a doctor's prescription. It is therefore universally available, and it is the most frequently used opioid analgesic used in labour in the United Kingdom, in up to 38% of women. However, it may not be the best opioid for women, and if physicians prescribed for midwives the woman's choice might include other opioids, such as those acting on κ-opioid rather than μ-opioid receptors [35], or diamorphine. Women using pethidine in the National Birthday Trust report complained of confusion and loss of control because of its sedative effects. Nitrous oxide was also available routinely and up to 75% of women used it, often in combination with other methods of analgesia such as pethidine, or while epidural analgesia was being set up. The availability of epidural analgesia was not universal among the 282 units surveyed, but more than two-thirds of the units provided this form of analgesia. However, at least one in five units lacked the staff and facilities for this service. This generated significant disappointment in labouring women. Women also reported reluctance among midwives to recommend epidural analgesia. A mother's choice is enhanced by providing a full range of methods for analgesia, and women wish to be prepared realistically. Epidural analgesia for labour was used in one in five of the women surveyed. If any method of pain relief is not available in a unit, the parturients attending it should be informed of its unavailability.

18.2.5 Systemic opioids

Pethidine

Despite the well-known lack of analgesic effect in labour [36,37] and its placental transfer with a long neonatal half-life [38], pethidine is commonly administered. Its main side effects in the mother are opioid-induced. In the gastrointestinal system, these effects include nausea, vomiting and slowing of gastrointestinal motility, which may increase the risk of acid aspiration and is not fully counteracted by metoclopramide. Hypotension and hypoventilation may occur through central depression. These may not occur during contractions, but maternal pulse oximetry has demonstrated more frequent hypoxic episodes with pethidine than with epidural analgesia [39]. Pethidine is usually administered as a dose of 150 mg intramuscularly together with a phenothiazine as anti-emetic (in spite of the antanalgesic effect of some phenothiazines). The combined effect of these drugs on maternal sedation is observed between contractions.

The depressant effects on the fetus are greater when the dose-to-delivery interval is two to three hours [40]. They are at their lowest when delivery is within an hour [41]. Pethidine is protein-bound (about 54% [42]) mainly to α1-acid glycoprotein. This globulin is in a higher concentration in the mother than the fetus. Initially, the fetal-to-maternal plasma concentration ratio is greater than 0.5, but with fast equilibration the plasma concentration in the mother decreases, whereas that in the fetal plasma decreases more slowly. The plasma half-life in the mother is three to four hours, compared with the fetus, in which it is 18 hours. This effect is magnified by fetal acidosis, because pethidine is a basic drug and becomes more ionized at the lower pH of the fetus. The fetal-to-maternal plasma concentration is maximal at two to three hours. Norpethidine, one of the important metabolites of pethidine, has a much longer half-life in the mother of about 20 hours. Its effects can therefore peak later in the fetus. It has convulsant activity, and is not readily reversed by naloxone. Norpethidine may be responsible for the long-term neurobehavioural abnormalities seen in babies born after maternal pethidine administration [43]. The safety of pethidine relies on pharmacological antagonism—for the mother, prophylactic ranitidine to protect her from aspiration and for the baby, naloxone.

Other opioids

Morphine and diamorphine have been used in obstetric practice for many years, but they have more depressant effects on the fetus than fentanyl. If a recent death *in utero* has occurred, there is a preference by obstetricians to use these drugs, because they provide a better quality of analgesia. Meptazinol is no longer advocated for pain relief in labour, because it produces more vomiting than pethidine.

Fentanyl is another μ-opioid, which is usually administered systemically by the intravenous route. It has been advocated either for a single dose to be used (25–50 μg i.v.) to allow the placement of an epidural catheter if a woman is in extreme pain and difficult to manage [44], or as the analgesia of choice in an intravenous infusion. Patient-controlled analgesia is an alternative system for women in whom epidural analgesia is contraindicated [45]. Fentanyl is highly lipid-soluble, binding mainly to albumin, and it rapidly crosses the placenta in minutes. It has the potential to produce respiratory depression in the fetus, but no measurable long-term neurobehavioural effects have been observed [46]. Alfentanil and sufentanil are both highly bound to α1-acid glycoprotein, whose concentration is greater in maternal than fetal plasma. Their use as systemic analgesics for labour has not been explored.

Opioid partial agonists and κ-agonists such as pentazocine, nalbuphine, buprenorphine and butorphanol are not controlled drugs, and are used in labour. The κ agonist activity of nalbuphine is reported to produce greater maternal and fetal sedation than pethidine [47].

18.2.6 Inhalational analgesia

Equipment development

Subanaesthetic doses of inhalational anaesthetic agents have been popular in obstetric anaesthesia since chloroform was administered to Queen Victoria in 1853. The first report of the use of nitrous oxide for the relief of labour pain appeared in 1880 in the *St Petersburg Medical Weekly,* where Klikovich described his use of a mixture of 80% nitrous oxide and 20% oxygen in obstetric patients. Self-administration of nitrous oxide and oxygen become available in 1910, when McKesson (United Kingdom) and Guedel (United States) independently introduced complicated machines for this purpose. Widespread use was delayed until 1933 when Minnitt developed a simple 'Gas and Air' apparatus in response to an invitation from the Clinical Investigation Subcommittee of the Medical Board of Liverpool Maternity Hospital. The first report of its use was read at the Liverpool Medical Institution on 22 February 1934, and this was followed by a paper read by Dr Minnitt at a meeting of the Royal Society of Medicine Section of Anaesthetics on 4 May 1934. Patient-controlled intermittent inhalational analgesia (PCIIA) became and remains a popular and widely used method of analgesia, almost unique to obstetrics and midwifery in the United Kingdom.

Simple draw-over vaporizers, which accurately administered fixed low concentrations of trichloroethylene or methoxyflurane in air, were then produced. These were used from 1952 to 1984 by parturients being cared for by unsupervised midwives. In 1984, the Central Midwives' Board in Britain withdrew its approval of the use of the Emotril and Tecota inhalers, although not the Cardiff inhaler. This decision effectively ended 32 years of PCIIA with volatile anaesthetic agents.

Entonox

In 1961, Tunstall described the use of a 50% nitrous oxide/oxygen mixture in a single cylinder for the production of pain relief in labour [48]. The 50 : 50 mixture of oxygen and nitrous oxide system (Entonox) used for obstetric patients consists of a single Entonox cylinder, a combined pressure-reducing and demand valve, standard length tubing connected to a one-way expiratory valve and a face mask or mouthpiece. The demand system provides minimal inspiratory resistance and can deliver gas flows in excess of those required in labour (> 40 L/min). The demand system and the 50% nitrous oxide concentration are the inherent safety features of PCIIA. Where only continuous flow of nitrous oxide and oxygen is available, an anaesthetist should administer it. PCIIA has a number of overwhelming advantages. It is simple, rapidly effective and has an impressive safety record. The physical properties of nitrous oxide—in particular, its low blood solubility and rapid diffusion characteristics—ensure that analgesia will be established after 15 seconds or seven breaths. The degree of pain relief can increase to a maximum if inhalation is continued for 90 seconds. The effects disappear as quickly. A concentration of 50% nitrous oxide was chosen to provide analgesia instead of the higher 70% concentration, because although the latter may improve analgesia, in a small number of women it may cause loss of airway control.

Safety depends on the patient using and controlling the breathing system without assistance. Inhalation of Entonox from the standard breathing system is only possible if the patient opens the demand valve attached to the cylinder by creating a negative pressure within the breathing system. Creation of the negative pressure requires the face mask to be firmly applied, producing an airtight seal. If the patient's level of consciousness becomes depressed, she will be unable to maintain the seal, administration of Entonox will cease, and the patient will begin to breath room air. Full consciousness will return rapidly. Any attempt by an attendant to hold the mask in place will override this safety feature. The patent may then be anaesthetized and may regurgitate gastric contents whilst her airway is unprotected.

Volatile anaesthetic agents

In spite of the safety and flexibility of this method, PCIIA with Entonox alone will only provide adequate analgesia in 50% of mothers who use it [37]. This can be increased with adequate explanation of use. A small concentration of a volatile anaesthetic agent with analgesic properties, such as trichloroethylene, methoxyflurane or isoflurane, can further increase the efficacy of the technique. In 1984, Levack and Tunstall [49] described a modification to the Entonox demand system that incorporated an Oxford Miniature Vaporizer filled with trichloroethylene. Trichloroethylene and methoxyflurane are no longer used. They accumulate in obstetric analgesia, and progressive maternal sedation occurs.

Studies omitting nitrous oxide and substituting a volatile anaesthetic with oxygen as the carrier gas have all encountered problems of maternal sedation. Abboud's group [50] described continuous administration of isoflurane in oxygen during the second stage of labour. Sedative effects limited its use. Isoflurane 0.75% in oxygen has been compared with Entonox [51] in the first stage of labour. A PCIIA system was devised from a continuous flow machine that filled a large reservoir system, from which the patient breathed. Patients receiving isoflurane rather than Entonox had significantly lower pain scores, but the scores for drowsiness were higher in the isoflurane group. A PCIIA crossover study with administration of Entonox drawn from a standard demand breathing system was compared with Entonox plus 0.2% isoflurane [52]. The isoflurane was obtained from an Ohmeda Isotec Drawover Vaporizer placed in line in the system, and the inspired concentration was measured. All women were studied for one-hour periods over three hours during the first stage of labour. Significantly lower linear analogue pain scores were recorded with the Entonox/isoflurane mixture, and drowsiness was not a clinical problem.

Maternal and fetal effects from inhalational agents

The reduction in the functional residual capacity of the lungs and the increase in minute ventilation encourages rapid uptake and equilibrium between the concentration of agent in the inspired gas and the alveoli. In addition, the minimum alveolar concentrations of inhaled volatile anaesthetic are reduced during pregnancy [53], so that mothers are more sensitive to the same dose given to non-pregnant women. All inhalational agents have the potential for overdosage, producing unconsciousness. The loss of protective airway reflexes could lead to maternal and fetal hypoxia.

Another mechanism for hypoxia is the reduced respiratory reserve in late pregnancy. A significantly greater number, duration and severity of hypoxic episodes (oxygen saturation less than 90%) were observed in mothers breathing Entonox during contractions compared with mothers receiving epidural analgesia (although hypoxic episodes still occurred). This reduction in oxygen saturation occurred after Entonox administration had stopped [54]. One explanation for this is that hyperventilation with Entonox during a contraction reduces carbon dioxide tension, and ventilatory drive is reduced. This effect, combined with a reduced respiratory reserve of oxygen in the functional residual capacity, may cause hypoxia. Another consideration is the potential for diffusion hypoxia that may occur as nitrous oxide is rapidly eliminated from the body.

Women will complain of feeling light-headed and nauseated when using Entonox. Often, Entonox is used after the administration of pethidine, and their effects may be combined, as may the effect on respiration. The main deleterious effect on the fetus is from maternal hypoxaemia. Washout of nitrous oxide from the blood is fast, provided that the baby is ventilating, so the neonate will show little, if any, effect following maternal entonox use.

Both enflurane and isoflurane are available for analgesic use in obstetrics. They are fluorinated ethers and release inorganic fluoride on metabolism. However, only a small amount is metabolized. The fetal/maternal ratio of enflurane is about 0.7 and that of isoflurane is 0.9, suggesting that the fetus may be more sensitive to prolonged maternal exposure to isoflurane [55].

18.2.7 Regional nerve blockade

The choices here are discussed in Chapter 15.

18.2.8 Paracervical block

A paracervical block is the infiltration of local anaesthetic around the rim of the cervix. By definition, this can only be used in the first stage of labour. The onset of analgesia is immediate, and the method does not produce a sympathetic blockade. The major disadvantage that prevents its use is the development of fetal bradycardia. This effect is multifactorial and related to a decrease in uterine artery flow and drug effects on the fetus.

References

1. Gardosi J, Hutson NB, Lynch C. Randomised control trial of squatting in the second stage of labour. *Lancet* 1989; **ii**: 74–7.
2. Stewart P, Hillan E, Calder AA. A randomised trial to evaluate the use of the birth chair for delivery. *Lancet* 1983; **i**: 1296–8.
3. Turner MJ, Romney NL, Webb JB, Gordon H. The birthing chair: an obstetric hazard? *J Obstet Gynecol* 1986; **6**: 232–5.
4. World Health Organization Maternal Health and Safe Motherhood Programme. World Health Organization partogram in management of labour. *Lancet* 1994; **343**: 1399–404.
5. Rogers J, Wood J, McCandlish R *et al.* Active versus expectant management of third stage of labour: the Hinchingbrooke randomised controlled trial. *Lancet* 1998; **351**: 693–9.
6. McDonald SJ, Prendiville WJ, Blair E. Randomised controlled trial of oxytocin alone versus oxytocin and ergometrine in active management of third stage of labour. *Br Med J* 1993; **307**: 1167–71.
7. Hytten FE, Thomson AM, Taggart N. Total body water in normal pregnancy. *J Obstet Gynaecol Br Commonw* 1966; **73**: 553–61.
8. Dumoulin JG, Foulkes JEB. Ketonuria during labour. *Br J Obstet Gynaecol* 1984; **91**: 97–8.
9. Philipson EH, Kalhan SC, Riha MM, Pimental R. Effects of maternal glucose infusion on fetal acid–base status in human pregnancy. *Am J Obstet Gynecol* 1987; **157**: 866–73.
10. Whipple B, Josimovich JB, Komisaruk BR. Sensory threshold during the antepartum, intrapartum and postpartum periods. *Int J Nurs Stud* 1990; **27**: 214–21.
11. Gintzler AR. Endorphin-mediated increases in pain threshold during pregnancy. *Science* 1980; **210**: 193–5.
12. Sander HW, Gintzler AR. Spinal cord mediation of the opioid analgesia of pregnancy. *Brain Res* 1987; **408**: 389–93.
13. Medina VM, Wang L, Gintzler AR. Spinal cord dynorphin: positive region-specific modulation during pregnancy and parturition. *Brain Res* 1993; **623**: 41–6.

14 Sander HW, Portoghese PS, Gintzler AR. Spinal κ-opiate receptor involvement in the analgesia of pregnancy: effects of intrathecal norbinaltorphimine, a κ-selective antagonist. *Brain Res* 1988; **474**: 343–7.
15 Dawson-Basoa MB, Gintzler AR. 17β-oestradiol and progesterone modulate an intrinsic opioid analgesia system. *Brain Res* 1993; **601**: 241–5.
16 Leng G, Mansfield S, Bicknell RJ *et al.* Endogenous opioid actions and effects of environmental disturbance on parturition and oxytocin secretion in rats. *J Reprod Fertil* 1988; **84**: 345–56.
17 Danforth DN. The fibrous nature of the uterine cervix and its relation to the isthmic segment in gravid and non-gravid uteri. *Am J Obstet Gynecol* 1947; **53**: 544–60.
18 Danforth DN, Buckingham JG, Roddick JW. Connective tissue changes incident to cervical effacement. *Am J Gynecol* 1960; **80**: 939.
19 Danforth DN. The distribution and functional activity of cervical musculature. *Am J Obstet Gynecol* 1954; **68**: 1261–71.
20 Melzack R. Labour pain as a model of acute pain. *Pain* 1993; **53**: 117–20.
21 Hellman LM, Tricomi V, Gupta O. Pressures in the human amniotic fluid and intervillous space. *Am J Obstet Gynecol* 1957; **74**: 1018.
22 Javert CT, Hardy JD. Measurement of pain intensity in labour and its physiological, neurologic and pharmacologic implications. *Am J Obstet Gynecol* 1950; **60**: 552–63.
23 Cousins M. Acute and postoperative pain. In: Wall PD, Melzack R, eds. *Textbook of Pain*. 3rd edn. Edinburgh: Churchill Livingstone 1994: 375.
24 Giamberardino MA, Berkley K, Iezzi S, de Bigentino P, Vecchiet L. Pain threshold variations in somatic wall tissues as a function of menstrual cycle, segmental site and tissue depth in non-dysmenorrheic women, dysmenorrheic women and men. *Pain* 1997; **71**: 187–97.
25 Bonica JJ. Labour pain. In: Wall PD, Melzack R, eds. *Textbook of Pain*. 3rd edn Edinburgh: Churchill Livingstone, 1994: 615–41.
26 Fields HL. *Pain*. New York: McGraw-Hill, 1987.
27 Bannister LH, Berry MM, Collins P *et al*. *Gray's Anatomy: The Anetomical Basis of Medicine and Surgery*. 38th edn. London: Churchill Livingstone, 1995: 1289.
28 Reynolds DV. Surgery in the rat during electrical analgesia induced by focal brain stimulation. *Science* 1969; **164**: 444–5.
29 Fields HL, Basbaum AI. Brain stem control of spinal pain transmission neurones. *Ann Rev Physiol* 1978; **40**: 217–48.
30 Sandler HW, Gintzler AR. Spinal cord mediation of the opioid analgesia of pregnancy. *Brain Res* 1987; **408**: 389–93.
31 Berkley KJ, Hubscher CH. Are there separate central nervous system pathways for touch and pain? *Nature Med* 1995; **1**: 766–73.
32 Chamberlain G, Wraight A, Steer P. *Pain and its Relief in Labour: Report of the 1990 NBT Survey*. Edinburgh: Churchill Livingstone, 1993.
33 Harrison RF, Woods T, Shore M, Mathews G, Unwin A. Pain relief in labour using transcutaneous electrical nerve stimulation (TENS): a TENS/TENS placebo-controlled study in two parity groups. *Br J Obstet Gynaecol* 1986; **93**: 739–46.
34 Alderdice IF, Renfrew M, Marchant SH *et al.* Labour and birth in water in England and Wales. *Br Med J* 1995; **310**: 837.
35 Gear R, Miaskowski C, Gordon NC, *et al.* Kappa-opioids produce significantly greater analgesia in women than in men. *Nat Med* 1996; **2**: 1248–50.
36 Olofsson CH, Ekblom A, Ekman-Ordeberg G, Hjelm A, Irestedt L. Lack of analgesic effect of systemically administered morphine or pethidine on labour pain. *Br J Obstet Gynaecol* 1996; **103**: 968–72.
37 Holdcroft A, Morgan M. An assessment of the analgesic effect in labour of pethidine and 50% nitrous oxide in oxygen (Entonox). *Br J Obstet Gynaecol* 1974; **81**: 603–7.

38 Caldwell J, Wakile LA, Snedden W. Maternal and neonatal disposition of pethidine in childbirth: a study using quantitative gas chromatography mass spectrometry. *Life Sci* 1978; **22**: 589–96.

39 Reed PN, Colquhoun AD, Hanning CD. Maternal oxygenation during normal labour. *Br J Anaesth* 1989; **62**: 326–18.

40 Morrison JC, Wiser WL, Rosser SI *et al*. Metabolites of meperidine related to fetal depression. *Am J Obstet Gynecol* 1973; **115**: 1132–7.

41 Belfrage P, Boreus LO, Hartvig P, Irestedt L, Raabe N. Neonatal depression after obstetrical analgesia with pethidine. *Acta Obstet Gynecol Scand* 1981; **60**: 43–9.

42 Szeto HH. Pharmacokinetic studies in experimental animals. In: Reynolds F, ed. *The Effects on the Baby of Maternal Analgesia and Anaesthesia*. London: Saunders, 1993: 29–45.

43 Kuhnert BR, Kuhnert PM, Philipson PM, Syracus CD. Disposition of meperidine and normeperidine following multiple doses in labor, 2: fetus and newborn. *Am J Obstet Gynecol* 1985; **151**: 410–15.

44 Hughes SC. Analgesic methods during labor and delivery. *Can J Anaesth* 1992; **39**: R18–R23.

45 Rosaeg OP, Kitts JB, Koren G, Byford LJ. Maternal and fetal effects of intravenous patient-controlled fentanyl analgesia during labour in a thrombocytopenic parturient. *Can J Anaesth* 1992; **39**: 277–81.

46 Rayburn W, Smith CV, Parriot JE, Woods RP. Randomised comparison of meperidine and fentanyl during labor. *Obstet Gynecol* 1989; **74**: 604–6.

47 Wilson CM, McClean E, Moore J, Dundee JW. A double-blind comparison of intramuscular pethidine and nalbuphine in labour. *Anaesthesia* 1986; 41: 1207–13.

48 Tunstall ME. Use of a fixed nitrous oxide and oxygen mixture from one cylinder. *Lancet* 1961; **ii**: 964.

49 Levack ID, Tunstall ME. Systems modification in obstetric analgesia. *Anaesthesia* 1984; **39**: 183–5.

50 Abboud TK, Gangolly J, Mosaad P, Crowell D. Isoflurane in obstetrics. *Anesth Analg* 1989; **68**: 388–91.

51 McLeod DD, Ramayya GP, Tunstall ME. Self-administered isoflurane in labour. *Anaesthesia* 1985; **40**: 424–6.

52 Wee MYK, Hasan MA, Thomas TA. Isoflurane in labour. *Anaesthesia* 1993; **48**: 369–72.

53 Palahnuik RJ, Shnider SM, Eger EI II. Pregnancy decreases the requirement for inhaled anesthetic agents. *Anesthesiology* 1974; **41**: 82–3.

54 Arfreen Z, Armstrong PJ, Whitfield A. The effects of Entonox and epidural analgesia on arterial oxygen saturation of women in labour. *Anaesthesia* 1994; **49**: 32–4.

55 Clyburn P, Rosen M. The effect of opioid and inhalational analgesia on the newborn. In: Reynolds F, ed. *The Effects on the Baby of Maternal Analgesia and Anaesthesia*. London: Saunders, 1993: 169–90.

19: Complications in Labour

19.1 Identification of obstetric anaesthetic complications

Women can be screened for obstetric anaesthetic problems in the antenatal clinic, parentcraft classes, or as hospital in-patients on the antenatal ward during obstetric anaesthetic ward rounds. Not all women can be screened before parturition—for example, if they have been managed in the community or are transferred between hospitals, or do not present for antenatal assessment. It is therefore still necessary to make an anaesthetic assessment during labour.

A list of expected difficulties can be found in Table 1.3, p. 10. This can be used by obstetricians and midwives as a reminder of those areas of particular interest to anaesthetists, but can be changed according to the type of patient population. In addition, a file card system has been described [1] in which individual patient details are filed on the labour ward, so that out-of-hours duty anaesthetic staff have access to defined problems and the plan of anaesthetic management for them. The card should include details such as previous anaesthetic history, especially difficulties with regional anaesthesia, estimated date of delivery, the relevant anaesthetic history and a consultant anaesthetist's assessment.

Women with a complicated pregnancy in whom there is a high risk of Caesarean section, such as maternal disease (e.g. renal failure), previous uterine scar (e.g. Caesarean section, myomectomy), abnormal fetal presentation (e.g. twins, breech), or a fetus at risk (e.g. intrauterine growth retardation) need planned induction of labour if a Caesarean delivery is not directly indicated. Induction of labour should be planned to occur when the whole team is informed and available. There is some encouragement to allow a woman a trial of labour if the indicators for the Caesarean delivery no longer apply. A large trial comparing women who selected vaginal or abdominal delivery for a second confinement recorded a rate of 1.6% of major complications (i.e. hysterectomy, uterine rupture or other trauma) in those who chose vaginal delivery, compared with 0.8% in the elective Caesarean section group. There was no difference in the fetal outcome [2]. An obstetric anaesthetist must therefore anticipate anaesthetic involvement during these labours.

19.2 Obstetric complications

19.2.1 Preterm labour

Preterm delivery is defined as that occurring in women who have not completed 37 weeks of gestation. Preterm labour and intrauterine growth retardation have recently become major obstetric problems, because facilities for neonatal intensive care are required for babies weighing less than 1500 g (3.5 lb). The perinatal mortality rate rises sharply below this weight, so that preterm delivery accounts for nearly 70% of perinatal deaths. Usually, babies delivered between 34 and 37 weeks' gestation can be nursed in district general hospitals. About 6% of babies in the United Kingdom are born before 37 weeks, and risk factors for preterm labour that have been identified include the mother's age, parity, socio-economic class, nutrition, smoking, medical and obstetric history, reproductive history and complications. *In utero* transfers of women preterm are common and pose some difficulties for anaesthetists.
- The anaesthetic risk factors may not have been identified antenatally.
- Childbirth preparation may be incomplete, or unrelated to events.
- Pain relief during transfer in labour is difficult.
- Patient expectations may not be met.
- There are incomplete hospital records.

About 10% of all babies are of low birth weight. Fetal abnormalities are the main cause of perinatal mortality in this group, followed by difficulties with preterm delivery.

The diagnosis of premature labour is usually retrospective. Rupture of the membranes is common, with associated cervical changes and regular uterine contractions. The main causes of premature labour are infection, fetal abnormalities, antepartum haemorrhage, cervical incompetence and overdistension of the uterus, as may occur in multiple pregnancies. The initial treatment of premature labour is usually tocolysis—especially if the gestational age is less than 32 weeks—together with bed rest, and antibiotics if infection is present. However, other treatment may have to be instituted if the mother becomes hypotensive, if she has an antepartum haemorrhage, or if there is known fetal abnormality. Tocolysis usually prolongs the pregnancy for a few days, during which time treatment with corticosteroids, especially dexamethasone, can promote fetal lung maturation, while transfer of the baby *in utero*, if necessary, can be organized.

Tocolytics

Tocolytics are drugs that inhibit uterine action, and they can be classified according to their mechanism of action.
- Prostaglandin synthesis inhibitors.
- β-Adrenoreceptor agonists.

Table 19.1 Tocolytics and anaesthesia.

Drug	Anaesthetic implications
Prostaglandin synthesis inhibitors, e.g. indometacin	Check for bleeding problems prior to initiating regional block
β-Adrenoreceptor agonists, e.g. ritodrine, turbutaline, salbutamol	Monitor fluid balance to avoid overload Caution when using sympathomimetic drugs, e.g. a tachycardia followed by ephedrine Delay anaesthesia to allow elimination Potential for dysrrhythmias with halothane and ephedrine
Oxytocin inhibitors, e.g. atosiban	None known
Calcium antagonists, e.g. nifedipine	Myocardial depression, especially with volatile anaesthetic agents Reduced uterine response to oxytocin and increased risk of hypotension from haemorrhage
Nitrates: glyceryl trinitrate	Dose 50–100 µg i.v. Hypotension if hypovolaemic

- Oxytocin inhibitors.
- Direct smooth-muscle relaxants.
- Calcium antagonists.

Most of the tocolytic drugs in common use have potential complications and interactions with anaesthetic drugs and techniques. They are summarized in Table 19.1.

Prostaglandin synthesis inhibitors. This is the mechanism of action of non-steroidal anti-inflammatory analgesic drugs, among which indometacin is the one most commonly used. It is a competitive inhibitor of the enzyme cyclo-oxygenase. It has fewer maternal side effects than the β-adrenoreceptor agonists, but it can reduce platelet aggregation. Its effects on the fetus are not so mild, and it has been implicated in causing necrotizing colitis and premature closure of the ductus arteriosus [3].

β-Adrenoreceptor agonists. There are a number of β-adrenoreceptor agonists that are used for tocolysis. They all have cardiovascular side effects, with potential morbidity [4]. They have positive chronotropic activity, and maternal tachycardia is common. Some inotropic effects can also increase the maternal blood pressure. Mothers also complain of headache and some mild sweating. Pulmonary oedema has been associated with the use of β-adrenoreceptor agonists in about 5% of cases [5]. It is therefore important to monitor fluid balance in these patients and to avoid the use of these drugs when a mother has cardiac disease, hyperthyroidism and diabetes. The β-adrenoreceptor agonists have metabolic effects, increasing the basal metabolic rate, and hyperglycaemia is associated with their use. It is the maternal effects that predominate as unwanted side effects, but in the fetus necrotizing colitis has been reported with the use of ritodrine. Salbutamol, terbutaline and ritodrine are the three main β-adrenoreceptor agonists used for tocolysis. Ritodrine was developed solely for obstetric use, and acts on uterine $β_2$-adrenoreceptors, producing relaxation of smooth-muscle cells.

The mechanisms for the formation of pulmonary oedema associated with adrenoreceptor use are multiple. Fluid overload is common, especially where saline-containing solutions have been used. Ritodrine also stimulates antidiuretic hormone (vasopressin) and renin release, producing additional sodium and water retention. The increase in heart rate may itself cause cardiac failure, and although there is no direct evidence for altered pulmonary capillary membrane permeability, this has also been suggested as the mechanism for pulmonary oedema in tocolysis with β-adrenoreceptor agonists.

Oxytocin inhibitors. The oxytocin inhibitor atosiban is presently being investigated. It is thought to act peripherally by competing with oxytocin receptors in the myometrium, and side effects are minimal.

Calcium antagonists. Calcium antagonists such as nifedipine are also drugs that are being investigated for use in tocolysis. They are hypotensive agents, and can induce tachycardia.

Glyceryl trinitrate (nitroglycerine, GTN). GTN is a short-term uterine relaxant used at the time of delivery of the premature fetus or the second twin, or to help to treat uterine inversion or facilitate removal of the retained placenta. It is thought to work as a nitric oxide donor, and hypotension is a predictable side effect.

Magnesium sulphate has been used as a tocolytic agent in the past. It has dose-related effects, but also causes generalized muscle weakness, a reduction in deep tendon reflexes and depression of respiration secondary to muscle weakness. When used as a tocolytic agent, it has also been associated with pulmonary oedema and cardiac failure.

Preterm delivery and anaesthesia

The preterm fetus at delivery is not mature, and may be showing signs of distress. Anaesthetic drugs crossing the placenta may have enhanced effects because of immature liver enzyme systems and alterations in receptor sites. Placental perfusion may be critical, and alterations in maternal blood flow and

Table 19.2 Suggested care for preterm infants.

Gestation at delivery (weeks)	Survivors (%)	Resuscitation
22	0	Comfort care
23	15	Flexible (predicted severe handicap > 50%)
24	56	Flexible (predicted severe handicap > 40%)
25	80	Full resuscitation

oxygenation therefore have to be monitored. Aortocaval compression must be avoided, and full attention should be given to prophylaxis against acid aspiration. Whenever possible, regional nerve blocks are preferred. However, most studies in obstetric anaesthesia involve parturients at term, so the optimal management of regional nerve block in preterm delivery is speculative.

Infants between 22 and 25 weeks' gestation have very different survival rates (Table 19.2) [6], and this can determine resuscitation care. Wherever possible, paediatric consultation with the mother prior to delivery should be achieved, and the maternity team should be aware of maternal choices for resuscitation of such low birth weight infants.

19.2.2 Breech

About 3–4% of parturients reach term with a singleton fetus in the breech position. It is common practice to perform an elective Caesarean section for delivery of these babies, although there are no adequate outcome studies of both the mother and infant to support advantages of this practice over planned vaginal deliveries [7]. Diagnosis and planned delivery should be the aim of good antenatal care. An undiagnosed breech can lead to neonatal morbidity and mortality in mothers presenting in advanced labour with the breech presentation, when Caesarean section is not possible.

A breech delivery requires good analgesia to allow full dilation of the cervix without the mother feeling the breech and having an overwhelming urge to push it out while the cervix is not fully dilated. Once full dilation is achieved, descent of the breech should be gradual. Too precipitate a delivery can move the baby into a difficult position for delivery. The perineum will not be stretched as much as in a cephalic presentation, so that when the head descends after the body, a larger than normal episiotomy will be required. Adequate analgesia is therefore required, not only to the perineum but also to the abdominal segments if the obstetrician needs to carry out manipulations. Occasionally, an emergency Caesarean section is required, in which case the anaesthetist will need to extend and make denser a regional nerve block.

19.2.3 Multiple pregnancies

Multiple pregnancy may develop as a result of division of the oocyte fertilized by one sperm into two separate bodies (i.e. identical or monozygotic twins), or the fertilization of more than one egg by separate sperm (non-identical offspring), which may occur either naturally or as a result of *in vitro* fertilization or assisted reproduction. The natural prevalence of twin births is one in 100, triplets one in 10 000, and quadruplets one in half a million deliveries. The incidence of multiple pregnancies has increased with greater maternal age and with the availability of fertility-enhancing treatments. Diagnosis of multiple pregnancies is usually made on the ultrasound scan at 16–18 weeks' gestation, when babies should also be screened for congenital abnormalities. Management of delivery is by Caesarean section for a primiparous woman, or when more than two fetuses are present. Vaginal delivery is initially discussed by the mother with the obstetrician.

The physiological changes associated with multiple pregnancies are greater than with singleton pregnancies; for example, blood volume increases correlate with fetal number and size. Symptomatic problems will increase, such as varicose veins, backache, oedema and increased pressure on the vena cava. The risk factors for a mother with multiple pregnancy that make anaesthetic involvement more likely, and which may complicate anaesthesia, include:
- increased incidence of pregnancy-induced hypertension;
- increased incidence of Caesarean section;
- anaemia (increased blood volume relative to red blood cell volume, demands of fetus);
- antepartum haemorrhage (larger surface bed of the placenta);
- aortocaval occlusion;
- physical size (pressure on the stomach and lungs).

Vaginal delivery

Perinatal mortality for the second twin can be much higher than the first, depending on the skills of the obstetrician. In the 10 years from 1974 to 1983, only 0.6% of deliveries of the second twin after vaginal delivery of the first were by Caesarean section in Birmingham (England). In the subsequent three years, this figure increased 10-fold, and today it is even higher [8]. The skills needed to carry out internal version and breech extraction are diminishing, while those needed for fast extraction by Caesarean section with epidural analgesia, electronic fetal heart rate monitoring, effective uterine stimulation and tocolysis, as well as real-time ultrasound scanning, can help manage the delivery of the second twin.

The increase in combination deliveries (e.g. cephalic/breech) requires an obstetric anaesthetist to have a regional block present for vaginal twin delivery, which can be readily used also during Caesarean section.

19.3 Unexpected anaesthetic interventions during labour

19.3.1 Umbilical cord prolapse

The risk factors for umbilical cord prolapse (UCP) are a non-cephalic presentation or a high presenting part, or both. Multiparity, preterm labour and multiple gestations are additional factors. The increased use of Caesarean section for the non-cephalic or unengaged presenting part may have been responsible for the reduction in the incidence of UCP from 0.6% of all births in 1932 to 0.2% in 1995 [9,10]. Perinatal mortality rates associated with UCP have also declined, and are related to prematurity and low birth weight. A more rapid and frequent use of Caesarean section has probably helped this reduction.

Obstetric management requires the elevation of the presenting part and rapid delivery by Caesarean section. The risk to the baby increases with the time from diagnosis to delivery. This will be greater if the parturient is outside hospital. Timely vaginal examination is of paramount importance. The fetal heart rate should be continuously monitored during all procedures and transfers. The presence of significant cardiotocographic abnormality is an indication that urgent delivery is needed. The absence of such changes allows a more planned approach to delivery, provided that monitoring is maintained. Anaesthetic management requires a fast, accurate anaesthetic assessment. If already sited, epidural anaesthesia can be extended, provided that the woman is kept lying in the lateral position slightly head-down, with vaginal access to the presenting part. Spinal anaesthesia can be achieved rapidly with the mother in the lateral position, but care must be taken to elevate the head, neck and shoulders, while the pelvis is also tilted if high nerve blocks are to be avoided (see Chapter 15). Where there is fetal compromise, oxygen should be given to the mother, haemodynamic stability should be checked, and if necessary general anaesthesia should be induced, provided that conditions for safety are followed. Access to the vagina still has to be maintained, but not with the mother's legs in the lithotomy position, since this increases pressure on the abdominal wall, which is transferred to the stomach and may precipitate regurgitation during the induction of anaesthesia.

19.3.2 Uterine hyperstimulation

An intense uterine contraction may be induced by an oxytocin infusion, causing blood supply to the uterus to be severely reduced. Fetal distress should be treated immediately with maternal oxygen and a lateral position. Salbutamol can be given by inhaler or by slow intravenous injection. Close maternal observation, preferably by an anaesthetist, and electrocardiographic (ECG) monitoring of the heart rate is required. Salbutamol infusion should stop if the maternal heart rate increases above 120 beats/min. The anaesthetist should be prepared for an emergency Caesarean section to be performed.

19.3.3 Subcutaneous emphysema and pneumothorax

During a Valsalva manoeuvre (forced expiration against a closed glottis), the intrathoracic pressure may increase to pressures above 50 cmH$_2$O. The pressure gradient between the air, the alveoli and the connective tissues is greatly increased, and traumatic rupture of the tissues can occur, forcing air into the tissues. The air may pass along blood vessel sheaths, or may rupture the alveoli directly into the pleural cavity if there are pre-existing bullae. The diagnosis can be made by feeling crepitus, eliciting chest pain and observing dyspnoea. Massive subcutaneous emphysema or a large pneumothorax can severely compromise the airway and cause haemodynamic instability. The majority of patients require conservative management [11]. Entonox is contraindicated, because the nitrous oxide can diffuse into the air cavity spaces and expand them further. Epidural anaesthesia will prevent the bearing-down reflex, which can initiate the Valsalva manoeuvre. General anaesthesia should be avoided, because the airway may be compromised and further barotrauma to the lungs may be induced by intermittent positive-pressure ventilation. Facilities for a chest drain should be immediately available in all cases. Inhalation of 100% oxygen should be used so that rapid absorption of gas from the pleural cavity can occur.

19.3.4 Critical care

Immediate access to a high-dependency unit and intensive-care and resuscitation facilities must be available in areas where parturition occurs. All hospital units should be able to provide resuscitation and some level of high-dependency care, including cardiovascular monitoring, rapid infusion of fluid or blood, and intermittent positive-pressure ventilation for up to six hours while the patient awaits transfer to the intensive-care unit [12]. Medical and midwifery staff should be trained in the management of emergency care and the necessary monitoring equipment available: ECG, oximeters, capnographs and direct blood pressure monitoring. The same chart documentation is used as in intensive-care units.

High-dependency care is appropriate when a single organ has failed or is failing, except for the respiratory system. Immediate postoperative care is of a similar nature. Intensive care is required for advanced respiratory support and when two or more organ systems are failing. An average high-dependency unit workload would be more than one in 100 deliveries, and intensive care may be required in between one in 100 and one in 1000 deliveries [13]. It is necessary for anaesthetists to train and maintain the expertise of midwives or other nursing staff in managing the sick mother.

References

1. Uncles DR, Carrie LE. Antepartum assessment for anaesthesia [letter]. *Br J Anaesth* 1993; **70**: 116.
2. McMahon MJ, Luther ER, Bowes WA, Olshan AF. Comparison of a trial of labor with an elective second Cesarean section. *N Engl J Med* 1996; **335**: 689–95.
3. Naughton ME, Merrill J, Cooper BAB, Kuller JA, Clyman RI. Neonatal complications after the administration of indomethacin for preterm labor. *N Engl J Med* 1993; **329**: 1602–7.
4. Hibberd BM, Department of Health. *Report on Confidential Enquiries into Maternal Deaths in the United Kingdom, 1991–1993.* London: HMSO, 1996: 200.
5. Clesham GJ, Scott J, Oakley CM *et al.* Beta adrenergic agonists and pulmonary oedema in pre-term labour. *Br Med J* 1994; **308**: 260–2.
6. Allen MC, Donohue PK, Dusman AE. The limit of viability: neonatal outcome of infants born at 22–25 weeks' gestation. *N Engl J Med* 1993; **329**: 1597–601.
7. Hannah M, Hannah W. Caesarean section or vaginal birth for breech presentation at term: we need better evidence as to which is better. *Br Med J* 1996; **312**: 1433–4.
8. [Editorial.] The second twin. *Lancet* 1990; **336**: 284.
9. Murphy DJ, MacKenzie IZ. The mortality and morbidity associated with umbilical cord prolapse. *Br J Obstet Gynaecol* 1995; **102**: 826–30.
10. Kurzrock J. Prolapsed umbilical cord: an analysis of one hundred cases. *Am J Obstet Gynecol* 1932; **23**: 403–7.
11. Jayran-Nejad Y. Subcutaneous emphysema in labour. *Anaesthesia* 1993; **48**: 139–40.
12. Royal College of Obstetrics and Gynaecologists Working Party. *Minimum Standards of Care in Labour.* London: Royal College of Obstetricians and Gynaecologists, 1994.
13. Umo-Etuk J, Lumley J, Holdcroft A. Critically ill parturient women and admission to intensive care: a five-year review. *Int J Obstet Anesth* 1996; 5: 79–84.

Section 6
The Fetus and Neonate

20: Fetal Medicine

Pregnancy makes many physiological demands on the mother. When maternal diseases affect fetal development, or when the fetus itself is diseased, the anaesthetist should be involved as early as possible in management of both the mother and fetus, as these problems can influence the choice of anaesthetic drugs and techniques. The search continues for methods of detecting fetal distress. The anaesthetist is also concerned with the effects of fetal drug exposure, either in pregnancy or during labour.

Advances in diagnosis and fetal therapy have made the fetus a person in its own right. Fetal disease can be detected and sometimes treated *in utero*. Conflicts of interest will arise between fetal and maternal autonomy. The fetus is legally registrable after 24 weeks' gestation in the United Kingdom and United States. Termination for serious fetal abnormality can be sanctioned later in pregnancy in the United Kingdom.

Antepartum fetal monitoring helps the obstetrician in considering timely delivery of the fetus before asphyxia and death occur, or in deferring delivery in a high-risk pregnancy until fetal maturity develops and induction of labour becomes easier. Biochemical and ultrasound monitoring are also used for diagnostic purposes.

Intrapartum monitoring of the fetus during labour assesses the effects of labour on fetal well-being. Indirect monitoring will be subject to technical difficulties, such as a restless mother, while direct monitoring is invasive and may not always be available.

20.1 Fetal pathophysiology

Organ maturity at birth is the ultimate determinant of fetal outcome. Options for delivery have to be weighed against an infant's chance of survival and normal life if it is to be born preterm. Babies of less than 32 weeks' gestation normally require initial intubation and ventilation. Aggressive resuscitation and improved obstetric and neonatal interventions have lowered the limit of viability. Studies of mortality and outcome based on birth weight are useful in counselling parents. Ultrasonographic estimates of weight may be inaccurate, and for prenatal counselling it is difficult to interpret outcome studies. Gestational age provides a guide. Infants born at 25–26 weeks require full resuscitation [1]. There is currently a poor prognosis for infants born before this, although fetal therapy may change this in future.

Antepartum and intrapartum stress affects fetal physiology in the following ways. The fetal response to hypoxia is metabolically similar to that of an adult, such that metabolic acidosis results from an excess of lactic acid produced by anaerobic metabolism. This occurs when the placental blood flow decreases. Oxygenation and carbon dioxide excretion are both affected, so that a respiratory acidosis develops. Fetal movements decrease, including breathing movements.

Cardiovascular responses develop, with redistribution of blood to the brain by adrenergic activity. Systemic hypertension occurs, as well as reflex bradycardia. A deterioration in cardiac output may particularly affect the response to labour of a fetus with intrauterine growth retardation [2].

Amniotic fluid can be regarded as an extension of fetal extracellular fluid until the fetal skin keratinizes at about 20 weeks' gestation. It is essential for normal lung development, especially in the second trimester. It allows the fetus to grow and move, while protecting it from localized pressures. If this protective function does not occur, fetal abnormalities can develop. The passage of urine changes its composition in relation to the maturity of the kidneys, and in a compromised fetus blood is diverted away from the kidneys, leading to a decrease in urine output and oligohydramnios. The fluid is swallowed by the fetus, and conditions such as oesophageal atresia are associated with polyhydramnios. Gastrointestinal activity results in the discharge of meconium into this fluid.

In preterm and term fetuses, cerebral autoregulation is maintained, but in the preterm fetus the range is considerably narrower, so that even small increases in mean arterial blood pressure may result in increased cerebral perfusion, leading to an increased risk of cerebral haemorrhage. Beta-sympathomimetic drugs or beta blockers such as atenolol can induce significant haemodynamic effects [3].

Breathing movements *in utero* decrease in frequency with the onset of labour, as well as with chronic fetal hypoxia.

20.2 Methods of fetal assessment

20.2.1 Fetal activity

Mothers can usually identify fetal movements from 16 to 18 weeks onwards, but counting them over extended periods can be burdensome. A 'kick count to 10' is taken, i.e. the time it takes for the fetus to make 10 movements. Fewer than 10 movements over 12 hours should be reported by a mother to her obstetric team. This is a subjective score and clinically not very significant.

20.2.2 Fetal growth/weight

Fetal growth is a good measure of fetal well-being. The comparison of weight and gestation is a standard that is measured in a normal healthy population of defined ethnic origin. Conventional subdivisions of gestational age are 'term', which includes 37–41 completed weeks, 'preterm' for babies of less than 37 weeks, and 'post-term' for all gestations of more than 41 weeks [4]. 'Intrauterine growth retardation' (IUGR) is diagnosed when the growth rate falls significantly from an established norm—for example, a fetus who remains on the 10th centile will probably be at less risk than one that changes from the 50th to the 5th centiles.

Gestational age is estimated from the mother's menstrual dates or ultrasound scan, e.g. biparietal diameter. Gestational age can only be measured at birth by techniques such as the Dubowitz score [5]. All fetal weight curves have been derived from cross-sectional data, because a baby can only be measured (rather than estimated prior to delivery) once. There is no way of knowing whether or not it followed the average growth rate to reach that point. The fetal growth curve is sigmoid (Fig. 20.1) [6–8], with apparent slowing of fetal growth during the final weeks of pregnancy.

Physiological variations in fetal weight occur with sex (males being, on average 150 g heavier than females), maternal size, ethnic origin and parity. Deleterious effects on birth weight occur from smoking, alcohol and drug abuse, and reduced oxygen supply to the fetus. Congenital fetal abnormalities or intrauterine infections can also affect fetal weight and growth. Fetuses of diabetic mothers may be macrosomic and therefore large for gestational age.

Mothers whose fetuses are at greater risk of growth retardation will often have several ultrasounds in later pregnancy. These are either mothers with a bad obstetric history, hypertensive disorders, intrauterine infection, and genetic abnormalities, or those with oligohydramnios. Amniotic fluid volume is a good indicator of fetal well-being, with oligohydramnios occurring with ruptured membranes or placental insufficiency.

20.2.3 Biochemistry

Urinary oestrogens

Most of the maternal oestrogen comes from the placenta in all but early pregnancy. Serial determination in late pregnancy has been used to detect a change in placental function that could be detrimental to the fetus [9]. Diurnal variation occurs, so 24-hour urinary collections are preferred to plasma concentrations. This method does not detect acute alterations in placental function, and is a poor predictor of fetal compromise. Placental protein hormones have also not been found helpful in measuring signs of fetal distress that require acute intervention.

Maternal blood sampling for Down syndrome and open neural tube defects

Chromosomal abnormalities increase with maternal age (Table 20.1). Biochemical screening tests for alpha-fetoprotein are carried out to identify those

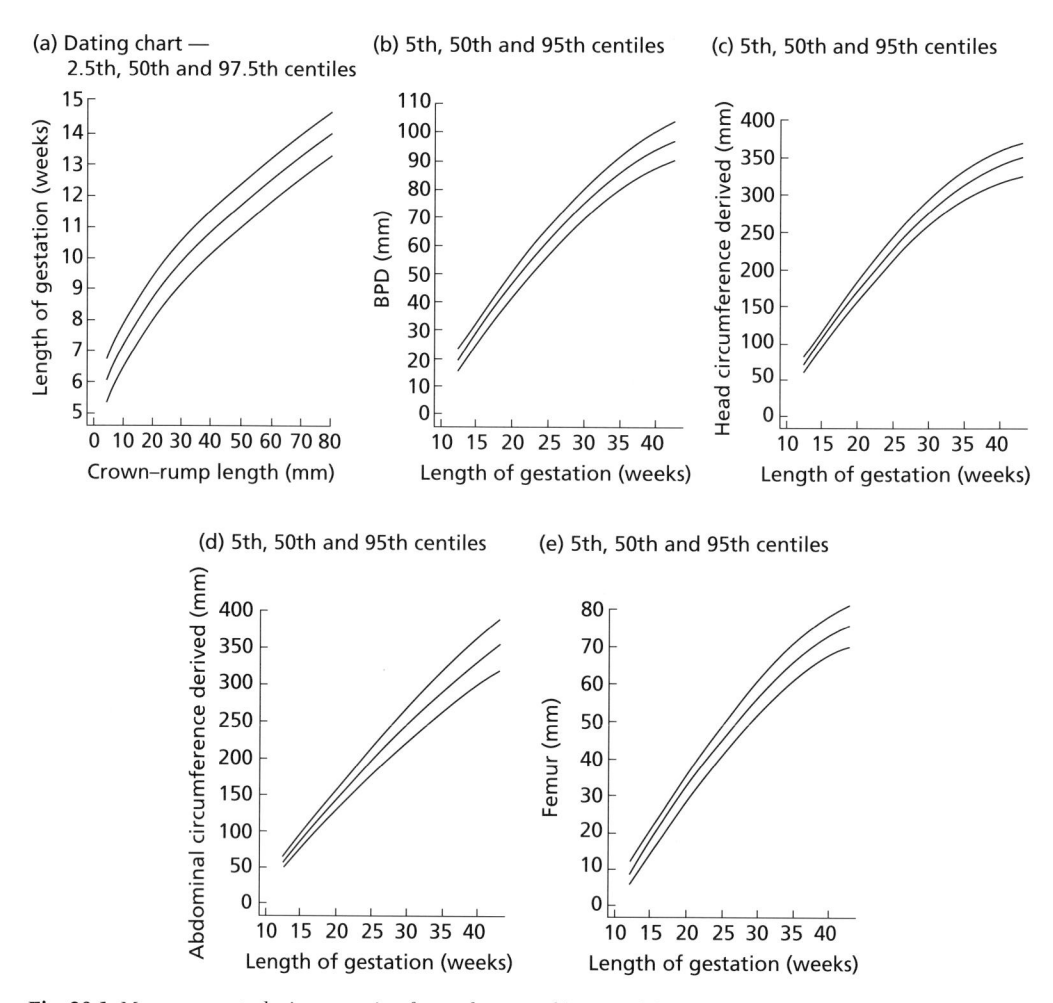

Fig. 20.1 Measurements during gestation from ultrasound images. (a) Crown–rump length and length of gestation. (b) Biparietal diameter (BPD) and length of gestation [6]. (c) Head circumference and length of gestation [6]. (d) Abdominal circumference and length of gestation [7]. (e) Femur length and length of gestation [8].

Table 20.1 Maternal age and chromosomal abnormalities.

	Rate per 1000 live births	
Age (years)	Down syndrome	All chromosomal abnormalities
25–29	0.9	2.2
30–34	1.4	3.1
35–39	4.2	8.1
40–44	14.2	24.0
45–49	50.0	65.0

women who are at high enough risk to warrant the hazards and costs of more invasive procedures [10]. The two abnormalities commonly screened for at present are Down syndrome and open neural tube defects. Both can be carried out between 15 and 18 weeks on a maternal blood sample.

20.2.4 Ultrasound

Physical principles

Real-time ultrasound. Ultrasound images depend on the computerized interpretation of the time delay between sending a pulse of sound into tissues and receiving the echo. The frequency difference will depend on the tissue reflecting the sound, so that a map of the sounds returned can build up a picture of the tissues. Real-time pictures are obtained, and hard copies or videos can be made. Abdominal ultrasonography can detect embryonic tissue at six to eight weeks. A vaginal probe will show it earlier. A scan at booking will confirm fetal viability, fetal number and gross abnormality (e.g. anencephaly), and establish gestational age (to help in the correct timing of other tests) [11–13]. The applications for this type of scanning are listed below.

- *Crown–rump length* (Fig. 20.1a). The length of the fetus from the crown of the head to the tip of the rump can be measured precisely from seven to 12 weeks. After this time, the measurement becomes less reliable, because the fetus flexes and extends to variable amounts.
- *Biparietal diameter* (Fig. 20.1b, c). The biparietal diameter is the maximum diameter of the fetal skull at the level of the parietal eminences. It is used in the assessment of gestational age and fetal growth rate. In a breech presentation, the head may be dolichocephalic, and head circumference is a more accurate measurement. At 18 weeks' gestation, it has 95% confidence limits of 10 days, and this increases with gestation.
- *Abdominal circumference* (Fig. 20.1d). The measurement of a cross-section of the trunk with a short section of the umbilical vein at its proximal end provides an assessment of the size of the fetal liver. A lack of nutrients from the placenta, i.e. placental insufficiency, will prevent normal growth of the liver.
- *Femur length* (Fig. 20.1e). Femur length can be easily measured. It is not subject to moulding, and is almost always accessible.
- *Amniotic fluid volume/index.* This has to be an assessment based on the height of the largest vertical column of fluid seen on ultrasonography. A column of less than 2 cm near term indicates oligohydramnios (poor production of amniotic fluid), and the fetus becomes at risk. The amniotic fluid volume is reduced in the presence of placental insufficiency, and may be associated with an impaired outcome. The amniotic fluid index is the sum of the maximum pool in the four quadrants of the uterus.
- *Placental scan.* Localization of the placenta is useful in the management of mothers with antepartum haemorrhage, in case there is a placenta praevia, and prior to an amniocentesis.

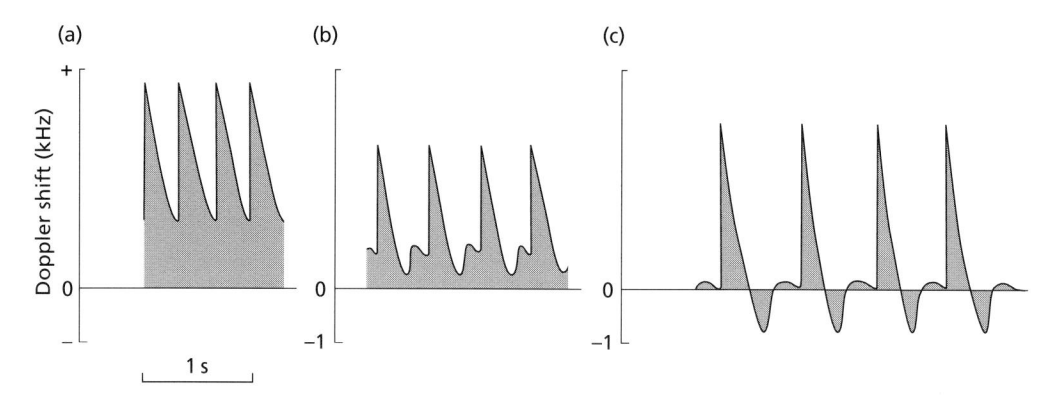

Fig. 20.2 A diagram of the flow velocity waveform in an umbilical artery. (a) Normal flow, (b) almost absent end-diastolic velocity, and (c) reversed end-diastolic velocity.

Doppler ultrasound. When ultrasound is directed at a blood vessel, the moving blood cells alter the frequency of the reflected beam. The change in frequency depends on the velocity of the blood in the vessel. The frequency change will increase or decrease, depending on the movement of blood in the vessel towards or away from the beam. The frequency of the initial ultrasonic wave (incident wave) and the reflected wave are compared.

It is difficult to quantify the velocity of blood in the vessel, so velocity ratios are used instead of measuring actual velocity. Errors would affect both systolic and diastolic measurements, and so they can be cancelled out in a ratio. The simplest ratio is the systolic to diastolic (S/D) ratio. It is normally less than 3.0. If the diastolic velocity is low, the value tends towards infinity. The pulsatility index (PI) does not have this limitation. It is the peak systolic frequency minus the end-diastolic frequency, divided by the mean maximum frequency over one cardiac cycle.

Continuous-wave Doppler is inexpensive and simple to use. Its main limitation is that it cannot identify a particular place on a vessel. The inability to target a vessel allows interference from other vessels. Pulsed-wave Doppler is expensive, but allows a small area to be identified and its depth to be calculated, because the speed of ultrasound through tissues is relatively constant. A simultaneous display of the cross-sectional image with the sampled area allows the recording of localized velocities. In practice, in antepartum mothers, no differences in S/D ratios were found between these methods [14].

Sampling site location can have an effect on these measurements. The ratios for umbilical artery velocity were significantly higher at the fetal than at the placental end [15].

Blood flow in the major fetal and uterine vessels can be measured using Doppler techniques [16]. Vessels that have been used with this technique include the umbilical artery (Fig. 20.2), fetal middle cerebral artery, ductus arteriosus and uterine artery. The measurement of umbilical artery flows is used to help gauge fetoplacental well-being. The use of Doppler techniques in the prediction of pregnancies affected by conditions such as pre-eclampsia and intrauterine growth retardation is still being assessed.

More recently, colour flow Doppler has been incorporated into obstetric practice. This allows the identification of the direction of flow in vessels (red for blood flowing towards the transducer and blue for blood flowing away). This technique helps in the identification of specific vessels and in the diagnosis of cardiac anomalies.

Doppler velocity wave forms in maternal and fetal arteries. The maintenance of blood flow on either side of the placenta is important in maintaining fetal oxygenation. The flow through vessels from the direction of the mother to the fetus is described below. Unfortunately, Doppler velocity waveforms do not detect the cause of any observed reduction in flow.

- External iliac artery. This is too far from the placental site.
- Uterine arteries. Although the total flow through these arteries at term is high—about 700 mL/min, there is a significant variation between flow in individual vessels. These arteries are under α-adrenergic control (endogenous or exogenous), and can vasoconstrict. Decreased flow occurs with hypotension; with hypertension due to an increase in systemic vascular resistance; and with each uterine contraction in labour.
- Arcuate arteries. Abnormal waveforms may predict mothers who develop severe hypertension [17].
- Umbilical artery. If absent or reversed, perinatal mortality increases to almost 100% with reverse flow [18]. Waveforms from an umbilical artery can distinguish a fetus that is progressing well, but is small for gestational dates, from one that is becoming compromised. Positive end-diastolic velocity is usually present, and when this is absent or reversed it is associated with a perinatal mortality of 28%. The quantity of blood flow relates to the size of the fetus, and is 120 mL/kg/min. This amount decreases with the liberation of catecholamines and with cord compression, but the two different causes cannot be distinguished by looking at the trace.
- Middle cerebral artery. The percentage of the cardiac output through a middle cerebral artery remains constant throughout gestation, with a range between 3% and 7%. In fetal vessels, the pulsatility index from the middle cerebral artery is most useful to predict adverse fetal outcome.
- Fetal aorta. Alterations in the velocity waveform in the descending fetal aorta may occur with a reduction in fetal cardiac output or when diversion of blood to the fetal brain takes place.

20.2.5 Telemedicine

Telemedicine is telecommunication that connects a mother and a health-care provider by live transmission across distances and allows effective diagnosis, treatment and other health-care activities to be carried out at a distance [19]. Movement of monitoring information affects the pregnant woman in a number of ways. Transfer of information can occur antenatally or intrapartum from a person's home to hospital, between hospitals and within rooms of a hospital. Telemetry allows a woman to be mobile in labour and yet carefully monitored. Images can be transferred and fetal heart rate can be monitored.

Labour ward telemetry

The connections between a piece of monitoring equipment and the mother in labour may prevent her from mobilizing and seeking a position that is comfortable in labour. Telemetric monitoring would support her choice, provided that she does not need to be confined to bed for other reasons.

20.2.6 Sampling techniques

Amniocentesis

This is the oldest and most commonly performed sampling technique [20]. This test is usually carried out after 15 weeks' gestation. Under ultrasound guidance (to avoid the placenta and fetus), a fine needle is inserted via the mother's abdomen into the amniotic cavity, and up to 20 mL of fluid is removed. This fluid contains amniotic fluid cells, which are combinations of cells shed from the fetus, amnion and umbilical cord. The cells are then cultured, and a result is usually available within three or four weeks. The fetal loss rate from amniocentesis is approximately 0.5–1.0% [21].

From the cells cultured, the fetal karyotype can be obtained, allowing diagnosis of chromosomal conditions such as Down syndrome [22]. In addition, many inborn errors of metabolism can be diagnosed by demonstrating protein or enzyme deficiencies in the cultured cells. There are also a number of other constituents of amniotic fluid that can be measured and give information about the fetus [23].

In the amniotic fluid, the concentration of bilirubin has been used as an index of the severity of rhesus isoimmunization [24], but more specific tests directly sampling fetal blood are now used. Maternal complications such as infection and rhesus isoimmunization are rare (provided that anti-D immunoglobulin is given to all rhesus-negative mothers at the time of the procedure).

Later in pregnancy, the amniotic fluid can be analysed for surfactant activity in order to assess the maturity of the fetus's lungs. The ratio of the major phospholipids—lecithin and sphingomyelin (the L/S ratio)—should be greater than 2. More rapid tests are the foam stability index and the phosphatidylglycerol radioimmunoassay. The use of steroid therapy given to the mother to enhance fetal lung maturity [25] has reduced the need for this test. However, when a clinical or ultrasonographic gestational age is not available, analysis of amniotic fluid for lung maturity may be the only option.

Chorionic villus sampling

This is a newer technique for identifying abnormalities, which can be carried out either transabdominally or transcervically [26]. It is carried out earlier than amniocentesis, after 10 weeks' gestation, thereby allowing earlier and safer termination of pregnancy. Under ultrasound guidance, a small portion of chorion frondosum is biopsied and cultured. Chromosomal abnormalities, some inherited conditions and certain inborn errors of metabolism can be diagnosed from the cultured cells. The risk of complications limits the use of this method [27].

Fetal blood sampling

Ultrasound-guided fetal blood sampling is usually carried out after 18 weeks' gestation. Under local anaesthesia and sometimes under sedation, a fine needle is passed through the maternal abdominal wall to sample fetal blood. The two most common sites of sampling are the umbilical vein or artery at the cord insertion into the placenta [28] and the fetal intrahepatic vein [29]. This technique allows more rapid diagnosis than amniocentesis and chorionic villus sampling. The main indications are in the prenatal diagnosis of chromosomal abnormalities, fetal infections, certain genetic disorders (e.g. haemoglobinopathies) and autoimmune thrombocytopenia. It is also commonly used to gauge the severity and in treating fetomaternal alloimmunization, and if the fetus is anaemic an intrauterine intravascular blood transfusion can be given.

The main complication is an early fetal loss rate of about 1.0–2.0% [30]. Other complications include chorioamnionitis, premature rupture of the membranes and premature labour.

Fetal tissue sampling

This is rarely carried out, and is either done under direct vision or ultrasound guidance to diagnose various conditions. The more common tissues biopsied are skin (e.g. for harlequin ichthyosis), liver (e.g. for ornithine carbamoyltransferase deficiency), lung (e.g. for congenital adenomatoid malformation), muscle (e.g. for Duchenne's muscular dystrophy) and kidney (e.g. for congenital Finnish nephrosis) [31].

20.3 Fetal therapy

Only a small number of fetal therapies have been developed satisfactorily enough so far to obtain widespread acceptance (Table 20.2) [32]. Most

Table 20.2 Examples of fetal therapy.

Intervention	Condition treated
Maternal administration of corticosteroids and/or thyrotrophin-releasing hormone	Maturation of fetal lungs
Maternal administration of digoxin	Fetal supraventricular tachycardia
Intrauterine intravascular blood transfusion	Red blood cell alloimmunization
In utero bladder decompression	Obstructive urinary anomaly, e.g. posterior urethral valves
Amnioreduction in polyhydramnios	Twin transfusion syndrome

therapies are still at the experimental stage, and these include intrauterine or open surgery (e.g. for congenital diaphragmatic hernia), gene therapy and *in utero* bone marrow transplantation. The fetus develops a hormonal stress response to invasive procedures [33], and analgesia and anaesthesia may be desirable. It is recommended that fetal analgesia and sedation should be considered for invasive procedures after 23 weeks' gestation.

Selective fetal reduction is also carried out to either reduce the number of fetuses in a high-order multiple pregnancy (more than three fetuses) in an attempt to benefit the remaining fetuses; or to terminate an abnormal fetus or fetuses in a multiple pregnancy. This is carried out under ultrasound guidance by giving the selected fetus an intracardiac injection of potassium chloride.

20.4 Fetal abnormalities

20.4.1 Screening

There is no universal agreement concerning which tests should be carried out to assess the fetus in a low-risk pregnancy. Apart from taking a comprehensive pregnancy and family history, the following tests are generally carried out.

Ultrasound

The earlier in gestation an ultrasound scan is carried out, the more accurate the dating; and the later it is carried out, the more likely it is that fetal abnormalities will be visualized.
• Booking scan: gross abnormality can be excluded.
• At 18–20 weeks: this is a compromise, so that fetal abnormalities can be found early enough to allow termination of pregnancy. An ultrasound at this gestational age is accurate for dating to within ±10 days, and it picks up approximately 40% of major abnormalities [34]. The most common abnormalities found include those of the cardiovascular system (e.g. hypoplastic left heart), central nervous system (e.g. hydrocephaly and neural tube defects),

musculoskeletal system (e.g. abdominal wall defects and diaphragmatic hernia), renal system (e.g. hydronephrosis), skeleton (e.g. achondroplasia) and some recognizable syndromes [35]. It must be remembered that ultrasound looks at structure rather than function, and many abnormalities cannot therefore be diagnosed by this method.

Biochemical screening

Down syndrome, or trisomy 21, is the commonest surviving chromosomal abnormality (one in 650 live births), with a life expectation of about 60 years [36]. The incidence of the condition increases with maternal age (Table 20.1), and it is associated with mental retardation and malformations of the heart, gastrointestinal system and eyes and ears. Down syndrome is associated with a raised maternal serum human chorionic gonadotrophin, low maternal serum unconjugated oestriol, and low maternal serum alpha-fetoprotein.

The risk of a pregnancy with Down syndrome can be calculated from the above parameters together with maternal age [37]. This is the basis of the 'triple test' or 'Bart's test'. A positive test is usually set at the level of a risk higher than one in 250 of having an affected child. This test picks up about 60% of Down pregnancies and has a false-positive rate of about 5% (that is, 5% of pregnancies will have a positive result, but the vast majority of these will have an unaffected child; for example, 199 of 200 women recalled with a risk of one in 200 will not have a child with Down syndrome) [38]. The results are discussed with women who have a positive test, and they will be offered a more definitive test such as amniocentesis to determine whether the fetus is affected or not. Women with an affected fetus have the option of termination of pregnancy.

Open neural tube defects, such as anencephaly and spina bifida, are associated with raised maternal serum concentrations of alpha-fetoprotein. This forms the basis of screening for open neural tube defects [39]. Alpha-fetoprotein is an oncofetal antigen that crosses the placenta in small amounts. Women with increased serum alpha-fetoprotein concentrations are offered ultrasound to diagnose the presence of any defects. There are a number of less common, although equally important, conditions that are also associated with a raised maternal alpha-fetoprotein concentration, including intrauterine growth retardation, exomphalos, gastroschisis and congenital nephrosis [40].

Future trends in the diagnosis of fetal abnormality

Molecular cytogenetics. Molecular cytogenetics has undergone rapid changes in the last few years. An increasing number of DNA probes have been developed to help in the rapid diagnosis of a number of chromosomal defects.

Preimplantation diagnosis. This technique involves the biopsy of one or a few cells from an embryo (produced by *in-vitro* fertilization methods) and the use of highly sensitive methods for analysis at the single-cell level to diagnose various disorders [41]. Although the method is still in the developmental stages, an increasing number of disorders are being diagnosed with this technique.

Fetal nucleated cells in the maternal circulation. Molecular cytogenetic techniques, including polymerase chain reaction amplification, are being developed to identify abnormal genes [42] in fetal nucleated cells, such as lymphocytes recovered from maternal blood.

20.4.2 Common fetal abnormalities

Congenital malformations

Craniosubarachnoid malformations. The more common malformations include anencephaly, hydrocephalus, spina bifida, holoprosencephaly, microcephaly and facial clefts [43]. Of those diagnosed prenatally, most are discovered at routine ultrasound (e.g. anencephaly) or by biochemical screening (e.g. spina bifida). Many are lethal abnormalities (e.g. holoprosencephaly), for which termination of pregnancy may be offered. The presence of hydrocephalus may make delivery difficult, and may warrant an elective Caesarean section. Some abnormalities require surgical attention at birth (e.g. facial clefts), and babies should therefore be delivered where there are adequate paediatric facilities.

Urinary tract abnormalities. These occur in approximately two to three per 1000 pregnancies. There is a wide range of abnormalities, including renal agenesis, various forms of polycystic and multicystic kidneys, obstructive uropathies and tumours. Ultrasound is the method of diagnosis [44]. Most of these conditions are not in themselves lethal (unlike renal agenesis), but it is important to investigate for the presence of other associated abnormalities, since a urinary tract lesion may be part of a more serious syndrome, including chromosomal abnormalities. Karyotyping is therefore often warranted in the presence of a urinary tract abnormality (and in fact in the presence of any other single-system abnormality).

Cardiovascular malformations. Most structural heart malformations can be diagnosed prenatally with fetal echocardiography [45]. The importance of diagnosing congenital heart disease prenatally is that approximately 16.5% of cases are associated with chromosomal abnormality; some are lethal (e.g. hypoplastic left heart) and some may need surgical correction soon after birth (transposition of the great arteries).

Abdominal wall defects. Abdominal wall defects such as omphalocele, gastroschisis, and bladder exstrophy can be diagnosed prenatally by ultrasound. It is important that affected fetuses should be delivered where there is an immediate paediatric surgical facility.

Inherited disorders

Cystic fibrosis. This is the most common serious autosomal recessive disorder in Caucasian populations, with a gene frequency of one in 20. The early diagnosis of a homozygous fetus [46] has been made possible by the cloning of the cystic fibrosis gene and techniques such as polymerase chain reaction. Tissue for analysis is collected at chorionic villus sampling.

Blood disorders. DNA analysis techniques have also been developed for the identification of the mutations responsible for sickle-cell anaemia, as well as α- and β-thalassaemia.

Chromosomal abnormalities

Cytogenetic abnormalities are believed to play a role in a wide range of human morbidity and mortality, ranging from early unrecognized miscarriage to normal but infertile individuals. The vast majority of these defects cannot be recognized prenatally. The incidences of the more common and potentially lethal autosomal abnormalities, such as trisomy 21 (Down syndrome), trisomy 18 and trisomy 13, increase with increasing maternal age (Table 20.1). Because of this increase, older mothers (over 35 years) are often offered prenatal diagnosis by amniocentesis or chorionic villus sampling.

References

1. Allen MC, Donohue PK, Dusman AE. The limit of viability: neonatal outcome of infants born at 22–25 weeks' gestation. *N Engl J Med* 1993; **329**: 1597–601.
2. Rizzo G, Arduini D. Fetal cardiac function in intrauterine growth retardation. *Am J Obstet Gynecol* 1991; **165**: 876–82.
3. Montan S, Ingemarsson I, Marsal K, Sjoberg NO. Randomised controlled trial of atenolol and pindolol in human pregnancy: effects on fetal haemodynamics. *Br Med J* 1992; **76**: 580–7.
4. Neligan GA, Ballabriga A, Beutnagel C *et al*. Working party to discuss nomenclature based on gestational age and birth weight. *Arch Dis Child* 1970; **45**: 730.
5. Dubowitz LM, Dubowitz V, Goldberg C. Clinical assessment of gestational age in the newborn infant. *J Pediatr* 1970; **77**: 1–10.
6. Chitty LS, Altman DG, Henderson A, Campbell S. Charts of fetal size, 2: head measurements. *Br J Obstet Gynaecol* 1994; **101**: 35–43.
7. Chitty LS, Altman DG, Henderson A, Campbell S. Charts of fetal size, 3: abdominal measurements. *Br J Obstet Gynaecol* 1994; **101**: 125–31.
8. Chitty LS, Altman DG, Henderson A, Campbell S. Charts of fetal size, 4: femur length. *Br J Obstet Gynaecol* 1994; **101**: 132–5.
9. Kochenour NK. Estrogen assay during pregnancy. *Clin Obstet Gynecol* 1982; **25**: 659–72.
10. Mant D, Fowler G. Mass screening: theory and ethics. *Br Med J* 1990; **300**: 916–18.

11 Bennett MJ, Little G, Dewhurst J, Chamberlain G. Predictive value of ultrasound in early pregnancy: a randomized controlled trial. *Br J Obstet Gynaecol* 1982; **89**: 338–41.
12 Altman DG, Chitty LS. Charts of fetal size, 1: methodology. *Br J Obstet Gynaecol* 1994; **101**: 29–34.
13 Dewbury K, Meire H, Cosgrove D. *Ultrasound in Obstetrics and Gynaecology.* Edinburgh: Churchill Livingstone, 1993.
14 Brar HS, Medearis AL, DeVore GR, Platt LD. Fetal velocimetry using continuous-wave and pulsed-wave Doppler ultrasound in high-risk pregnancies: a comparison of systolic to diastolic ratios. *Obstet Gynecol* 1988; **72**: 607–10.
15 Mehalek KE, Rosenberg J, Berkowitz GS, Chitkara U, Berkowitz RL. Umbilical and uterine artery flow velocity waveforms: effect of the sampling site on Doppler ratios. *J Ultrasound Med* 1989; **8**: 171–6.
16 Kurjak A, Alfirevic Z, Miljan M. Conventional and colour Doppler in assessment of fetal and maternal circulation. *Ultrasound Med Biol* 1988; **14**: 337–54.
17 Chamberlain G. Checking for fetal well-being, 1. *Br Med J* 1991; **302**: 837–9.
18 Karsdorp VHM, van Vugt JMG, van Geijn HP *et al.* Clinical significance of absent or reversed end-diastolic velocity waveforms in umbilical artery. *Lancet* 1994; **344**: 1664–8.
19 McLaren P, Ball CJ. Telemedicine: lessons remain unheeded. *Br Med J* 1995; **310**: 1390–1.
20 Bevis DCA. Composition of liquor amnii in haemolytic disease of the newborn. *J Obstet Gynaecol Br Commonw* 1953; **60**: 244–51.
21 Tabor A, Philip J, Madsen M. Randomised controlled trial of genetic amniocentesis in 4606 low-risk women. *Lancet* 1986; **i**: 1287–93.
22 Steele MW, Berg WT. Chromosome analysis of human amniotic cells. *Lancet* 1966; **i**: 383–5.
23 Connor JM. Diagnosable Mendelian disorders. In: Brock DJH, Rodeck CH, Ferguson-Smith MA, eds. *Prenatal Diagnosis and Screening.* Edinburgh: Churchill Livingstone, 1992: 515–47.
24 Queenan JT. Amniotic fluid analysis. *Clin Obstet Gynecol* 1971; **14**: 505–36.
25 Garite TJ, Rumney PJ, Briggs GG, Harding JA. A randomised, placebo-controlled trial of betamethasone for the prevention of respiratory distress syndrome at 24–28 weeks' gestation. *Am J Obstet Gynecol* 1992; **166**: 646–51.
26 Old JM, Ward RHT, Karagozlu F. First-trimester fetal diagnosis for haemoglobinopathies: three cases. *Lancet* 1982; **ii**: 1413–16.
27 Canadian Collaborative CVS-Amniocentesis Clinical Trial Group. Multicentre randomized clinical trial of chorion villous sampling and amniocentesis. *Lancet* 1989; **i**: 1–6.
28 Daffos F, Capella-Pavlovsky M, Forestier F. Fetal blood sampling via the umbilical cord using a needle guided by ultrasound: report of 66 cases. *Prenat Diagn* 1983; **3**: 271–7.
29 Bang J, Bock JE, Trolle D. Ultrasound-guided fetal intravenous transfusion for severe rhesus haemolytic disease. *Br Med J* 1982; **284**: 373–4.
30 Daffos F. Fetal blood sampling. In: Harrison MR, Golbus MS, Filly RA, eds. *The Unborn Mother.* Philadelphia: Saunders, 1990: 75–81.
31 Nicolini U, Rodeck CH. Fetal blood and tissue sampling. In: Brock DJH, Rodeck CH, Ferguson-Smith MA, eds. *Prenatal Diagnosis and Screening.* Edinburgh: Churchill Livingstone, 1992: 46–9.
32 Kuller JA, Golbus MS. Fetal therapy. In: Brock DJH, Rodeck CH, Ferguson-Smith MA, eds. *Prenatal Diagnosis and Screening.* Edinburgh: Churchill Livingstone, 1992: 703–17.
33 Giannakoulopoulos X, Sepulveda W, Kourtis P, Glover V, Fisk NM. Fetal plasma cortisol and beta-endorphin response to intrauterine needling. *Lancet* 1994; **344**: 77–81.
34 Saari-Kemppainen A, Karjalainen O, Ylostalo P, Heinonen OP. Ultrasound screening

and perinatal mortality: controlled trial of systemic one-stage screening. *Lancet* 1990; **336**: 387–91.
35 Chitty LS, Hunt GH, Moore J, Lobb MO. Effectiveness of routine ultrasonography in detecting fetal structural abnormalities in a low-risk population. *Br Med J* 1991; **303**: 1165–9.
36 Baird PA, Sadovnik AD. Life expectancy in Down syndrome adults. *Lancet* 1988; **ii**: 1354–6.
37 Wald NJ, Cuckle HS, Densem JW *et al.* Maternal screening for Down syndrome in early pregnancy. *Br Med J* 1988; **297**: 883–7.
38 Wald NJ, Cuckle HS, Densem JW, Kennard A, Smith D. Maternal serum screening for Down syndrome: the effect of routine ultrasound scan determination of gestational age and adjustment for maternal weight. *Br J Obstet Gynaecol* 1992; **99**: 144–9.
39 Wald NJ, Cuckle HS. Biochemical detection of neural tube defects and Down syndrome. In: Turnbull A, Chamberlain G, eds. *Obstetrics*. Edinburgh: Churchill Livingstone, 1989: 269–89.
40 Brock DJH. Mechanisms by which amniotic fluid alpha-fetoprotein may be increased in fetal abnormalities. *Lancet* 1976; **ii**: 345–6.
41 Monk M. Preimplantation diagnosis: a comprehensive review. In: Brock DJH, Rodeck CH, Ferguson-Smith MA, eds. *Prenatal Diagnosis and Screening*. Edinburgh: Churchill Livingstone, 1992: 627–38.
42 Adinolfi MC. Fetal nucleated cells in maternal circulation. In: Brock DJH, Rodeck CH, Ferguson-Smith MA, eds. *Prenatal Diagnosis and Screening*. Edinburgh: Churchill Livingstone, 1992: 651–60.
43 Chervenak FA, Isaacson G, Streltzoff J. Craniosubarachnoid defects. In: Brock DJH, Rodeck CH, Ferguson-Smith MA, eds. *Prenatal Diagnosis and Screening*. Edinburgh: Churchill Livingstone, 1992: 189–226.
44 Romero R, Cullen M, Jeanty P *et al.* The diagnosis of congenital renal anomalies with ultrasound, 2: infantile polycystic kidney disease. *Am J Obstet Gynecol* 1984; **150**: 259.
45 Allan LD, Crawford DC, Anderson RH, Tynan MJ. Echocardiographic and anatomical correlations in fetal congenital heart disease. *Br Heart J* 1984; **54**: 542–8.
46 Farrall M, Law HY, Rodeck CH *et al.* First-trimester prenatal diagnosis of cystic fibrosis with linked DNA probes. *Lancet* 1986; **i**: 1402–4.

21: The High-Risk Fetus: Labour and Delivery

21.1 The high-risk fetus

21.1.1 Fetal heart rate changes

Fetal heart rate monitoring has been used to help to identify periods of fetal compromise that may be associated with fetal damage, especially neurological sequelae. Unfortunately, fetal heart rate patterns are fairly predictive of a good outcome, but not of a poor outcome. Because of this, other more predictive tests of poor outcome should be used in conjunction with abnormal heart rate patterns. It is not surprising that such an association has not been found. The majority of fetal neurological damage occurs antepartum and not intrapartum. Fetal heart rate monitoring may identify times of increased fetal risk, and other methods of evaluation should be used in conjunction with it.

Methods of measurement

Assessments can be made externally using a phonocardiogram or Doppler ultrasound, or internally using electrocardiography (ECG) or an oximeter. The ECG accurately measures the R–R interval for heart rate changes, and S–T segment variability can be studied [1]. In the antepartum period only external methods can be used. Internal measurements can only be made when the membranes are ruptured and the cervix is dilated. Infection can be introduced by the insertion of instruments, and structures can be perforated [2]. External measurements are disturbed by maternal movements and obesity, and frequent adjustments may have to be made, all of which limit maternal mobility. Telemetric methods have been used to try to reduce some of these difficulties.

Beat-to-beat variability

The fetal heart rate fluctuates at each beat by 3–8 beats/min. This variability is a characteristic of fetal well-being and is a measure of normal central sympathetic nervous system control in a fetus. A reactive fetus accelerates the fetal heart rate during movement or external stimuli [3]. The normal reactive pattern shows a baseline variability greater than 6 beats/min (Fig. 21.1a see below). If the fetus is not reactive it may just be resting, or it may be unwell. Another check should be performed after waking the baby up by asking the mother to move around and then repeating the test after about an hour. If it is resting at one time, it should be reactive at the other. This method is not, however, a sensitive

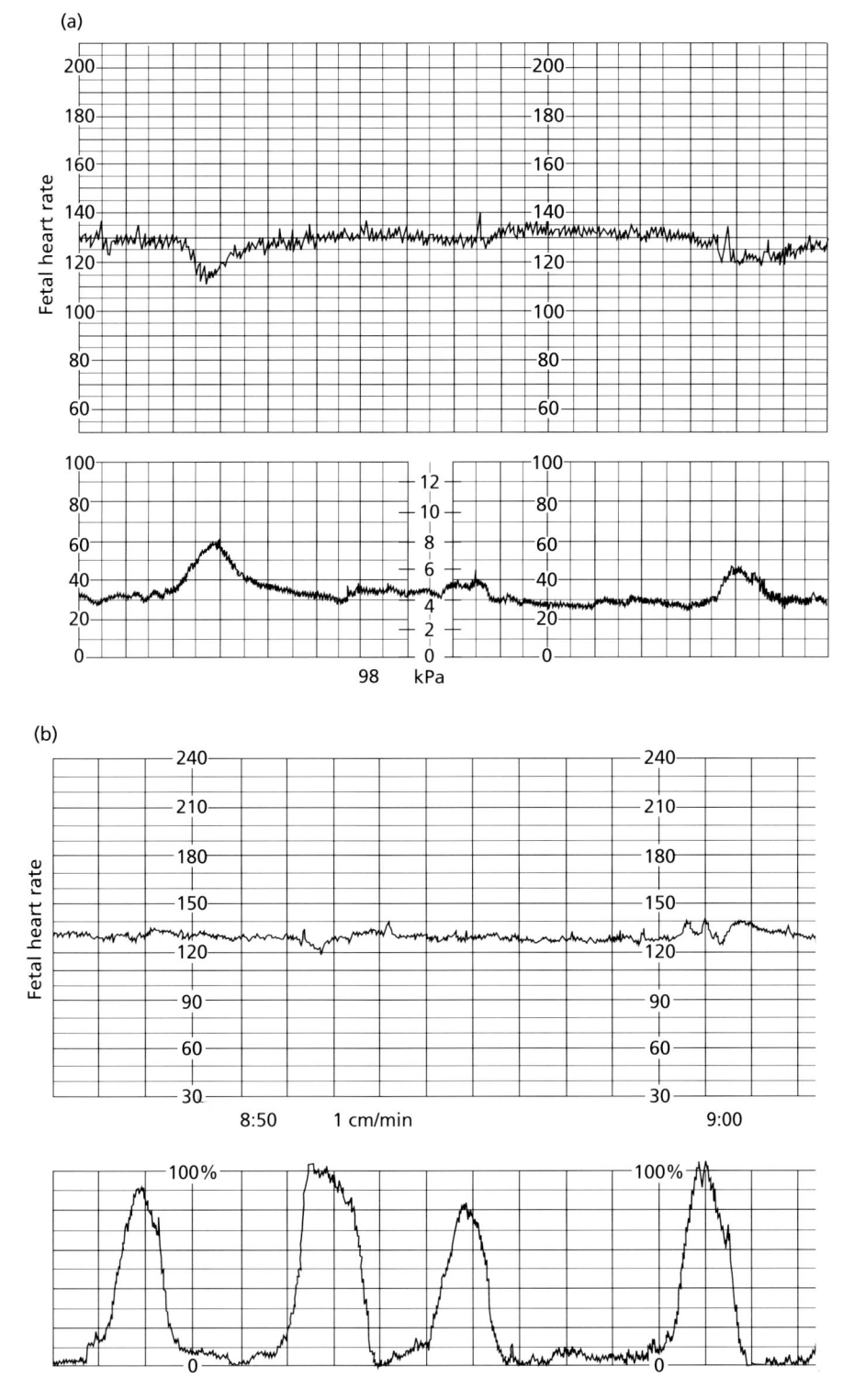

Fig. 21.1 Fetal heart beat-to-beat variability and uterine contractions record: (a) normal; (b) reduced.

indicator of impending fetal death [4]. When a fetus becomes compromised, such as occurs when the oxygen supply to the brain decreases [5], a damping of this normal response occurs until the variability disappears (Fig. 21.1b) [6]. Sleep, drugs (especially central nervous system depressants) and congenital abnormalities of the heart and central nervous system can also have this effect.

Bradydysrhythmia and tachydysrhythmia

The fetal heart rate range between contractions is 120–160 beats/min (Fig. 21.2). Fetal tachycardia and bradycardia are defined as rates higher or lower than this range. Continuous tachydysrhythmias or bradydysrhythmias are caused by:
- *Fetal tachycardia:*
  - Infection (e.g. chorioamnionitis).
  - Anaemia.
  - Maternal fever.
  - Maternally administered drugs:
    sympathomimetics.
    anticholinergics.
  - Fetal hypoxia.
- *Fetal bradycardia:*
  - Fetal hypoxia: central; umbilical cord compression.
  - Heart block, e.g. in maternal systemic lupus erythematosus.
  - Maternally administered drugs: beta blockers.
  - Maternal hypotension.

Periodic changes

These refer to the relation between heart rate decelerations and uterine contractions. When the changes mirror the contraction, the decrease in heart rate is thought to be mediated by vagal reflexes. This is called 'early deceleration'. When the changes start some time after the beginning of a contraction and do not return to normal baseline until some time after the end of the contraction (Fig. 21.2b), they are termed 'late decelerations', and are always pathological. They may be caused by uteroplacental insufficiency as a result of maternal conditions such as hypertension, diabetes or hypotension. Variable changes can occur that are neither early nor late, and are caused by cord compression.

It is important to recognize changes that are pathological and treat them quickly. Initially, oxygen should be administered to the mother, and her position should be changed to remove aorto-caval occlusion. Her blood pressure must be measured to exclude hypotension (especially if she has an epidural block), and any oxytocin being given should be stopped. There is then usually time to examine the heart rate trace for beat-to-beat variability and to take a fetal scalp sample for pH measurement if necessary.

21.1.2 Biophysical profile

The biophysical profile assesses several variables [7].
- Fetal breathing.
- Fetal movements.
- Fetal tone.
- Fetal heart rate.
- Amniotic fluid volume.

Each variable has a maximum score of 2, with a total of 10. A score of less than 4 is associated with a 50–100 times increase in perinatal mortality. Although the five components each receive equal weighting, a decrease in amniotic fluid is a critical risk factor. It represents a chronic fetal condition, whereas the other components can be changed acutely. The biophysical profile attempts to evaluate the different signs of fetal distress. It is indicated as a method of monitoring pregnant women who have hypertension, diabetes and intrauterine growth retardation.

The relation between the fetal biophysical profile and fetal acidosis, as measured by direct analysis of umbilical blood drawn under ultrasonographic guidance, was studied in severely ill fetuses [8]. A poor biophysical profile, i.e. score 0, was always associated with a pH < 7.2, whereas a high score of 10 was always associated with a pH > 7.2. Scores of 1 to 9 were of unreliable significance.

21.1.3 Monitoring the fetus in labour

Reports on a number of methods of detecting fetal distress indicate that none of the methods provide good markers. Methods need to be developed to distinguish chronic hypoxia from an acute situation. Delivery by Caesarean section because of abnormal fetal monitoring results has not been followed by a decrease in perinatal mortality. For example, electronic monitoring of the fetal heart rate in labour does not identify the majority of infants at risk of cerebral palsy.

Fetal heart rate monitoring in labour

The monitoring of the fetal heart rate is an essential part of intrapartum care, and an instrument capable of monitoring twins should be available on each unit. Basic care requires quarter-hourly monitoring and recording throughout labour. Simple auscultation with a Pinard stethoscope can miss periodic decelerations [9]. A 30-minute cardiotocography study should be recorded for all women on admission in labour and reviewed by an obstetrician. If this is normal and the woman is not in a high-risk category, she can be intermittently monitored for 20 minutes every three hours; otherwise continuous monitoring should be used. Continuous monitoring is also required when a woman is receiving epidural analgesia.

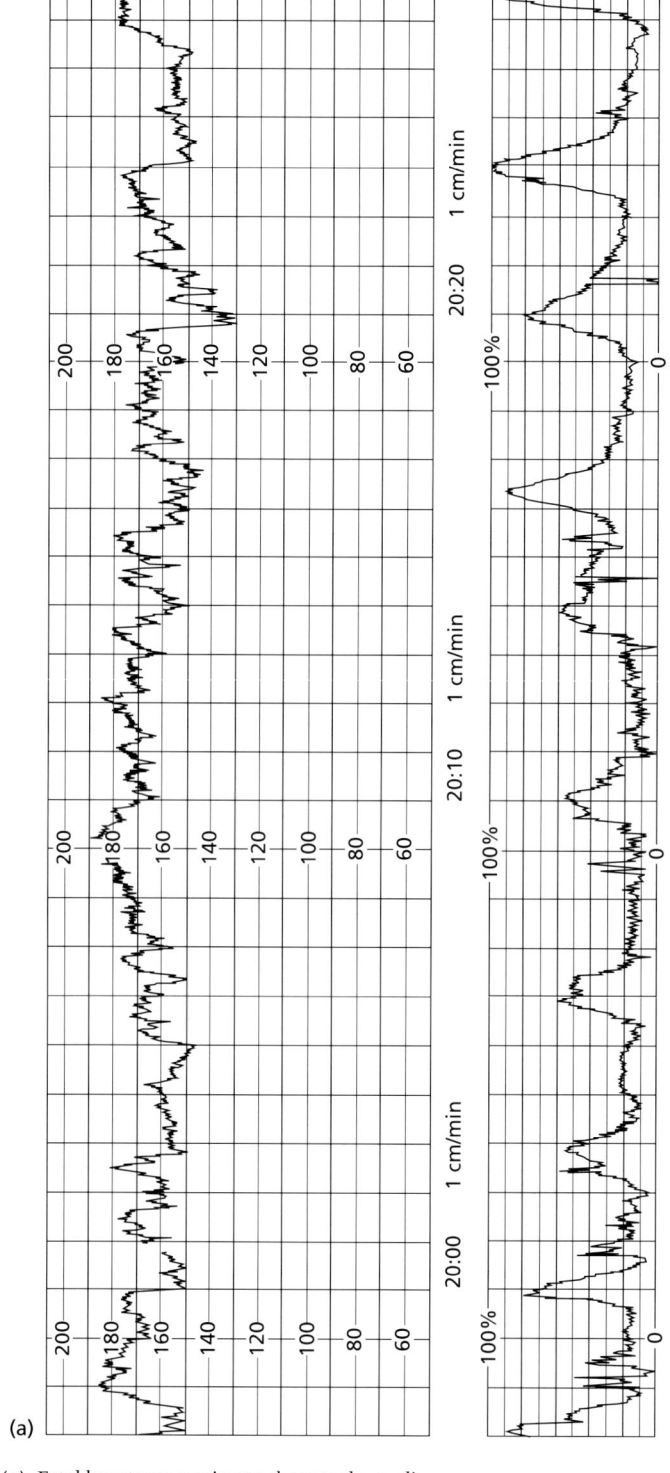

Fig. 21.2(a) Fetal heart rate tracing to show tachycardia.

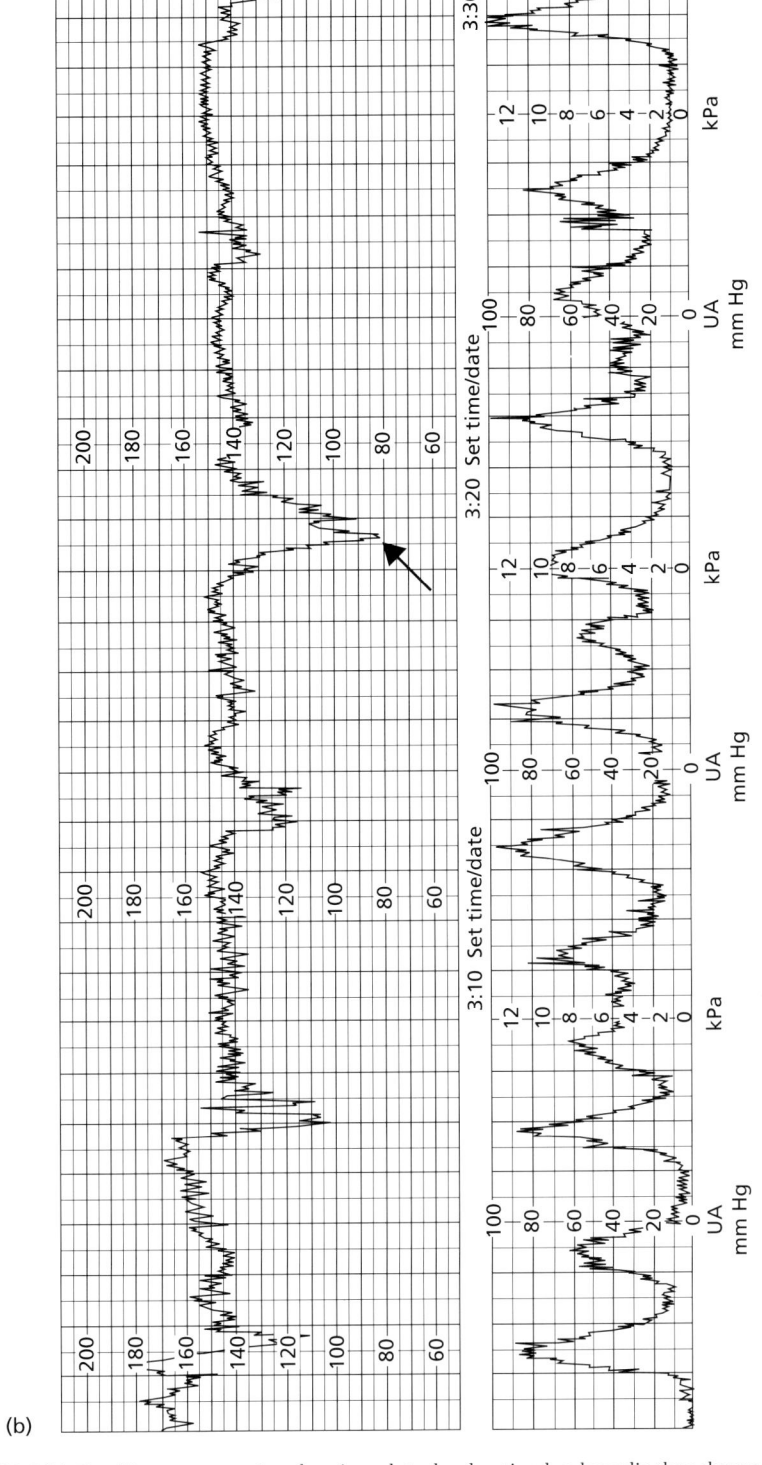

Fig. 21.2(b) Fetal heart rate tracing showing a late deceleration bradycardia thus shown by the arrow.

The obstetric anaesthetist should view the tracing prior to insertion of an epidural catheter, and if possible maintain monitoring during the procedure. This may be difficult with external electronic monitoring. If the fetus is compromised, the use of internal monitoring should be discussed with the obstetrician, since otherwise a fetal heart trace may not be available for 20–30 minutes. The obstetric anaesthetist should also routinely request fetal heart rate measurements prior to operative delivery, before and after induction of anaesthesia for Caesarean section.

Blood gas and pH analysis

Fetal pH sampling. The predictive value of an abnormal fetal heart rate trace in diagnosing fetal distress is only about 30–50%. This can be improved by sampling the pH of the capillary blood of the presenting part, usually the scalp. A reduction in gas exchange across the placenta from the mother to the fetus will reduce the available oxygen to the fetus and prevent the elimination of carbon dioxide. A combined respiratory and metabolic acidosis develops, which produces a small progressive decline in pH during labour, especially in the second stage. If the fetal circulation is adequate, fetal scalp blood will exhibit this generalized acidosis. Local changes in scalp pH can arise if there is prolonged pressure on the area of the fetal scalp being assessed. Fetal pH sampling can only be performed if the membranes are ruptured and the cervix is dilated more than 3–4 cm.

Normal pH values exceed 7.25. Values of 7.20 or below require immediate delivery of the fetus. If blood gases indicate a metabolic component, a pH between 7.20 and 7.25 requires rechecking within a few minutes to determine a trend. Fetal scalp capillary blood pH can be highly correlated with cord blood pH when the fetus is delivered immediately [10] but other factors may affect the result. The acidosis may be temporary—for example, respiratory acidosis can occur from cord compression. Similarly, scalp sampling should not be performed during transient decelerations. Misleading results can also be obtained from sample contamination with amniotic fluid, or during maternal acidosis.

Cord blood sampling. Reduced oxygen delivery to the fetus, which occurs in placental insufficiency, for example, initiates an adrenergic response in the fetus that switches blood flow to high-priority areas and away from the cerebral cortex, leading to an encephalopathic state. In chronic hypoxia, this results in reduced muscle bulk and renal blood flow, leading to a small-for-dates baby with oligohydramnios. When tissues lack oxygen, energy is provided to maintain viability of cells by anaerobic metabolism. Lactic acid accumulates, and metabolic acidosis is produced.

The umbilical vein transfers blood from the placenta to the baby. Acute hypoxia will be diagnosed from a cord blood sample. If chronic hypoxia is present, the problem exists at fetal tissue level. The acidosis cannot be corrected by placental exchange. In this condition, the umbilical vein/artery base deficit ratio is reduced. Measurement of blood in the umbilical vein, and when possible in the umbilical artery, should be made for each delivery when the fetus is at risk.

Time of cord clamping. Cord blood sampling may not be possible if cord clamping is performed late. A 30-second delay in cord clamping may help to reduce mortality in preterm infants, although this delay may cause a temperature loss and hypothermia in the baby. More evidence is needed as to the best time to clamp the cord. Early cord clamping may present hazards of hypovolaemia, but would prevent excessive placental transfusion. Obviously, if cord clamping is performed late, then cord blood samples will provide an erroneous estimation of the baby's acid–base status at birth.

The method of cord blood sampling is as follows:
1 a blood gas machine must be available, calibrated and subject to quality control;
2 isolate 10 cm of the cord before the baby takes the first breath;
3 if the cord is to be kept at room temperature, the cord blood should be sampled within 30 minutes of delivery. If it is in ice, this can be extended up to four hours;
4 care should be taken not to confuse the umbilical arteries and vein during sampling. There are two small-diameter umbilical arteries and one large umbilical vein;
5 it is necessary to heparinize the sample, but too much heparin can affect the acid–base results.

Oxygen saturation monitoring of the fetus (Sao_2). Oxygen tension in the fetal circulation is low, but left shift of the fetal haemoglobin dissociation curve results in high oxygen saturation at these tensions. The spectral absorptions of fetal and adult haemoglobin, reduced or oxygenated, are similar, but the oxygen binding curves are quite different. Calibrations have to be performed on the whole range of saturation, because fetal values can be as low as 30% [11]. Both reflectance and transmission photometry have been tried [12,13]. At present, a device for reflectance measurements is available and is being developed in clinical practice. A mean oxygen saturation value is 82% (SD ± 6%) for scalp probes. Although artefacts and failure are common with this method—for example, high intrauterine pressures can disturb local perfusion—it is becoming a useful non-invasive method to provide evidence of trends.

Near-infrared spectroscopy can supplement current methods of detecting fetal hypoxia by measuring the change in the concentration of oxyhaemoglobin and deoxyhaemoglobin. Desaturation has been observed in association with early fetal heart rate decelerations [14]. Limited access to the fetus is a major problem for quantification of data. At present, this is a research tool for measuring changes following specific events, such as epidural analgesia [15].

Meconium-stained amniotic fluid. Meconium from the bowel of the fetus is passed into the amniotic fluid in about 10% of labours. Changes in meconium concentration seem to correlate with known stressful stimuli. A flexible optical uterine probe has been developed to study this [16].

21.2 Fetal and neonatal resuscitation

21.2.1 Intrauterine resuscitation

When late decelerations or loss of beat-to-beat variations occur and persist prior to blood sampling and delivery, the following measures should be taken.
- Oxygen administration 15 L/min via a non-breathing system with a reservoir bag.
- Left lateral position, but if fetal heart deceleration persists move to another position, e.g. right lateral.
- Stop oxytocin (Syntocinon).
- Intravenous crystalloid if fluid intake is not restricted (up to 1000 mL).
- If hypotensive, give ephedrine.

21.2.2 Neonatal resuscitation

The priority for all staff working in a delivery suite is to be prepared and ensure that resuscitation facilities are available. These include drugs and equipment, with one resuscitation trolley per baby (Table 21.1), a warm environment (above 24°C) and trained staff.

Normal procedure at delivery

Pharyngeal suction is rarely necessary unless the amniotic fluid is stained with meconium or blood. Once the baby is delivered, the clock is started and the baby is dried with a warm towel to reduce evaporative heat loss, while at the same time an examination for congenital abnormalities is carried out. A neutral neck position must be maintained. Most babies will start breathing, since the median time of onset of spontaneous respiration is 10 seconds. If the baby is not breathing and does not respond to gentle tactile stimulation, e.g. by flicking the baby's feet, resuscitation starts. Basic resuscitation guidelines have been published [17], but a satisfactory algorithm has yet to be agreed.

Resuscitation

1 If secretions are contributing to impaired respiration, aspirate the nose and mouth (5 cm maximum distance) and then the pharynx directly using a laryngoscope. This is important where meconium aspiration is suspected (see below).

Table 21.1 Resuscitation equipment and drugs.

Equipment
Padded shelf/resuscitation trolley
Overhead heater
Overhead light
Oxygen supply
Clock
Stethoscope
Airway pressure manometer and pressure relief valve
Face mask
Oropharyngeal airway 00 + 0
Resuscitation system (face mask/T piece/bag and mask)
Suction catheters (sizes 5, 8, 10 Fr)
Mechanical and/or manual suction with double trap
Two laryngoscopes with spare blades
Endotracheal tubes 2, 2.5, 3, 3.5 and 4 mm, introducer (approx. 2.5 mm < 1000 g, 3.5 mm > 4000 g)
Umbilical vein catheterization set
Umbilical artery catheterization set
Intraosseous needle
2, 10 and 20 mL syringes with needles
ECG and transcutaneous oxygen saturation monitor (capnometer as optional extra)

Drugs
1 : 10 000 epinephrine (1 mL = 100 μg)
Naloxone hydrochloride (200 μg/mL)
Alkalizing agent e.g. sodium bicarbonate
Sodium chloride 0.9%
Dextrose (10–20%)
Immediate access to plasma expanders
Access to group O rhesus-negative blood

ECG, electrocardiography.

2 Check for respiratory efforts. If they are present but producing no tidal exchange, the airway is obstructed. This may be overcome by extending the baby's head or inserting an airway if the baby has congenital airway abnormalities. If respiratory efforts are feeble or absent, count the heart rate for 10–15 seconds with a stethoscope. When the heart rate is above 80 beats/min, repeat the skin stimulation, and if this fails, proceed to face mask resuscitation.

3 If the heart rate is below 80 beats/min, intubate, ventilate and start gentle chest compression (three compressions/one ventilation) at a rate of 100–120 compressions per minute. The compression is started by pressing over the junction of the lower and middle third of the sternum with the tips of two fingers, or by placing a hand around the chest and compressing it between the thumb and fingers.

4 If there is no dramatic improvement within 10–15 seconds, the umbilical vein should be catheterized with a 5-Fr catheter and epinephrine 10 μg/kg should be administered. Alternatively, epinephrine 10 g/kg can be given down the endotracheal tube. If the baby is pink with a satisfactory circulation but no

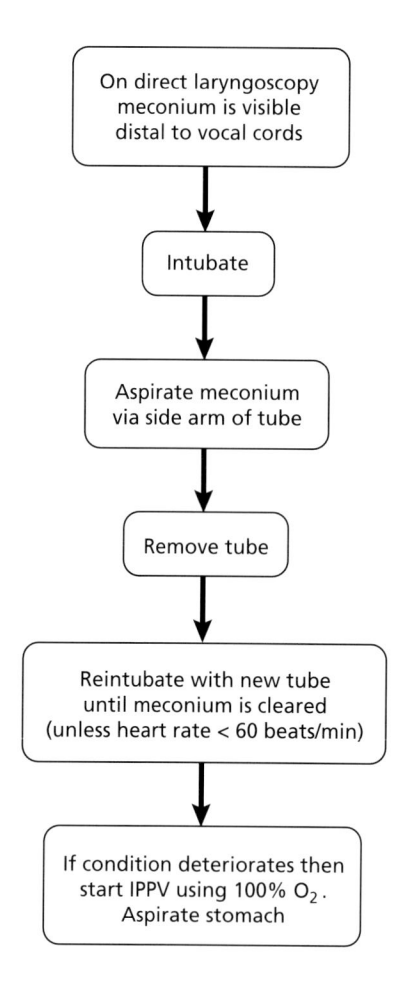

```
On direct laryngoscopy
meconium is visible
distal to vocal cords
         ↓
      Intubate
         ↓
  Aspirate meconium
  via side arm of tube
         ↓
     Remove tube
         ↓
  Reintubate with new tube
  until meconium is cleared
  (unless heart rate < 60 beats/min)
         ↓
  If condition deteriorates then
  start IPPV using 100% O₂.
  Aspirate stomach
```

Fig. 21.3 Management of meconium aspiration (IPPV, intermittent positive-pressure ventilation).

respiratory efforts and there is a history of maternal opioid administration, naloxone 100 µg/kg can be given intravenously or through the endotracheal tube.

In addition

Intubation and ventilation. The breathing system must incorporate a 30 cmH$_2$O blow-off valve in the inspiratory limb. Ventilation is at a rate of about 30 breaths/min with a flow of 4–6 L/min. Usually, an oxygen–air mixture is used (40% oxygen). During the first few inflations after intubation, look for chest wall movement and confirm by auscultation that oxygen is entering both lungs. If there is no air entry, check that the endotracheal tube is not in the oesophagus, and if there is no improvement consider other causes, such as a pneumothorax or diaphragmatic hernia.

Meconium aspiration (Fig. 21.3). If direct laryngoscopy for meconium staining reveals meconium in the pharynx and trachea, the neonate should be

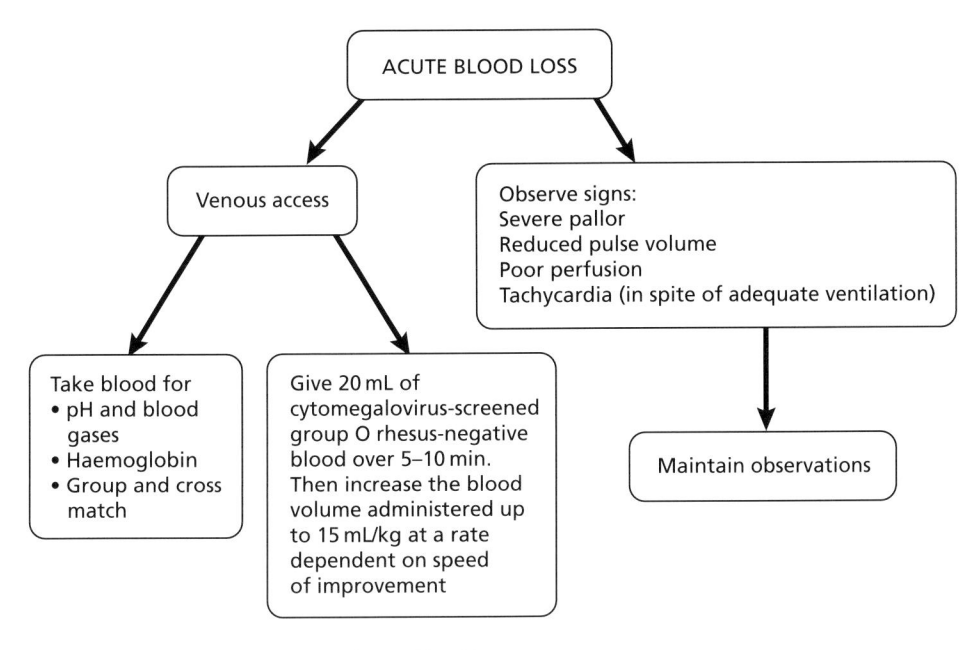

```
                    ┌─────────────────────┐
                    │  ACUTE BLOOD LOSS   │
                    └──────────┬──────────┘
              ┌────────────────┴──────────────────┐
              ▼                                   ▼
     ┌────────────────┐              ┌──────────────────────────┐
     │ Venous access  │              │ Observe signs:            │
     └───────┬────────┘              │ Severe pallor             │
             │                       │ Reduced pulse volume      │
     ┌───────┴────────┐              │ Poor perfusion            │
     ▼                ▼              │ Tachycardia (in spite of  │
┌──────────┐  ┌──────────────────┐   │ adequate ventilation)     │
│Take blood│  │Give 20 mL of     │   └───────────┬──────────────┘
│for       │  │cytomegalovirus-  │               │
│• pH and  │  │screened group O  │               ▼
│  blood   │  │rhesus-negative   │   ┌──────────────────────┐
│  gases   │  │blood over 5–10   │   │ Maintain observations│
│• Haemo-  │  │min. Then increase│   └──────────────────────┘
│  globin  │  │the blood volume  │
│• Group   │  │administered up   │
│  and     │  │to 15 mL/kg at a  │
│  cross   │  │rate dependent on │
│  match   │  │speed of          │
│          │  │improvement       │
└──────────┘  └──────────────────┘
```

Fig. 21.4 Management of acute blood loss.

intubated immediately and the side port of the tracheal tube should be attached to the suction at 100 cmH$_2$O (70 mmHg). Suck up the free fluid while the endotracheal tube is removed, and then re-intubate. This procedure can be repeated if the fetal heart rate is above 60 beats/min.

Choice of drugs and fluid. Once the heart rate is less than 80 beats/min and intubation with intermittent positive-pressure ventilation (IPPV) is started.
1 Epinephrine.
   • Intravenous (i.v.) or intraosseous (i.o.), first dose 10 μg/kg (0.1 mL/kg of 1 : 10 000); second dose 100 μg/kg (1 mL/kg of 1 : 10 000).
   • Endotracheal tube (if i.v. or i.o. access is not established in 90 seconds): 100 μg/kg (1 mL/kg of 1 : 10 000).
2 Sodium bicarbonate. This requires a central venous catheter, e.g. an umbilical vein catheter, and is not in routine use for resuscitation. Consider the administration of sodium bicarbonate before a second dose of epinephrine (1 mmol bicarbonate/kg, i.e. 2 mL/kg of 4.2% sodium bicarbonate) with measurement of base deficit from the umbilical artery in a cord blood sample.
3 Glucose: use an i.v. bolus of 500 mg/kg (2.5 mL/kg of 20% glucose) through an umbilical venous catheter to treat hypoglycaemia.
4 Fluid therapy: in hypotension or shock, give 20 mL/kg intravenously or intraosseously of 50% human albumin preferably, or crystalloid or artificial colloid. Repeat as necessary. If blood loss is suspected, e.g. placental abruption, use the management outlined in Fig. 21.4.

398   CHAPTER 21

5 Naloxone: intravenous naloxone 100 µg/kg, an opioid antagonist, should be used if appropriate. It can also be given down the endotracheal tube. An additional 200 µg can be given intramuscularly to prevent relapse. Naloxone must not be given to infants of mothers addicted to opioids, as it can evoke severe withdrawal symptoms.

21.3 The fetus at delivery: scoring systems

21.3.1 Apgar score (Table 21.2)

In 1953, Virginia Apgar developed a scoring system for newborn babies. It required close observation—at defined times of one, five and 10 minutes—of five clinical signs: heart rate, respiratory effort, reflex irritability, muscle tone, and colour. The maturity of the infant affects reflex responses, muscle tone and respiratory effort. Subjective errors arise during resuscitation when there is no independent observer to score, and faulty recall occurs.

An improved Apgar score that excluded the colour score and worked to a maximum of 8 was introduced by Crawford *et al.* [18]. Exclusion of colour from the score removes the least useful of the assessments. Today, the usefulness of the Apgar score lies in its ready availability and familiarity. It can measure the changing condition of the neonate, particularly in the one-minute and five-minute scores. The Apgar score correlates poorly with the degree of neonatal acidosis, unless the latter is severe [19]. An infant can cope with an asphyxial insult by increasing catecholamine levels, which modify the Apgar score. The Apgar score does not detect those infants who require active resuscitation. It was not designed to do this, and the object of the score was instead to predict long-term morbidity and mortality. An accurate predictor of outcome could be useful, but with improved neonatal interventions, the prognostic value of an initial assessment at delivery is questionable. Neither the decision to resuscitate nor the prediction of survival is based on the Apgar score.

Table 21.2 Assessment of the fetus by Apgar score.

	Score 0	Score 1	Score 2
Heart rate beats/min	0	< 100	> 100
Respiratory effort	0	Slow/irregular	Good, crying
Muscle tone	Flaccid	Some flexion	Active
Reflex response to stimulation	0	Grimace	Cough, sneeze
(Colour)	(Pale blue/white)	(Body pink/ extremities blue)	(All pink)

21.3.2 Neurobehavioural scores

Measurement of the effects of drugs given to the mother or the neonate after birth has led to the development of clinical scores that measure aspects of neurological function and interactive behaviour and the response to stress. In the test described by Brazelton [20] the initial assessment took 45 minutes.

A shorter form of the test was described by Scanlon *et al.* [21], but it lacked the quality of the behavioural observations. The score now in use is the Neurologic and Adaptive Capacity Score (NACS). This was developed by Amiel-Tison *et al.* [22], and was designed to distinguish between drug-induced depression and perinatal asphyxia or birth trauma, in full-term neonates. In simple terms, global effects are more likely to be drug-related than focal effects. Twenty items are scored: including four for passive tone, five for active tone, three for primitive reflexes and five for behavioural items from the Brazelton test. A normal score ranges from 35 to the maximum of 40. The score takes five minutes to measure.

NACS tests have demonstrated an absence of neonatal effects of bupivacaine [23], and even when up to 100 µg fentanyl is administered with bupivacaine into the epidural space, no effect on neurobehaviour scores has been detected [24]. Sufentanil in doses of less than 50 µg in association with epidural anaesthesia for Caesarean section does not depress the fetus, but in doses above this, low NACS scores at four and 24 hours have been reported [25]. The administration of epidural morphine in a 2-mg dose causes no depression of the NACS score [26].

References

1 Westgate J, Harris M, Curnow JS, Greene KR. Randomised trial of cardiotocography alone or with S–T waveform analysis for intrapartum monitoring. *Lancet* 1992; **340**: 194–8.
2 Ledger WJ. Complications associated with invasive monitoring. *Semin Perinatol* 1978; **2**: 187–94.
3 Lee CY, DiLoreto FC, O'Lane JM. A study of heart rate acceleration patterns. *Obstet Gynecol* 1975; **45**: 142–6.
4 Thacker SB, Berkelman RL. Assessing the diagnostic accuracy and efficacy of selected antepartum fetal surveillance techniques. *Obstet Gynecol Surv* 1986; **41**: 121–41.
5 Paul RH, Suidan AK, Yeh S, Schifrin BS, Hon EH. Clinical fetal monitoring, 7: the evaluation and significance of intrapartum baseline FHR variability. *Am J Obstet Gynecol* 1975; **123**: 206–10.
6 Martin CB Jr. Physiology and clinical use of fetal heart rate variability. *Clin Perinatol* 1982; **9**: 339–52.
7 Manning FA, Morrison I, Lange IR, Harman C. Antepartum determination of fetal health: composite biophysical profile screening. *Clin Perinatol* 1982; **9**: 285–96.
8 Manning FA, Snijders R, Harman CR *et al.* Fetal biophysical profile score, 6: correlation with antepartum umbilical venous fetal pH. *Am J Obstet Gynecol* 1993; **169**: 755–63.

9 Mohamed K, Nyouni R, Mulambo T, Kasuli J, Jacobus E. Randomised controlled trial of intrapartum fetal heart rate monitoring. *Br Med J* 1994; **308**: 497–500.
10 Miller FC. Prediction of acid–base values from intrapartum fetal heart rate data and their correlation with scalp and funic values. *Clin Perinatol* 1982; **9**: 353–61.
11 Peat S, Booker M, Lanigan C, Ponte J. Continuous intrapartum measurement of fetal oxygen saturation. *Lancet* 1988; **ii**: 213.
12 Gardosi JO, Schram CM, Symonds EM. Adaption of pulse oximetry for fetal monitoring during labour. *Lancet* 1991; **338**: 1265–7.
13 Buschmann J, Rall G, Knitza R. Fetal oxygen saturation measurement by transmission pulse oximetry [letter]. *Lancet* 1992; **339**: 615.
14 Peebles DM, Edwards AD, Wyatt JS *et al.* Changes in human fetal cerebral hemoglobin concentration and oxygenation during labor measured by near infrared spectroscopy. *Am J Obstet Gynecol* 1992; **166**: 1369–73.
15 Doyle PM, O'Brien PMS, Wickramasinghe YABD, Houston R, Rolfe P. Near infrared spectroscopy used to observe changes in fetal cerebral haemodynamics during labour. *J Perinatal Med* 1994; **22**: 265–8.
16 Genevier ES, Danielian PJ, Steer PJ. Continuous meconium monitoring during labour using an intrauterine probe. *Physiol Meas* 1993; **14**: 337–46.
17 Zideman D. Paediatric and neonatal life support. *Br J Anaesth* 1997; **79**: 178–87.
18 Crawford JS, Davies P, Pearson JF. Significance of the individual components of the Apgar score. *Br J Anaesth* 1973; **45**: 148–58.
19 Sykes GS, Johnson P, Ashworth F *et al.* Do Apgar scores indicate asphyxia? *Lancet* 1982; **i**: 494.
20 Brazelton TB. *Neonatal Behavioral Assessment Scale*, 2nd edn. London: Blackwell Scientific/Spastics International Medical Publications, 1984. (Clinics in developmental medicine, 88.)
21 Scanlon JW, Brown WU, Weiss JB, Alper MH. Neurobehavior responses of newborn infants after maternal epidural anesthesia. *Anesthesiology* 1974; **40**: 121–8.
22 Amiel-Tison C, Barrier G, Shnider SM *et al.* A new neurological and adaptive capacity scoring system for evaluating obstetric medications in full term newborns. *Anesthesiology* 1982; **56**: 340–50.
23 Abboud TK, Afrasiabi A, Sarkis F *et al.* Continuous infusion epidural analgesia in parturients receiving bupivacaine, chloroprocaine or lidocaine: maternal, fetal and neonatal effects. *Anesth Analg* 1984; **63**: 421–8.
24 D'Athis F, Macheboeuf M, Thomas H *et al.* Epidural analgesia with bupivacaine–fentanyl mixture in obstetrics: comparison of repeated injection and continuous infusion. *Can J Anaesth* 1988; **35**: 116–22.
25 Copogna G, Celleno D, Tomasetti M. Maternal analgesia and neonatal neurobehavioral effects of epidural sufentanil for Cesarean section [abstract]. *Reg Anesth* 1989; **14**: 24.
26 Abboud TK, Avfrasiabi A, Zhu J *et al.* Epidural morphine or butorphanol augments bupivacaine analgesia during labor. *Reg Anesth* 1989; **14**: 115–20.

Section 7
Obstetric Complications

22: Hypertensive Disorders in Pregnancy

The increase in cardiac output in pregnancy is the result of an increase in pulse rate, stroke volume and cardiac output, while there is a reduction in peripheral vascular resistance, so that diastolic blood pressure normally decreases in the first half of pregnancy. The definition of hypertension is therefore difficult, and many diagnostic criteria have been proposed. The use of Korotkoff sound phase V (KV) is discussed in Chapter 3. This is the preferred method, and it should be measured with the woman seated and with an appropriate cuff size chosen. In women with hypertensive disease, the use of direct arterial pressure measurements or automated blood pressure measuring machines, such as the Dinamap, introduces further confounding factors into the assessment. Sphygmomanometry in comparison with direct measurements has been shown to overestimate both the systolic and Korotkoff V diastolic pressure by about 6 and 15 mmHg, respectively [1]. Dinamap measurement underestimates diastolic blood pressures when compared with a midwife/sphygmomanometer reading by approximately 10 mmHg [2]. Such differences may delay the introduction of therapy unless appropriate corrective factors are applied when considering blood pressure results from automated blood pressure recordings in the hypertensive pregnant woman.

Blood pressure increases during labour in response to pain, and repeated autotransfusion of boluses of blood from the uterine circulation add to these normal changes in cardiovascular physiology. A mean blood pressure of 80–85 mmHg at the start of labour and 90 mmHg at the end of the first stage should be considered as normal [3]. Some forms of hypertensive disease complicating parturition are of considerable pathological significance, but interpretation of absolute blood pressure measurements requires a consideration of gestation and/or stage of labour.

22.1 Hypertension in pregnancy

22.1.1 Chronic hypertension

A diastolic pressure greater than 90 mmHg before 20 weeks' gestation suggests chronic hypertension. It is only with resolution of hypertension after delivery that pregnancy-induced hypertension can be differentiated from chronic hypertension. The diagnosis may be based on a history of hypertension before delivery, and can be associated with renal or cardiovascular disease. Therapy to control hypertension, which is started prior to conception, should be continued. Drugs such as angiotensin-converting enzyme inhibitors and atenolol, which may have adverse effects on the fetus, should be replaced by methyldopa or labetalol [4].

22.1.2 Pregnancy-induced hypertension

Pregnancy-induced hypertension, or gestational hypertension, occurs after 20 weeks' gestation. It affects up to a quarter of primiparous women and 10% of multiparous women. The degree of hypertension is usually mild (e.g. two readings of > 90 mmHg diastolic or > 140 mmHg systolic at least six hours apart) [5], with no associated symptoms.

22.1.3 Anaesthetic management of women with hypertension but not pre-eclampsia

When antihypertensive medication is given regularly to a mother, it should be maintained, but the cardiovascular responses to anaesthesia, hypotension and haemorrhage may be obtunded. However, the risks of a hypertensive reaction to labour or intubation and surgery, with secondary cerebrovascular haemorrhage or other vascular disorders, outweigh the risks inherent in maintenance of normotension. Pain relief in labour with epidural analgesia should be advocated, mainly to reduce catecholamine release, as there is little additional risk to the mother or fetus.

22.2 Pre-eclampsia

Pre-eclampsia has been described as a syndrome of hypertension, proteinuria and oedema that occurs during pregnancy. The term was adopted because the condition could herald eclamptic seizures. However, eclampsia is only one of a number of dangerous crises that can occur rapidly and unpredictably—the syndrome of acute *h*aemolysis, *e*levated *l*iver enzymes and *l*ow *p*latelet count (HELLP) being another. These crises of convulsion and pulmonary, liver and renal dysfunction can occur without hypertension. As a result, women without an increase in blood pressure may be mismanaged. For example, some of the conditions listed in Table 22.1 can present as emergencies with severe abdominal pain requiring anaesthesia, or with rapid clinical deterioration requiring resuscitation and intensive care [6]. Early diagnosis is essential, and delivery is the ultimate cure. The ultimate goals are first the safety of the mother, and secondly the delivery of a live infant who will not require intensive and prolonged neonatal care.

The categorization of pre-eclampsia as a hypertensive disorder has led to research attempting to clarify the causes of the hypertension. However, in more general terms, pre-eclampsia is really a disorder of pregnancy, since that is the only common factor in the various conditions covered by the term.

Table 22.1 Conditions mimicked by pre-eclampsia.

Acute pancreatitis
Acute fatty liver of pregnancy
Cholecystitis
Viral hepatitis
Appendicitis
Renal stones
Glomerulonephritis
Haemolytic–uraemic syndrome
Thrombocytopenia
Cerebral vein thrombosis
Cerebral haemorrhage
Encephalitis

22.2.1 Clinical presentation

Pre-eclampsia affects 5% of women in their first pregnancy. Women are at higher risk if they have hypertensive disease or coexisting vascular disease, in association with obstetric factors such as obesity, diabetes and age over 40 years. The criteria for pregnancy-induced hypertension apply, together with proteinuria > 300 mg/24 h. Oedema is not essential for diagnosis. The rate of progression can vary from days to minutes. Routine surveillance includes blood tests for hyperuricaemia, thrombocytopenia and changes in liver function tests, and clinical monitoring of central nervous system symptoms and signs such as headache and clonus. These are summarized in Table 22.2.

22.2.2 Pathophysiology

There is evidence from epidemiological and molecular biology sources that pre-eclampsia has a genetic basis. The targeting of first pregnancies has suggested immune mechanisms. The widespread presence of haemorrhage and necrosis presents a different pathology from that of mechanical damage and vasoconstriction effects in severe hypertension in non-pregnant patients. Multiorgan endothelial damage is the distinguishing feature.

The focus of origin of these changes, which only occur in pregnancy, is the placenta [7]. The vascular changes on trophoblastic invasion are similar to those seen with allograft rejection. Normal implantation is not complete until about 20 weeks' gestation. If this process is impeded, fetal hypoxia can develop, and the placenta may produce substances that alter endothelial cell integrity (Table 22.3). For example, plasma from pre-eclamptic women can reduce prostacyclin and nitric oxide production [8]. This in turn affects platelet aggregation and blood vessel size. Abnormal lipid metabolism occurs early in pregnancy in women who develop pre-eclampsia [9]. The majority of endothelial changes can be reproduced by lipid peroxidation. The failure of antioxidants to protect cells from the destructive effects of peroxides

Table 22.2 Signs and symptoms in pre-eclampsia.

Central nervous system	Cerebral oedema
	Hyperreflexia
	Convulsions
	Cerebral haemorrhage
Respiratory system	Upper airway oedema
	Pulmonary oedema
Cardiovascular system	Increased systemic vascular resistance leading to increased left ventricular work
	Cardiac failure
	Hypertension
	Increased cardiac output
	Increased vascular permeability (oedema)
	Hypoproteinaemia
Renal system	Decreased renal blood flow (oliguria) and glomerular filtration rate
	Endothelial damage
	Proteinuria
	Decreased urea clearance
Haematological system	Thrombocytopenia
	HELLP syndrome
	Increased bleeding time
Hepatic system	Periportal haemorrhage (abdominal pain)
	Increased bilirubin
	Increased liver enzymes (HELLP syndrome)
	Subcapsular haematoma
Placenta	Placental abruption

HELLP, haemolysis, elevated liver enzymes and low platelet count.

Table 22.3 Proposed stages in the pathogenesis of pre-eclampsia.

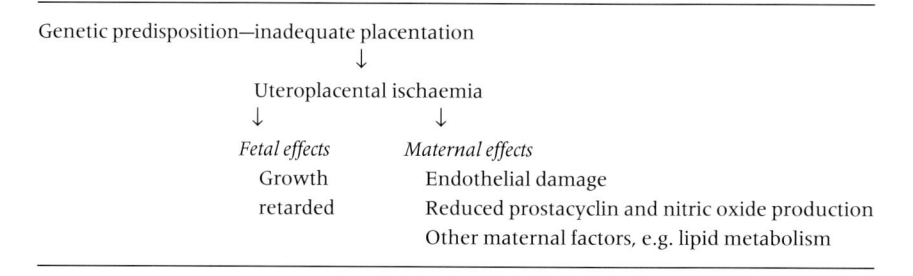

Genetic predisposition—inadequate placentation
↓
Uteroplacental ischaemia
↓   ↓
Fetal effects   *Maternal effects*
Growth   Endothelial damage
retarded   Reduced prostacyclin and nitric oxide production
                     Other maternal factors, e.g. lipid metabolism

may result in decreased prostacyclin synthesis or platelet damage and production of thromboxane. The loss of normal endothelial depressor functions results in increased sensitivity to normal circulatory pressor agents, such as angiotensin and epinephrine. Microthrombi further compromise organ perfusion.

In addition to the abnormalities of fatty acid constituents of the blood, uric acid concentrations are high. This elevation is not simply due to renal dysfunction, but may indicate an increased xanthine dehydrogenase/oxidase activity and imbalance. Uric acid is formed by the breakdown of purines into xanthine, which is metabolized by xanthine oxidase into uric acid, and by direct synthesis from phosphate compounds and glutamine. Uric acid production by xanthine oxidase is coupled with the formation of reactive oxygen species and decreased concentrations of antioxidants. Confirmation of altered oxidative products has been reported in a study showing that serum from women with pre-eclampsia had an antioxidant activity only half as great as that from serum from normal pregnant controls [10]. The oxidative stress is compounded by effects in both maternal and placental tissues. It leads to endothelial dysfunction throughout the maternal vascular endothelium, activating the coagulation cascade with loss of vascular integrity and inducing vasoconstriction, so that the circulating blood volume may be reduced.

22.2.3 Prevention

The rationale for the use of daily low-dose aspirin is to reverse the production of thromboxane, a vasoconstrictor and promotor of platelet aggregation, in favour of prostacyclin, a vasodilator. The Collaborative Low-Dose Aspirin Study in Pregnancy (CLASP) concluded that while prophylactic aspirin was safe for the fetus—even though it crosses the placenta—it did not reduce the incidence of pre-eclampsia [11]. This result should be interpreted as confirming that only part of the pathogenesis relates to the balance between thromboxane and prostacyclin effects.

To date, no treatment instituted after recognition of clinical disease has reduced the prenatal morbidity, since many of the pathophysiological changes antedate clinical disease.

22.2.4 Management

Early diagnosis, close medical supervision and timely delivery are the requisites for management. Severe hypertension, in which the blood pressure is 160/110 mmHg or above, affects about 1% of all nulliparous women. The goal of antihypertensive therapies is to prevent maternal stroke. Antihypertensive medication does not prevent eclampsia nor change the pathology in pre-eclampsia. However, the fetus may remain *in utero* for a sufficient number of days to allow pharmacological induction of lung maturity with corticosteroid.

Mild pre-eclampsia

There is no clear benefit of drug treatment in this condition. However, methyldopa may prevent progression to severe hypertension [12]. Methyldopa is the drug of choice for long-term therapy. It reduces blood pressure by a central effect, and extensive use suggests it is safe for the fetus.

Severe pre-eclampsia/eclampsia

Guidelines for the management of severe pre-eclampsia must be available to all obstetric units. The discussion as to the timing and mode of delivery will be made by the consultant obstetrician, but the plan of management outlined below should be conducted on a team basis.

Monitoring. Monitoring a stable patient will include (from the more frequent to the less frequent observation): four-hourly blood pressure record; fluid balance chart; daily urinalysis; daily or more frequent review of symptoms and/or signs; twice-weekly full blood count, especially platelets; uric acid, urea and electrolytes; creatinine; liver function; 24-hour urinary protein estimation if there is more than a trace of proteinuria; and weekly weighing. If platelet numbers are above 100×10^9, no further clotting studies need be sought, but if their number is less than 100×10^9, a prothrombin time and activated thrombin time should be measured. If these are abnormal, the haematology department should be alerted and blood should be sent for fibrinogen concentration and fibrin degradation product assessments.

All women should have the clinical and laboratory details of this monitoring recorded, preferably on a 'pre-eclampsia chart', and coordinated by a designated obstetrician. The frequency with which investigations are repeated will be deter-mined by the consultant obstetrician and anaesthetist after review of the patient. More severe pre-eclampsia will require quarter-hourly blood pressure recordings and central venous pressure monitoring for accurate fluid balance. The diagnosis of severe pre-eclampsia alerts staff to the possibility of complications which can occur many hours later. Monitoring of blood presure, symptoms, signs and investigations should continue for a minimum of 72 hours post-partum for the severe form of disease. Transfer from this level of care to more normal ward care should be made after discussion between the obstetrician and anaesthetist.

Antihypertensive drugs. Treatment should be given if the blood pressure is more than 160/110 mmHg (mean 125 mmHg) on three consecutive readings. Parenteral hydralazine is administered as 5 mg intravenously, with similar bolus doses every 15 minutes until the blood pressure is less than these values or the heart rate is > 120 beats/min or 15 mg of hydralazine has been given. Alternatively, after the initial bolus, hydralazine can be infused at the rate of 5–20 mg/h, with the infusion rate titrated against the blood pressure response. Hydralazine is a direct arteriolar vasodilator. It is associated with a number of problems: its side effects of headache, tremulousness and vomiting mimic the symptoms of impeding eclampsia; it has a slow and often unpredictable onset; it may accumulate and cause hypotension with continuous infusion; and it reflexly causes maternal tachycardia.

Sublingual nifedipine may offer some advantages. This is a calcium channel blocker that acts rapidly. An immediate dose of 10–20 mg can be given repeatedly every 8 hours. It is not yet licensed for use in this situation. It can also induce maternal tachycardia, and should be used cautiously with magnesium therapy, since potentiation occurs.

Labetalol is an α_1 and β-adrenergic blocker that decreases maternal systemic vascular resistance and arterial blood pressure without increasing heart rate or decreasing uterine flow. However, the dose range is very variable between patients. Intravenous therapy should start at 20 mg, followed at 10-minute intervals by 40, 60 and 80 mg, up to a cumulative dose of 220 mg. A β-adrenergic blocking drug such as oxprenolol may be useful in the rare circumstance of iatrogenic tachycardia.

Diazoxide is no longer used, and the use of esmolol, a cardioselective β-adrenergic blocker, is controversial because it is transferred to the fetus. Nitroglycerine has been used as a single intravenous dose to cause smooth-muscle relaxation of the uterus. It is also predominantly a venodilator, and it should not be used until other antihypertensive drugs have been attempted without avail. Use of vasoactive doses of nitroglycerine would necessitate direct monitoring of arterial blood pressure.

As diuretics reduce intravascular blood volume, they are contraindicated in the treatment of pre-eclampsia in pregnancy, unless the start of administration (in consultation with a renal physician) predated the pregnancy. They are only recommended for use if fluid overload has occurred.

Fluid balance. Accurate control of fluid input and output is required [13]. Assessments must not only include urine volume measurement, but should also take into account losses of other fluids, such as vomitus. Early placement of a central venous pressure (CVP) line is required, since changes in blood coagulation can occur. It is best to access a central line as soon as the coagulation screen is returned as normal. If the coagulation screen is abnormal, peripheral siting of a long central venous catheter may be required, with a clinical check on its positioning by observing the CVP waveform on an oscilloscope screen. Pressure on the internal jugular veins will produce a rise in the measured pressure if the catheter has migrated cranially rather than passing into the superior vena cava/right atrium.

The woman will have both an intravenous infusion and access to oral fluids. Before delivery, since she is at high risk of obstetric intervention, oral fluids must be restricted to the minimum required for oral drug therapy. If pre-eclampsia occurs after delivery, oral fluid allowances should be discussed with her obstetric team. The intravenous fluids available are:

- balanced salt solution administered as a maintenance of 85 mL/h (Hartmann's);
- colloid solutions if the serum albumin is less than 30 g/dL, or if the central venous pressure is less than normal;
- blood if red blood cell replacement is necessary;
- blood products to correct abnormalities.

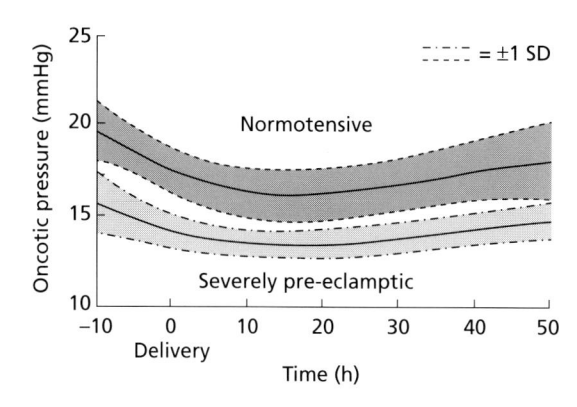

Fig. 22.1 Plasma oncotic pressures at parturition in normotensive and severely pre-eclamptic women. (With permission by The Lancet Ltd, 1985 [14].)

Any fluids used to dilute drugs must be monitored, and it is preferred that volume restriction for drug administration is practised.

If urine output per hour is less than 25 mL, the CVP must be measured. There are three alternative findings and responses.

1 *CVP below normal* (check zero reference point and catheter tip position). A fluid challenge with 200 mL of colloid, should be given rapidly. This may not be enough to correct a fluid deficit unmasked by vasodilation resulting from antihypertensive therapy, so titration of 200 mL boluses should be given until the CVP returns to normal. In the case of hypovolaemia, a transient increase in CVP will be observed during the bolus infusion, but it will not persist. If more than 500 mL is required, consider the occurrence of a concealed haemorrhage.

2 *CVP above normal* (again, make sure that the measurement has the correct zero and that the catheter tip is positioned freely in a central vein). Examine the patient for signs of pulmonary oedema and the oxygen saturation on air. If the saturation is < 92%, give furosemide 10 mg intravenously and wait for a diuresis in 10–15 minutes. If no diuresis has occurred and the CVP remains high, give 40 mg of furosemide intravenously. If there is no response, stay with the woman and request advice and critical care facilities. A direct arterial catheter will at this stage provide direct arterial pressure monitoring and blood gas analysis.

3 *CVP normal* (depends on the zero reference point). Continue maintenance fluids and recheck blood urea, creatinine and electrolytes. Assess hydration, as additional fluids may be required. If the oliguria persists, request advice and consider the use of dopamine.

Fluid loading must be considered hazardous in the management of epidural analgesia in severe pre-eclampsia. Fluid retention and proteinuria have effectively reduced the plasma oncotic pressure (Fig. 22.1) [14], so that any additional fluid load may precipitate pulmonary oedema and congestive cardiac failure. These cardiopulmonary effects can initiate acute respiratory distress syndrome, and obstetric anaesthetists must therefore closely monitor the effects of any fluid given, preferably using direct CVP.

CVP measurement is used more to restrict i.v. fluid administration than to encourage it. Pressures over 5–6 mmHg should alert the anaesthetist to the possibility of over hydration and pulmonary oedema.

Anticonvulsant therapy. Women with severe pre-eclampsia do not require routine anticonvulsant prophylaxis. The use of magnesium sulphate prophylactically in this group of parturients is still being investigated.

22.2.5 Eclampsia

This is an emergency situation. The woman should be treated with an intravenous bolus of Diazemuls 10 mg for the first fit. The resuscitation team called needs to assess the ABC of basic resuscitation: airway, breathing and circulation. The woman should then receive a magnesium sulphate infusion as prophylaxis to prevent recurrent convulsions. In a large-scale trial, magnesium sulphate [15] was superior to both phenytoin and diazepam for the treatment and prevention of recurrent convulsions in women with eclampsia. Magnesium is a normal intracellular ion, and its excretion relies on normal renal function. It can compete with free calcium ions, and this effect is particularly noticeable with regard to neuromuscular function. Contraindications to magnesium therapy include renal impairment, cardiac disease, neuromuscular disease and myasthenia gravis. An ampoule of calcium gluconate (1 g) should always be available by a mother's bedside as an antidote. If magnesium is contraindicated, Diazemuls should be administered as an infusion of 2.5 mg/h.

The loading dose for magnesium sulphate is 4 g given slowly intravenously (preferably by infusion) over 15–20 minutes. This almost always causes nausea, vomiting and flushing. Metoclopramide 10 mg intravenously can be given to counteract these effects. Magnesium sulphate is stocked in different concentrations, e.g. 10% and 50% so care must be taken when preparing diluted solutions. More than 6 g over 20 minutes, or 8 g in the first hour of therapy, or 6 g/h in subsequent hours, can cause respiratory arrest. The intravenous maintenance dose is 2 g/h, and this should be continued for 24–48 hours after delivery. The volume of the solution needs to be deducted from the calculated fluid input. During the loading dose and maintenance infusion, the following monitoring must be recorded so that toxicity is detected early and dosages can be altered.

- Tendon reflex: the biceps or patella reflex (hourly). NB, the patella reflex cannot be used in a patient with an epidural *in situ*. When the reflex activity is lost, the magnesium infusion must be stopped.
- Electrocardiography (ECG): this is mandatory during and for one hour after the loading dose.
- Oxygen saturation: this is required continuously. Respiratory muscle weakness can occur with inadequate ventilation. The magnesium infusion must be stopped if the oxygen saturation is less than 90%.

Table 22.4 Magnesium dose adjustments based on extremes of therapeutic range.

Mg concentration > 4 mmol/L	Decrease maintenance dose by 0.5–1 g/h, depending on concentration
Mg concentration < 1.7 mmol/L	Consider further 2 g i.v. bolus over 20 min. Increase maintenance dose by 0.5–1 g/h
Mg concentration 1.7–2.0 mmol/L	Although this is strictly 'subtherapeutic', provided the patient is stable and levels are not persistently < 1.7 mmol/L, it is reasonable to continue on 2 g/h maintenance dose

Table 22.5 Toxicity of magnesium and clinical management.

	Magnesium concentration mmol/L	Management
Loss of tendon reflexes, double vision, slurred speech	5	Stop infusion until Mg^{2+} concentration known
Muscle paralysis, respiratory arrest	6.0–7.5	Give oxygen, stop infusion, call anaesthetist
Cardiac arrest	> 12	Stop infusion, institute resuscitation, i.v. calcium gluconate 1 g as antidote Intubate and ventilate, determine Mg^{2+} concentration

- Magnesium concentration: the therapeutic range is between 2 and 4 mmol/L (4.0–8.0 mg/dL). Monitor blood concentration at one hour after the start of the maintenance dose and six-hourly thereafter. Recurrent seizures may occur due to subtherapeutic doses. The risk factors for loss of magnesium include protracted vomiting and diuretic administration.

Dose alterations are required if oliguria develops, if the plasma urea is over 10 mmol/L, or liver function deteriorates. A maintenance dose of 1 g/h should be used in these situations, with magnesium concentrations being measured every two to four hours. A subtherapeutic or toxic magnesium concentration also requires dose adjustment (Table 22.4). The plasma levels for toxicity are shown in Table 22.5.

22.2.6 Recurrent convulsions

Treat the second convulsion with a bolus of magnesium 2–4 g over five minutes, and take blood for magnesium concentration prior to the bolus. If further convulsions occur despite the magnesium bolus, consider Diazemuls 10 mg i.v. and then an infusion of thiopental (on an intensive-care unit). Transfer to an intensive-care unit will be required if the woman is unconscious or fits recur after delivery.

22.2.7 Anaesthetic management of pre-eclampsia and eclampsia

The choice of local anaesthetic agent, mainly for epidural use, is of some significance, since the pharmacokinetics of lidocaine in pre-eclampsia differ from those in normotensive patients. Bupivacaine and ropivacaine have been used without adverse effect [16–18], but total body clearance of lidocaine is prolonged in pre-eclampsia, and higher blood concentrations are achieved for any given dose. Theoretically, the addition of epinephrine may mitigate these effects, but in pre-eclampsia epinephrine is usually avoided because it can contribute further to an already high plasma catecholamine concentration. When epidural analgesia is used for pain relief in labour, or for Caesarean delivery, bupivacaine is the agent of choice, and should be mixed with an opioid so that the dose of bupivacaine can be minimized and effectiveness maximized. When rapid regional nerve block is required, the choice lies between bupivacaine with bicarbonate (if time allows) for epidural analgesia or subarachnoid block with hyperbaric bupivacaine or general anaesthesia.

Labour

A regional nerve block is the preferred method of analgesia. It produces an improvement in placental perfusion in pre-eclamptic women [19], probably due to a decrease in uterine vascular resistance [20], and helps to control blood pressure. The beneficial effects are in part due to sympathetic blockade and in part due to a reduction in maternal responses to pain. A clotting screen and platelet count is required. A platelet count of $< 80 \times 10^9$/L, abnormal clotting results, or maternal refusal are contraindications to the technique. The thromboelastogram (TEG) has been advocated for use in such patients to provide a rapid test (about 30 minutes) for patients at risk [21]. It is not routinely available. The absolute value of the platelet count may not be as important as whether or not the platelets are functioning normally. The TEG requires further evaluation. A clinical history of coagulation problems should also be used in patient assessment, and the risks and benefits should be discussed with the woman. Often, however, she is sedated and wider consultation may be required, with documented records. The risks and benefits are summarized in Table 22.6.

The management of an epidural nerve block requires close monitoring of fluid balance, to maintain intravascular volume, and of position, to avoid aortocaval compression. An additional intravascular catheter separate from the infusion lines for magnesium or oxytocin provides rapid access without compromising drug therapies.

Table 22.6 Risks and benefits of epidural analgesia in labour in women with severe pre-eclampsia.

Risks	Benefits
Hypovolaemia unmasked	Reduced stress response (catecholamines)
Epidural haematoma	Maintains/improves uteroplacental blood flow
Revealed inferior vena caval occlusion	Prevents administration of systemic opioids, which may further depress the mother or fetus
	Available for operative delivery if necessary

Caesarean section

A regional nerve block is preferred to general anaesthesia for operative intervention. Contraindications would be similar to those in labour, plus: a failed epidural in labour, unless circumstances change and it can be sited by a more senior person; unconsciousness; an emergency; and a need for unrestricted surgical and anaesthetic access.

Coagulation abnormalities require treatment before surgery, since surgical and anaesthetic trauma will predispose to haemorrhage. In severe pre-eclampsia and eclampsia, a central venous pressure line is required prior to a regional nerve block. For urgent—rather than emergency—Caesarean section, fluid can be given incrementally, and the principles outlined in the fluid balance section should be followed.

Management of epidural nerve block requires fractional doses of local anaesthetic solution to be given while maintaining arterial and venous blood pressures. The fetal heart rate must also be monitored. Ephedrine (3–5 mg i.v.) is administered if hypotension develops. Once a stable haemodynamic state has been achieved with a dermatomal sensory block to T8–T10, further increments are given until the T4 dermatome is reached. The use of epinephrine with local anaesthetic solutions is not recommended, because it may decrease uteroplacental flow. Opioids may be added to the local anaesthetic solution. Their central effects may be exaggerated by drugs given to treat pre-eclampsia, and respiration and sedation levels must therefore be closely monitored. Spinal anaesthesia should also be considered if there is no epidural catheter *in situ*. There has been controversy about its use in preference to epidural anaesthesia, because prolonged and profound maternal hypotension has been said to occur, compromising fetal and maternal well-being. However, the evidence for this is slight and provided the systolic arterial pressure is maintained at more than 80% of baseline, the neonate demonstrates no change in Apgar score or umbilical artery pH [22]. Spinal anaesthesia is indicated in women in whom a difficult intubation is predicted. The risks for the latter are compounded by fluid retention in the tissues, especially around the larynx. A subarachnoid nerve block only requires a small volume of local anaesthetic solution, in contrast to the large volume used in epidural anaesthesia, where there is always a significant risk of total spinal anaesthesia. The combined spinal–epidural technique may be useful as a compromise.

The two major problems faced by anaesthetists using general anaesthesia in this situation focus on the larynx [23]. Signs of upper body oedema, especially facial oedema, should alert the anaesthetist to a greatly increased risk of airway oedema and difficulty with endotracheal intubation. There is a technical problem, not only during intubation but also at extubation, in maintaining airway patency, and there is a pathophysiological problem of the pressor response to intubation. The hypertensive response to intubation involves risks to the cerebral and pulmonary circulations (such as stroke, cardiac dysrhythmias, pulmonary oedema), and must be pharmacologically controlled. The choice of drug will be influenced by existing therapy. Magnesium, opoids, beta blockers and lidocaine have all been used. Labetalol 10–20 mg can be used, as it is short-acting and can be rapidly discontinued if blood loss occurs. The quantity of this bolus dose should be assessed on the basis of previous antihypertensive therapies and any maintenance infusion. A repeat dose should be given on extubation. In addition, a short-acting opioid can also be administered. However, opioid drugs pass to the fetus, and the attending paediatrician should be warned of opioid use so that antagonists are available to the neonate on delivery and preparations can be made to support ventilation of the baby. An alternative to both of these drugs is a slow bolus dose of 2 g magnesium sulphate (over 5 minutes). The interaction between magnesium and suxamethonium may extend suxamethonium's duration of action. Neuromuscular monitoring is required to detect the offset of action of suxamethonium in this situation. Another notable difference for anaesthetists is the reduction in fasciculation when suxamethonium is administered to a mother who is receiving magnesium therapy. Non-depolarizing drugs should be used in reduced dosage, and the dose response must be measured using a nerve stimulator.

Postoperative care will continue the management plan for pre-eclampsia and eclampsia in all respects except fetal monitoring. Postoperative analgesia can be provided by epidural opioids, patient-controlled intravenous opioid analgesia, or patient-controlled epidural opioid and dilute local anaesthetic infusion. The maternal outcome will depend on the resolution of the pathology rather than on the postoperative analgesia. Improvement after delivery is usual, but may take days. Convulsions can occur postoperatively, and vigilant nursing care and monitoring are therefore essential until evidence of resolution occurs, such as spontaneous diuresis and normalization of blood pressure.

22.2.8 Complications of pre-eclampsia

Maternal complications of pre-eclampsia can interfere with organ function. They are listed in Table 22.7.

Table 22.7 Complications of pre-eclampsia.

Convulsions
Central nervous system—focal and generalized lesions
Placental abruption
Renal failure
Pulmonary oedema
Disseminated intravascular coagulation (DIC)
Haemolysis, elevated liver enzymes and low platelet count

Placental abruption

Premature separation of the placenta can vary in degree, and has a high level of prenatal mortality. It is associated with hypertensive disorders, uterine abnormalities, multiparity, previous abruptions and cocaine abuse. It presents as abdominal pain, which may be masked by epidural analgesia in labour. This is one of the rarer differential diagnoses of hypotension during epidural analgesia in labour. Vaginal bleeding may be manifest, but it underestimates the hidden blood loss around the placenta and fetus, and in the myometrium or broad ligaments. The diagnosis can be made by ultrasound.

A clotting screen and platelet count must be obtained prior to epidural or SAB analgesia. Fetal distress or cardiovascular instability may be present, and an emergency Caesarean section may be preferred. Initial management will be to check that the woman is in the left lateral position and has oxygen and antacid prophylaxis. A large-bore intravenous catheter must be sited and blood for cross-matching taken. A general anaesthetic is usually required for this type of emergency Caesarean section, and cardiovascular stability must be maintained. Ketamine should be avoided, as it can increase uterine muscle tone and increase fetal distress.

Disseminated intravascular coagulation (DIC)

The causes of DIC are listed in Table 22.8. Treatment should be directed to removing the trigger [24]. Prevention is the best management. Early appraisal by a consultant obstetrician and haematologist is required, so that haematological therapy is aimed both at maintaining the blood volume and at correcting any coagulation defects, using the appropriate blood products. Regular assessment of the clotting screen will be required: full blood count, platelets, prothrombin time (PT), activated partial thromboplastin time (APTT), thrombin time, fibrinogen and fibrin degradation products. The diagnosis of DIC is made by the presence of hypofibrinogenaemia, thrombocytopenia, increased PT and APTT, decreased factors V and VIII, and increased fibrin degradation products. The presence of fibrin degradation products can inhibit the action of oxytocin on the uterus and cause uterine atony, which can contribute to

Table 22.8 Causes of disseminated intravascular coagulation.

Chronic
Retained dead fetus
Acute
Severe pre-eclampsia
Severe haemorrhage
Antepartum and postpartum haemorrhage
Placental abruption
Amniotic fluid embolism
Liver disease (e.g. acute fatty liver of pregnancy)
Septicaemia
Abortion
Postpartum
Transfusion with ABO-incompatible red blood cells

further haemorrhage. Cytokine release can cause tachycardia, oedema and hypotension, with resultant renal and respiratory failure.

Haemolysis, elevated liver enzymes and low platelet count (HELLP)

This is described in Chapter 7, Section 7.2.2, p. 112. The syndrome is of anaesthetic interest, as the woman may require delivery by Caesarean section. There is increased maternal and fetal morbidity and mortality. By definition, the syndrome has low platelets; general anaesthesia is therefore necessary, and haemorrhage control may require a hysterectomy as the last resort. The most severe morbidity occurs in the early puerperium after the Caesarean section, and elective admission to an intensive-care unit should be considered.

References

1 Ginsburg J, Duncan S. Direct and indirect blood pressure measurements in pregnancy. *J Obstet Gynaecol Br Commonw* 1969; **76**: 705.
2 Hassan MA, Thomas TA, Prys-Roberts C. A comparison of automatic oscillometric blood pressure measurement with conventional auscultatory measurement in the labour ward. *Br J Anaesth* 1993; **70**: 141–4.
3 Robson SC, Dunlop W, Boyes RJ, Hunter S. Cardiac output during labour. *Br Med J* 1987; **295**: 1129.
4 Sibai BM. Treatment of hypertension in pregnant women. *N Engl J Med* 1996; **335**: 257–65.
5 American College of Obstetricians and Gynecologists. *Hypertension in Pregnancy.* Washington, DC: American College of Obstetricians and Gynecologists, 1996.
6 Barry C, Fox R, Stirrat G. Upper abdominal pain in pregnancy may induce pre-eclampsia. *Br Med J* 1994; **308**: 1562–3.
7 Roberts JM, Redman CW. Pre-eclampsia: more than pregnancy-induced hypertension. *Lancet* 1993; **311**: 1447–54.
8 Baker PN, Davidge ST, Barankiewicz J *et al.* Plasma from pre-eclampsia women stimulates then inhibits endothelial prostacyclin. *Hypertension* 1996; **27**: 56–61.

9 Lorentzen B, Drevon CA, Endersen MJ *et al.* Fatty acid pattern of esterified and free fatty acids in sera from women with normal and pre-eclamptic pregnancy. *Br J Obstet Gynaecol* 1995; **102**: 530–7.
10 Davidge ST, Hubel CA, Braden RD, Capeless EC, McLaughlin MK. Sera antioxidant activity in uncomplicated and pre-eclamptic pregnancies. *Obstet Gynecol* 1992; **79**: 897–901.
11 CLASP (Collaborative Low-dose Aspirin Study in Pregnancy) Collaborative Group. CLASP: a randomised trial of low-dose aspirin for the prevention and treatment of pre-eclampsia among 9364 pregnant women. *Lancet* 1994; **343**: 619–29.
12 Redman CWG, Beilin LJ, Bonnar J. Treatment of hypertension in pregnancy with methyldopa: blood pressure control and side effects. *Br J Obstet Gynaecol* 1977; **84**: 419–26.
13 Robson SC, Redfern N, Walkinshaw SA. A protocol for the intrapartum management of severe pre-eclampsia. *Int J Obstet Anesth* 1992; **1**: 222–9.
14 Zinaman M, Rubin J, Linsheimer MD. Serial plasma oncotic pressure levels and electro-encephalography during and after delivery in severe pre-eclampsia. *Lancet* 1985; **4**: 1245–7.
15 Eclampsia Trial Collaborative Group. Which anticonvulsant for women with eclampsia? Evidence from the Collaborative Eclampsia Trial [published erratum in *Lancet* 1995; **346**: 258]. *Lancet* 1995; **345**: 1455–63.
16 Abboud T, Artal R, Srakis F, Henriksen EH, Kammula RK. Sympatho-adrenal activity: maternal, fetal and neonatal responses after epidural anesthesia in the pre-eclamptic patient. *Am J Obstet Gynecol* 1982; **144**: 915–18.
17 Jouppila R, Jouppila P, Hollmen AI, Koivula A. Lumbar epidural analgesia to improve intervillous blood flow during labour in severe pre-eclampsia. *Obstet Gynecol* 1982; **59**: 158–61.
18 Ramanathan J, Bottorff M, Jeter JN, Khalil M, Sibai BM. The pharmacokinetics and maternal and neonatal effects of epidural lidocaine in pre-eclampsia. *Anesth Analg* 1986; **65**: 120–6.
19 Jouppila R, Jouppila P, Hollmen AI *et al.* Epidural analgesia and placental blood flow during labour in pregnancies complicated by hypertension. *Br J Obstet Gynaecol* 1979; **86**: 696–8.
20 Ramos-Santos E, Devoe LD, Wakefield ML, Sherline D, Metheny WP. The effects of epidural anesthesia on the Doppler velocimetry of umbilical and uterine arteries in normal and hypertensive patients during active term labor. *Obstet Gynecol* 1991; **77**: 20–6.
21 Bushnell TG. A survey of coagulation screening practices in preeclampsia and low-dose aspirin prophylaxis. *Int J Obstet Anesth* 1994; **3**: 13–15.
22 Karinen J, Rasanen J, Alahuhta S, Joupilla R, Joupilla P. Maternal and uteroplacental haemodynamic state in pre-eclamptic patients during spinal anaesthesia for Caesarean section. *Br J Anaesth* 1996; **76**: 616–20.
23 Rocke DA, Scoones GP. Rapidly progressive laryngeal oedema associated with pregnancy-aggravated hypertension. *Anaesthesia* 1992; **47**: 141–3.
24 Baglin T. Disseminated intravascular coagulation: diagnosis and treatment. *Br Med J* 1996; **312**: 683–7.

23: Haemorrhage, Thromboembolism and Amniotic Fluid Embolism

23.1 Major obstetric haemorrhage

Haemorrhage from the genital tract is defined by the amount (> 500 mL) and the time when it occurs: *Antepartum haemorrhage* occurs after 24 weeks of pregnancy and before delivery of the baby. *Postpartum haemorrhage* is (i) primary, in the first 24 hours after delivery of the baby, or (ii) secondary, after the first 24 hours postpartum until six weeks after the birth.

It is not easy to assess blood loss from the genital tract unless it is overt. Often, it is concealed. The measured blood loss plus an estimate of the concealed loss should be added together (Table 23.1), and a prediction of the continuing risk and extent of blood loss should be made in order not to delay treatment.

If the uterus is contracted after delivery, a mother's effective blood volume will have increased by approximately 500 mL. She will have a larger blood volume than in the non-pregnant state, so that a blood loss of up to 1000 mL can usually be tolerated without physiological compromise. This loss may occur in one episode, or over several hours. Major obstetric haemorrhage is therefore defined as a loss (concealed and revealed) in excess of 1000 mL.

It is necessary in view of the preceding observations to assume that blood loss measurements are an underestimation. Any blood clots represent red blood cells without plasma, and their measured volume can be doubled to estimate actual loss. In addition, warning clinical signs must be observed, such as skin pallor and cold peripheries, hypotension < 90 mmHg systolic, and tachycardia (> 100 beats/min), as shown in Table 23.2. Other vital signs should be sought,

Table 23.1 Estimation of overt and concealed blood loss.

Total blood volume loss
Weigh swabs (1 g = 1 mL)
Suction volume (minus estimations for amniotic fluid volume)
Visual assessment of bedding, floor etc.
Inspect vagina
Palpate uterus for intrauterine collection

Clinical signs
Tachycardia
Appearance: pallor, air hunger
Syncope, hypotension
Low jugular venous pressure, central venous pressure
Urine output

Table 23.2 Determination of blood loss when fluid replacement has not occurred.

Blood loss (mL)	< 750	750–1500	1500–2000	> 2000
Blood loss (% blood volume)	< 15%	15–30%	30–40%	
Pulse rate	< 100	100–120	120–140	> 140
Blood pressure	Normal	Normal	Decreased	Decreased
Pulse pressure	Normal or increased	Decreased	Decreased	Decreased
Respiratory rate	14–20	20–30	30–40	30–40
Urine output (L/h)	> 30	20–30	5–15	Negligible
Central nervous system	Slightly anxious	Mildly anxious	Anxious and confused	Confused and lethargic
Fluid replacement	Crystalloid	Crystalloid	Crystalloid and blood	Crystalloid and blood

such as the urine output and central venous pressure, if available. Haemorrhage must also be correlated with the woman's medical condition, e.g. anaemia, when deciding on the most appropriate intravenous fluid therapy.

The aims of treating major obstetric haemorrhage are to:
1 restore the circulating blood volume and oxygen-carrying capacity of the blood (red blood cells) *rapidly*;
2 treat the cause of haemorrhage;
3 restore normal blood circulation.

The immediate management is to:
1 secure two venous access lines with 14-gauge cannulae;
2 provide a fast intravenous infusion of colloid and/or blood using a pressure infusing device;
3 provide oxygen 15 L/min by mask using a breathing system that delivers 100% oxygen;
4 send blood for urgent laboratory investigations:
   Cross-match.
   Full blood count and platelets.
   Coagulation screen.

By definition, blood replacement must be given, so it is necessary to cross-match six units of group-specific blood. Where possible, the woman's own blood group should be used in preference to uncrossmatched O rhesus-negative blood. However, two units of uncrossmatched screened O negative blood must be immediately available on all labour wards at all times for treatment of major haemorrhage. The group-specific blood sent urgently by the blood transfusion unit should be supplied in less than 20 minutes without a full cross-match. The mechanisms for this and the supply of blood products, e.g. fresh frozen plasma, should be agreed jointly between the consultant haematologist, anaesthetist and obstetrician, and should be maintained as a labour ward policy. The role of the staff on call for a major obstetric haemorrhage should also be defined, so that there is no repetition of work and thus delay. The staff to be assembled through a predetermined callout system include:

obstetric staff: resident, senior trainee, consultant;
anaesthetic staff: resident, senior trainee, consultant;
midwifery staff: patient's midwife, midwife in charge;
laboratory staff: haematologist, Medical Laboratory Scientific Officer;
porters.

It is necessary not only to have a major obstetric haemorrhage policy document, as recommended by the *Report on Confidential Enquiries into Maternal Deaths in the United Kingdom* [1], but also to improve training by staging regular drill scenarios. All the items required to treat haemorrhage should be together in a trolley, so that a complete set of matching and complementary equipment can be brought immediately for use by a team trained to use it. A suggested list is itemized in Table 23.3.

23.1.1 Continuing management

Central venous cannulation

The choice of peripheral or central cannulation depends on the experience of the anaesthetist. The angle of Louis can be established as a zero reference point, and the central venous pressure can be measured. A pressure below 3 cmH$_2$O indicates that continuing infusion of fluids is required. A pressure above 7 cmH$_2$O must be avoided, to reduce the risk of pulmonary oedema. The rate of infusion should equal the rate of continuous blood loss once the initial blood loss has been adequately replaced. Peripheral access to a central vein is preferred, unless experienced staff and facilities for treating complications of internal jugular or subclavian line insertion are readily available.

Monitoring

The bedside monitors should display the electrocardiogram (ECG), pulse rate, oxygen saturation and arterial and venous pressures as pressure waveforms. An indwelling arterial catheter should be sited soon after the central venous catheter, so that baseline measurements of acid–base balance and blood gases can be made and any abnormalities corrected. Care should be taken that an obsession with monitoring does not interfere with timely treatment of the patient's problem.

Urine output should be monitored half-hourly in the initial stages, and peripheral perfusion, particularly the change in temperature along the limbs, should be noted.

Table 23.3 Items for inclusion in a haemorrhage trolley.

Vascular access and infusion
Gloves
Skin preparation
Tourniquet
Venous cannulae: peripheral 14-gauge, 8-gauge (e.g. exchange kit), central venous pressure (e.g. drum cartridge, multiple lumen)
Lidocaine
3-way tap
Extension tube
Plaster
Surgical blades/cut-down set
Syringes
Needles
Razor
Sterile towels
Swabs
Stitches
Pressure bags
Blood giving sets
Blood warmers
Arm splint
Colloid solutions

Record
Clipboard and pencil

Laboratory investigations
Specimen bottles (two complete sets)

Oxygen therapy
Breathing system to deliver 100% oxygen by mask
Oxygen supply and flowmeter

Monitoring
Urine output: catheterization pack, urinary catheters and bag

Cardiovascular: ECG, oxygen saturation, direct arterial and venous pressures

ECG, electrocardiography.

Uterine contraction

Major haemorrhage may be caused by a failure of uterine contraction. The consequences of major haemorrhage, such as increased concentrations of fibrin degradation products and hypotension, may cause uterine relaxation. Successful treatment of the haemorrhage will make the maintenance of uterine tone easier. In the absence of known vascular haemorrhage, e.g. tears of

Table 23.4 Pregnancy complications that predispose to disseminated intravascular coagulation.

Pre-eclampsia and eclampsia
Placenta praevia
Placental abruption amniotic fluid embolism
Intrauterine death
Amniotic fluid embolism
Severe rhesus disease
Septic abortion

the pelvic blood vessels, uterine contraction is usually maintained pharmacologically, after expelling any blood clot. Oxytocin in intravenous boluses of 5 IU may suffice, but a fast intravenous bolus can cause transient vasodilation and hypotension. Many parturients will need an infusion of 40 IU oxytocin in one to two hours to maintain good uterine contractions. Prostaglandins such as carboprost (Hemabate) are now widely used to stimulate uterine contractions when oxytocin is not fully effective. Since the 1940s, ergometrine has been used to stimulate uterine contractions, but it is now used much less frequently due to its side effects of nausea, vomiting and vasoconstriction. Ergometrine is a long-acting vasoconstrictor, and its use is contraindicated in hypertensive disorders. General anaesthesia can reverse this profound vasoconstriction, but it recurs postoperatively and may precipitate pulmonary oedema through rapid rises in peripheral resistance that increase the preload and afterload on the heart.

Fluid balance

A complete record of the initial fluids infused and an hourly record of fluid intake and output is a vital part of major haemorrhage management. A urine output of 30 mL/h is acceptable. If renal function is normal and urine output is less than this, blood volume, cardiac output or blood pressure may be decreased. These can be assessed by both clinical observation and cardiovascular monitors. If cardiovascular function is not impaired, furosemide 10–40 mg i.v. should be administered. Osmotic diuretics are not indicated. If cardiac output is depressed—for example, by acidosis—correction of any respiratory component should be effected and inotropic support may be indicated, e.g. dopamine, provided there is no pre-existing disease or drugs that might contraindicate its use.

Coagulation

After the initial resuscitation, hourly checks of haemoglobin, platelets and coagulation status must be made. Disseminated intravascular coagulation (DIC) may manifest as obstetric haemorrhage, or may complicate it. It should be considered in the group of conditions listed in Table 23.4. Estimation of cross-linked fibrin degradation products is usually made only when other indices of coagulation are abnormal. In pregnancy, they normally have slightly increased values. One of the most sensitive indicators of continuing DIC is a decrease in the platelet count. Treatment of this disorder should be coordinated by the consultant haematologist. There is no place for the use of heparin. Prevention of secondary DIC is best achieved by maintaining circulating blood volume. The liver will then rapidly clear the fibrin degradation products and manufacture the necessary clotting factors to reverse the situation. Fresh frozen plasma will assist this process—especially if many units of optimal additive bank blood are being transfused, since they contain little more than red blood cells and normal saline.

23.1.2 Management of obstetric haemorrhage in women who refuse blood transfusion

Management of haemorrhage in those who refuse blood transfusion is difficult. There is a higher mortality rate among women who refuse blood transfusion on grounds of personal or religious beliefs than among those who will accept transfusion if it proves advisable. Women are normally asked their religious beliefs on antenatal booking, and this information is recorded. If the woman decides against accepting blood transfusion after receiving information about the risks she may incur, her haemoglobin should be checked regularly and haematinics should be given to maximize iron stores. During antenatal care and labour, consultant staff must be available if complications occur. The management of the immediate postpartum period requires vigilance with oxytocics given when the baby is delivered.

If unusual bleeding occurs at any time, a consultant obstetrician and consultant anaesthetist must be informed. Intravenous crystalloid and plasma expanders, except for dextran, should be used to maintain blood volume. If this standard treatment is not controlling the effects of haemorrhage, the woman should be counselled that blood transfusion is strongly recommended. It is reasonable to ask accompanying persons to leave the room to ensure that the woman is allowed to consider her decisions and their consequences fully, and that she has an opportunity to change the decision if she should wish to. Consultant staff must be involved with this procedure and thereafter. Watching a parturient bleed to death knowing that a transfusion might save her is not a duty that can be left with trainee staff. If the haemorrhage is antepartum, the baby should be delivered promptly by Caesarean section. A hysterectomy is the last resort, and in some cases internal iliac artery ligation may be preferred. General anaesthesia will be required for such interventions, and direct arterial and central venous pressure monitoring should be in place prior to induction. Acid–base measurements will assist in the management of tissue acidosis. If the woman survives the acute episode, she can be transferred (preferably being ventilated to maintain oxygenation to the tissues) to

Table 23.5 Prophylaxis and risk assessment for thromboembolism in Caesarean section.

Low risk
Prophylaxis: mobilization and hydration
Elective/scheduled Caesarean section with no other risk factors

Moderate risk
Prophylaxis: heparin
Age > 35 years
Obesity (> 80 kg)
Para 4 or more
Gross varicose veins
Current infection
Pre-eclampsia
Immobility prior to surgery (> 4 days)
Major current illness
Emergency Caesarean section in labour

High risk
Prophylaxis: heparin + compression leg stockings
3 or more 'moderate' risk factors
Extended surgery, e.g. Caesarean hysterectomy
History of deep venous thrombosis, pulmonary embolism, thrombophilia or paralysis of the lower limbs
Antiphospholipid antibody (e.g. SLE)

SLE, systemic lupus erythematosus.

the intensive-care unit, where facilities to improve haemoglobin synthesis should be available.

23.2 Thromboembolism

Maternal deaths from cerebral thrombosis and pulmonary thromboembolism have been one of the top three causes of maternal mortality for nearly 50 years [1]. The majority of these cases are caused by pulmonary embolism. If this is massive, the woman may have a sudden cardiac arrest, but increasingly women are resuscitated and transferred to intensive-care units, where they may die from multiple organ failure. Bedrest and immobilization in pregnancy, e.g. for pre-eclampsia, are risk factors for the development of deep venous thrombosis, and prophylaxis must be considered, particularly if other risk factors such as age, smoking and obesity exist. Caesarean section, whether elective or emergency, is also a risk factor.

23.2.1 Prophylactic heparin therapy and anaesthesia

Anaesthetic involvement in women at low risk of thromboembolism, as defined in Table 23.5, is to provide adequate pain relief so that early mobilization

Table 23.6 Summary of safe use* of regional nerve block for obstetrics in the presence of anticoagulants.

Drug	Precautions
Prophylactic low-dose unfractionated heparin	Site block before first dose or 4–6 hours after last dose
Prophylactic low molecular weight heparin	Site block before first dose or 12 hours after last dose
Therapeutic anticoagulation	Block contraindicated

* Alternatives may be considered for individual cases after consultation with a consultant haematologist.

is possible and to maintain hydration. In addition, anaesthetists should be aware that aspirin (75 mg daily) may also be used by obstetricians as prophylaxis in low-risk cases. Heparin prophylaxis is required for women at moderate and high risk. When prophylaxis is planned to start in labour and if an epidural is to be used, the catheter is best sited one to two hours before the first heparin injection [2]. There is a lack of a clinically useful method of determining the actual anticoagulant activity of low molecular weight heparins such as enoxaparin. Each case should be referred to a consultant anaesthetist and a haematological opinion should be sought on the clotting screen and platelet count. This time delay may also assist in the normal elimination of heparin, and a period of four to six hours between the administration of low-dose unfractionated heparin and regional anaesthesia has been recommended [3]. A longer period is required for low molecular weight heparins (Table 23.6). However, such events should be planned in advance, with adequate anaesthetic consultation. Catheter removal in women receiving heparin thromboprophylaxis should be timed by the anaesthetist to be 20–30 minutes before the next heparin dose.

There have been rare reports in the literature of haematomas following thromboprophylaxis, usually with warfarin, and most of these cases occur spontaneously. The contrast between the rarity of an epidural haematoma, as described in a recent case report of a bloody tap [4], with the mortality rate from thromboembolism should be discussed with the mother. The only treatment for a compressing spinal haematoma is a decompression laminectomy. The final neurological outcome depends on the time span between haematoma formation and surgical decompression. To be effective, this must be within six to eight hours. Regular neurological assessments in the postpartum period are therefore required in any woman who has received thromboprophylaxis and a regional nerve block, and must be particularly meticulous if a bloody tap has occurred. The spinal route may be preferable if a one-shot technique is possible, but radicular vessels can still be traumatized.

It should be emphasized to obstetricians that regional analgesia in itself reduces the tendency to thrombosis in lower limb veins. The evidence for this has been reviewed [5], and the reduction may be due not only to vasodilatation but also to an effect on the coagulation process. Prolonged pain relief with spinal opioids also assists postoperative and postdelivery mobility, especially after Caesarean section.

23.2.2 Pulmonary embolism

A history of dyspnoea or chest pain that may have been treated previously as a respiratory infection now generates a barrage of investigations to exclude pulmonary embolism. Thrombosis frequently begins in the veins in the legs or iliofemoral segment of the venous system. Swelling and discomfort in the legs is not an uncommon symptom in pregnancy. Non-invasive methods of diagnosing venous thrombosis include Doppler ultrasonography and impedance plethysmography in pregnancy, whereas venography can be used after delivery. The uterus must be displaced in the pregnant woman to avoid venous compression.

The diagnosis of pulmonary embolism requires ECG, a chest radiograph, and arterial blood gas measurements to exclude other causes. The ventilation/perfusion scan is the primary screening tool for pulmonary embolism in both pregnant and non-pregnant patients, but it is only diagnostic in about 30% of cases [6]. If there is doubt, pulmonary angiography is necessary [7]. Heparin is the anticoagulant of choice. Where there are contraindications to anticoagulant therapy, filters in the inferior vena cava have been used effectively in pregnant women. In antenatal women, it is usual to stop heparin at the onset of regular contractions. However, low molecular weight heparins are being introduced to replace unfractionated heparin. Their half-lives are longer, the dose response is more predictable, and in laboratory animals they cause less bleeding for the same antithrombotic effect. They also allow outpatient treatment, and there is evidence that, like unfractionated heparin, they do not cross the placenta.

23.2.3 Aspirin and regional nerve blockade

Aspirin and other antiplatelet therapies, such as dipyridamole administration, are used in thromboprophylaxis for both low-risk venous thrombosis and arterial thrombosis. The daily dose of aspirin used is low, 60–75 mg, and this preferentially and irreversibly inhibits platelet cyclo-oxygenase and reduces thromboxane A_2 production. This is a potent vasoconstrictor and platelet aggregation stimulator. Since platelets are devoid of a cell nucleus and thus do not have the genetic material for protein synthesis, the effect of aspirin lasts for the lifetime of the platelet. The bleeding time is the only test capable of providing information about platelet aggregation, and it is associated with operator errors. If the bleeding time is normal, it should be interpreted together with physical examination for bruising, platelet count and the patient's history. Since there is no documented evidence [8,9] of an increase in vertebral canal haematomas after aspirin in pregnant women, the routine use of bleeding times is not advocated, and regional anaesthesia is not contraindicated. The combination of aspirin and heparin therapy should alert an anaesthetist to avoid a regional nerve block, as perioperative heparin is the most frequently reported factor implicated in spinal haematoma formation [2].

23.3 Amniotic fluid embolism

Amniotic fluid embolism accounted for 8% of direct maternal deaths in the United Kingdom from 1991 to 1993 [1], and its incidence has not changed over many years. No consistent risk factors have been identified, and the condition can occur in all trimesters. Amniotic fluid embolism is a postmortem histological diagnosis. It is made by examining the lung tissues for amniotic squames. The clinical definition is by exclusion (the differential diagnoses are listed in Table 23.7), and the condition is associated with the presentation of a sudden collapse and respiratory distress followed rapidly by cyanosis and then by the development of a coagulopathy with consequent bleeding (Table 23.8). Convulsions from hypoxia are not uncommon. It is not known how many women have been successfully resuscitated after a postpartum haemorrhage in whom there was a less severe presentation of amniotic fluid embolism. The reporting of suspected cases without mortality might help to identify successful management protocols. This has been assisted in the United States by the establishment of a national registry [10].

The embolization of amniotic fluid triggers disseminated intravascular coagulation. The fluid may enter through the endocervical veins or the placental bed. Experimentally, clear amniotic fluid when injected is benign. However, the fluid also contains particles that plug the pulmonary vessels and

Table 23.7 Differential diagnosis of amniotic fluid embolism.

Eclampsia
Uterine rupture or laceration
Anaphylaxis
Anaesthetic mishap
Sepsis
Uterine atony and haemorrhage

Table 23.8 Presenting features among women collapsing with amniotic fluid embolism before delivery ($n = 30$) [10].

Convulsion	30%
Dyspnoea	27%
Fetal bradycardia	17%
Hypotension	13%
Cyanosis	3%

cause the release of vasoactive substances. These induce vasospasm in the pulmonary circulation, which results in pulmonary hypertension and hypoxaemia. This effect occurs early. It is possible to aspirate blood from the right side of the heart and examine it for fetal squames, but this is unnecessary because these cells can be found in the absence of amniotic fluid embolism [11]. Evidence of right ventricular strain on the ECG and the presence of perihilar infiltrates on the chest radiograph suggest the diagnosis.

Initial management is the ABC of resuscitation, and includes rapid delivery of the fetus if still *in situ*. Administration of 100% oxygen by positive-pressure ventilation is required. Blood should be removed for coagulation studies as soon as possible, and a consultant haematologist should be involved in treatment. The factors generating the coagulopathy are poorly understood. Late sequelae, such as acute respiratory distress syndrome and renal failure, may be prevented by appropriate monitoring and treatment in an intensive-care unit.

References

1. Hibberd BM, Department of Health. *Report on Confidential Enquiries into Maternal Deaths in the United Kingdom, 1991–1993.* London: HMSO, 1996.
2. Vandermeulen EP, Van Aken H, Vermylen J. Anticoagulants and spinal–epidural anesthesia. *Anesth Analg* 1994; **79**: 1165–77.
3. Wildsmith JAW, McClure J. Anticoagulant drugs and central nerve blockade. *Anaesthesia* 1991; **46**: 613–14.
4. Sterno JE, Hybbinette CH. Spinal subdural bleeding after attempted epidural and subsequent spinal anaesthesia in a patient on thromboprophylaxis with low molecular weight heparin. *Acta Anaesthesiol Scand* 1995; **39**: 557–9.
5. Bullingham A, Strunin L. Prevention of postoperative venous thromboembolism. *Br J Anaesth* 1995; **75**: 622–30.
6. Fennerty T. The diagnosis of pulmonary embolism. *Br Med J* 1997; **314**: 425–9.
7. Toglia MR, Weg JG. Venous thromboembolism during pregnancy. *N Engl J Med* 1996; **335**: 108–14.
8. CLASP (Collaborative Low-dose Aspirin Study in Pregnancy) Collaborative Group. CLASP: a randomised trial of low-dose aspirin for the prevention and treatment of pre-eclampsia among 9364 pregnant women. *Lancet* 1994; **343**: 619–29.
9. De Swiet M, Redman CWG. Aspirin, extradural anaesthesia and the MRC collaborative low dose aspirin study in pregnancy. *Br J Anaesth* 1992; **69**: 109–10.
10. Clark SL, Hankins DV, Dudley DA, Dildy GA, Porter TF. Amniotic fluid embolism: analysis of the national registry. *Am J Obstet Gynecol* 1995; **172**: 1158–69.
11. Clarke SL. Amniotic fluid embolism. *Crit Care Med* 1991; **7**: 877–82.

24: Other Complications

24.1 Maternal resuscitation (Fig. 24.1)

Survival from cardiac arrest in late pregnancy is exceptional. The main causes of collapse are listed in Table 24.1. Cardiac arrest is rare in pregnancy, and regular staff training with practical drills is essential. There are particular difficulties in pregnancy that obstruct basic resuscitation measures. The most important problem is compression of the inferior vena cava by the gravid uterus, particularly in the supine position. Other factors are: (a) anatomical changes that make intubation difficult—large breasts, an expanded rib cage in anteroposterior diameter, raised diaphragm, oedema, obesity and full dentition; and (b) physiological changes that reduce oxygen delivery to the tissues, increase ventilation difficulties and increase acidosis. These include an increase in oxygen consumption, decreased lung compliance, and increased susceptibility to regurgitation and pulmonary aspiration.

A speedy response is essential. Remove any obstruction to inferior vena cava blood flow.

- *Activate position:*
  Either use a left lateral tilt;
  or tilt the pelvis to the left (using wedge, blanket, pillows, etc.);
  or manually displace the uterus to the left.
- *Breathing:*
  Apply cricoid pressure until intubated. Use a cuffed endotracheal tube for ventilation.

Table 24.1 Factors precipitating cardiac arrest.

Respiratory	
Hypoxia	Failed intubation
Embolism	Pulmonary
	Amniotic fluid
Cardiovascular	
Reduced preload	Haemorrhage
	Vasodilatation, e.g. general anaesthetic drugs
	Severe inferior vena caval occlusion
Spinal anaesthesia	Severe hypotension
	Severe bradycardia
Patient transfer	Repositioning patients can cause sudden, profound hypotension

OTHER COMPLICATIONS 431

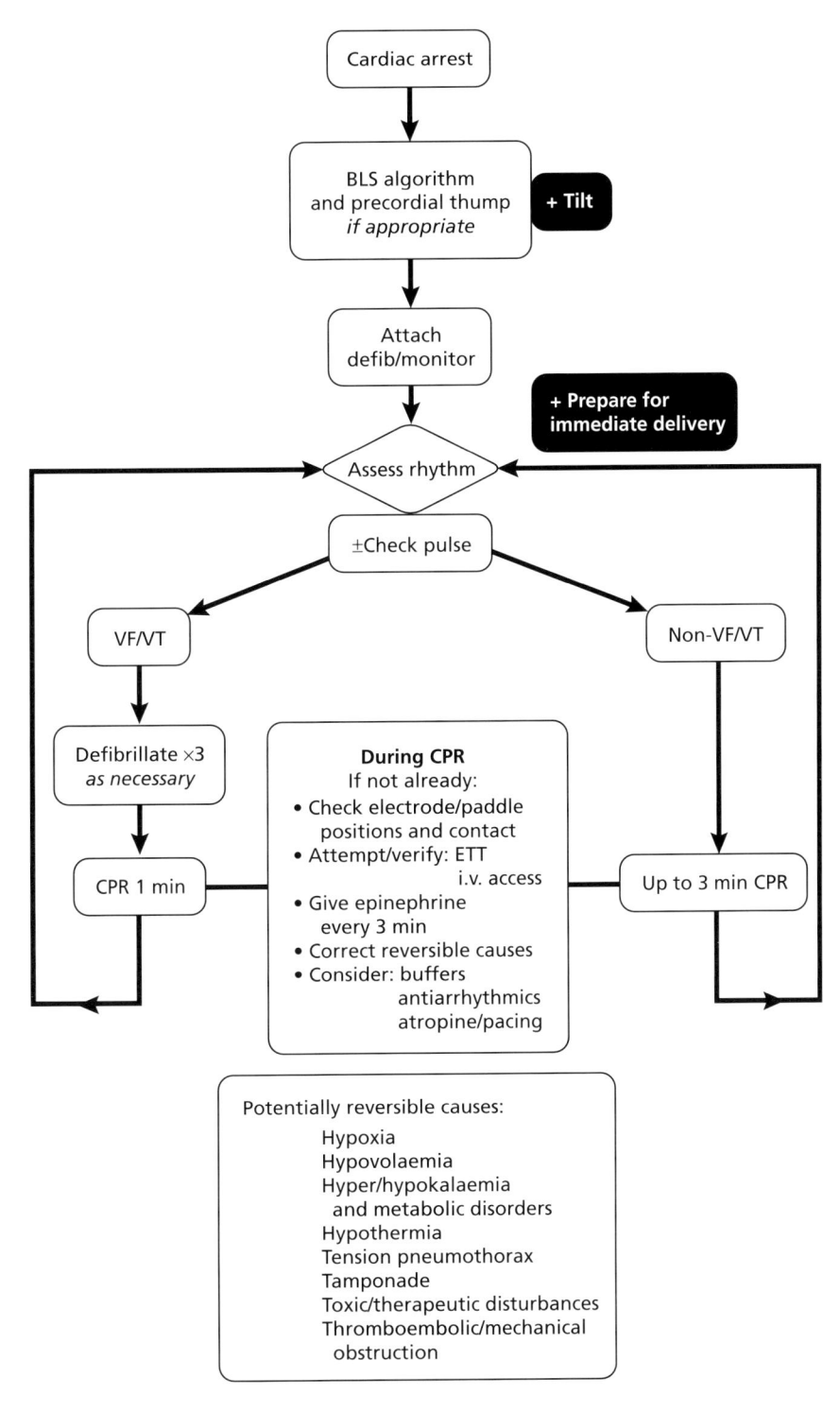

```
            ┌─────────────────┐
            │  Cardiac arrest │
            └────────┬────────┘
                     ▼
            ┌─────────────────┐
            │  BLS algorithm  │    ┌────────┐
            │and precordial thump├──│ + Tilt │
            │  if appropriate │    └────────┘
            └────────┬────────┘
                     ▼
            ┌─────────────────┐
            │     Attach      │
            │  defib/monitor  │   ┌──────────────────┐
            └────────┬────────┘   │  + Prepare for   │
                     ▼            │immediate delivery│
            ┌─────────────────┐   └──────────────────┘
            │  Assess rhythm  │◄──────────
            │  ±Check pulse   │
            └──┬───────────┬──┘
               ▼           ▼
         ┌─────────┐  ┌──────────┐
         │  VF/VT  │  │ Non-VF/VT│
         └────┬────┘  └─────┬────┘
              ▼              │
      ┌──────────────┐       │
      │Defibrillate ×3│   During CPR
      │ as necessary │   If not already:
      └──────┬───────┘   • Check electrode/paddle
             ▼             positions and contact
      ┌──────────┐       • Attempt/verify: ETT
      │CPR 1 min │                       i.v. access
      └──────────┘       • Give epinephrine
                           every 3 min
                         • Correct reversible causes
                         • Consider: buffers
                                    antiarrhythmics
                                    atropine/pacing

         Potentially reversible causes:
            Hypoxia
            Hypovolaemia
            Hyper/hypokalaemia
             and metabolic disorders
            Hypothermia
            Tension pneumothorax
            Tamponade
            Toxic/therapeutic disturbances
            Thromboembolic/mechanical
             obstruction
```

Fig. 24.1 Algorithm for maternal resuscitation, modified from the European Resuscitation Council's recommendations [1]. BLS: basic life support. ETT, endotracheal tube; CPR, cardiopulmonary resuscitation, VF, ventricular fibrillation; VT, ventricular tachycardia.

- *C*aesarean section:
  Chest compression must be started at 80 beats/min, but it is often ineffective due to poor venous return until the uterus is emptied. Vaginal or Caesarean delivery should be performed as soon as possible, preferably within five minutes. Continue with advanced life support [1].
- *D*efibrillation and drugs:
  Use of epinephrine: epinephrine should be used as advised in resuscitation guidelines, even though it may constrict uterine blood vessels. The fetus in a cardiac arrest is already compromised.
- *E*quipment:
  Cardiopulmonary resuscitation equipment must be available in labour wards and obstetric operating theatres.

24.2 Obstetric complications presenting for anaesthetic management

24.2.1 Placenta praevia

The choice of anaesthesia for a woman who has a placenta praevia that is obstructing normal delivery and in whom Caesarean section is planned depends on the position of the placenta and the risk of haemorrhage. The sympathetic blockade induced by a regional nerve block impairs the normal cardiovascular responses to haemorrhage, and treatment of major haemorrhage can be difficult in a conscious woman. An anterior placenta praevia, as it lies over the lower segment, will be approached by the obstetrician before delivery of the baby, and haemorrhage can result. Blood flow to the uteroplacental unit can be disrupted if there is operator difficulty, or if maintenance of circulating blood volume is not optimal. Additional factors for haemorrhage include a previous scar, either from Caesarean section or uterine surgery. The risk factor is increased by five times [2] if a previous scar is present, because the placental site may occur within the scar and placenta accreta may be present. After delivery, when uterine contraction tends to obliterate the bleeding placenta site, the scar cannot contract, and bleeding from this area continues. Four units of cross-matched blood must be in the theatre and two large-bore cannulae sited and attached to fluid administration sets with blood warmers. A central venous pressure line is best sited prior to blood loss, and a direct arterial line should be considered. Caesarean section in a woman with placenta praevia and a history of a uterine scar should only be undertaken by very experienced anaesthetists and obstetricians. A Caesarean hysterectomy may be required. The mother requires information about the risks of the procedure, but the choice of anaesthetic lies with the anaesthetist.

24.2.2 Uterine rupture

Uterine rupture can occur at any time, but it is associated with excessive oxytocin stimulation, a uterine scar, multiparity and operative trauma through the vagina. It presents as abdominal pain or fetal distress. The pain may stimulate a demand for epidural analgesia, which may be a disastrous event. If there is an epidural nerve block in place, the pain often breaks through the epidural, and an anaesthetist should be alerted to this complication by the continuous persistence of the pain, an associated change in fetal heart rate, or by shoulder tip pain caused by subdiaphragmatic irritation by blood. Sympathetic blockade may aggravate hypotension, and if cardiovascular instability occurs, conversion to general anaesthesia is therefore necessary.

24.2.3 Septic shock

Septic shock in obstetrics mainly occurs after surgical procedures such as abortion, or in the puerperium. It is an important cause of maternal mortality; it can be fulminating. When the woman has systemic manifestations, urgent and repeated bacteriological specimens, including blood cultures, must be obtained. When serious intra-abdominal sepsis is present, collaboration with a consultant microbiologist is necessary.

The general systemic response to infection is hypoxia and hypotension of non-cardiac origin. Secondary changes in many organs can result in multiple organ failure and death. Septic shock is the end result of the interaction of numerous inflammatory mediators released mainly from macrophages, neutrophils and endothelial cells in response to bacterial stimulation. These mediators include cytokines, arachidonic acid metabolites, kinins, phospholipid mediators, complement and nitric oxide. Some of these mediators may be targets for therapeutic intervention. The endothelium is damaged by these processes, so that profound vasodilation, hypotension and capillary leakage occurs, resulting in organ damage. The usual processes controlling inflammation, such as inhibiting cytokines and cytokine inhibitors, may be altered by the pathogen or by host circumstances.

Invasive monitoring is helpful in women who develop septic shock, both as an aid to the diagnosis of hypotension and to assist management decisions. Typically, the cardiac output is elevated (above pregnancy values) and the systemic vascular resistance reduced (below pregnancy values). The prevailing metabolic acidosis and myocardial depression from inflammatory mediators often reduce the cardiac output that would be expected from the reduced vascular resistance. The aim of treatment is to maintain tissue oxygenation. These aspects of management can only be combined in an intensive-care unit, where organ support is available.

Measurement of central venous pressure followed by pulmonary artery pressure will be needed to manage fluid administration. Initially, fluid replacement is with colloid to prevent fluid overload and pulmonary oedema. If this fails to correct the hypotension, vasopressors and inotropes should be added. No therapy for septic shock has so far been able to specifically antagonize the inflammatory mediators that are released. There are strategies either to limit bacterial interaction and activation of host cells or to inhibit the secondary mediators. However, these focus on limiting the organ damage by maintaining adequate oxygen delivery [3], nutritional requirements [4] and organ support.

24.2.4 Backache

Acute back pain may be simple backache, nerve root pain, or a symptom of serious spinal pathology. The characteristics of each are described in Table 24.2. Backache is a very common symptom, particularly in women of childbearing years in whom ligamentous laxity and added mechanical stress can exacerbate the symptoms. It occurs in about half of pregnant women and there is anecdotal evidence that multiple fetuses can cause more discomfort. Management of simple backache over the years has changed from recommending inactivity to recommending activity together with analgesics such as paracetamol. Simple back pain can be severe; it can interfere with normal daily life and work, and it contributes to the insomnia suffered in late

Table 24.2 Characteristics of acute low back pain in child bearing age group.

Simple backache
20 > years of age
Lumbosacral, buttock and thighs
Mechanical
Woman well

Nerve root pain
Unilateral leg pain worse than low back pain
Radiates to feet or toes
Numbness and paraesthesia in the same distribution
Straight leg raising reproduces leg pain
Local neurological signs

Serious spinal pathology (non-specific)
Non-mechanical
Thoracic pain
Medical symptoms
Widespread neurology
Structural deformity

Cauda equina syndrome
Sphincter disturbance
Gait disturbance
Saddle anaesthesia

Table 24.3 Management of women with a positive history of backache.

Positive history of backache pre-pregnancy/during pregnancy
Refer for obstetric physiotherapy advice and therapy antenatally
Antenatal classes
Advise on stopping smoking, analgesia: paracetamol

Discuss options for analgesia in labour
Position during labour
Use of low-dose epidural local anaesthetics with opioids to minimize muscle weakness

Epidural analgesia chosen for pain relief in labour
Avoid multiple attempts to site catheter
Support: avoid flexion and overstretching ligaments
Monitor muscle weakness and change solution according to pain and muscle weakness

Postpartum prevention
Advise on posture, lifting, feeding position
Physiotherapy advice on exercises, swimming, etc.
Examine back for bruising and record details
Encourage mobilization with analgesia; TENS if necessary
Provide follow-up advice/care if symptoms persist

TENS, transcutaneous electrical nerve stimulation.

pregnancy. It is therefore not a minor symptom of pregnancy to many women. A number of risk factors have been associated with back pain, but none repeatedly: parity, older age and a past history of back pain. Relaxin is the hormone that regulates collagen activity and softens ligaments in preparation for parturition. Younger women may have sensitivity to this hormone, and parous women will have had more exposure. There is also an increase in abnormalities of lumbar discs on magnetic resonance images, with almost a third of older childbearing women having an abnormal pattern of disc hydration. These findings can be imaged in women with histories of back trauma, but also occur in asymptomatic women [5].

It is against the background of this high prevalence of symptoms, plus the effects of hormones and age-related lumbar disc changes, that the complication of backache after lumbar regional nerve block has to be assessed. Local tenderness from tissue bruising may persist for a few days. Acute tissue injury around the vertebral canal and ligaments has not been observed on magnetic resonance imaging [6], and none of the studies of postpartum and epidural-related backache have found any correlation between the local bruising reported to anaesthetists and longer-term problems. Women with a previous history of back pain have a significantly increased risk of postpartum back pain. This information should now generate preventative measures to avoid long-term problems using cognitive and physiotherapy methods (Table 24.3) [7].

Although the symptom of postpartum backache has been reported in a number of studies, the first retrospective study on the topic—reviewing information collected by postal questionnaire was completed by 11 701 women who gave birth in a single maternity hospital between 1978 and 1985—and published in 1990 [8]. Of the women who had received epidural anaesthesia 18.9% complained of new-onset backache, compared with 10.5% of those who had not had an epidural. The difference was significant ($P < 0.05$). The authors concluded that a causal relationship existed, and speculated that the cause was postural, resulting from a combination of stressed positions for labour and delivery as well as muscle relaxation and a lack of mobility. The study is open to several criticisms. It was a retrospective review of only 39% of the target population; selection bias may have occurred, and poor recall over the years would tend to add to the unreliability of the relationship claimed between backache and epidural analgesia. However, publication of the report stimulated prospective studies. A study of one group of 1042 women interviewed on admission for delivery and again two months later found no difference in the incidence of new postpartum back pain between those who received analgesia for labour (44%) and those who did not (45%) [9]. These groups were not randomized. There is controversy regarding whether or not women can be genuinely randomized into one group that receives epidural analgesia in labour and one that does not. In another study 515 primiparous women had a 36% incidence of back pain whether or not an epidural was used [10]. Another prospective, randomized and controlled trial using either bupivacaine or low-dose bupivacaine with opioid in order to avoid significant muscle weakness collected follow-up data by questionnaire after three months. The incidence of long-term backache was not increased above 34% in either group [11].

References

1 Robertson C, Steen P, Adgey J *et al*. The 1998 European Resuscitation Council guidelines for adult advanced life support. *Resuscitation* 1998; **37**: 81–90.
2 Arcario T, Green M, Ostheimer GW, Datta S, Naulty JS. Risks of placenta previa/accreta in patients with previous Cesarean deliveries. *Anesthesiology* 1988; **68** (3A): A659.
3 Hayes MA, Timmins AC, Yau EH *et al*. Evaluation of systemic oxygen delivery in the treatment of critically ill patients. *N Engl J Med* 1994; **330**: 1717–22.
4 Bower RH, Cerra FB, Bershadsky B *et al*. Early enteral administration of a formula (Impact) supplemented with arginine, nucleotides, and fish oil in intensive care patients: results of a multicentre, prospective, randomised, clinical trial. *Crit Care Med* 1995; **23**: 436–49.
5 Holdcroft A, Baudouin C, Fernando R, Samsoon G, Oatridge A. Postpartum magnetic resonance imaging: lumbar tissue changes are unrelated to epidural analgesia or mode of delivery. *Int J Obstet Anesth* 1995; **4**: 201–6.
6 Holdcroft A, Samsoon G, Fernando RA, Baudouin C. Acute tissue damage following epidural cannulation: a comparison between the midline and paramedian approach in obstetric patients. *Int J Obstet Anaesth* 1994; **3**: 35–9.

7 MacEvily M, Buggy D. Back pain and pregnancy: a review. *Pain* 1996; **64**: 405–14.
8 MacArthur C, Lewis M, Knox EG, Crawford JS. Epidural analgesia and long-term backache after childbirth. *Br Med J* 1990; **301**: 9–12.
9 Breen TW, Ransil BJ, Groves PA, Oriol NE. Factors associated with back pain after childbirth. *Anesthesiology* 1994; **81**: 29–34.
10 Loughnan BA, Gordon H, Frank AO. Long-term backache after childbirth: study should have been randomised. *Br Med J* 1996; **313**: 755.
11 Russell R, Dundas R, Reynolds F. Long-term backache after childbirth: prospective search for consecutive factors. *Br Med J* 1996; **312**: 1384–8.

Section 8
Appendices

Appendix 1: Reference values

These are reference values for normal healthy Caucasian women [1].
NB: Control, non-pregnant data will vary between laboratories. Check your own laboratory values and then calculate the percentage changes in pregnancy.

	Non-pregnant	Term	Comments
Sodium	136–142	131–140 mmol L^{-1}	Net retention 3 mmol day^{-1}
Potassium	3.7–4.8	3.7–4.9 mmol L^{-1}	Net retention 1 mmol day^{-1}
Chloride	101–108	100–109 mmol L^{-1}	Unchanged
Bicarbonate	22–29	17–25 mmol L^{-1}	Compensates for CO_2
Urea	2.5–6.5	1.4–5.3 mmol L^{-1}	Significantly lower
Creatinine	50–90	22–94 mmol L^{-1}	
Uric acid	154–325	141–429 µmol L^{-1}	Decreased until 28 weeks
Total calcium	2.17–2.43	2.02–2.46 mmol L^{-1}	
Ionized calcium	1.10–1.36	1.16–1.36 mmol L^{-1}	Daily intake 1200 mg
Phosphate	0.82–1.37	0.73–1.34 mmol L^{-1}	
Magnesium	0.67–0.92	0.52–0.87 mmol L^{-1}	Renal failure can precipitate toxicity
Glucose (plasma)	3.9–5.5	3.4–5.5 mmol L^{-1}	4 h postprandial
Fasting blood glucose	(plasma 10–15% lower)	3.3–3.9 mmol L^{-1}	
Unconjugated bilirubin	4–20	4–10 µmol L^{-1}	Decrease in albumin
Alanine aminotransferase	5–29	0–36 U L^{-1}	
Alkaline phosphatase	38–98	102–328 U L^{-1}	Placental production
Amylase	28–82	10–82 U L^{-1}	Higher in Asian and Afro-Caribbean
Creatine kinase	20–137	0–227 U L^{-1}	Low values until start of 3rd trimester
Gamma-glutamyl transferase	14–33	9–34 U L^{-1}	Used to diagnose liver dysfunction
Lactate dehydrogenase	250–525	342–686 U L^{-1}	Transient increase at delivery
Total protein	63–78	50–67 g L^{-1}	Total circulatory protein is increased in pregnancy
Albumin	36–46	26–28 g L^{-1}	Mainly dilutional effects
Colloid osmotic pressure	22–33	19–27 cmH$_2$O	Albumin is major determinant
Haemoglobin	11.5–14.7	10.4–14.8 g dL^{-1}	Haemoglobin < 10 g dL^{-1} is abnormal
Haematocrit	0.34–0.43	0.31–0.44	
Osmolality	290	280 mosm kg^{-1}	
Mean corpuscular volume (MCV)	83.3–96.8	79.5–100.3 fl	Influenced by deficiencies of iron and folate
Mean corpuscular haemoglobin Concentration (MCHC)	314–360	319–351 g L^{-1}	

(Cont'd on p. 442)

(Cont'd)

	Non-pregnant	Term	Comments
White blood cell count	3.1–8.7	4.2–22.2 × 10^9 L^{-1}	Increased neutrophils
Platelet count	166–381	121–397 × 10^9 L^{-1}	
Prothrombin time	9.4–12.0	7.9–12.7 s	Mild decrease in clotting times
Activated partial thromboplastin time	26.6–35.5	23.0–34.9 s	
Fibrinogen	1.76–3.64	2.48–6.60 g L^{-1}	Interpret with haematologist

Reference

[1] Lockitch G. *Handbook of Diagnostic Biochemistry and Haematology in Normal Pregnancy.* London: CRC Press, 1993.

Appendix 2: Pharmacology

Principles of prescribing in pregnancy

Prescribing in pregnancy is necessary for three reasons: (1) when a pre-existing medical condition exists; (2) when a medical condition is diagnosed during pregnancy, e.g. infection; (3) when pregnant-specific disorders exist, e.g. hypertension, preterm labour. Some of the physiological changes in pregnancy influence drug disposition. Renal blood flow increases so that clearance of renally excreted drugs is increased, e.g. ampicillin has a clearance increased by 100%. However, in a systemic infection the dose should be increased to compensate for renal losses. Some metabolic reactions are also increased, e.g. anticonvulsant drugs.

Drugs can harm the fetus mainly in the first trimester when organogenesis occurs. It is during this period (18–55 days) that teratogenesis can occur. The choice of general anaesthetic agents is discussed in Chapter 17, p. 326. Few drugs have been confirmed as human teratogens [1]. Later in pregnancy, drugs can affect fetal growth and development.

Principles of prescribing postpartum

The anaesthetist may prescribe drugs either for pain relief or for anaesthesia. Physiological changes in the puerperium are described in Chapter 12, together with the anaesthetic management related to breast feeding. This section considers the excretion of anaesthetic drugs in breast milk. A full review is presented by Lee and Rubin [2].

Many mothers wish to breast feed and expect information on the use of drugs at this time. It is the free, unbound drug that is available for diffusion into breast milk. The breast tissues act as a semipermeable lipid membrane between the non-ionized drug in the plasma and breast milk. The mean pH of human milk is 7.1 and weak bases can achieve a higher concentration in milk lipid. This is a drug diffusion phenomenon magnifying that of the placenta. The total dose of a drug ingested by a baby depends on the total concentration present in the milk and the volume of milk taken. The drug then passes into the digestive system of the baby where oral bioavailability and clearance will determine its effects.

Considerations should be given to the type of anaesthetic drug used, its physical characteristics and the dosage. For example, the only opioid to be contraindicated is pethidine, especially if used repeatedly for postoperative pain relief by injection or patient controlled analgesia. The active metabolite has a long half-life in the infant. Of the non-opioid analgesics, aspirin is contraindicated because it is excreted in breast milk and the infant can develop platelet dysfunction and possibly Reye's syndrome. Other non-steroidal anti-inflammatory analgesics and paracetamol are in routine use. General anaesthetic agents for induction of anaesthesia, inhalational agents and muscle relaxants are theoretically safe. Glycopyrrolate is the anticholinergic drug of choice because it is a quaternary ammonium compound. No adverse effects have been reported from midazolam or temazepam use in single doses prior to anaesthesia. Prophylactic use of H_2 antagonists warrants the avoidance of cimetidine because it is concentrated in milk. Ranitidine is not known to be harmful. Data on anti-emetic drugs are sparse and their routine use, with postoperative opioid analgesia, is not recommended. They should only be used as required for clinical indications. Local anaesthetics do not pass into breast milk in any significant amounts [3].

Central nervous system drug effects in response to the passage of an opioid drug have been reported for epidural buprenorphine with bupivacaine [4]. Buprenorphine passes into the fetus through the breast milk and its effects are manifest as a decrease in milk fed and infant weight comparing a control group who only received bupivacaine. The epidural bupivacaine and buprenorphine were given for three postoperative days by continuous infusion. Neonatal weight gain significantly decreased by day 7 post delivery with a total dose of 800 μg buprenorphine. This effect would be difficult to detect in a typical UK hospital because of the rapidity of discharge of patients. It may be one of the more subtle effects of opioids which so far have been undetected.

Local anaesthetic toxicity

The local toxicity of local anaesthetics describes their irreversible action on nerves. Systemic toxicity relates to the dose of drug which reaches either the cerebral or coronary circulation. An alert to bupivacaine cardiotoxicity was given in 1979 [5]. This is a rare event but precipitated the withdrawal of concentrated 0.75% solutions and the search for less toxic local anaesthetics which has resulted in S(−)bupivacaine (levobupivacaine) and ropivacaine as alternatives to the racemic mixture of bupivacaine.

Local neurotoxicity

High concentrations of local anaesthetics are directly toxic to nerves, even when there are no preservatives in the solution [6]. The addition of 7.5% dextrose could increase toxicity.

In vitro after 3 min exposure to 5% lidocaine in 7.5% dextrose, a sciatic nerve preparation did not recover its activity. The use of microcatheters for spinal anaesthesia has highlighted the problem of local toxicity with cases of cauda equina syndrome developing, particularly related to the absence of mixing between the injected drug and cerebrospinal fluid [7].

Cardiac toxicity

Local anaesthetics are sodium channel blockers but vary in potency. Lidocaine is used as an antiarrhythmic agent but bupivacaine in toxic concentrations causes dysrhythmias, QRS widening, heart block and ventricular tachycardia. Local anaesthetics cross into the cell (intracellular pH 6.9–7.1) as non-ionized compounds, but because of the pH difference inside and outside the cell, bupivacaine probably remains ionized and dissociation from the receptor is slower. Bupivacaine also is more soluble in lipids than lidocaine and this physical attribute changes in the ionized form. Reversal of bupivacaine cardiotoxicity requires the wash-out of bupivacaine, and provided that coronary blood flow is maintained (by cardiac massage), it should eventually wash away from the sodium channels where it is active [8].

Central nervous system toxicity

It is necessary to maintain verbal contact with a parturient during the onset of an epidural block because the initial symptoms of toxicity can be reported to the anaesthetist. The woman may complain of numbness of the tongue and mouth, slurred speech, tinnitus, vision disturbances, muscle twitching, convulsions, anxiety or feeling of impending doom! These symptoms are followed by hypotension, dysrhythmias, convulsions and cardiovascular collapse, not necessarily in that order. Immediate treatment is that of basic resuscitation: Airway, Breathing and Circulation, with additional items relating to a pregnant woman if a fetus is *in situ*: position laterally and prepare for immediate Caesarean section. CALL THE RESUSCITATION TEAM.

Additional pharmacology of drugs used in obstetric anaesthesia

Clonidine

The α_2-adrenoreceptor agonists have been used in anaesthesia since the 1980s. They have properties of anxiolysis, analgesia, reduction in anaesthetic requirements and maintenance of haemodynamic stability. Their use has not developed because (1) they are hypotensive agents and the margin between effective analgesia and hypotension is small, and (2) there are no antagonists to their use, unlike the opioids with which they share many actions.

At present the only clinically available drug is clonidine but there is an injectable preparation suitable for regional nerve blockade. Clonidine was originally used as an antihypertensive drug and it is not a pure α_2-adrenoreceptor agonist. It possesses α_1 properties (ratio 220 : 1). It has a relatively long half-life of 9–12 hours. Dexmedetomidine is a more specific agent with a shorter duration of action.

Clonidine can reduce opioid requirements for postoperative and labour pain relief [9]. Epidural clonidine in a dose of 75 µg improved labour analgesia without adverse effects on the mother or fetus, and systemic clonidine has been used to treat mothers with pregnancy-induced hypertension [10], again with a lack of toxicity.

Intrathecal clonidine does not provide the expected benefit of improved analgesia and the mode of action of epidural clonidine requires further investigation.

Desflurane

Desflurane and sevoflurane offer potential advantages over existing volatile agents in obstetrics because of a faster onset and offset of action which may assist in preventing awareness during general anaesthesia for operative delivery and have less depressant effects on the fetus. The favourable physicochemical properties are shown in Table 16.6. However, clinical recovery from these agents has not proved to be faster than isoflurane in all but the early phase of recovery [11].

The action of desflurane on the sympathetic nervous system may involve a central nervous system mechanism and pharmacological blockade of this effect was achieved by clonidine rather than fentanyl [12,13]. The triggering of the sympathetic nervous system could be harmful in parturients with a tendency to hypertension.

Desflurane has been investigated as both an analgesic agent in labour and for anaesthesia during Caesarean section. A concentration of 3% desflurane plus nitrous oxide was comparable with 0.6% enflurane for Caesarean section, but 6% desflurane resulted in neonatal respiratory depression [14]. When desflurane was used in the second stage of labour in concentrations between 1 and 4.5% for analgesia, compared with 30–60% nitrous oxide, similar analgesia was achieved but 23% of the group of mothers who had received desflurane had amnesia for the birth of their baby [15].

Ketamine

Ketamine is used in obstetrics in rare circumstances because it can induce anaesthesia without depressing the cardiovascular system. It is also a potent analgesic agent. It acts as a non-competitive antagonist of the N-methyl-D-aspartate receptor. However, ketamine does not act on one receptor. It has anticholinergic effects (i.e. bronchodilation, salivation, mydriasis and amnesia) and this is mediated through activity on the M1 muscarinic receptor. These effects can be inhibited by atropine.

Ketamine is a racemic mixture of S(+) and R(−) enantiomers. It is the R(−) enantiomer which is associated with psychomimetic emergence reactions and agitation. Ketamine causes central sympathetic stimulation so that the use of vasoconstrictions such as ergometrine and epinephrine should be avoided.

When ketamine is used in its present form, its cataleptic side-effects have to be obtunded. Benzodiazepines given prophylactically can prevent post-operative reactions but are best not given with a fetus *in utero*.

Nitrous oxide

Nitrous oxide continues to be used in obstetric anaesthesia and analgesia because it is a good analgesic, it causes no airway irritation and no cumulation over time. If nitrous oxide is used, the use of other drugs may be reduced or avoided. Its particular use in obstetrics follows from an extensive safety record for both the mother and baby. No metabolites are produced and because of its low anaesthetic potency, it is a mild hypnotic. Its physical characteristics ensure a fast onset and offset, however long it is used for. Nitrous oxide has an exceptionally low solubility in brain and body tissues which is equivalent to desflurane and sevoflurane. It differs from them in potency. It therefore has a fast onset of analgesic action with a very rapid rise of nitrous oxide partial pressure in the brain which produces its analgesic and hypnotic effects.

Nitrous oxide, however, is not without its side-effects. Unwanted pressure and volume effects occur when air-containing cavities develop such as a pneumothorax and air embolism, because nitrous oxide diffuses rapidly into these spaces and expands them. Cardiodepressive effects have been reported [16] which are usually compensated for by endogenous sympathetic stimulation and may be of importance in obstetric patients with heart failure [17]. Nitrous oxide is a gas and has the potential for toxic effects mediated through non-reversible inhibition of methionine synthetase when given for long periods in a highly polluted environment (above 400 ppm [18]), or when abused by health personnel [19]. The main danger in the use of nitrous oxide in midwifery occurs when a gas cylinder of a mixture of nitrous oxide and oxygen, such as Entonox, is left exposed at temperaures below freezing, such as may occur outside in winter in the United Kingdom. Liquefaction of the nitrous oxide can allow separation of the two gases and the development of a hypoxic mixture, especially towards the end of a cylinder's contents. The gas nitrous oxide has a critical temperature of 36.5°C. A 'pseudocritical temperature' describes a similar effect in a mixture of oxygen and nitrous oxide when separation of the gases can occur by nitrous oxide forming a liquid. A temperature below −7°C is required for this effect to occur in cylinders. All Entonox cylinders should therefore be kept in environments above this temperature. The Entonox pipelines have a lower pseudocritical temperature as a result of different pressures in the pipeline than in the cylinder (4.1 bar and 117 bar, respectively).

Remifentanil

Remifentanil is a μ-opioid agonist that incorporates a methyl ester group at position 1 of the piperidine ring. This makes it susceptible to rapid hydrolysis by non-specific esterases. It has a very rapid onset of action, comparable with that of alfentanil, and with similar cardiovascular effects. Remifentanil is not a substrate for pseudocholinesterase and is not associated with the release of histamine. Its advantages in obstetric anaesthesia would be to rapidly control stressful events during general anaesthesia and surgery without the risk of respiratory depression. The precise effect of remifentanil on opoid receptors is still under investigation. Its role in obstetric anaesthesia and analgesia remains unclear. The dose for this effect is not known at present [20].

Sevoflurane

Sevoflurane and desflurane have yet to be studied widely in obstetrics to establish their safety and efficacy. They are both fluorinated ethers. Sevoflurane is defluorinated by hepatic cytochromes P450 to fluoride and hexafluoroisopropanol. Serum fluoride levels of greater than 50 µmol L^{-1} have produced nephrotoxicity with methoxyflurane administration, but serum fluoride ions are not a marker of clinical significance with sevoflurane anaesthesia. No clinical evidence of renal dysfunction has been associated with the use of the drug [21], but patients with renal disease require further study. Sevoflurane has provided satisfactory anaesthesia for Caesarean section [22] but no advantages in recovery characteristics were measured.

Tramadol

Tramadol is a centrally acting synthetic analgesic with a weak affinity for opioid receptors and inhibitory actions on neuronal monoamine reuptake. It has a high oral bioavailability (> 70%) and low protein binding. It passes into breast milk and has been used to treat postCaesarean section pain [23].

References

1 Rubin PC (ed.). *Prescribing in Pregnancy*, 2nd edn. London: BMJ Publishing Group, 1995.
2 Lee JJ, Rubin AP. Breast feeding and anaesthesia. *Anaesthesia* 1993; **48**: 616–25.
3 Spigset O. Anaesthesia agents and excretion in breast milk. *Acta Anaesthesiol Scand* 1994; **38**: 94–103.
4 Hirose M, Hosokawa T, Tanaka Y. Extradural buprenorphine suppresses breast feeding after Caesarean section. *Br J Anaesth* 1997; **79**: 120–1.
5 Albright GA. Cardiac arrest following regional anesthesia with etidocaine and bupivacaine. *Anesthesiology* 1979; **51**: 285–6.
6 Lambert LA, Lambert DH, Strichartz GR. Irreversible conduction block in isolated nerve by high concentrations of local anesthetics. *Anesthesiology* 1994; **80**: 1082–93.
7 Rigler ML, Drasner K, Krejcie TC *et al.* Cauda equina syndrome after continuous spinal anesthetic. *Anesth Analg* 1991; **72**: 275–81.
8 Mazoit JX, Orhant EE, Boico O, Kantelip JP, Samii K. Myocardial uptake of bupivacaine: 1. Pharmacokinetics and pharmacodynamics of lidocaine and bupivacaine in the isolated perfused rabbit heart. *Anesth Analg* 1993; **77**: 469–76.

9. Cigarini I, Kaba A, Bonnet F et al. Epidural clonidine combined with bupivacaine for analgesia in labor. *Reg Anesth* 1995; **20**: 113–20.
10. Boutroy MJ, Gisonna C, Legagneur M, Vert P. Hypertensive crisis in infants born to clonidine treated mothers [letter]. *Clin Exp Hypertens* 1987; **6**: 261.
11. Eriksson H, Haasio J, Kortila K. Recovery from sevoflurane and isoflurane anaesthesia after outpatient gynaecological laparoscopy. *Acta Anaesthesiol Scand* 1995; **39**: 377–80.
12. Devcic A, Muzi M, Ebert TJ. The effects of clonidine on desflurane-mediated sympathoexcitation in humans. *Anesth Analg* 1995; **80**: 773–9.
13. Pasentine GG, Muzi M, Ebert TJ. Effects of fentanyl on sympathetic activation associated with the administration of desflurane. *Anesthesiology* 1995; **82**: 823–31.
14. Abboud TK, Zhu J, Richardson M, Da Silva EP, Donovan M. Desflurane: a new volatile anesthetic agent for cesarean section: maternal and neonatal effects. *Acta Anaesthesiol Scand* 1995; **39**: 723–6.
15. Abboud TK, Swart F, Zhu J, Donovan MM, Da Silva EP, Yakal K. Desflurane analgesia for vaginal delivery. *Acta Anaesthesiol Scand* 1995; **39**: 259–61.
16. Houltz E, Caidahl K, Hellstrom A, Gustavsson T, Miocco I, Ricksten SE. The effects of nitrous oxide on left ventricular systolic and diastolic performance before and after cardiopulmonary bypass: evaluation by computer-assisted two-dimensional and Doppler echocardiography in patients undergoing coronary artery surgery. *Anesth Analg* 1995; **81**: 243–8.
17. Hohner P, Reiz S. Nitrous oxide and the cardiovascular system. *Acta Anaesthesiol Scand* 1994; **38**: 763–6.
18. Donaldson D, Meechan JG. The hazards of chronic exposure to nitrous oxide: an update. *Br Dent J* 1995; **178**: 95–100.
19. Hadzic A, Glab K, Sanborn KV, Thys DM. Severe neurologic deficit after nitrous oxide anesthesia. *Anesthesiology* 1995; **83**: 863–6.
20. Hughes SC, Kan RE, Rosen MA et al. Remifentanil: ultra-short acting opioid for obstetric anesthesia. *Anesthesiology* 1996; **V85**: A894.
21. Kharasch ED, Hankins DC, Thummel KE. Human kidney methoxyflurane and sevoflurane metabolism: intrarenal fluoride production as a possible mechanism of methoxyflurane nephrotoxicity. *Anesthesiology* 1995; **82**: 689–99.
22. Gambling DR, Sharma SK, White PF, Van Beveren T, Bala AS, Gouldson R. Use of sevoflurane during elective Cesarean birth: a comparison with isoflurane and spinal anesthesia. *Anesth Analg* 1995; **81**: 90–5.
23. Sunshine A, Olson NZ, Zighelborn I, De Castro A, Minn FL. Analgesic oral efficacy of tramadol hydrochloride in postoperative pain. *Clin Pharmacol Ther* 1992; **51**: 740–6.

Index

Page numbers in **bold** refer to tables; those in *italics* to figures.

abdominal circumference *374*, 375
abdominal wall defects 382–3
abortion
   induced, anaesthesia for 327–8
      maternal mortality **23**
      rates 22
   selective, in multiple pregnancy 380
   spontaneous 326
abruptio placentae 151, 205, 416
abscess, epidural 131
acetylcholinesterase 153
acid aspiration pneumonitis 91, 95–6
   see also aspiration of gastric contents
acidosis, fetal *see* fetal acidosis
acquired immune deficiency syndrome (AIDS) 170, **181**
   see also human immunodeficiency virus
activated partial thromboplastin time (APTT) *34*, 408, 442
acute fatty liver of pregnancy **110**, 114
acute respiratory distress syndrome (ARDS) 76–7, 78–81
   in acid aspiration 91, 96
   complications 80–1
   management 79–80
   maternal deaths 25, 57
acyclovir 178, 183
Adamkiewicz, artery of 222–4
adolescent pregnancy 16–17
adrenaline *see* epinephrine
age, maternal 16–18
   chromosomal abnormalities and *374*
   maternal mortality and 17, 22
airway
   artificial, for difficult intubation 313
   emergency techniques of establishing 317–18
   fat deposition 59
   obstruction
      during sleep 64–5
      in neonates 394–5
   preoperative assessment 310–12
   resistance 61
   suction 95–6, 394, 396–7
   upper, changes in pregnancy 57–9
albumin, plasma 37–8, 109, **138**, 441
   fetal 192
   in pre-eclampsia 39
alcohol abuse 198, 201–3, 205
   anaesthetic problems 202–3
   detection **200**
alcoholic cirrhosis 110

alfentanil
   for analgesia in labour 353
   in early pregnancy 328
   epidural 252
   on induction of anaesthesia 300
   for perioperative analgesia 306
   placental transfer 192
alkaline phosphatase, plasma 109, **110**, 441
alkalinization, local anaesthetic solutions 262–3
allergic reactions 171–5
α_1-acid glycoprotein 192
α_2-adrenoceptor agonists 245–6, 445–6
alpha-fetoprotein 168
   maternal serum 373–5, 381
aminophylline 70, 72
aminotransferases, plasma 109, 441
   in liver disease **110**, 112, 113
amniocentesis 378–9
amniotic fluid 372
   embolism **23**, 76, 428–9
   index/volume 375, 389
   meconium-stained 394
   surfactant activity 378–9
amphetamine abuse 199, **200**, 207–8
anaemia, physiological, of pregnancy 32
anaesthesia
   for antepartum surgery 326–9
   care recommendations 25–6
   complications 359
   depth, measurement 319–20
   in ectopic pregnancy 329–31
   for fetal surgery 329
   maternal mortality 20, **23**, 24–6, 285
   for postpartum surgery 329
   support services 7–8
   see also general anaesthesia; regional anaesthesia
anaesthetic assistants 25, 231
   in general anaesthesia 287, 288
anaesthetic services 5–8
   facilities 6–8, 230
   guidelines 6
   staffing 6, 25, 26, 230
anaesthetists, obstetric 5–6, 25–6
analgesia
   fetal 380
   patient-controlled 308, 353
   postpartum 195–6
   see also epidural analgesia; labour, analgesia for; postoperative analgesia
anaphylactoid reactions 171, 172–5

anaphylaxis 167, 172–5
anatomy 213–25
  applied 224–5
  perivertebral 213–15
  spinal cord arteries 222–4
  vertebral canal 215–24
angiotensin-converting enzyme inhibitors 404
antacids 91–2, *295*
antenatal assessment 5, 8–9, **10**
  anaesthetic complications 359
  in diabetes 149
  perinatal mortality and 27
antenatal classes 344
antenatal screening, fetal abnormalities 380–2
antibiotics 131, 177
  in cystic fibrosis 74
  hypersensitivity reactions 173
anticholinergic agents
  in aspiration prophylaxis 95
  in cystic fibrosis 75
  in hypotension 272
  in nausea and vomiting 309
anticoagulants 49, 425–7
anticonvulsant drugs
  in epilepsy 119–20, 121
  in pre-eclampsia 411
  teratogenesis 120
antidiuretic hormone (arginine vasopressin, AVP) 102
anti-emetic drugs 308–10, 328, 444
antihistamines
  in anaphylactic reactions 173, **174**
  anti-emetic **309**
  in opioid-induced pruritus 272
antihypertensive therapy 404
  in heart disease 51
  in induction of anaesthesia 299, 300, 415
  in pre-eclampsia 407–9
  in renal disease 105
antioxidants 405–6, 407
antithrombin III (At III) 33–5
aorta
  aneurysms 49, 50
  coarctation 49, 51
  compression 44
  fetal, Doppler ultrasound 377
aortic stenosis 51, 285–6
aortocaval compression 43–5, 265
Apgar score 398
apnoea
  in labour 63
  obstructive sleep 64–5, 158
  suxamethonium 155, 305
appetite, in labour 342
arachnoid mater 216, 218
  immune function 224–5
arcuate arteries, Doppler ultrasound 377
ARDS *see* acute respiratory distress syndrome
asepsis, regional nerve block 224–5, 232–3
aspiration of gastric contents 86
  in antepartum surgery 328
  in asthma 72

clinical signs 96
  in dystrophia myotonica 130
  management 95–6
  maternal mortality 25, 91
  in postpartum surgery 329
  prophylaxis 91–5
  cricoid pressure 294–6
  high-risk pregnancies **89**, 94
  in obesity 159
  postoperative 95
  recommendations 25, 88
aspirin 407, 426
  postpartum use 443–4
  regional anaesthesia and 427–8
asthma 65–73
  acute severe, management 69–70
  anaesthesia for Caesarean section 72–3
  chronic, management 68–9
  clinical assessment 68
  fetal effects 67
  intensive care 71
  labour and delivery 71–2
  management guidelines 68–70
  pathophysiology 66–7
  severity classification **68**
atelectasis, in ARDS 80
atosiban **361**, 362
atracurium 288, 305–6
  in asthma 72
  in myasthenia gravis 129
  in renal disease 107
atrial natriuretic peptide (ANP), plasma 194
atrial septal defect 52
atropine 66, 95, 96, *295*
  in awake fibre-optic intubation 318
  in general anaesthesia 288
  in total spinal block 278
audit
  clinical 11
  maternal deaths 20–2
auditory evoked response 320
autoimmune diseases 169, 171, 175–6
autonomic hyperreflexia 126
awareness, anaesthetic 292, 301, 319–20
  detection methods 319–20
azathioprine 170, 176

back pain (backache) 434–6
  in labour 346–7, 348–9
  postpartum 195, 435–6
barbiturates
  abuse 199
  induction of anaesthesia 297–8
  in porphyria **153**
  see also thiopental
Batson, system of 224
beclomethasone, in asthma 68
benzodiazepines *295*
  abuse 199, **200**, 207
  postpartum use 444
  see also diazepam
bereavement, perinatal 27–8

β-adrenergic agonists
  in asthma 68–9, 70, 71
  in maternal diabetes 149
  in preterm labour 361–2
β-adrenergic blocking drugs 50–1, 206, 300
Bezold–Jarisch reflex 46, 265
bicarbonate, serum 62, 103
bilirubin
  amniotic fluid 378
  placental transfer 190
  plasma 109, **110**, 111–12
biochemistry, maternal 373–5, 381
biophysical profile, fetal 389
biparietal diameter *374*, 375
birth chairs 335, 336
birthing pool 351
birth weight 26, 373
bladder
  anatomy *131*
  dysfunction 130
    after regional nerve block 273
    in multiple sclerosis 127
  pain, in subarachnoid block 269
bleeding time 427–8
blood disorders, inherited 383
blood loss
  estimation 419–20, **420**
  neonatal, management 397
blood patch, epidural 274, 276–8
  in HIV infection 181
blood pressure, arterial 40–1, 403
  causes of variations 40, **42**
  in labour 403
  measurement 40–1, 403
    in epidural analgesia **258**
    in fetal distress 388
    intra-arterial 40–1, 403
    in labour 337
    in subarachnoid block 268
  regulation in pregnancy 42–3
  in renal disease 105, 107
  see also hypertension; hypotension
blood transfusion
  Caesarean section and 307
  facilities required 7–8
  in major obstetric haemorrhage 420–1
  in pre-eclampsia 409
  reducing need for 32
  refusal 424–5
blood volume 31–3
  postpartum changes 193–4, 419
body mass index (BMI) 157
Bohr effect 188–90
bradycardia
  fetal 356, 388, *390–1*
  regional analgesia-induced 46, 272
  in total spinal block 278
breast feeding 195, 443
  after Caesarean section 308
  in epilepsy 120
breast milk, drugs in 195, 308, 443–4

breathing movements, fetal 372
breech presentation 363
Broca index 157
Bromage scoring system **244**, 254–5
bronchodilators
  in acute asthma 70
  in chronic asthma 68, 69
  uterine tone effects 73
Budd–Chiari syndrome 110
bupivacaine
  combined spinal–epidural 270–1
  epidural 243, 244, 249–50
    for Caesarean section 262–3
    doses 241–2, 243, **245**
    fetal effects 260, 399
    infusions 254–5
    onset 264
    postpartum 444
    top-up doses 254, 257
  hyperbaric 266, 267
  in inadvertent dural puncture *238*
  minimum local analgesic concentration (MLAC) 249–50
  placental transfer **191**, 192
  in pre-eclampsia/eclampsia 413
  S isomer 263, 444
  subarachnoid 266, 267–8
  toxicity 444, 445
buprenorphine 353, 444
butorphanol 353
butyrophenones **309**

C1 esterase deficiency 170
Caesarean section 195–6, 285–320
  in cerebrovascular disorders 123
  combined spinal–epidural (CSE) nerve block 271
  consent 5
  in diabetes 148, 150–1
  epidural anaesthesia 260–4
    testing height of block 256–7
  general anaesthesia 285–320
  in HIV infection 180
  induction–delivery interval 301
  in multiple pregnancy 364
  patient positioning 44, 45
  perioperative analgesia 306–7
  in placenta praevia 432
  postmortem 121
  postoperative care 307–10
  in pre-eclampsia/eclampsia 414–15
  preoperative assessment 289, **290**
  rates 3–5
  subarachnoid block 266, 268–9
caffeine 119, **276**
calcium-channel blockers
  in induction of anaesthesia 300
  in pre-eclampsia 408–9
  in preterm labour **361**, 362
calcium gluconate 411, **412**
cannabis 198, 199, 200, 207
capnography (end-tidal carbon dioxide monitoring) 25, 291, 294, 299

carbohydrates 139–42
  dietary 138, 146
  metabolism 139–42
carbon dioxide
  end-tidal, monitoring 25, 291, 294, 299
  placental transport 188–90
  tension in arterial blood (Pa_{CO_2})
    in asthma **68**, 70
    maternal–fetal gradient 103
carboprost 423
cardiac function 40–6
  in labour 45–6
cardiac output 42–3
  in labour 45, 46
  monitoring 50
  postpartum 194
cardiomyopathy, hypertrophic 51
cardiopulmonary resuscitation, maternal 430–2
cardiotocography 389–92
  see also fetal heart rate (FHR), monitoring
cardiovascular system 31–53
  in laryngoscopy and intubation 299–300
  in obesity 158
  in puerperium 193–4
  stability, in epidural analgesia 263–4
cardioversion, direct current 52
carpal tunnel syndrome 132
cauda equina syndrome 126–7, **434**
caudal nerve block 213
central venous pressure (CVP) 43
  monitoring
    in heart disease 50
    in labour 43, 337
    in major obstetric haemorrhage 421
    in pre-eclampsia 409, 410–11, 414
cerebral venous sinus thrombosis 122
cerebrospinal fluid (CSF) 218
  flow
    in epidural cannulation 237, 240
    in subarachnoid anaesthesia 265–6
  leakage 276
cerebrosubarachnoid fluid shunts 123–4
cerebrovascular disorders 121–3
cervix, pain from 269, 346–7, 348
chest radiography
  in asthma 70
  changes in pregnancy 59
  in heart disease 48
chest wall compliance 60–1
chlorhexidine 172, 233
chloroform 353
chloroprocaine, epidural 261–2
chlorpheniramine 173, **174**
cholestasis, intrahepatic, of pregnancy **110**, 111–12
cholesterol, plasma 109, **138**
cholestyramine 112
cholinergic crisis 129
cholinesterase, plasma 153–5, 205, 305, 306
chorionic villus sampling 379
chromosomal abnormalities 374, 379, 381, 383
  see also Down syndrome

cimetidine 72, 93, **153**, 444
cisatracurium 306
clonidine 245–6, 445–6
coagulation 33–7
coagulopathies
  epidural analgesia in 229, 413
  in major obstetric haemorrhage 423–4
  in pre-eclampsia/eclampsia 413, 414
cocaine
  abuse 198, 199, 204–7
    anaesthesia in 205–7
    complications 199–200, 205
    detection 200
    heart disease 51
    malignant hyperthermia 156
  alcohol/drug interactions 203, 205
  metabolism 154, 199, 205
  topical, for awake intubation 319
codeine 196, 308
cold temperature discrimination testing 255–6, **258**
colloid osmotic pressure 38–9, 441
combined spinal–epidural (CSE) nerve block 213, 227, 269–71
  for Caesarean section 271
  for labour 246, 269–71
  in obesity 161
  in pre-eclampsia/eclampsia 415
  versus subarachnoid block 264
common peroneal nerve 134
community services 14–16
congenital heart disease 46, 47, 52, 382
congenital malformations 120, 145–6, 382–3
consent
  informed 8, **9**, 289–90
  to epidural analgesia 228–9, 230–1
constipation 97, 195
convulsions 119–21
  in amniotic fluid embolism 428
  in eclampsia 411–12, 415
  treatment 121
corticosteroids see steroids
cortisol, serum 66, 168
craniotomy, after Caesarean section 123
C-reactive protein (CRP) 165, 167, 229
creatine kinase (isoenzymes) 195, 441
creatinine 101–2, 104–5, 194
cricoid pressure 294–7
  in difficult/failed intubation 316, 317
cricothyrotomy 313, 316, 317–18
critical care see high-dependency/intensive care
cromoglycate 68, 174–5
crown–rump length 374, 375
Cumberledge report 11–14
cystic fibrosis 73–5, 383
cytokines 165, 167, 417

dantrolene 130, 156
depression 134
dermatomes 345, 348
desflurane **302,** 446
dexmedetomidine 245–6, 445

dextrose solutions 121, 147–8, 231, 341
  in neonatal resuscitation **395**, 397
diabetes mellitus 74, 142–51
  anaesthetic management 149–51
  combined specialist care 146–7
  complications 144–5, 149, 151
  gestational 139, 141, 142–3, **144**
    risk factors **144**
  infants of mothers with 139, 148, 373
  labour in 147–8
  management 145–51
  peripartum transfer 15
diabetic ketoacidosis 146–7, 149
diamorphine (heroin) **243**
  abuse 203
  for analgesia in labour 352
  combined spinal–epidural 271
  epidural *238*, 243, **245**, 252, 254, 262
  subarachnoid 251–2, 266
Diazemuls 121, 411, 412
diazepam
  abuse 207
  in eclampsia 411, 412
  in epilepsy 120, 121
diazoxide 409
diclofenac 308
diet
  in gestational diabetes 146
  in labour 87, 88, 342
digoxin 51
Dinamap 40–1, 403
disseminated intravascular coagulation (DIC) 36, 416–17
  in amniotic fluid embolism 428–9
  in major obstetric haemorrhage 423–4
diuresis
  postpartum 194
  recumbent, in normal pregnancy 38
diuretics 39–40, 50–1, 409
domiciliary obstetrics 14–16
dopamine 410, 423
Doppler ultrasound 376–7
dorsal columns *223*, 349
Down syndrome 383
  age-related risk 17, *374*
  maternal blood sampling 373–5, 381
  prenatal diagnosis 378
dressing packs, for epidural analgesia 246
droperidol 300, **309**
drug abuse 198–209
drugs 443–8
  in breast milk 195, 308, 443–4
  pK_a values 191–2, 262
  placental transfer 191–2
  prescribing in pregnancy 443
  unlicensed 227
dural puncture
  inadvertent 275–8
    detection 237, 241
    epidural catheters 240
    management plan 237, *238*
  needle bevel orientation 219, 238
dural sac 216, 218–19

dura mater 216, 224–5
dynorphin 344
dysrhythmias
  fetal 388, *390–1*
  in pregnant women 52, 286
dystrophia myotonica 129–30, 155

eating, in labour 87, 88, 342
echocardiography
  in heart disease 48
  transoesophageal (TOE) 48, 50
eclampsia 119, 404, 411–12
  anaesthetic management 413–15
  recurrent convulsions 412–13
  transfers 16
ectopic pregnancy 327, 329–31
  maternal mortality **23**, 329
  ruptured 330–1
edrophonium 129
Eisenmenger's syndrome 52
elderly parturient 17–18
electrocardiography (ECG)
  in eclampsia 411
  fetal 386
  in general anaesthesia 291
  in heart disease 48, 50
  in labour 337
electrolytes 102–3, 190, **191**, 441
embolism
  air 77, 291–2
  amniotic fluid **23**, 76, 428–9
  see also pulmonary embolism; thromboembolism
emergency services 12
emphysema, subcutaneous 77, 366
endocarditis 47
endothelial dysfunction, in pre-eclampsia 405–6, 407
endotoxin 176–7
endotracheal intubation 72, 299–300
  awake fibre-optic 318–19
  cardiovascular responses 299–300, 415
  difficult 310–13, 315–18
  extubation **316**
  failed 24–5, 313–18
  in obesity 159, 161, 311
  in pre-eclampsia/eclampsia 311, 415
  in rapid-sequence induction 293–4
endotracheal tubes 299
  confirming position 294, 299
  for difficult intubation 313, 316
energy requirements 137, 138
enflurane 72, **153**, 181, **302**, 303
  for analgesia in labour 356
Entonox 161, 260, 354, 355
  maternal and fetal effects 355
  storage at low temperatures 447
  see also nitrous oxide
ephedrine 153, 263–4, 268, 272, 288
  in anaphylaxis 173, 174
  in cocaine abuse 205, **206**, 207
  in fetal distress 394
  in heart disease 49, 51

INDEX   455

in pre-eclampsia/eclampsia 414
in reflex bradycardia 46
in renal disease **106**, 107
risks 81
in total spinal block 278
epidural abscess 131, 229
epidural anaesthesia
   for Caesarean section 260–4
   in eclampsia/pre-eclampsia 414
epidural analgesia 213, 227, 242–60, 351
   ambulatory 335
   anticoagulant therapy and 426–7
   asepsis 232–3, 246
   in back pain **435**
   back pain after 436
   cardiovascular effects 46
   complications 271–8
   consent 228–9, 230–1
   contraindications 228–30
   extension for Caesarean section 261–4
   fetal effects 260
   fetal heart rate monitoring 259–60, 389–92
   in heart disease 49, 230
   in herpes simplex infections 184
   history 243–4
   in hypertension 404
   indications in labour 228
   infusions 253–5, **258**
   maintenance in labour 259–60
   onset time 263, 264
   patient-controlled (PCEA) 245, 246
   patient position 116, 231–2
   pharmacological adjuvants 245–6
   physiological changes and 116
   in pre-eclampsia/eclampsia 404, 413, **414**
   preparation for 230–42
   regimens 245–6
   in spinal cord injury 126
   technique 233–42
   test doses 241–2, 243
   testing height of block 255–7, **258**
   top-up injections 254, 257, **258**
   see also combined spinal–epidural (CSE) nerve block
epidural blood patch *see* blood patch, epidural
epidural catheters 240–1, 248–9
   checking position 260
   closed- and open-ended 248–9
   insertion 44, 239–41
   removal **258**, 273, 426
   re-siting, in dural puncture 275
epidural haematoma 229, 426, 427–8
epidural needles 247
   bevel orientation 238
   for combined spinal–epidural block 270
   insertion techniques 233–9
epidural space
   anatomy 215–16, *217*, 218–19, *220*
   catheterization 239–41
   crystalloid infusions 275
   identification 234, 236–7, 239

lateral approach 233
midline approach 233–5
paramedian approach 239
pressures 116
venous plexus (of Batson) 224
   inadvertent puncture 240–1
epilepsy 22, 119–21, 303
epinephrine (adrenaline) 327
   in anaphylaxis 173, 174, 175
   in cocaine abuse **206**, 207
   in epidural anaesthesia/analgesia 242, 252, 262, 263
   in maternal resuscitation 432
   in neonatal resuscitation 395, 397
   in pre-eclampsia/eclampsia 413, 414
   in sickle-cell disorders 33
episiotomy 195–6, 363
epoprostenol 52
equipment
   for difficult intubation 312–13
   for epidural analgesia 246–9
   for general anaesthesia 287, 288
   haemorrhage trolley **422**
   for inhalational analgesia 353
   neonatal resuscitation **395**
   operating theatre 7
   for regional anaesthesia 231
   universal precautions 182
ergometrine 340
   in major obstetric haemorrhage 423
   pulmonary oedema risk 81
   in renal disease **106**
esmolol 409
ethyl chloride spray 255, **258**
etomidate **120**, 298
exercise, respiratory function during 62–3

face masks
   protective 233
   for ventilation 315, 317
fat
   airway deposition 59
   body 157
   vertebral canal 218
fatty acids, free, plasma **138**
fatty liver of pregnancy, acute **110**, 114
feeding, in labour 88, 342
femoral nerve lesions 133
femur length *374*, 375
fentanyl
   abuse 203
   for analgesia in labour 353
   combined spinal–epidural 270–1
   in early pregnancy 328
   epidural 244, **245**, 252
      for Caesarean section 262
      fetal effects 260, 399
      infusions 254
   on induction of anaesthesia 300
   in opioid drug abusers 204
   for perioperative analgesia 306
   pharmacokinetics **243**
   placental transfer 191–2

fetal abnormalities 380–3
  see also chromosomal abnormalities; congenital malformations
fetal acidosis 389, 392–3
  drug transfer in 191–2
fetal alcohol syndrome 201
fetal blood sampling 379, 392–3
fetal heart rate (FHR)
  beat-to-beat variability 386–8
  decelerations 388
  dysrhythmias 388, *390–1*
  monitoring 386
    in epidural analgesia 259–60, 389–92
    in labour 389–92
    in umbilical cord prolapse 365
fetal hypoxia 45, 67, 371–2
  intrapartum diagnosis 392–3
fetal surgery 329
fetal therapy 371, 379–80
fetus
  activity (movements) 372
  assessment methods 372–9
  biophysical profile 389
  growth/weight 372–3
  high-risk 386–94
  intrauterine resuscitation 394
  monitoring 371, 389–94
fever 177–8
fibrin 33, 37
fibrin degradation products (FDPs) 33, 36, 416–17, 424
fibrinogen 36, 155, 167–8, 442
fibrinolysis 33, 35–6
filters
  bacterial 241
  inferior vena cava 427
fluids
  body 31–40
  extracellular 37–40
  intravenous
    in fetal distress 394
    in hypotension 272
    in major obstetric haemorrhage 423
    in pre-eclampsia 409–11
    pulmonary oedema risk 39, 81
    in regional analgesia 231
    in renal disease 107
  in labour 88, 341–2
  in neonatal resuscitation 397
  in pre-eclampsia 409–10, 414
fluoride ions 448
folic acid 138, 326
foot drop 134
fungal infections, oral 181
furosemide (frusemide) 39, 123, 410, 423

gastric emptying 86–8
  physical methods 94–5
  postpartum 88–9, 329
gastric secretions 89, 93–5
gastrointestinal system 86–97
  changes in obesity 158
  symptoms in pregnancy 96–7

gastro-oesophageal reflux 72, 90, 328
general anaesthesia 285–320
  aspiration prophylaxis 91
  in asthma 72–3
  awareness during *see* awareness, anaesthetic
  complications 310–20
  in eclampsia/pre-eclampsia 415
  equipment, staff and facilities 287–8
  in heart disease 49
  indications 285–7
  induction–delivery interval 301
  maternal mortality 24–5, 285
  monitoring during **288**, 291–2
  in obesity 160
  oxygenation 300–1
  preoperative evaluation 289, **290**
  preoxygenation 292–3
  preparation for 287–92
  risk information 289–90
  see also endotracheal intubation
general practitioners 14, 15
genetic disorders 383
  see also chromosomal disorders
genital tract trauma 340
globulins, plasma **138**
glomerular filtration rate (GFR) 101–2
gloves 182, 184, 275
glucocorticoids 167, 170
  see also steroids
glucose 139–41
  blood 441
    control in diabetes 146
    measurements 143, 146
    regulation 140, 142
  CSF 237
  renal threshold 141
  solutions *see* dextrose solutions
  tolerance test 143–4
glyceryl trinitrate (nitroglycerine)
  in acute inversion of uterus 340
  in constriction of cervix 341
  in induction of anaesthesia 300
  in pre-eclampsia 409
  in preterm labour **361**, 362
glycopyrrolate 72, 95, 444
glycosuria 141, 143
guidelines, clinical 6

haematocrit 32, 441
haemodialysis, long-term 105–6
haemoglobin (Hb) 32, 441
  C 32
  glycosylated (HbA1c) 141, 146
  oxygen affinity, fetal 188–90
  see also sickle-cell disorders
haemolysis, elevated liver enzymes and low platelet count *see* HELLP syndrome
haemolytic anaemia, autoimmune 169
haemorrhage
  antepartum 419
  blood transfusion refusal 424–5
  in Caesarean section 307
  cerebrovascular 122

INDEX 457

facilities/equipment for 7–8, **422**
  in HELLP syndrome 113
  major obstetric 23–4, 419–24
  maternal mortality 22–4
  neonatal resuscitation 397
  in older women 17
  in placenta praevia 432
  postpartum 36–7, 194, 340–1, 419
  in ruptured ectopic pregnancy 330
haemorrhoids 97, 195
haemostasis, at delivery 36–7
Haldane effect *189*, 190
hallucinogens 208–9
halothane 116, 302, 303
  in asthma 71, 72
  in cocaine abuse 206
  in obesity 158
hanging drop technique 236
Hartmann's solution 409
head, intubation and 299, 311, 315
headache 117–19
  causes **117**
  postdural puncture 117–18, 275
    clinical features **277**
    in HIV infection 180–1
    pathophysiology 219, 238
    prophylaxis 275–8
  postpartum 117–18, 195
heart and lung transplantation 74
heartburn 90
heart disease 31, 46–53
  congenital 46, 47, 52, 382
  cyanotic 52, 53
  epidural analgesia 49, 230
  general anaesthesia 285–6
  ischaemic 47, 51
  labour in 337
  obstetric anaesthesia 49–53, 285–6
  prevalence 46–7
  risk assessment 47–8
heart failure
  congestive 410
  right-sided, in cystic fibrosis 74–5
heart rate
  in epidural analgesia 242
  in labour 45, 46
  in neonatal resuscitation 395
  postpartum 194
  in pregnancy 42, 49
heart valves, prosthetic 49
HELLP syndrome **110**, 112–14, 148, 404, 417
heparin 424, 428
  low molecular weight 426, 427
  in pulmonary embolism 427
  thromboembolism prophylaxis 425–7
hepatic vein thrombosis 110
hepatitis, viral 109, **110**, 182–3
  hepatitis B 178, 182–3
  hepatitis C 183
  hepatitis E 183
hepatobiliary system 109–14
heroin *see* diamorphine

herpes simplex 183–4
high-dependency/intensive care 25, 366
  in acute respiratory failure 76–7
  in asthma 71
  in drug abuse 199, **201**
  in heart disease 52–3
high-frequency oscillatory ventilation 71
high-risk fetus 386–94
high-risk pregnancies **89**, 288
  aspiration prophylaxis 94
  Caesarean section 359
histamine H_2-receptor antagonists 91, **92**, 93–4
  recommendations 25, 88
HIV *see* human immunodeficiency virus
home births 12, 14
Huber tip 247
human immunodeficiency virus (HIV) 170, 178, 179–82
  high-risk patients 179–80
  infection
    anaesthesia in 180–1
    clinical features 180, **181**
  prevention of occupational exposure 181–2
  vertical transmission 180
hydralazine **153**, 408
hydrocephalus 123–4
hydrocortisone
  in anaphylactic reactions 173, **174**
  in asthma 70, 72
hydrostatic pressure, interstitial 39
5-hydroxytryptamine type 3 (5-HT) antagonists 309
hyoscine 95, 309
  for awake fibre-optic intubation 318
  in early pregnancy 328
hyperemesis gravidarum 96, 111
hyperglycaemia 141
hyperkalaemia
  in haemodialysis patients 106
  in malignant hyperthermia 156
  in neurological disorders 125
hypersensitivity reactions 167–8, 171–5
hypertension 403–4
  chronic pre-existing 303, 403–4
  in cocaine abuse 206
  pregnancy-induced 404
  in renal disease 105, 107
  response to intubation 299, 300, 415
hypertensive disorders in pregnancy 31, 403–17
  management **23**
  maternal mortality 22, **23**
  in older women 17
  see also pre-eclampsia
hyperthermia, malignant 155–6
hyperthyroidism 152
hypertrophic cardiomyopathy 51
hyperventilation 61, 63, 350
hypoalbuminaemia 39, 109
hypoglycaemia
  maternal 148
  neonatal 148

hypotension
    in anaphylactic reactions 172–3
    contraindicating epidural analgesia 230
    definition 272
    oxytocin-associated 340
    in regional nerve block **258**, 263–4, 265, 268, 271–2
    spinal cord ischaemia 222–4
    supine 43–5
    in total spinal block 278
    treatment, pulmonary oedema risk 81
hypothyroidism 151, 152–3
hypoxia/hypoxaemia
    in ARDS 78
    fetal *see* fetal hypoxia
    in inhalational analgesia 355
    in labour 63–4
    in sleep 65
hysterectomy, in obstetric haemorrhage 424

ibuprofen 308
iliac crests, superior border 213, *214*
immunity 165–78
    clinical disorders 170–8
    fetomaternal relationships 168–70
    spinal meninges and 224–5
immunoglobulins 67, **166**, 169, 171–2
immunosuppressive therapy 170, 176
incontinence, stress 130, 196
indomethacin 361
induction agents, intravenous 297–9
infections 178–84
    autologous blood patch and 181
    epidural analgesia risk 229
    fetal 178
    precautions for staff 182
    see also sepsis
inferior vena cava
    compression 43–4, 265
    filters 427
information
    for informed consent 8, **9**
    risk 26, 289–90
inhalational agents 301–3
    in asthma 72
    in failed intubation 315
    fetal effects 302–3, 326, 355–6
    malignant hyperthermia 156
    minimum alveolar concentration (MAC) 116, 292, 302
    monitors 292
    postpartum use 444
    see also individual agents
inhalational analgesia 353–6
    equipment 353
    maternal and fetal effects 355–6
    patient-controlled intermittent (PCIIA) 353, 354–5
    volatile anaesthetic agents 354–5
    see also Entonox
insulin 142
    administration 147–8
    resistance, peripheral 139, 141
    secretion 139, 141

intensive care *see* high-dependency/intensive care
interleukins 165, 167
intermittent positive pressure ventilation (IPPV)
    in acid aspiration 95–6
    in asthma 71
    in neonatal resuscitation 396, 397
    in prolonged neuromuscular blockade 305
    in pulmonary oedema 81
internal jugular vein **50**
interspinous ligament 214, *215*
    local anaesthetic infiltration 233
    Tuohy needle resistance 234
intra-arterial catheters 50, 337, 421
intracranial pressure, increases in 123, **124**
intrahepatic cholestasis of pregnancy **110**, 111–12
intrathecal anaesthesia *see* subarachnoid block
intrauterine growth retardation 64, 372, 373
intravenous access *see* venous access
intravenous anaesthesia, total 328–9
intravenous fluids *see* fluids, intravenous
intravenous induction agents 297–9
introducers, endotracheal tube 313
intubation *see* endotracheal intubation
IPPV *see* intermittent positive pressure ventilation
ipratropium 70
iron 138
ischaemic heart disease 47, 51
isoflurane 302, 303, 326
    anaesthetic awareness and 319
    for analgesia in labour 354, 355, 356
    in asthma 72
    minimum alveolar concentration (MAC) 116
    properties **302**
    in renal disease 107
isolated forearm technique 319
itching *see* pruritus

jaundice 109, 111–12
jaw mobility, intubation and 311, **312**

ketamine 298, 446–7
    in asthma 72
    in cocaine abuse **206**
    in epilepsy **120**
    in HIV infection 181
    malignant hyperthermia 156
    in placental abruption 416
    in ruptured ectopic pregnancy 330
ketonuria, in labour 341
kidneys
    anatomical changes 100
    plasma osmolality and 102
Korotkoff phases 40

labetalol 404
    in cocaine abuse 206
    in induction of anaesthesia 300
    in pre-eclampsia 409, 415
laboratory facilities 8

labour 335–56
  active management 337–41
  analgesia for 342–56
    choice 350–1
    combined spinal–epidural (CSE) nerve
      block 269–71
    during transfers 360
    epidural nerve block 242–60
    inhalational analgesia 353–6
    methods **343**
    in obesity 161
    in opioid drug abusers 204
    paracervical block 356
    in pre-eclampsia/eclampsia 413–14
    systemic opioids 352–3
  carbohydrate metabolism 142
  cardiac function changes 45–6
  complications in 359–66
  diet in 87, 88, 342
  fetal monitoring 371, 389–94
  fluid balance 341
  gastric emptying 87–8
  induction 71, 147, 359
  informed consent during 8
  in maternal diabetes 147–8, 149–50
  mobility 335–6
  monitoring during 336–7
  nausea and vomiting 96, 274
  pain 344–50
    intensity 344–5
    mechanisms 344–9
    pathophysiological responses 349–50
  preterm 360–3
  respiratory physiology 63–4
  third stage, active management 340–1
  trial of 359
labour ward
  obstetric anaesthesia services 6–7
  support services 7–8
  telemetry 378
lactate 139
laminectomy, decompression 426
laparoscopic surgery 329, 330–1
laryngeal mask airways (LMA) 313
  blind intubation via 317
  cricoid pressure application 297
  in failed intubation 315, 317
laryngoscopes, for difficult intubation 312–13
laryngoscopy
  cardiovascular responses 299–300
  Cormack–Lehane (C & L) scale 316
  in difficult intubation 315, 316
larynx
  changes in pregnancy 57–9
  local anaesthesia 319
lateral decubitus position
  in failed intubation 316
  in fetal distress 394
  in labour 335
  regional nerve block 214, 231–2
  in umbilical cord prolapse 365
lateral position, subarachnoid block 266–7
lateral tilt position 44, 45
latex allergy 172

laudanosine 306
lecithin/sphingomyelin (L/S) ratio 378
levobupivacaine 262, 263
lidocaine 73, 250
  in cocaine abuse 206
  epidural, for Caesarean section 262, 263
  on induction of anaesthesia 300
  placental transfer **191**
  in pre-eclampsia/eclampsia 413
  topical, for awake intubation 318–19
  toxicity 444, 445
ligamentum flavum 214, *215*, 234
  see also supraspinous ligament
lignocaine see lidocaine
lipids
  peroxidation, in pre-eclampsia 405–6
  plasma **138**
lipid solubility, placental transfer and 192
liver
  physiological changes 109
  rupture 112, 113
  transplantation 110
liver disease 109–14
  chronic 110
  pre-eclampsia-associated 112–14
  pregnancy-specific 111–12
liver function tests 109, **110**, 112, 441
local anaesthetics
  alkalinization of solutions 262–3
  allergic reactions 173
  epidural 244, 245, 249–50
    test doses 241–2
  infiltration, for epidural analgesia 233, 239
  mechanisms of action 348
  minimum local analgesic concentration
    (MLAC) 249–50
  physicochemical properties **262**
  placental transfer 192
  topical, for awake intubation 318–19
  toxicity 127, 444–5
  see also bupivacaine; lidocaine; prilocaine;
    procaine; ropivacaine
loss of resistance 236–7, 239
low birth weight infants 17, 360, 363
  see also intrauterine growth retardation
Luer–Lok syringe 246–7, 266
lumbar disc prolapse, acute 126–7
lumbar interspaces 213, 231–2
lung
  acute injury 78
  maturity, fetal, estimation 378–9
  volumes 59–60
lung function
  in obesity 158, 159
  peak expiratory flow (PEF) rates 66–7, *69*,
    70
  postpartum 194
  in pregnancy 57, 59–63
lysergic acid diethylamine (LSD) **200**, 208–9

magnesium sulphate
  in eclampsia 411–12, 415
  hazards in myasthenia gravis 129
  in induction of anaesthesia 300

magnesium sulphate (*cont.*)
  in preterm labour 362
  in renal disease **106**
  toxicity **412**
magnesium trisilicate 91
malignant hyperthermia 155–6
Mallampati score 310, 311
mandible, receding **312**
mannitol 123
Marfan syndrome 49
maternal health 3
maternal mortality 20–6
  anaesthesia 20, **23**, 24–6, 285
  aspiration of gastric contents 25, 91
  definition of terms **21**
  in developing countries 3, 20
  ectopic pregnancy **23**, 329
  late **21**, 25
  in obesity 158
  in older women 17, 22
  rates 21–2
maternity services 3–18
  adolescent pregnancy 16–17
  elderly parturient 17–18
  international issues 3–5
  maternal choices 11–14
  UK policies 5–16
measles 178
meconium aspiration 396–7
meconium-stained amniotic fluid 394
membranes, artificial rupture 337
Mendelson's syndrome 91, 95
meninges 224–5
meningitis 225, 274–5
meptazinol 352
meralgia paraesthetica 132
metabolism
  disorders 142–61
  inborn errors 378, 379
  in pregnancy 137–42
metaraminol 51
methadone 199, 203–4
methionine synthetase 326, 447
methohexital **120**, 298
methoxamine 49, 52, 268
methoxyflurane 353, 354
methyldopa 404, 407
metoclopramide 94, *295*
  aspiration prophylaxis 91, **92**
  in early pregnancy 328
  in obesity 159
  suxamethonium interaction 155, 305
micturition, disturbances of 130
midazolam 444
middle cerebral artery, fetal 377
midwives 14, 15
  domiciliary care 14
  in epidural analgesia 253, 273
    care guidelines **258**, 259
    top-up injections 257, **258**
  pethidine injections 351
mini-tracheostomy *see* cricothyrotomy
mitral stenosis 47, 50–1, 285–6

mivacurium 154, 306
monitoring
  fetal *see* fetus, monitoring
  in general anaesthesia **288**, 291–2
  in labour 336–7
  in major obstetric haemorrhage 421
  operating theatre 7
  in pre-eclampsia 408
  recommendations 25, 26
mood disorders 134
morphine
  for analgesia in labour 352
  epidural 244, **245**
  fetal effects 399
  in herpes simplex infections 184
  for perioperative analgesia 306–7
  pharmacokinetics **243**
  postoperative analgesia 308
  subarachnoid 251
motor function, abnormal **124**, 125–30
motor nerve blockade
  Bromage scoring system **244**, 254–5
  in combined spinal–epidural block 270
  in epidural analgesia 244, 254–5
mouth
  breathing 59
  opening 310–11
multiple pregnancy 364
  plasma volume 31
  selective fetal reduction 380
  vaginal delivery 364
multiple sclerosis 125, 127–8
muscle relaxants 303–6
  in asthma 72
  depolarizing 304–5
  hypersensitivity reactions 172
  in myasthenia gravis 129
  non-depolarizing 305–6
  placental transfer 192, 306
  postpartum use 444
  in renal disease **106**, 107
muscle weakness **124**, 125, 128
muscular dystrophies 125, 155
musculoskeletal disorders 9, 196, 305
myasthenia gravis 128–9, **176**
  neonatal 129, 169
myasthenic crisis 129
myocardial infarction 47
myotonic dystrophy 129–30, 155

nalbuphine 353
naloxone
  in neonatal resuscitation **395**, 396, 398
  in opioid-induced pruritus 272
narcotics *see* opioids
nasal stuffiness 57, 64
nasogastric tubes 59
nasopharyngeal airways 313
nausea and vomiting 96
  in labour 96, 274
  opioid-associated 274
  in patient-controlled analgesia 308
  postoperative 308–10

INDEX

neck
  position, for intubation 299
  short **312**
needle-stick injuries 181–2
needle-through-needle technique 270
neonatal deaths 26
neonates
  of cocaine-abusing mothers 207
  of diabetic mothers 139, 148, 373
  of epileptic mothers 120
  neurobehavioural scores 399
  opioid withdrawal effects 203, **204**
  resuscitation 394–8
  scoring systems 398–9
neostigmine 128, 153–4
  in asthma 72
  placental transfer 192
nerve damage
  in subarachnoid block 265
  traumatic 132–4
nerve roots
  connective tissue coverings 220–1, *222*
  lesions 132–4
  pain **434**
nerve stimulator 292, 306
neural tube defects 373–5, 381
neurobehavioural scores, neonates 399
neuroleptic-like syndrome, malignant 156
neurological disorders 116–24
  classification **117**
  epidural analgesia and 230
  general anaesthesia 286–7
neuromuscular blockade
  evaluating recovery 292
  prolonged 154, 155, 305
  reversal 72, 305, 306
neuromuscular blocking drugs *see* muscle relaxants
nifedipine
  in induction of anaesthesia 300
  in porphyria **153**
  in pre-eclampsia 408–9
  in preterm labour **361**, 362
nitrogen washout 293
nitroglycerine *see* glyceryl trinitrate
nitrous oxide 301–2, 303, 447
  in air embolism 77
  anaesthetic awareness and 319
  for analgesia in labour 351, 353, 354
  in pneumothorax/subcutaneous emphysema 77
  properties **302**
  side-effects 447
  teratogenesis 326
  see also Entonox
nociceptive threshold, in pregnancy 344
nocturia, pregnancy-related 38
non-steroidal anti-inflammatory agents
  hazards 71, 104, **106**, 119, 275
  mechanisms of action 348
  perioperative analgesia 307
  postoperative analgesia 308–9
  postpartum analgesia 196, 444

norpethidine 352
nutrition 138
  in cystic fibrosis 73

obesity 157–61
  anaesthesia in 159–61
  endotracheal intubation 159, 311
  epidural analgesia 234–5, 239
  measures 157
  perivertebral anatomy 213–14
  physiology and pharmacology 157–9
obstetric anaesthetists 5–6, 25–6
Obstetric Anaesthetists' Association, minimum data set 11, **12–13**
obstetric interventions, international comparisons 3–5
obturator nerve lesions 132, 133
occupational risks 181–2, 246
oedema
  airway 311, 415
  in normal pregnancy 38–9
  in pre-eclampsia 405
  susceptibility 102
oesophagus
  rupture 297
  sphincters 90–1, 294–6
oestrogens 35, 42, 57, 373
  metabolic effects 141, 154–5
oligohydramnios 372
omeprazole **92**, 94
oncotic pressure, plasma 410
ondansetron 309
opioids
  abuse 199, **200**, 203–4
  analgesia in labour 352–3
  combined spinal–epidural 270–1
  in dystrophia myotonica 130
  endogenous 344, 349
  epidural 243, 244, 250–3
    for Caesarean section 262
    complications 272–3
    fetal effects 260
    regimens **245**, 246
  fetal effects 260, 299–300
  gastric motility and 87, 88
  in herpes simplex infections 184
  immune effects 167
  on induction of anaesthesia 300, 415
  mechanisms of action 348
  in myasthenia gravis 129
  in obesity 161
  perioperative analgesia 306–7
  pharmacokinetics **243**
  postoperative analgesia 308
  postpartum use 443–4
  in renal disease **106**, 107
  in sleep apnoea 65
  subarachnoid 250–3, 266
    complications 272–3
  withdrawal symptoms 203, **204**
  see also alfentanil; diamorphine; fentanyl; morphine; pethidine; sufentanil
oral contraceptives 35, 112, 154–5

oral fluids *see* fluids
orogastric tube **92**, 94–5
osmolality, plasma 102
oxprenolol 409
oxygen
 administration 70, 174, 394
 consumption 63
 partial pressure 61, **68**
 placental transport 188–90
 saturation, fetal blood (Sao$_2$) 393
oxygenation
 before induction of anaesthesia 292–3
 during general anaesthesia 300–1
 in eclampsia 411
 in sickle-cell disorders 33
 tissue, in ARDS 80
 see also oxygen, administration
oxytocin 288
 fluid therapy and 121, 231
 hypersensitivity reactions 173
 inhibitors **361**, 362, 416–17
 in labour management 337–40, 394
 in major obstetric haemorrhage 423
 pulmonary oedema and 39
 in third stage of labour 340
 uterine hyperstimulation 365

pain
 central pathways 348–9
 in epidural analgesia/anaesthesia 259–60, 264
 in epidural catheterization 235
 labour *see* labour, pain
 pathophysiological responses 349–50
 postpartum 195–6
 prolapsed/thrombosed haemorrhoids 97
 relief *see* analgesia
 sensation testing 261
 somatic, in labour 345–6, 348
 in subarachnoid block 265
 visceral 345–7, 348–9
pancreatic function, in cystic fibrosis 73, 74
pancuronium 305–6
paracervical block 356
paracetamol 88, 119, 434
 postoperative analgesia 308
 postpartum 196, 444
paravertebral space 216
partogram 336–7, *338–9*
patella reflex 411
patient-controlled analgesia 308, 353
patient-controlled epidural analgesia (PCEA) 245, 246
patient-controlled intermittent inhalational analgesia (PCIIA) 353, 354–5
periaqueductal grey 349
perinatal mortality 17, 26–8
peripheral nerve disorders 131–4
pethidine 351, 352
 adverse effects 172, 274
 in asthma 72
 in breast milk 308
 combined with Entonox 355
 gastric motility and 87

 in opioid drug abusers 204
 pharmacokinetics **243**, **245**
 placental transfer 191–2
 postpartum use 443–4
 risks with epidural/spinal opioids 273
pH
 blood 188, 191
  fetal 191, 392
 local anaesthetics 262
pharmacology 443–8
pharynx
 changes in pregnancy 57–9
 suction 95–6, 394, 396–7
phencyclidine **200**, 208
phenothiazines 309
phenylephrine 52, 268
phenytoin 120, 121
pia 224
pial blood vessels 222
pinprick sensation testing 255–6, 261
pK_a values 191–2, 262
placenta 188
 abruption 151, 205, 416
 accreta 432
 hormones 194, 373
 praevia 22–3, 432
 retained 340–1
 transport 188–92
 ultrasound scan 375
placental site
 continued bleeding 340–1
 haemostatic mechanisms 36–7
plasma
 fresh frozen 305, 424
 osmolality 102
 volume 31
plasmin 35
plasminogen activators 35–6
platelets 36
 counts 442
 in postpartum haemostasis 37
 in pre-eclampsia 405–6
plica mediana dorsalis (dorsal midline septum) *217*, 219
pneumomediastinum 77
pneumonia, viral 178
pneumothorax 77, 366
 in ARDS 80
polyhydramnios 372
porphyria, acute intermittent 153
position, patient
 aortocaval compression 43–5
 blood pressure variability and *41*
 in difficult/failed intubation 316, 317
 in endotracheal intubation 299
 in hypotension 272
 in labour 335–6
 in maternal resuscitation 430
 in obesity 160–1
 for regional analgesia 116, 214, 231–2
 respiratory function and 57, 60
 sodium excretion and 102–3
 for subarachnoid block 266–7
 see also lateral decubitus position

postoperative analgesia 307–8
   in opioid drug abusers 204
   in pre-eclampsia/eclampsia 415
postoperative care 307–10
postpartum period *see* puerperium
povidone iodine 233
pre-eclampsia 404–17
   anaesthetic management 413–15
   ARDS 78
   aspiration prophylaxis 94
   cardiovascular changes 31
   clinical presentation 405, **406**
   complications 415–17
   differential diagnosis **405**
   difficult intubation 311, 415
   general anaesthesia 286, 303
   liver disorders 112–14
   management 407–11
   mild 407
   pathophysiology 405–7
   peripartum transfer 16
   plasma cholinesterase activity 155
   prevention 407
   pulmonary oedema risk 39–40, 410
   severe 408–11
pregnancy, anaesthesia in 326–9
preimplantation diagnosis 381–2
preoperative assessment 289, **290**
preoxygenation 292–3
preterm infants 373
   adolescent pregnancy 17
   care 362–3
   pathophysiology 371, 372
preterm labour 360–3
   anaesthesia for delivery 362–3
   tocolytics 360–2
prilocaine, topical 318–19
procaine 154
prochlorperazine 96, 309
progesterone
   gastrointestinal effects 90
   metabolic effects 141
   protein binding of drugs and 110
   renal effects 102
   respiratory effects 62, 66
prokinetic drugs **92**, 94
   see also metoclopramide
propofol 298–9
   in early pregnancy 328–9
   in malignant hyperthermia 156
propranolol, in cocaine abuse 206
prostacyclin 52, 405–6, 407
prostaglandins 71, 167, 340
   cardiac output and 42
   in major obstetric haemorrhage 423
prostaglandin synthesis inhibitors 361
protein C 33–5
protein S 33–5
proteins
   dietary requirements 138
   plasma 37–40, **138**
      see also albumin, plasma; α1-acid
         glycoprotein
proteinuria 405

prothrombin time (PT) *34*, 408, 442
proton-pump inhibitors **92**, 94
pruritus 111–12
   after epidural/spinal opioids 272
   in herpes simplex infections 184
pubic symphysis 195
puerperium 193–6
   gastric motility 88–9, 329
   morbidity 195–6
   in obesity 161
   physiological changes 193–5
   prescribing in 443–4
   role of obstetric anaesthetist 5
   surgery in 329
pulmonary artery catheterization 50, 78
pulmonary blood flow 63
pulmonary capillary pressure 39, 63, 81
pulmonary circulation 63
pulmonary dynamics 60–3
pulmonary embolism 76, 425, 427
   maternal mortality 22, **23**, 158
pulmonary hypertension 47, 51–2
pulmonary mechanics 60–1
pulmonary oedema 81–2
   β-adrenergic-agonist induced 361–2
   in pre-eclampsia 39–40, 410
   tendency to develop 39, 63, 81–2
pulmonary vascular resistance 63
pulsatility index (PI) 376
pulse oximetry 25, 291–2
pulse pressure 40
pyrexia 177–8
pyridostigmine 128

Quetelet index 157
Quincke spinal needle 247, *248*, 265
   bevel orientation 219, 238
quinine 130

ranitidine 72, **92**, 93–4, 159, 444
   hypersensitivity reactions 173
   meningitis due to 275
records 11, **12–13**
   held by woman 14
red cell mass 32
reference values 441–2
regional anaesthesia 227–78
   anatomy 213–25
   anticoagulant therapy and 426–7
   aspirin therapy and 427–8
   in asthma 73
   back pain after 435–6
   in cocaine abuse 206–7
   complications 271–8
   contraindications 285, **286**
   in dystrophia myotonica 130
   in herpes simplex infections 184
   in HIV infection 180–1
   maternal mortality 24
   nausea and vomiting 96
   in obesity 160–1
   in pre-eclampsia/eclampsia 414–15
   in pregnancy 326–7
   service provision 6

regional anaesthesia (cont.)
  unlicensed drug use 227
  see also epidural anaesthesia; epidural analgesia; subarachnoid block
regurgitation
  cricoid pressure in prevention 294–6
  in early pregnancy 328
  factors affecting 295
  mechanisms 90–1
  see also aspiration of gastric contents
relaxin 435
religious beliefs 424
remifentanil 447–8
renal blood flow 45, 101–2
renal disease 103–7
  anaesthetic management 106–7
  diabetic 144, **145**
renal failure
  acute 103–4
  chronic 104–5
renal pelvis 100
renal system 100–7
renal transplantation 106
respiratory depression, opioid-induced 272–3
respiratory failure, acute 75–82
respiratory muscle function 59
respiratory rate
  in epidural analgesia **258**
  in exercise 62–3
respiratory system 57–82
  anatomy 57–60
  applied physiology 65–82
  physiology 63–5
  pulmonary dynamics 60–3
  see also lung function
respiratory tract infections 69
resuscitation
  intrauterine 394
  in local anaesthetic toxicity 445
  maternal 430–2
  neonatal 394–8
Rexed's laminae 223
Rhesus haemolytic disease 169, 378
rheumatoid arthritis **176**
ritodrine **361**, 362
rocuronium 306
ropivacaine 444
  epidural 243, 250, 262
  in pre-eclampsia/eclampsia 413

sacral nerve block 261, 269
sacroiliac joint pain 346–7
salbutamol
  in acute asthma 70
  in anaphylactic reactions **174**
  in preterm labour **361**, 362
  in uterine hyperstimulation 365
scalp, fetal, blood sampling 392
sciatic nerve lesions 134
seizures see convulsions
sensory function
  abnormal 125–30
  testing, in epidural analgesia 255–7, 261

sepsis **23**, 167, 176–7
  see also infections
septicaemia, epidural analgesia and 229
septic shock 433–4
sevoflurane **302**, 446, 448
shoulder girdle muscles, injuries 196
sickle-cell disorders 32–3, 383
sitting position 44
  in labour 335
  regional nerve block 214, 231, 232, 253, 268
skin
  preparation, regional nerve block 233
  puncture, in epidural needle insertion 233, 239
skin-to-epidural space distance 215, 234–5, 237
sleep
  apnoea, obstructive 64–5, 158
  disorders 64–5
smoking 64
sodium bicarbonate 262–3, **395**, 397
sodium citrate 92, 93, 94, 159
sodium nitroprusside 206
sodium retention 102–3
solvent abuse 208
sphygmomanometry 40, 403
spina bifida 381, 382
spinal anaesthesia see subarachnoid block
spinal block, total 278
spinal cord 215, 223
  arterial blood supply 222–4
  injury 125–6
  ischaemia, vulnerability 222–4
  pain pathways 348–9
  vascular disorders 121
  venous drainage 224
spinal needles 247–8, 265
  bevel orientation 219, 238
  for combined spinal–epidural block 270
  neural damage risks 265
spiral arterioles 188, 189
squatting, in labour 336
staffing
  anaesthetic services 6, 230
  for epidural analgesia 246
  for general anaesthesia 287–8
standards
  data collection 11, **12–13**
  maternity care 11–12
Starling's equation 38–9
steroids
  in anaphylactic reactions 174–5
  antenatal, in diabetes 149
  in asthma 65, 68–9, 70, 71, 72
  in dystrophia myotonica 130
  in HELLP syndrome 113
  immune effects 167, 170
  infection risks 177
  in multiple sclerosis 127
Stillbirth and Neonatal Death Society 27–8
stillbirths 17, 26
stress incontinence 130, 196

stroke 121, 122
stroke volume 42, 45, 194
subarachnoid anaesthesia *see* subarachnoid block
subarachnoid block (SAB) 213, 227, 264–9
  advantages and disadvantages 265–6
  after inadvertent dural puncture *238*
  asepsis 224–5, 232–3
  for Caesarean section 266, 268–9
  complications 46, 271–8
  doses and volumes 266–8
  extent of block 268–9
  history 264–5
  inadvertent, detection 241–2
  in lumbar disc prolapse 127
  in obesity 160–1
  patient positioning 266–7
  in pre-eclampsia/eclampsia 414–15
  preparation for 230–42
  in spinal cord injury 126
  testing the block 255–7
  see also combined spinal–epidural (CSE) nerve block
subarachnoid haemorrhage **122**
subarachnoid space *215*, 218
  connective tissue bands/septa 218, 219–21
  needle insertion 237
    bevel orientation 238
    midline approach 234–5
    paramedian approach 239
subdural haematoma 278
subdural space 216–18
substance abuse 198–209
sufentanil **243**
  for analgesia in labour 353
  epidural 243, **245**, 252
  fetal effects 399
supine hypotensive syndrome 43–5
supine position 43
  wedged 267, 317
supraspinous ligament 214, *215*
  local anaesthetic infiltration 233
  Tuohy needle resistance 234
suxamethonium 288, *295*, 304–5
  apnoea 155, 305
  contraindications 305
  hypersensitivity reactions 172
  magnesium sulphate interaction 415
  malignant hyperthermia 156
  metabolism 154, 155, 305
  in neurological disorders 123, **124**, 125, 128
  in neuromuscular disorders 129, 130
  postoperative morbidity 196, 305
  prolonged paralysis after 305
  in rapid-sequence induction 293
  in renal disease **106**, 107
sympathetic nervous system
  blockade 255, 256, 264, 265
  in blood pressure regulation 42–3
  desflurane actions 446
  responses in labour 45–6
syncytiotrophoblast 188
Syntocinon *see* oxytocin

Syntometrine 340
syringes
  for epidural analgesia 246–7
  loss-of-resistance 237
  for subarachnoid block 266
systemic lupus erythematosus (SLE) 168, 169, 175–6
systemic vascular resistance (SVR) 40, 42, 52
systolic/diastolic (S/D) ratio 376

tachycardia
  in anaphylactic reactions 172–3
  fetal 388, *390–1*
  in heart disease 49
  paroxysmal 52
  pulmonary oedema risk 81
  response to intubation 299, 300
teeth, prominent **312**
telemedicine 377–8
telemetry, labour ward 378
temazepam 444
temperature
  cerebrospinal fluid 237
  control
    central nervous system 225
    in dystrophia myotonica 130
    in spinal cord injury 126
  Entonox storage 447
  fetal–maternal difference 177
tendon reflexes 411, **412**
teratogens 120, 201, 326, 443
terbutaline
  in acute asthma 70
  in preterm labour **361**, 362
termination of pregnancy *see* abortion
thalassaemia 33, 383
theophylline 69, 70
thiopental 288, *295*, 297–8
  anaesthetic awareness and 319
  cricoid pressure and 294
  in eclampsia 412
  hypersensitivity reactions 172
  placental transfer 192
  precipitation test 237
thoracic cage, in pregnancy *58*, 59
thrombin time *34*
thrombocytopenia 36, 113, **176**
thromboelastogram (TEG) 413
thromboembolism 77, 425–8
  in heart disease 53
  maternal mortality 22
  prophylaxis 425–7
  recommendations 26
  risk assessment **425**
  see also pulmonary embolism
thromboxane A$_2$ 407, 427
thyroid function 151–3
  neonatal 152, 169
thyromental distance 310
tibial nerve lesions 134
tocolytics 360–2
topical anaesthesia, for awake intubation 318–19

touch, light, discrimination testing 255-6
tracheal suction 95-6, 396-7
tracheostomy 318
tramadol 448
transcutaneous electrical nerve stimulation (TENS) 351
transfers 8, 15-16
　in preterm labour 360
trichloroethylene 353, 354
triple test 381
trisomy 13 383
trisomy 18 383
trisomy 21 see Down syndrome
tuberculosis 178-9
d-tubocurarine 72, **120**
Tuohy needle 233, 247
　insertion 233-9
　withdrawal 240
　see also epidural needles

ultrasound
　antenatal 375-7
　screening for fetal abnormalities 380-1
umbilical artery 189
　Doppler velocity wave forms 376, 377
umbilical cord
　prolapse 365
　sampling 392-3
umbilical vein catheterization, in neonatal resuscitation 395
United Kingdom
　anaesthetic services 5-8
　Caesarean section rates 4, 5
　domiciliary obstetrics 14-16
　maternity services 5-16
urate, plasma 103
urea, serum 102
uric acid 103, 406-7
urinary tract 100-1
　congenital abnormalities 382
urine output, in major obstetric haemorrhage 421, 423
uterine arteries 188, 189
　Doppler velocity wave forms 377
　postpartum changes 195
uterine contractions 346-7, **350**
　effects of inhalational agents 303
　in major obstetric haemorrhage 422-3
　postpartum 195
　in postpartum haemostasis 36, 37
uterine hyperstimulation 365
uteroplacental unit 188, 189
uterus
　acute inversion 340
　anatomical changes 188
　manipulation, regional anaesthesia 269
　rupture 433

vaginal delivery
　in breech presentations 363
　in diabetes 147, 149-50

　in multiple pregnancy 364
　regional analgesia and 255, 274
Valsalva manoeuvre 45, 366
vascular disorders
　cerebral 121-3
　spinal cord 121
vecuronium 172, 288, 305-6
　in asthma 72
　phenytoin interaction **120**
venous access
　in Caesarean section 307
　in obesity 159
　in regional analgesia 231
　in ruptured ectopic pregnancy 330
venous thrombosis, deep 425, 427
　prophylaxis 161, 425-7
ventilation 62-3
　in asthma 72-3
　high-frequency oscillatory 71
　intermittent positive pressure see intermittent positive pressure ventilation (IPPV)
　mechanical
　　in acid aspiration 95, 96
　　after Caesarean section 286
　　in ARDS 78-9
　minute 62
　in neonatal resuscitation 395, 396
　transtracheal intermittent jet 318
ventilation/perfusion relations 76, 427
vertebral canal 213, 215-24
　connective tissue 218-21
vertebral column 225
　bony landmarks 213-14
　immunology 224-5
　thermal regulation 225
vertebral spines 213, 214, 215
vertebral venous plexus 218
viral infections 178
vitamin K
　deficiency 74
　therapy 112, 120
vitamin supplements 73-4
vomiting
　during cricoid pressure 297
　see also nausea and vomiting

warfarin 426
water
　intoxication 231
　retention 102, 341
weight
　in cystic fibrosis 73
　fetal 372-3
wheezing
　differential diagnosis **67**, 68
　intraoperative 72-3
white blood cell counts 177, 442
Wilson's score 310
women, attitudes to 3

zidovudine 180